PATHOLOGY
Understanding Human Disease

PATHOLOGY
Understanding Human Disease

ABNER GOLDEN, M.D.

Professor and Chairman
Department of Pathology
University of Kentucky
College of Medicine
Lexington, Kentucky

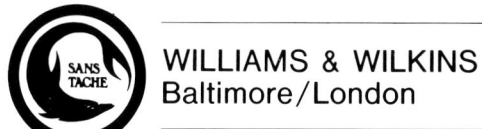

WILLIAMS & WILKINS
Baltimore/London

Copyright ©, 1982
Williams & Wilkins
428 East Preston Street
Baltimore, MD 21202, U.S.A.

All rights reserved. This book is protected by copyright. No part of this book may be reproduced in any form or by any means, including photocopying, or utilized by any information storage and retrieval system without written permission from the copyright owner.

Made in the United States of America

Library of Congress Cataloging in Publication Data

Golden, Abner, 1918–
   Pathology: understanding human disease.

   Includes index.
   1. Pathology, I. Title. [DNLM: 1. Pathology. QZ 4 G618p]
RB111.G64   616.07   81-11481
ISBN 0-683-03726-9   AACR2

Composed and printed at the
Waverly Press, Inc.
Mt. Royal and Guilford Aves.
Baltimore, MD 21202, U.S.A.

Dedication

*To 33 classes of medical students
who have done their best to educate me*

Preface

The role of the teacher is to create an environment that is conducive to learning. The principal ingredient of that environment is enthusiasm—enthusiasm for the subject matter, and enthusiasm for learning. I hope that this volume will convey some of my own enthusiasm as a teacher.

I approached writing this book with the firm conviction that we try to force too much detailed information into our students at a time when they are ill-prepared to accept or digest it. I did not want to write another large reference text, but rather a volume that could be read from cover-to-cover—one that presents pathology as an integral part of the study of medicine, and as a subject of lifelong learning. I hope that students reading the book will feel that they have gained a perspective, understanding, and a point of view, a sense that they have been introduced to the study of human disease. Each student can then expand his own personal education through his clinical experiences and by consulting reference texts and the current literature in pathology and the other clinical sciences.

I considered it highly desirable to limit the size of the volume to no more than 500 pages. Although most important disorders have been included, the contents and the treatment afforded them reflect my personal bias, and no attempt has been made to be "complete" in the sense required of reference texts. Except in a few specialized areas, reviews of normal anatomy and histology have not been included, and I have assumed that students reaching pathology have completed courses in basic immunology and genetics. Controversial topics have not been debated; rather the most reasonable statements, based on current thinking, have been given. Suggestions for further reading have been kept to a minimum, and include predominantly up-to-date review articles and summary editorials.

I am indebted to a great many people. My initial desire to teach was whetted and encouraged by exposure to many great teachers during my student and residency years, foremost among them Walter H. Sheldon, Eugene A. Stead, Jr., Paul B. Beeson, and John B. Hickam. I have learned a great deal from my colleagues and friends who have taught with me at Georgetown University and the University of Kentucky: Donald M. Kerwin, Heinz Bauer, Byungkyu Chun, Deborah E. Powell, Ralph D. Powell, William R. Markesbery, William N. O'Connor, Michael L. Cibull, and Norbert W. Tietz. I have made extensive use of my notes and the illustrations from their lectures. Most of them have reviewed individual chapters, and Don Kerwin has read and criticized most of the volume. Others who have reviewed chapters include John F. Maher, Ewa Marciniak, Barbara Markesbery, and Thomas L. Roszman.

The chapters on breast and the female genital tract were written by Deborah Powell, those on the central nervous system and disorders of muscle by William Markesbery.

John Furcolow, Michael Moran, Brenda Hoffman, Larry Munch, and Douglas Arnold, members of my student group of 1980–1981, reviewed most of the chapters and offered many constructive suggestions.

Charlotte C. Taraba did a very conscientious and painstaking job of manuscript typing. Dr. Powell's two chapters were prepared by Glenna Porter and Mary Luoma assisted in the preparation of the index. Most of the photographic work was done by Bernard F. Salb of Georgetown University, and many excellent additions were supplied by Richard Geissler at the University of Kentucky.

The help and encouragement offered by Nan C. Tyler, Sara A. Finnegan, Diana L. Welch, and the others at Williams & Wilkins helped make the planning and execution of this book an enjoyable experience for the author.

Finally, my thanks are due Rita and Bud James for making me so welcome in Stanley, Idaho, where most of the book was written.

Abner Golden, M.D.

Illustration Acknowledgments

Figures 5.1, 5.2, 7.7, 8.2, 8.3, 8.5, 8.6, 8.7, 8.8, 12.2, 17.1 through 17.10, 17.12, 17.13, 17.15 through 17.17, 18.1, 18.2, 18.4 through 18.6, and 26.1 are reprinted from Golden A, Maher JF. The kidney, 2nd ed. Williams & Wilkins, Baltimore, 1977.

Figures 25.14 through 25.17 are reprinted from Golden A, Kerwin DM. The parathyroid glands. In: Bloodworth JMB, ed. Endocrine pathology, 2nd ed. Williams & Wilkins, Baltimore, 1981.

Figures 15.16, 15.17, and 15.18 are reproduced with permission from Moller JH, Amplatz K, Edwards JE. Congenital heart disease. Universities Associated for Research and Education in Pathology, Bethesda, MD, 1971.

Contents

Preface vii

Illustration Acknowledgments ix

Chapter 1
Understanding Human Disease 1

Chapter 2
Mechanisms of Injury 3

Chapter 3
Reaction to Injury 14

Chapter 4
Host-Injurious Agent Interactions 28

Chapter 5
Patterns of Infection 42

Chapter 6
Disturbances of Fluid, Electrolyte, and Acid-Base Balance 55

Chapter 7
Hemostasis and Blood Coagulation 64

Chapter 8
Immunologic Mechanisms of Injury 75

Chapter 9
Nutrition and Disease 88

Chapter 10
Genetic Determinants of Disease 95

Chapter 11
Aging 104

Chapter 12
The Environment and Health 108

Chapter 13
Alterations of Cell Growth **121**

Chapter 14
Neoplastic Disease **128**

Chapter 15
The Heart **143**

Chapter 16
Vascular Disorders **167**

Chapter 17
The Kidneys **178**

Chapter 18
Hypertension **203**

Chapter 19
The Lungs **211**

Chapter 20
The Central Nervous System
By William R. Markesbery, M.D. **231**

Chapter 21
The Liver and Gall Bladder **258**

Chapter 22
The Exocrine Pancreas **279**

Chapter 23
The Digestive Tract **286**

Chapter 24
The Lymphoreticular and Hematopoietic Organs ... **308**

Chapter 25
The Endocrine Glands **329**

Chapter 26
Diabetes Mellitus **353**

Chapter 27
The Female Genital Tract
By Deborah E. Powell, M.D. **358**

Chapter 28
The Breast
By Deborah E. Powell, M.D. **391**

Chapter 29
The Urinary Bladder 406

Chapter 30
The Male Genital Tract 410

Chapter 31
Disorders of Bone 418

Chapter 32
The Joints 435

Chapter 33
Diseases of Skeletal Muscle
By William R. Markesbery, M.D. 444

Chapter 34
The Skin 451

Chapter 35
Pediatric Disorders 459

Index 469

Chapter 1

Understanding Human Disease

The proper study of mankind is Man.
—*Alexander Pope*

The practice of medicine, once predominantly empiric, has become deeply rooted in science. The contemporary physician, no longer able to get by solely on his concern for his fellow man, must, instead, understand the mechanisms and anatomic basis of his patient's disease if he is to interpret correctly the functional disturbances that constitute signs and symptoms, and if he is to approach therapy in a rational manner.

Pathology occupies a critical position in the education of the physician. Its methodology is that of the basic sciences, but its intellectual stimulus, and, in fact, its very reason for existence, derives from the study of human disease. It is the historic and continuous orientation of pathology to clinical medicine that has made it a discipline and science fundamental to the practice of medicine.

A pathologist is highly qualified by his training to demonstrate the structural consequences of disease. He must not stop there; he must, instead, build from his knowledge of structure an understanding of pathogenesis on the one hand, and functional consequences on the other. The recent and burgeoning development of the several disciplines of laboratory medicine has greatly broadened the scope of his contribution to the understanding of disease, and its therapy or prevention. Thus, the pathologist's role in medicine is highly integrative.

It is the educational responsibility of departments of pathology, then, to create a bridge that unites the basic sciences with clinical medicine. In studying pathology, one learns the language of medicine, acquires the ability to organize quantitative and qualitative data derived from disparate sources, and to use these data in gaining an understanding of both the mechanisms of disease and its manifestations in the individual patient. Pathology is the student's introduction to medicine, and his understanding of pathology becomes an essential part of the personal education that permits him to function as a physician. It promotes a way of thinking about disease and about patients. Pathologists, because of the breadth of their orientation, are perhaps singularly able to view disease as it affects the entire human organism, an ability often lacking in members of highly structured and subdivided clinical disciplines. In a sense, the pathologist may serve as the last "generalist" in the curriculum. With his background in pathology, the student will be prepared for the study of disease in individual patients during his clinical clerkships.

Pathology is a graduate course, and must be approached as such by both students and faculty. It is perhaps the first course in medical school in which the content cannot be defined with precision. Its scope will be determined by each individual for himself, and will reflect his educational background, commitment to the study of medicine, and hopes for the future. In the final analysis, each physician must complete his own bridge between basic science and clinical medicine, one that will best enable him to provide modern health care.

Chapter 2

Mechanisms of Injury

Our environment includes many forces and substances that have the capacity to injure or kill human cells. Some are natural and inherent in our surroundings; others are manmade. Among them are extremes of temperature, mechanical forces, ionizing radiation, electrical energy, bacterial, viral and other living organisms, toxic chemicals, and the effects of immunologic reactions. Cells and tissues may also be injured by alterations of our internal environment that result from a multitude of congenital and acquired disorders.

MECHANISMS OF INJURY

The mechanisms by which injury is produced are at times obvious; more often they are obscure. One readily understandable mechanism of injury is interference with the blood supply to an organ or part of an organ, depriving its cells and tissues of oxygen and nutrients. For example, a blood clot or *thrombus* may form in a vein of a lower extremity, break off, and travel through the systemic venous system to the right heart, and then lodge in and occlude one of the branches of the pulmonary artery. Unless the bronchial circulation is sufficient to maintain viability, there is death, or *necrosis,* of the tissue fed by the occluded arterial branch. This is clearly recognized with the naked eye as an area of lung, often triangular in shape, that is darkly hemorrhagic and airless (Fig. 2.1). Histologically, one can recognize the pulmonary architecture, but the cells have lost their nuclei and cytoplasmic detail. Such tissue necrosis resulting from the loss of blood supply is called *infarction*. Another, perhaps more familiar, example is infarction of the myocardium due to occlusive atherosclerosis of the coronary arteries (Fig. 2.2). Severe arterial disease of the lower extremities may result in necrosis of several toes or a large segment of the foot (Fig. 2.3). This is referred to as *gangrene.* Myocardial infarction and gangrene of toes are again lesions that are readily recognizable on gross inspection. Somewhat more subtle changes are observed in the liver when blood supply is deficient, as in congestive heart failure. The organ will appear grossly congested, but the microscope will further reveal the accumulation of droplets of triglyceride in the cytoplasm of hepatocytes in the central lobular areas. This is *fatty change.* Other liver cells may show intense staining of their cytoplasm, nuclear fragmentation, and lysis (Fig. 2.4).

Infarction, gangrene due to arterial disease, and the effects on the liver of congestive heart failure are all examples of *ischemia*. In ischemic injury, the

4   *Pathology: Understanding Human Disease*

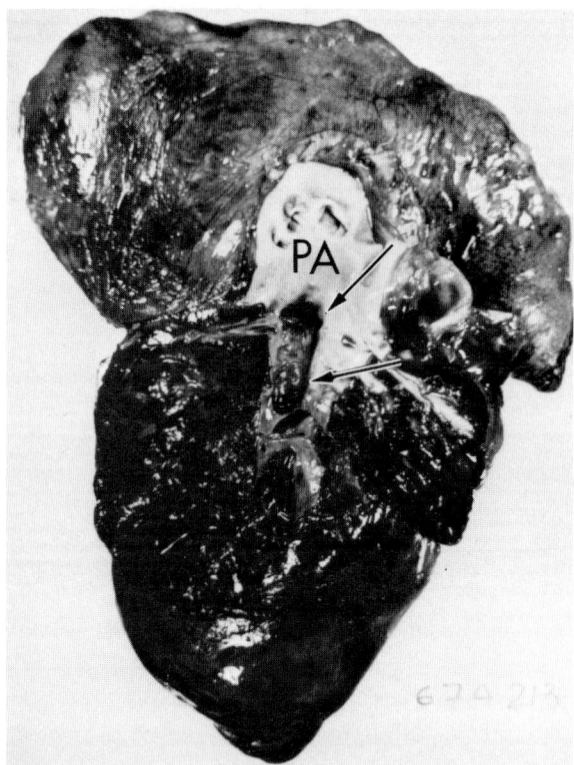

Figure 2.1. Pulmonary embolism and infarction. The pulmonary artery (*PA*) has been opened to reveal a large thrombotic embolus (*arrows*) in the main branch to the lower lobe. The entire lobe is deeply hemorrhagic and partially collapsed.

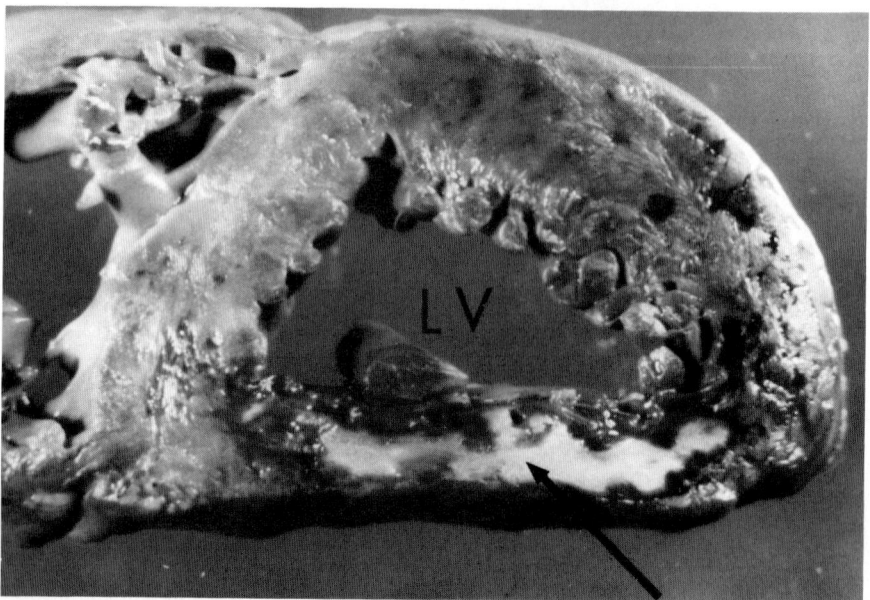

Figure 2.2. Acute myocardial infarction. This horizontal section shows a large area of necrosis in the free wall of the left ventricle (*arrow*). The affected wall is thinned. The necrotic area is soft, yellowish gray in color, and surrounded by a darker area containing congested and dilated blood vessels.

Mechanisms of Injury

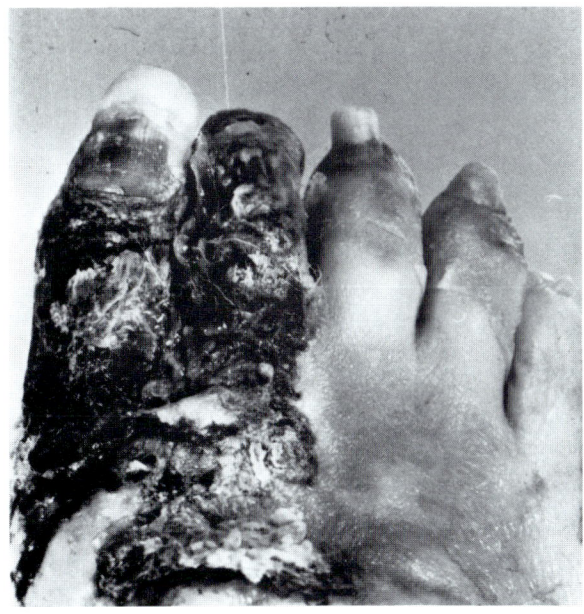

Figure 2.3. Gangrene. There is sharply demarcated gangrene of the first two toes, with extensive sloughing of superficial tissue. The patient had severe artherosclerosis of peripheral arteries.

earliest cellular changes that indicate irreversible injury appear to result from damage to cell membranes, including the membranes of cellular organelles. There is swelling of mitochondria and lysosomes, reflecting altered fluid balance and energy production, loss of cellular glycogen, and margination of nuclear chromatin.

Some other mechanisms of injury can be considered. Trauma can result in rupture of large numbers of cells. It may also lead to interference with, or disruption of, blood supply. Excessive heat greatly increases cellular metabolic needs, and, if severe, can cause coagulation of cellular proteins. Exposure to very cold temperatures can result in injury because of ice crystal formation that can mechanically rupture cells. Injury to the vascular endothelium can cause intravascular clotting and superimposed ischemic injury, as in frostbite. Ionizing radiation injures cells by either of two mechanisms. Direct chromosomal injury may alter the genetic material of the cell so as to prevent viable products of cell division or yield cells demonstrating highly abnormal patterns of growth, while ionization of water molecules may yield such abnormal products as peroxides which may become incorporated in cellular enzymes, or react with DNA, RNA, and cell membranes. Electrical energy can cause severe burns. Current passing through the body can also trigger fatal cardiac arrhythmias.

Pathogenic microorganisms injure through many mechanisms. Some bacteria produce powerful exotoxins that destroy cell membranes at the site of infection or act at remote locations of the body. Other bacterial organisms release endotoxins when they lose their integrity. These may have locally cytotoxic effects, but endotoxins may also produce widespread vascular injury leading to disseminated intravascular coagulation, consumption of coagulation factors, and hemorrhagic phenomena. Many viruses alter the genetic apparatus of cells, and

6   Pathology: Understanding Human Disease

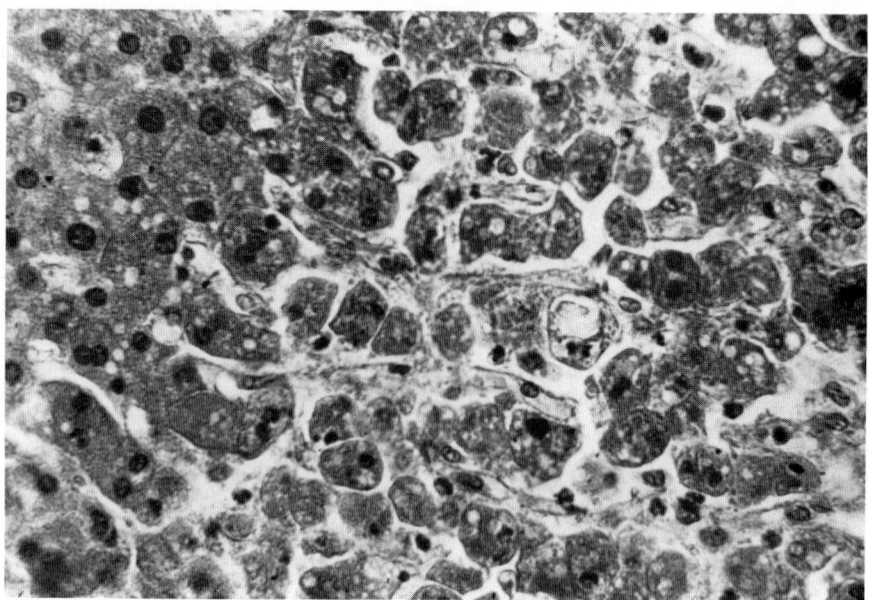

Figure 2.4.   Ischemic liver injury. The liver cells at the *left-hand margin* appear viable, although many small droplets of triglyceride can be seen. The cells in the *central* and *right areas* are necrotic. Many of the nuclei are shrunken, darkly staining masses; other cells have lost their nuclei and several cells are disrupted.

incorporation in the genome of the cell diverts its synthetic pathways to viral replication. Viruses may destroy the host cell, or have profound effects on its growth pattern. Either effect may be apparent only after prolonged periods of latency.

Several types of immunologic reactions are associated with host injury. Soluble antigen-antibody complexes, deposited in vascular walls or in the renal glomerular filter, attract polymorphonuclear leukocytes from the circulation, and these cells release damaging enzymes from their lysosomes. Antigen-antibody complexes may also activate complement, and some of its components and cleavage products are toxic to tissues. Other immunologic reactions liberate histamine from mast cells, inducing anaphylaxis. When antigens are attached to cell surfaces, antigen-antibody reactions can injure and disrupt the cell membrane. Finally, in cell-mediated immunity, sensitized lymphocytes may have the capacity to kill other cells.

Chemical substances act by many mechanisms. Such strong chemicals as phenol and formalin coagulate all cellular proteins. Others, in relatively low concentration, interfere with very specific cell functions. Carbon tetrachloride produces membrane injury and interferes with cellular synthetic mechanisms. In the liver cell, altered protein synthesis results in the accumulation of cytoplasmic triglyceride (fatty change). Much has been learned about chemical mechanisms of injury through the development of antineoplastic therapeutic agents. Alkylating substances, such as nitrogen mustard and cyclophosphamide, injure DNA throughout the cell cycle, and block cell proliferation at the premitotic phase.

Antimetabolites inactivate specific enzymes that provide precursors for the synthesis of the purine and pyrimidine bases of DNA. Thus, the folic acid antagonist methotrexate blocks folic acid reductase, and death takes place in the S phase of the cell cycle. Natural alkaloids, *e.g.*, colchicine, arrest cells in metaphase by binding specific proteins of cell microtubules, and such antibiotics as actinomycin D and mithramycin bind directly to DNA and prevent further DNA synthesis.

Although the causes of injury are many, and the specific mechanisms almost innumerable, it appears that most act through one or more common pathways:

1. *Interference with membrane function.* There is altered cellular osmotic balance, with failure to exclude sodium and calcium, and loss of potassium. Cellular enzymes may leave the cell and enter the extravascular space.

2. *Interference with energy production.* This is manifested by mitochondrial swelling, loss of their structural detail, and accumulation of calcium salts.

3. *Interference with protein synthesis.*

4. *Alteration of genetic behavior.* This may result from synthesis of an abnormal DNA incompatible with continued life of the cell or an altered DNA that results in disturbed cell growth.

Maintenance of osmotic balance, energy production, protein synthesis, and genetic integrity are interdependent functions, and any persistent injury to one function is likely to be followed soon by alteration of the others. Fatty change of the liver cell consists of an accumulation of triglyceride in its cytoplasm. It is observed in many circumstances, among them anemia, hypoxia, starvation, obesity, diabetic acidosis, alcoholism, and exposure to such toxic or potentially toxic substances as carbon tetrachloride, phosphorus, halothane, and tetracycline. Alcohol and carbon tetrachloride injure liver cell membranes. Tetracycline interferes with the mitochondrial energy production necessary for protein synthesis. Starvation is associated with increased mobilization from fat stores and deranged synthesis of lipoprotein complexes. Thus, there are various points of attack, but the end result is failure of fat transport from the liver cell, and the accumulation of cytoplasmic triglyceride.

MORPHOLOGIC MANIFESTATIONS OF CELLULAR INJURY

In view of the very limited cellular pathways through which injurious agents act, it is not surprising that the morphologic manifestations of cellular injury are relatively few. Very similar findings may result from very diverse causes of injury, and only occasionally are the morphologic changes indicative of a specific causative agent.

The early manifestations of injury are best observed on electron microscopy. They consist of dilatation of the endoplasmic reticulum and loss of ribosomes, a decrease in cellular glycogen, and swelling of mitochondria with accumlation of calcium. Myelin figures are thought to form from phospholipid released from injured membranes. Nuclear changes include condensation of nuclear material with separation from the nuclear membrane (Figs. 2.5 and 2.6).

Two cellular changes observed on light microscopy are considered to be evidence of reversible injury. *Cloudy swelling*, a very frequent finding, is char-

8 Pathology: Understanding Human Disease

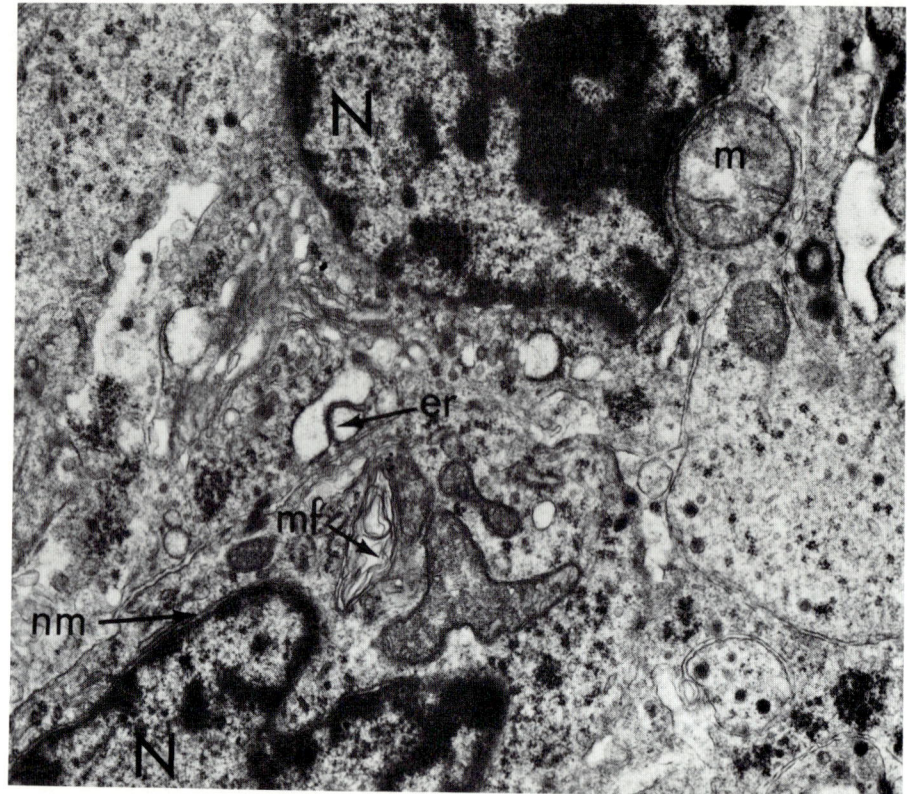

Figure 2.5. Electron micrograph showing manifestations of cellular injury. The nuclear chromatin is clumped, and the nuclear membrane (*nm*) is separating from the chromatin material. A mitochondrion (*m*) shows swelling and blurring of cristae. The endoplasmic reticulum (*er*) is dilated, and there is some loss of ribosomes. An early myelin figure (*mf*) is noted.

acterized by a swollen, pale granular cytoplasm, reflecting altered cellular osmotic behavior (Fig. 2.7). Corresponding changes on electron microscopy are swelling of mitochondria and dilatation of endoplasmic reticulum. A more advanced stage is *hydropic* or *vacuolar degeneration*, seen most dramatically in the renal tubules in the presence of hypokalemia. Marked cystic dilatation of the endoplasmic reticulum is seen on electron microscopy. Fatty change, seen most frequently in liver cells, is another example of reversible injury. Here the cytoplasm is enlarged by one or more droplets of fat, often of sufficient size to displace the nucleus. Changes observed on light microscopy that are evidence of irreversible cellular injury include intense cytoplasmic eosinophilia and nuclear condensation (*pyknosis*), fragmentation, and dissolution (Figs. 2.4 and 2.8).

MORPHOLOGIC MANIFESTATIONS OF TISSUE INJURY

The death of cells and tissues initiates a sequence of events that optimally leads to the removal of devitalized material and its replacement by the regeneration of normal tissue, or, when that cannot take place, by scar tissue formation. An important first step in this process is enzymatic digestion of necrotic debris.

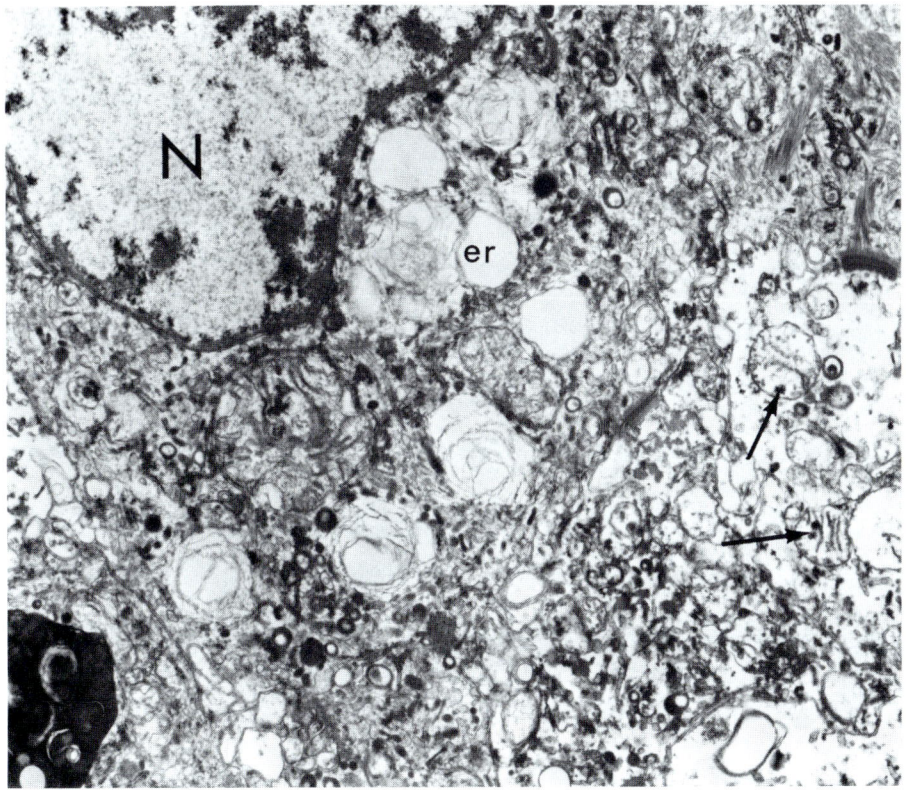

Figure 2.6. Electron micrograph showing advanced cellular degeneration. The nuclear chromatin is concentrated near the nuclear membrane. There is striking dilatation of endoplasmic reticulum (*er*). The mitochondria show varying stages of degeneration. Several show floccular densities (*arrows*).

This happens in part because of the release of lysosomal enzymes from the necrotic cells themselves, and in part from enzymes brought to the area of injury by circulating leukocytes.

The rapidity of digestion, and its thoroughness, have profound consequences on the appearance of dead tissue. Most infarcts tend to be digested very slowly, and, for a considerable time, the lesion remains firm and rather dry, with preservation of tissue landmarks (Fig. 2.9). This is designated *coagulation necrosis*. In contrast, the fluid center of an abscess is an example of rapid and complete digestion, or *liquefactive necrosis* (Fig. 2.10). When digestion is partial and incomplete, the tissue may have a cheesy appearance and consistency, called *caseation necrosis* (Fig. 2.11). *Fat necrosis* results from death of adipose tissue. It is firm and often chalky in appearance as a result of the binding of calcium salts to free fatty acids released in the breakdown of neutral fats.

SYSTEMIC MANIFESTATIONS OF INJURY

The presence of significant tissue necrosis may be expressed by a variety of clinical manifestations, some of a general systemic nature, others relating more

10 *Pathology: Understanding Human Disease*

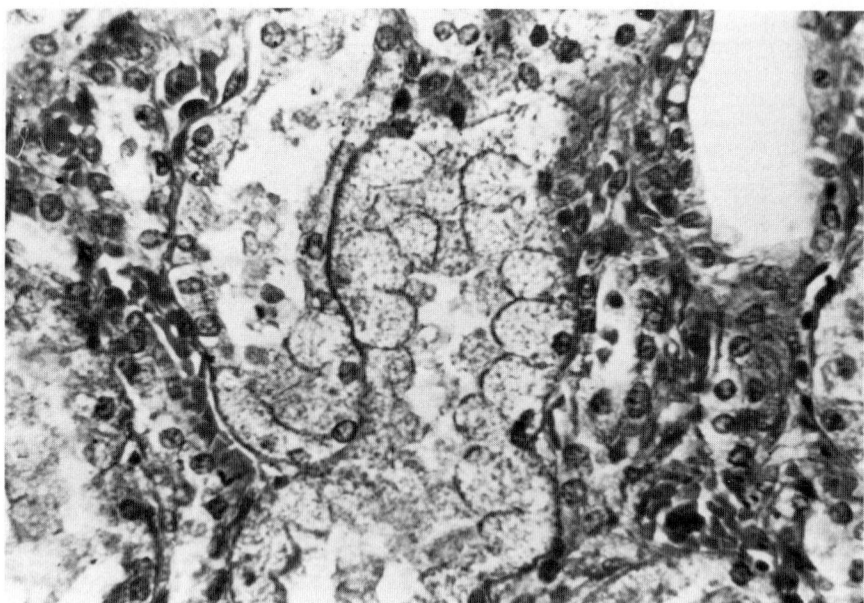

Figure 2.7. Cloudy swelling. The tubular epithelial cells in the *center* of the field are markedly swollen, and have pale, granular cytoplasm. These changes reflect increased water content, loss of potassium, and failure to exclude sodium.

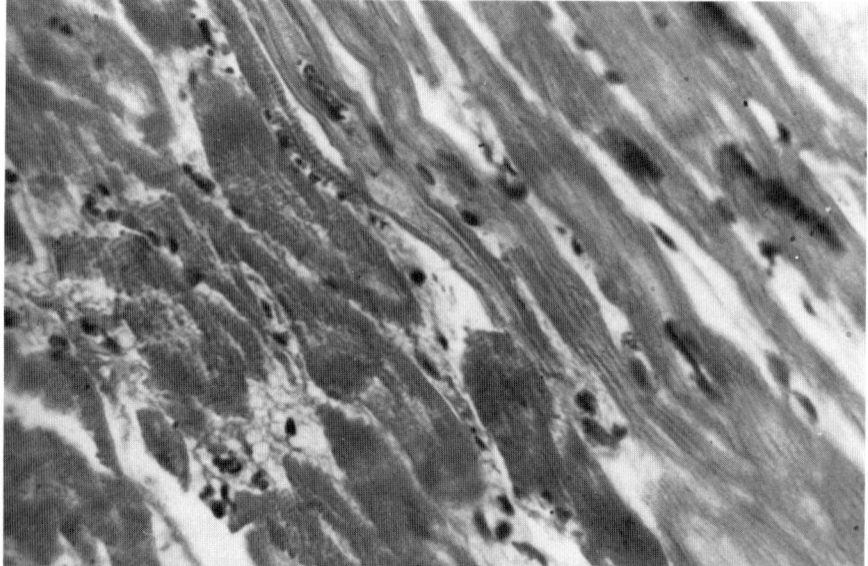

Figure 2.8. Necrosis of myocardial fibers. Normal fibers are seen to the *right*. The necrotic fibers at the *left* appear smudgy and are deeply staining. There is loss of nuclei and some cellular fragmentation.

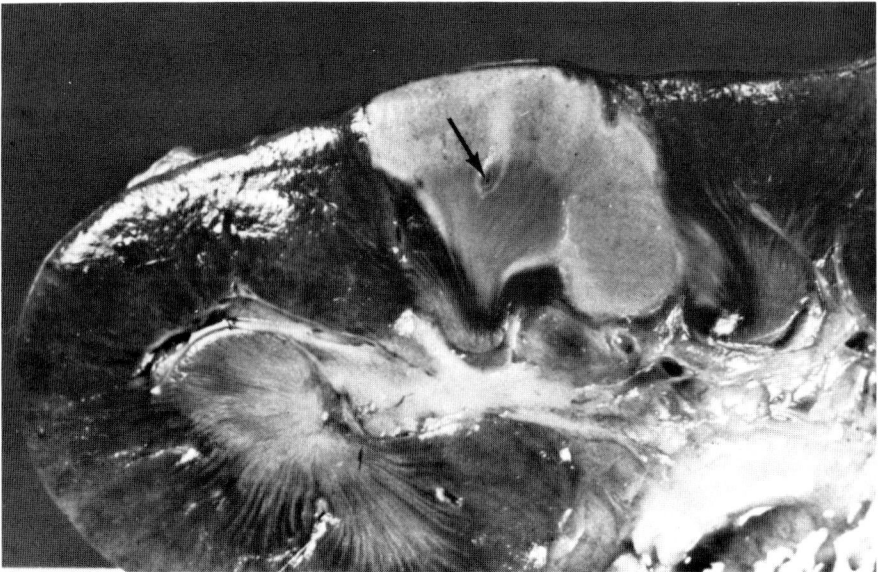

Figure 2.9. Kidney infarct. A large area of coagulation necrosis is seen along the upper margin of this specimen. It is sharply demarcated, and such normal landmarks as medullary striations remain clearly visable. The *arrow* points to a thrombosed arcuate artery.

specifically to the site and type of injury. Systemic manifestations include a generalized malaise, or sense of loss of well-being, lassitude, and altered appetite. Fever is often present, the result of release of endogenous pyrogens from fixed tissue cells or from circulating cells attracted to the area of injury, and possibly by the production of one or more prostaglandins. The pulse is often rapid. Tissue injury is most usually associated with an increase in circulating leukocytes (*leukocytosis*), although their number may be normal or depressed in certain circumstances. Other frequent manifestations of injury include an acceleration of the erythrocyte sedimentation rate and some elevation of blood glucose concentration.

Pain frequently points to the site of injury. Myocardial infarction, pulmonary infarction, and splenic infarction are each signaled by one or more characteristic patterns of pain. Loss of function is another manifestation of injury that indicates the area of involvement. Ischemic injury to the kidney can result in a cessation of all urine formation; injury to the brain is accompanied by loss of the specific functions of the injured area. Injury to certain tissues is reflected in altered electrical activity, monitored by such procedures as the electrocardiogram and the electroencephalogram.

A clinically important manifestation of injury is the increased release of cellular enzymes into the extracellular fluid. The rapidity of this transfer is a function of the molecular weight of the enzyme, and the concentration gradient across the cell membrane. Although most injured cells merely release their enzymes, some may increase their production. How long elevated levels of cellular enzymes may be detected in the blood is determined by the rates of metabolism and excretion.

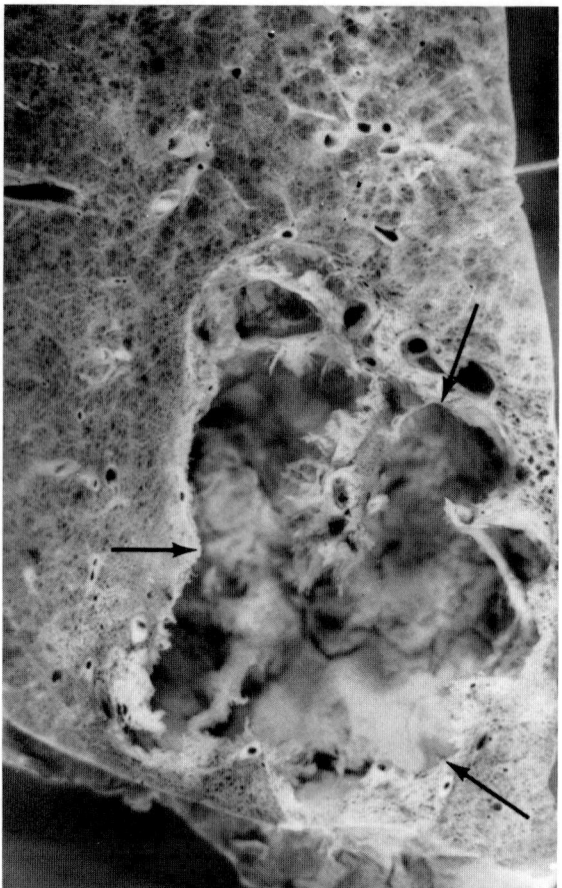

Figure 2.10. Lung abscess. A large abscess cavity is noted in the left lower lobe. It has ragged margins (*arrows*), and it is lined by an irregular membrane composed primarily of fibrin and polymorphonuclear leukocytes. An abscess is an example of liquefaction necrosis.

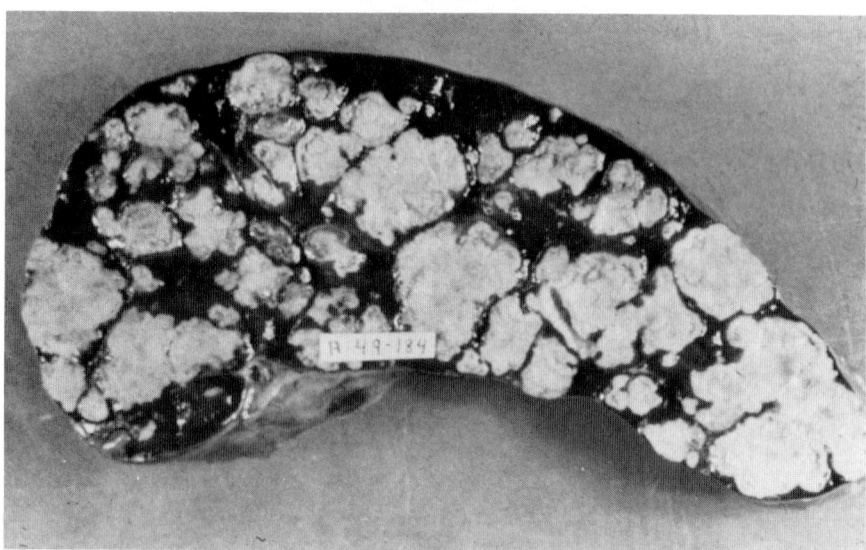

Figure 2.11. Caseation necrosis. This specimen is a cut surface of spleen showing multiple areas of cheesy necrosis due to tuberculosis.

Table 2.1
Some Clinically Important Tissue Enzymes and Their Principal Sources

Enzyme	Abbreviation	Sources
Lactate dehydrogenase	LDH	Liver, heart, red cells, kidney, skeletal muscle
Creatine phosphokinase	CPK	Skeletal muscle, brain, heart
Glutamate oxalacetate transaminase (aspartate transaminase)	GOT	Heart, liver, skeletal muscle, kidney, pancreas
Glutamate pyruvate transaminase (alanine transaminase)	GPT	Liver, kidney, heart
γ-Glutamyltransferase	GGT	Liver, kidney
Alkaline phosphatase	ALP	Liver, bone
Amylase		Pancreas
Aldolase		Skeletal muscle, heart

Determinations of blood levels of many enzymes have become important in clinical diagnosis and in evaluating the progress of disease. Some of the more important enzymes and their principal tissue sources are shown in Table 2.1. Many of these enzyme determinations are highly sensitive to the presence of tissue injury, but rather nonspecific to the site of injury. However, the determination of isoenzymes has, in many instances, added specificity. Thus, isoenzyme levels of CPK and LDH may, together with other clinical manifestations, permit the highly accurate diagnosis of myocardial infarction.

Suggested Reading

Jennings RB, Ganote CE, Reimer KA. Ischemic tissue injury. Am. J. Pathol. *81:* 179, 1975.

Trump BF, Berezesky IK, Collan Y, Kahng MW, Mergner WJ. Recent studies on the pathophysiology of ischemic cell injury. Beitr. Pathol. *158:* 363, 1976.

Trump BF, McDowell EM, Arstila AU. In: Hill RB Jr, LaVia MF, eds. Principles of pathobiology. New York, Oxford University Press, 1980.

Chapter 3

Reaction to Injury

The presence of necrosis, cellular or tissue death occurring in the living host, triggers a sequence of events that optimally results in healing, replacement of destroyed tissue, and restoration of function. This response to injury consists of vascular and cellular phenomena that permit the digestion and removal of dead cells and their products, and the repair of injury by regeneration of normal tissue components, when possible, or by the formation of a scar. Although somewhat complex and incompletely understood, it is remarkably constant regardless of the site of injury or the cause of injury. It is the fundamental body reaction that we call *inflammation*.

This chapter consists of a brief summary of inflammation, a more detailed description of each of its phases, a consideration of the chemical mediators known to play a determining or controlling role, and a discussion of some disorders that represent abnormalities or aberrations of the inflammatory response. Chapter 4 deals with modifications of the inflammatory sequence determined by host-injurious agent interactions, definitions of acute, chronic, and granulomatous inflammation, and a consideration of disturbances of host response resulting from disease and certain therapeutic substances.

THE MORPHOLOGY OF THE INFLAMMATORY RESPONSE

Inflammation occurs in and around an area of injury. It consists of a medley of overlapping events that can be separated sequentially into:

1. Altered vascular permeability that permits passage of a protein-rich plasma into the injured area.
2. Migration of circulating leukocytes from the vascular compartment to the interstitium of the injured tissue.
3. Phagocytosis and enzymatic digestion of dead cells and tissue elements.
4. Repair of injury by
    a. Regeneration of normal parenchymal cells, or
    b. Proliferation of granulation tissue and eventual scar formation

Each of these phases is now considered in some detail. Figures 3.1 to 3.11 illustrate each phase as it can be observed in the reaction to and healing of a myocardial infarct. Myocardial infarction is a particularly good circumstance in which to study the inflammatory response, because all elements of the reaction are clearly recognizable at varying times after infarction occurs.

Altered Vascular Permeability

The earliest observable changes of the inflammatory response consist of altered blood flow in the microcirculation and increased vascular permeability. These phenomena have been studied extensively in a variety of experimental injuries. Immediately following acute injury (*e.g.*, a thermal burn), there is a brief period of reflex arteriolar spasm, with reduction of blood flow. This is followed by dilatation of arterioles, capillaries, and venules, and a dramatic increase in blood flow in and around the injury site. As fluid leaves the vascular compartment, the viscosity of blood increases and there is progressive stasis of blood flow.

Increased vascular permeability permits fluid approaching the composition of plasma to escape into the area of injury (Fig. 3.1). This fluid, rich in protein, has a specific gravity above 1.020, and is called an *exudate*, as opposed to a *transudate* consisting of low protein content fluid (*e.g.*, the edema fluid of congestive heart failure). Several phases of altered permeability are defined in experimental injuries. An *immediate* and usually *transient* response occurs within seconds of a mild injury and lasts for only a few minutes. Fluid leaves the vascular compartment through openings that appear at endothelial cell junctions of postcapillary venules. These openings result from contraction of the endothelial cells.

When injury is severe, there is extensive, often necrotizing, injury to the endothelial lining of the entire microcirculation, and fluid escapes from arterioles, capillaries, and venules. The increased permeability is both *immediate* and *prolonged*.

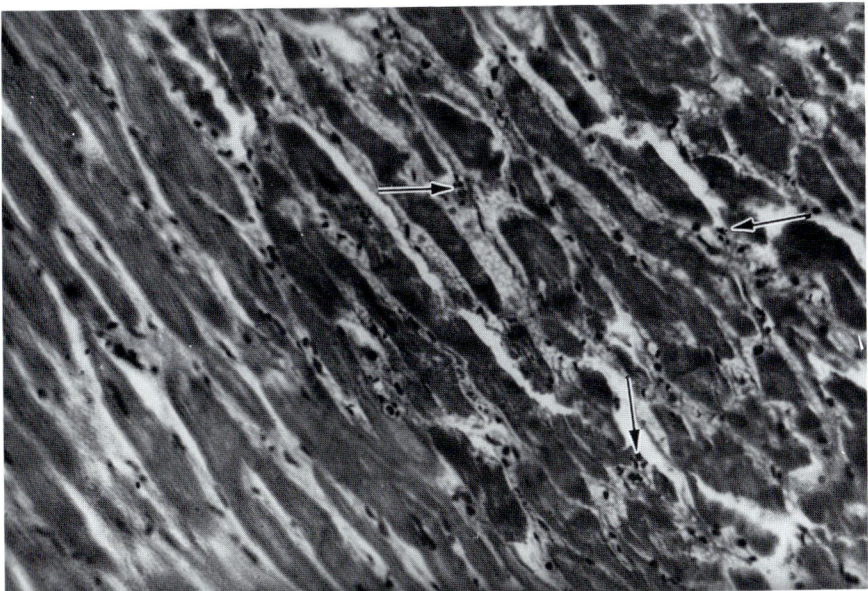

Figure 3.1. Acute myocardial infarction. The early response to the necrotic myocardial fibers at the *right* is seen as an accumulation of fluid between the fibers, congestion of small blood vessels, and early migration of a few polymorphonuclear leukocytes into the area of injury (*arrows*).

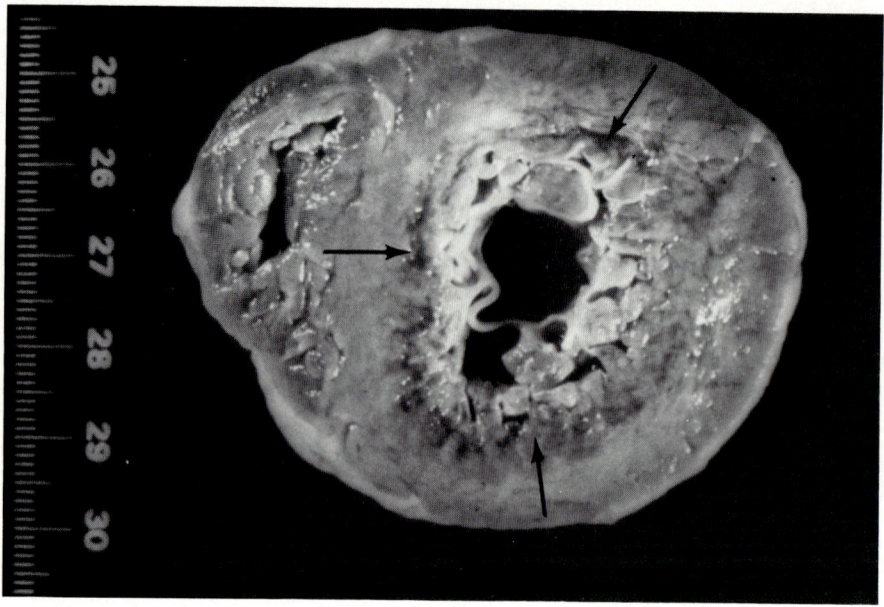

Figure 3.2. Acute subendocardial infarction. This horizontal section of heart shows a diffuse subendocardial infarction, corresponding to the lesion seen in Figure 3.1. The *arrows* point to the area of softening, and the darker color reflects vascular congestion.

Following many injuries, a second, and more prolonged increase in permeability is apparent. This response is *delayed*, occurring several hours after injury and lasting for hours or even days. Here again, it results from openings between endothelial cells, but capillaries as well as venules are involved. The delayed phase of vascular permeability is prominent in injuries resulting from various forms of radiant energy and in those associated with cell-mediated immunity, where latent periods characteristically precede the manifestations of injury.

Migration of Leukocytes

Very early in the inflammatory response, leukocytes of the circulating blood start migrating to the area of injury. The leukocytes, which usually occupy an axial position in the flow of blood through the microcirculation, begin to assume a more peripheral location, and give the appearance, on light microscopy, of sticking to the endothelial walls of postcapillary venules. They accumulate and form a "pavement" over the endothelial surfaces. Leukocytes move across surfaces by amoeboid motion, pseudopods are forced between endothelial cell junctions, and the flexible cell body pushes its way through the vessel wall (Fig. 3.3). It is slowed by the venular basement membrane, but temporarily disrupts the membrane to permit its passage and gains entrance into the interstitium of the injury site. The migration of leukocytes may begin during the phase of increased vascular permeability, but the ability of leukocytes to cross venular walls is independent of permeability.

The stimulus to this leukocytic migration is incompletely known, although

Reaction to Injury 17

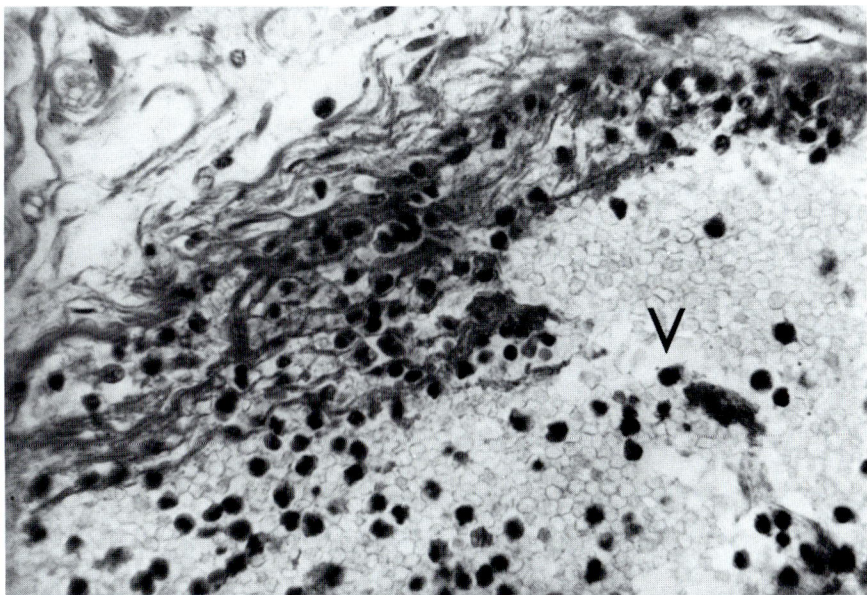

Figure 3.3. Leukocytic migration. This photograph shows a congested venule (*V*), with many polymorphonuclear leukocytes adhering to the endothelium, and working their way through the vessel wall by amoeboid motion. Several have reached the surrounding loose connective tissue.

substances that attract them are released in an area of tissue injury. Once through the vascular wall and free in the interstitium, however, leukocytes often demonstrate directional rather than random movement, and accumulate in areas of necrosis. This directional movement is called *chemotaxis*.

The polymorphonuclear leukocyte is, at first, the predominant cell of the inflammatory exudate. It appears within several hours of injury, and, although there may be great variations from one injury to another, it tends to dominate the scene for 24 to 48 hours (Figs. 3.4, 3.5, and 3.6). There is then a period when the mononuclear phagocyte (monocyte, macrophage) is dominant (Figs. 3.7 and 3.8). The reason for this shift in cell population is not clear. Polymorphonuclear leukocytes survive but a few hours after leaving the bloodstream, whereas mononuclear phagocytes may persist for months. This could provide a partial explanation, but it is also true that most cells leaving the vascular compartment early in inflammation are granulocytes, whereas later, increasing numbers of monocytes migrate. They appear to respond to different chemotactic stimuli.

Lymphocytes, when participating in an inflammatory reaction, also gain access to tissue spaces by working their way through endothelial junctions. Some reactions, particularly those involving certain types of allergy, are characterized by the inclusion of many polymorphonuclear eosinophils. These cells respond to separate chemotactic factors; they secrete histaminase, and may ingest certain soluble antigen-antibody complexes. Red blood cells may be passive participants in inflammation. A few red cells are commonly encountered, but a hemorrhagic inflammatory exudate usually signals severe injury to the microvasculature.

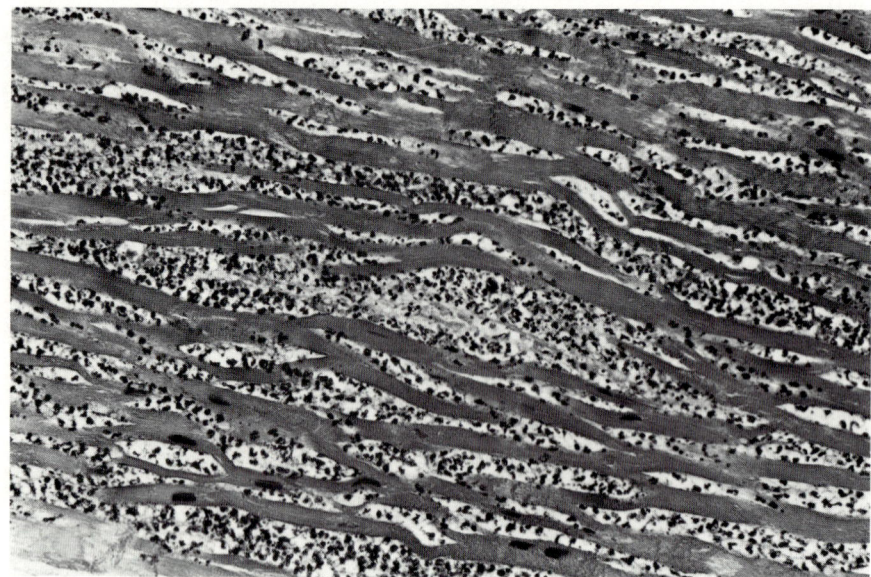

Figure 3.4. Acute myocardial infarction, showing massive infiltration by polymorphonuclear leukocytes.

Phagocytosis

When granulocytes and mononuclear phagocytes arrive at an area of tissue injury, they begin to ingest and digest particulate matter (Figs. 3.5 and 3.8). This consists primarily of necrotic debris, but in many circumstances also includes foreign particles such as bacteria. Soluble matter, such as protein aggregates and antigen-antibody complexes, may also be ingested. This process is called *phagocytosis*. Particulate matter is contacted by the phagocytic cell and is taken into the cell in a *phagosome* lined by cell membrane. The lysosomes of the granulocytes or mononuclear phagocytes, containing powerful hydrolytic and other enzymes, fuse with the phagosome and stimulate digestion of its contents. Phagocytosis of many bacteria may be difficult in the absence of *opsonins* (immunoglobins and the C3 component of complement) that facilitate the initial contact between cell and microorganism. Phagocytosis is an energy-consuming process, energy being derived to a considerable extent from anaerobic glycolysis. The ability of phagocytes to kill microorganisms appears related to the production of hydrogen peroxide in the phagosome, the presence of halide ions, and the release of myeloperoxidase from cellular lysosomes (the "hydrogen peroxide-halide-myeloperoxidase" system).

Microorganisms ingested by phagocytic cells may be destroyed, may persist in phagosomes for prolonged periods of time, or may destroy the host cell. In the latter event, lysosomal proteases will be released and can add significantly to the injury of surrounding tissue.

Mononuclear phagocytes unsuccessful in ingesting and digesting particulate matter may fuse with other mononuclear phagocytes to form giant cells. These

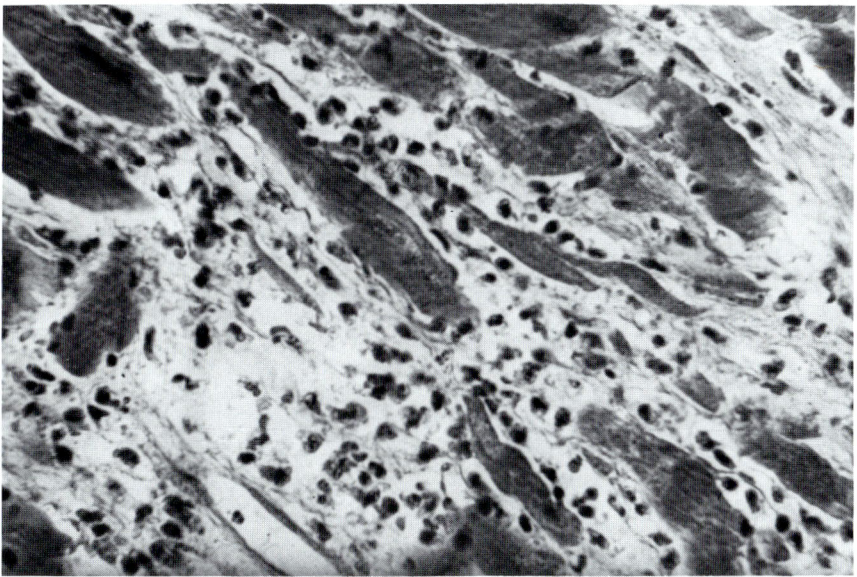

Figure 3.5. Acute myocardial infarction. At high magnification, polymorphonuclear leukocytes can be seen clustering around fragments of necrotic muscle fibers. They digest these fragments by phagocytosis or by releasing their proteolytic enzymes in the area of injury.

are frequently seen surrounding large fragments of foreign material, such as surgical sutures, but are also of frequent occurrence in fungus diseases, tuberculosis, and some other infections in which cell-mediated immunity is prominent.

Repair

The removal of necrotic debris and such injurious agents as bacteria makes possible the repair of the injury that triggered the inflammatory response. In many tissues, this can be accomplished by regeneration and reconstitution of an entirely normal anatomy. Pneumococcal pneumonia is an example of a dramatic inflammatory process diffusely involving one or more lobes of the lung but which usually heals with a complete return to normal structure and function.

A myocardial infarct cannot heal by regeneration. The area of destroyed myocardium is replaced by *granulation tissue* and eventually by a *scar* (Figs. 3.9, 3.10, and 3.11). Granulation tissue consists of young budding capillaries and actively proliferating fibroblasts. It makes its appearance as early as 8 or 10 days following a myocardial infarction, when many mononuclear phagocytes are still completing the removal of necrotic muscle fibers. The growing fibroblasts secrete collagen in ever increasing amounts, until the myocardial defect is replaced by strong connective tissue. The capillaries gradually recede and fibroblastic cells become less prominent, and the area gradually assumes the appearance of an amorphous scar. The ingrowth of granulation tissue and subsequent scar formation is called *organization*.

Many injuries heal by an admixture of regeneration and scar tissue formation. Repeated and persistent alcoholic injury to the liver destroys many liver cells

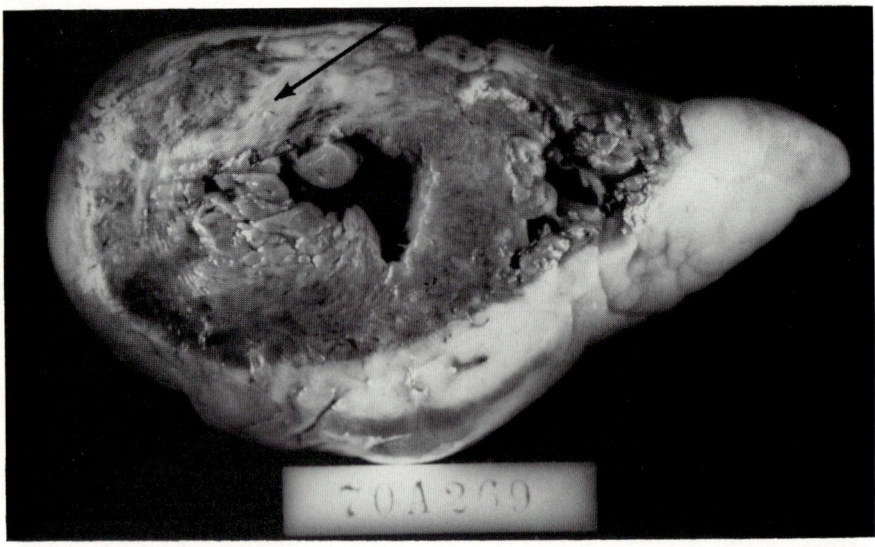

Figure 3.6. Acute myocardial infarction, corresponding to Figures 3.4 and 3.5. The area of infarction (*arrows*) is soft and yellowish gray in color. The area has the appearance of coagulation necrosis, although softening indicates considerable proteolytic digestion.

and injures the architectural framework of the liver lobule. There is extensive regeneration of liver cells, but there is also a proliferation of fibrous tissue, so that the liver comes to consist of irregular atypical lobules of regenerated liver cells traversed and surrounded by bands of scar tissue. This result is *cirrhosis*.

MEDIATORS OF THE INFLAMMATORY RESPONSE

Many chemical substances have been found capable of mediating the inflammatory response. Although a few, such as bacterial products, are from exogenous sources, the vast majority are endogenous, derived from normal components of plasma or circulating cells. Most of the mediators studied have their effects on vascular permeability and the chemotactic behavior of leukocytes. Only a few are discussed at this time, but most known mediators are summarized in Table 3.1.

Histamine

Histamine is the vasoactive amine generally accepted as the mediator of the immediate phase of increased vascular permeability. It is normally stored in the granules of mast cells, circulating basophil granulocytes, and platelets. The role of histamine is particularly significant in those allergic or hypersensitivity reactions mediated by IgE. Mast cells have receptor sites for IgE; interaction between allergens and IgE adherent to mast cells results in the release of histamine and other vasoactive amines.

Kinins

Kinins are vasoactive peptides released by the action of the enzyme kallikrein on the precursor kininogen. The initial step, activation of the precursor form of

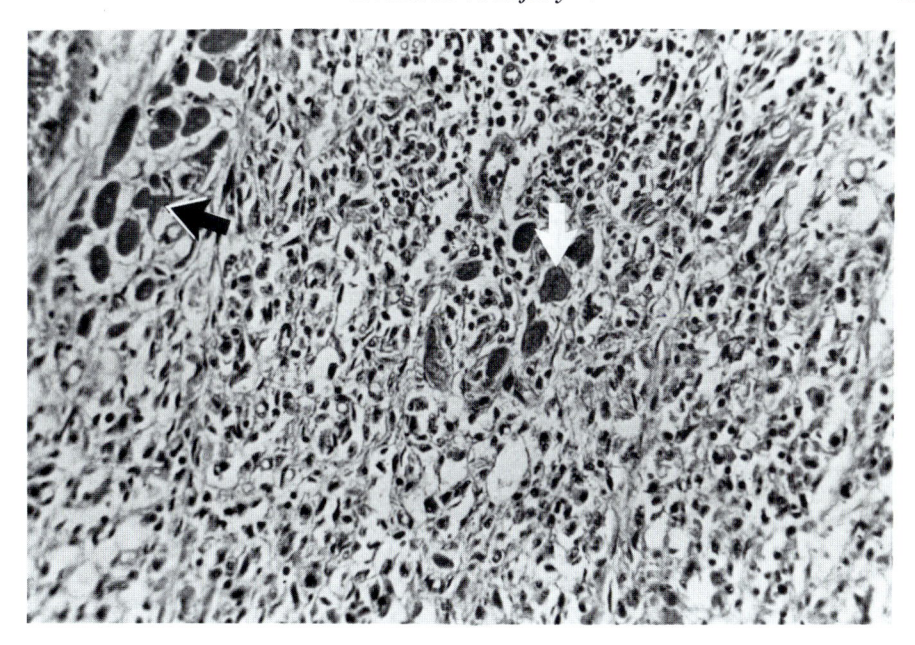

Figure 3.7. Myocardial infarction: mononuclear phase. Most of the necrotic fibers have been digested, although a few still remain (*arrows*). Most of the cells are mononuclear phagocytes, but some fibroblasts secreting collagen and a few capillaries can also be seen.

kallikrein, results from the action of Hageman factor, a β-globulin. Hageman factor, or clotting Factor XII, is key to the intrinsic coagulation mechanism of blood and to activation of the fibrinolytic system. Bradykinin is the principal kinin produced. It stimulates vasodilatation and increased vascular permeability, and is also related to the pain associated with the early phases of inflammation.

Complement

Complement consists of a series of nine proteins present in plasma. Activation of C1 (classical pathway), or C3 (alternative pathway), results in a cascade of activating events, with a progressive increase in the number of molecules involved, the splitting off of various fragments, and the formation of activated complexes. Many of these serve as mediators of various phases of the inflammatory reaction. A fragment derived from the second component, C2, stimulates vasodilatation, and is called C2-kinin. Fragments from C3 and C5 (C3a and C5a), called *anaphylotoxins*, promote the release of histamine from mast cells. C3 enhances phagocytosis, serving as an opsonin. A C5 fragment and the activated complex C567 are major chemotactic factors for polymorphonuclear leukocytes.

Blood Coagulation System

Several byproducts of the coagulation system may influence the inflammatory response. Plasmin, indirectly activated by Hageman factor, releases chemotactic fragments from the degradation of fibrin. It may also activate the complement cascade and stimulate kinin production.

Table 3.1
Some Mediators of Inflammation

Phase	Mediators	Related Disorders
Increased vascular permeability	Histamine Serotonin Bradykinin C2-kinin Anaphylotoxins, C3a, C5a Polymorphonuclear (PMN) cationic proteins Prostaglandins PGE_1, PGE_2	Urticaria pigmentosa Hereditary angioneurotic edema
Chemotaxis PMN	C5 fragment C$\overline{567}$ complex C3 fragment Fibrin degradation products Collagen fragments Plasminogen activator Bacterial products Viral products	 Complement deficiencies Chédiak-Higashi syndrome Lazy leukocyte syndrome
Monocyte	Bacterial products C3 and C5 fragments PMN cationic protein Lymphokines Plasminogen activator	Diabetes mellitus
Eosinophil	Eosinophil chemotactic factor of anaphylaxis (ECF-A)	
Lymphocyte	Lymphokines	Thymic aplasia Agammaglobulinemia (Swiss)
Phagocytosis	Immunoglobulins C3 fragment H_2O_2-halide-myeloperoxidase system	C3 deficiency Chronic granulomatous disease Sickle cell disease Immune deficiency states
Repair	Chalones Growth factors	

It is clear that the complement system, the clotting system, and the kinin-generating system are all interrelated in the inflammatory response. The activation of Hageman factor initiates the intrinsic clotting mechanism (see Chapter 7). It activates kallikrein, which catalyzes the production of bradykinin. Hageman factor also leads to the activation of plasmin. Plasmin releases fibrin degradation products from the lysis of fibrin, can trigger the complement cascade, and also stimulates the formation of subunits of Hageman factor which further enhance kinin generation.

Lymphokines

Stimulated sensitized lymphocytes can release a variety of substances called lymphokines that affect the inflammatory response. They are particularly note-

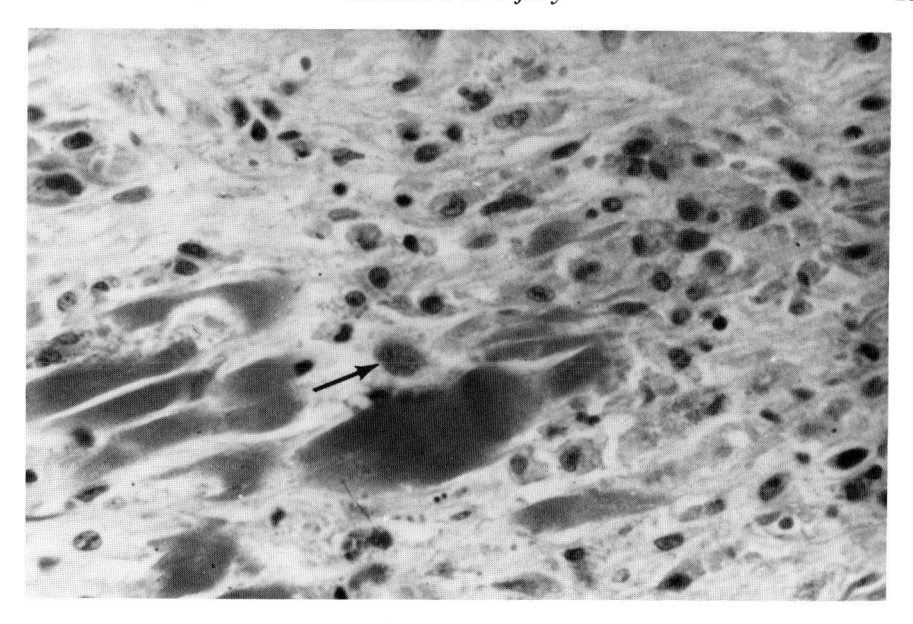

Figure 3.8. Mononuclear phase of myocardial infarction. Numerous mononuclear phagocytes are removing remaining fragments of necrotic muscle fibers by phagocytosis and digestion. The *arrow* points to a mononuclear cell containing golden brown hemosiderin pigment derived from the catabolism of bilirubin in tissue.

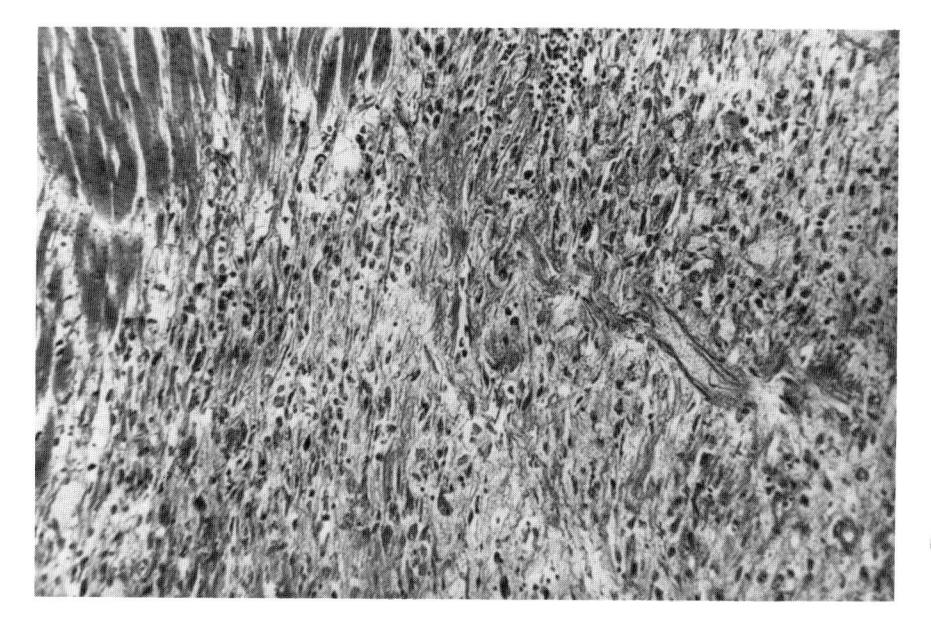

Figure 3.9. Myocardial infarction: reparative fibrosis. Many delicate collagen fibers can be seen, oriented from *top* to *bottom*. Most of the cells are fibroblasts or mononuclear phagocytes, although capillaries are numerous. See Figure 3.12 for a more dramatic example of capillary proliferation. A few necrotic muscle fibers remain at the *upper left*.

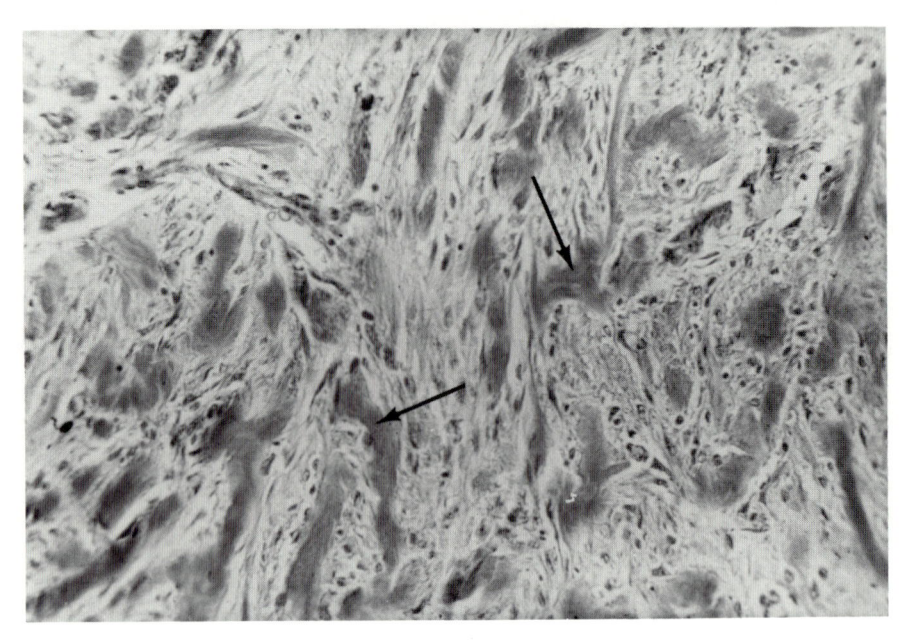

Figure 3.10. Myocardial infarction: scar formation. There has been extensive deposition of collagen, and many of the fibers are fused into dense collagen bundles (*arrows*). With further time, this scar tissue will lose its cellularity and blood vessels.

worthy in disorders characterized by cell-mediated immunity. Among the substances produced are chemotactic factors for mononuclear phagocytes and lymphocytes, a factor that inhibits migration of mononuclear phagocytes and activates them, a mitogenic factor, and a lymphotoxin that injures many cells.

Mediators Derived from Polymorphonuclear Leukocytes

Neutrophil lysosomes contain many substances that affect the inflammatory response upon their release. These include a kallikrein enzyme, proteases that promote formation of active products from complement, cationic proteins that release histamine from mast cells, and basic peptides that are chemotactic for mononuclear phagocytes.

Prostaglandins

Prostaglandins are synthesized as part of the inflammatory response, probably as a result of the release of lysosomal phospholipase from granulocytes and its interaction with arachidonic acid. Prostaglandins PGE_1 and PGE_2 influence vasodilatation and vascular permeability and may be chemotactic for neutrophils.

Control of Inflammation

It should be apparent that there are many mediators of inflammation, and that their uncontrolled activity would result in its perpetuation and progressive destruction of tissue. Most inflammatory responses, however, are controlled, and this is because many of the mediators discussed are effective for only very brief times before they are enzymatically inactivated, and because there are inhibitors

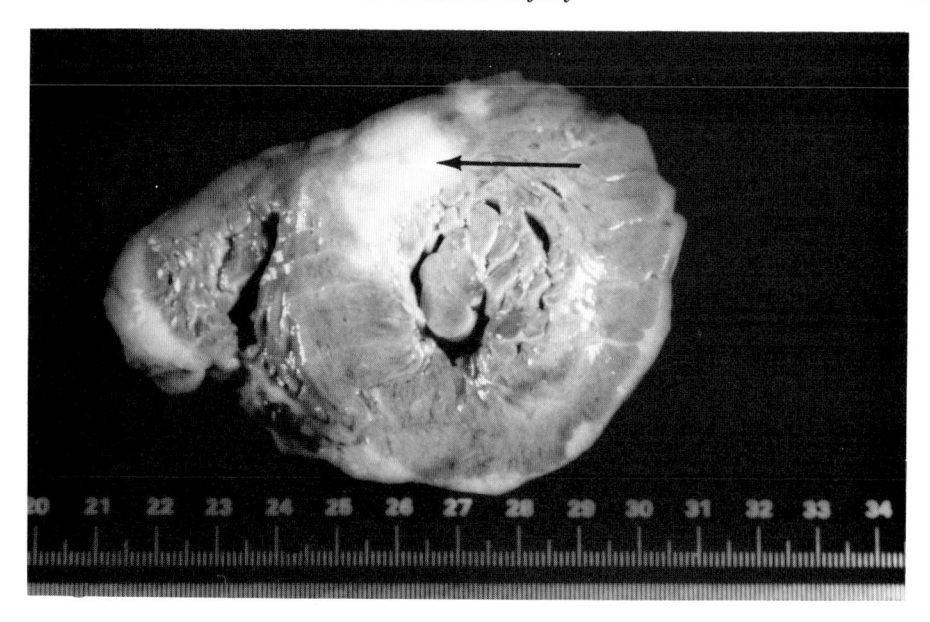

Figure 3.11. Healed myocardial infarction. The *arrow* points to an area of dense grayish white scar tissue, representing the end result of the inflammatory reaction to myocardial infarction.

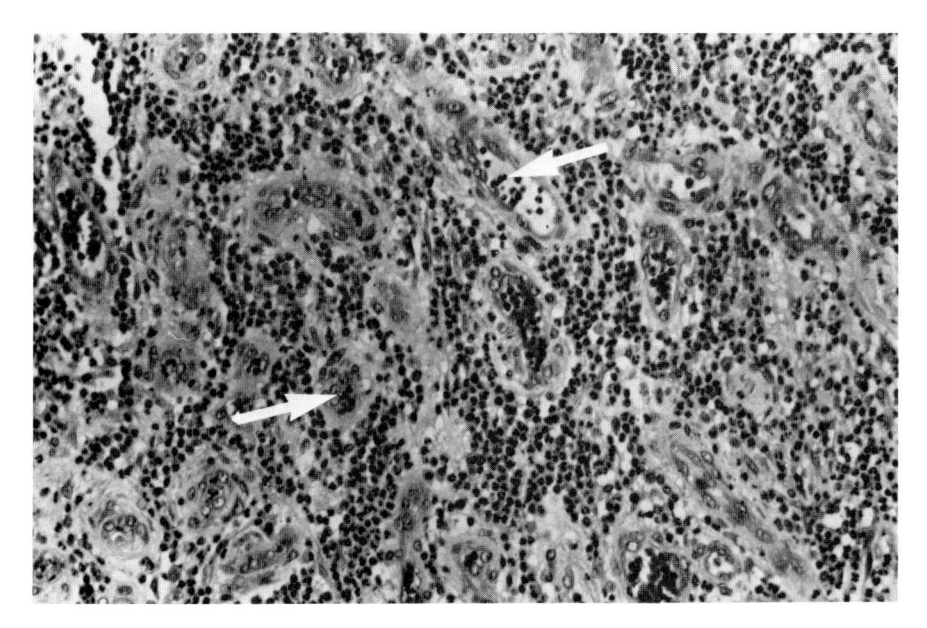

Figure 3.12. Granulation tissue. There are numerous proliferating small capillaries, recognized by the large numbers of endothelial nuclei. The intervening cells are predominately polymorphonuclear leukocytes and mononuclear phagocytes. Their numbers make recognition of fibroblasts difficult.

or antagonists for the mediators. Some disorders discussed below are the result of failure to control the mediators of inflammation.

Control of the repair process is poorly understood. Whether healing takes place by parenchymal regeneration or by organization, there must be a rapid increase in growth and multiplication rate of the appropriate cells, and then growth must return to normal when repair is complete. Increased growth may result from a temporary loss of inhibition by local tissue-specific *chalones* and by loss of *contact inhibition* in epithelial cells (Chapter 14). At the same time, stimulatory factors may play a role; a product of blood platelets may be important in promoting the proliferation of fibroblasts and endothelial cells.

CAUSES OF INFLAMMATION

The inflammatory response has been presented in this chapter as the sequence of events that follows cellular and tissue injury, as a defense mechanism that attempts to heal the injury and return function to normal. It must now be emphasized that the inflammatory response itself has the capacity to injure tissue, primarily through the release of lysosomal neutral proteases from leukocytes. Thus, any mechanism that can trigger the inflammatory response can potentially cause injury. Immune complexes can activate complement and induce an injurious inflammatory reaction. This is the basis of injury in poststreptococcal glomerulonephritis. Circulating antigen-antibody complexes consequent to a streptococcal pharyngitis are filtered by and lodge in the renal glomerulus. Complement is activated, releasing factors chemotactic for polyphonuclear leukocytes. When these granulocytes release their lysosomal enzymes, the glomerular apparatus is injured, and a further inflammatory response ensues. The inflammatory response is itself the principal cause of injury in disorders such as rheumatic fever and rheumatoid arthritis and the autoimmune diseases.

DISORDERS OF THE INFLAMMATORY RESPONSE

Many disorders result from congenital or acquired abnormalities of the inflammatory response. Only a few are mentioned here.

Hereditary angioneurotic edema is transmitted as an autosomal dominant. It is characterized by repeated bouts of edema, often associated with emotional stress, and tends to involve the skin, respiratory tract (larynx), and the gastrointestinal tract. This disorder results from a deficiency of C1 esterase inhibitor, an important substance in the control of complement. C1 esterase inhibitor also inhibits kinin generation, and the disorder may be a reflection of uncontrolled bradykinin synthesis.

The *Chédiak-Higashi syndrome* is a rare disorder inherited as an autosomal recessive trait. The principal manifestation is marked susceptibility to bacterial infections, but other findings include decreased pigmentation, hepatosplenomegaly, and pancytopenia. Giant lysosomes are seen in granulocytes, and the function of these cells is abnormal; they respond poorly to chemotactic factors, and do not discharge their granules normally. Abnormal organelles are also present in circulating monocytes.

Chronic granulomatous disease is a disorder of phagocytic function, inherited as a sex-linked recessive, and characterized by repeated persistent infections involving skin, lung, bones, and other organs. In this disease, leukocytes fail to increase their metabolic activity following phagocytosis, and do not produce hydrogen peroxide. This is, then, a failure of the hydrogen peroxide-halide-myeloperoxidase system, the principal basis of intracellular bactericidal activity.

Suggested Reading

Becker EL, Stossel TP, et al. Chemotaxis. Fed. Proc. *39:* 2949, 1980.
Ryan GB, Majno G. Acute inflammation. Am. J. Pathol. *86:* 183, 1977.
Ward PA. Inflammation. In: Hill RB Jr, LaVia MF, eds. Principles of pathobiology. New York, Oxford University Press, 1980.

Chapter 4

Host-Injurious Agent Interactions

The sequence of events that comprise the inflammatory response is remarkably constant regardless of the site of injury or its cause. All inflammatory reactions, however, are not identical. Striking quantitative variations occur and reflect a diversity of interactions between injurious agents and the defensive and reparative capacity of the host. The phases of the inflammatory response described in Chapter 3 were illustrated with examples from the evolution and healing of a myocardial infarct, since each phase was prominent and clearly recognizable. In many injuries, the relationship between host and injurious agent is such that the early part of the inflammatory sequence predominates in intensity, while in others the late phases are more dramatic. These differences in interplay between opposing forces are the basis for defining *acute* and *chronic* inflammation.

By way of introduction, the morphologic consequences of differing host-injurious agent relationships are illustrated by observing the consequences of introducing three different microorganisms into the lung. These are the pneumococcus (*Streptococcus pneumoniae*), *Staphylococcus aureus*, and the tubercle bacillus (*Mycobacterium tuberculosis*).

The Pneumococcus

The capacity of the pneumococcus to cause disease, or its *pathogenicity*, lies in its ability to grow rapidly, and, thanks to its thick polysaccharide capsule, to resist phagocytosis. It also produces hyaluronidase and a hemolysin. The classical disease resulting from pneumococcal infection is pneumococcal pneumonia, formerly one of our major killers. The disease is of rapid onset, heralded by chills and high fever, with cyanosis, cough productive of "rusty" sputum, and evidence of pleural inflammation. During this time, there is rapid spread through one or more lobes. At the spreading edge, one observes dilatation and congestion of alveolar capillaries and massive alveolar edema containing myriads of pneumococci (Fig. 4.1). Extensive fibrin deposition is seen in the exudate. Behind this wave, there is rapid migration of large numbers of polymorphonuclear leukocytes into the alveoli (Figs. 4.2 and 4.3), and these succeed in phagocytizing some organisms by trapping them against alveolar walls or strands of fibrin. A few mononuclear phagocytes are seen in the exudate. The involved lung is now airless and consolidated (Fig. 4.4).

Patients who recover tend to do so dramatically between the 5th and 10th days of illness by crisis. There is rapid defervescence and subsidence of symptoms.

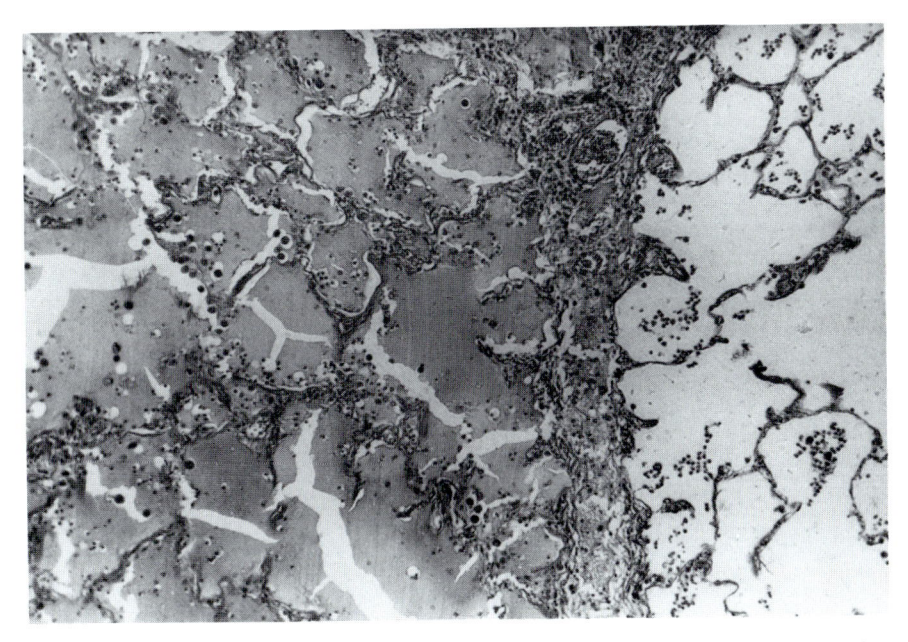

Figure 4.1. Pneumococcal pneumonia. This section shows the spreading edge of infection, characterized by an outpouring of edema fluid containing large numbers of microorganisms. The advance of the process has been temporarily slowed by the minor fissure to the right of center.

The patient's defenses have been successful. At the time of crisis, anticapsular opsonins have usually been produced and enhance greatly the ability of leukocytes to phagocytize and destroy the pneumococci. The pneumonic consolidation heals by *resolution;* the alveolar exudate is enzymatically digested and liquefied with the help of mononuclear phagocytes as well as polymorphonuclear leukocytes. It is expelled from the lung through the bronchial tree or absorbed. Superficial injury to the alveolar lining cells is readily repaired by regeneration, and there is return to completely normal structure.

In this disorder, a pathogenic organism has been able to spread rapidly through the lung and evoke an intense reaction in which the early phases of the inflammatory response are predominant. The host, however, has gained mastery over the organism in but a few days, and complete healing by resolution follows. This is an example of *acute inflammation.*

Occasionally, pneumococcal pneumonia, especially when due to Type III pneumococcus, fails to heal by resolution, and much cellular debris, some organisms, mononuclear phagocytes, and fibrin remain in the alveolar spaces. Granulation tissue begins to grow into the alveolar spaces from the septa, and there is gradual and progressive fibrosis of the alveoli (Fig. 4.5). The host-parasite relationship has changed. The organism now has only limited ability to injure host tissues, but the host has been only partially successful in controlling and destroying the organism. This is the host-injurious agent relationship that characterizes *chronic inflammation.*

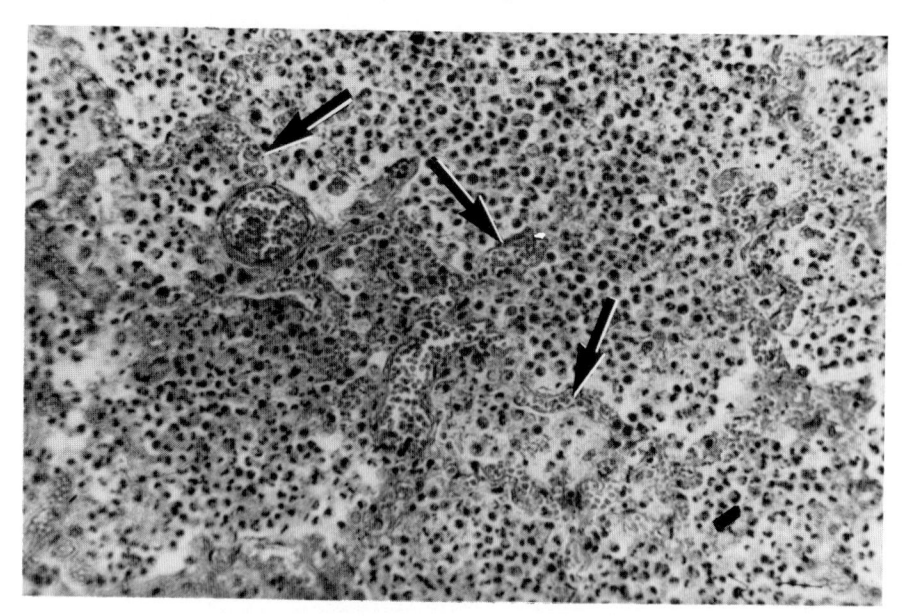

Figure 4.2. Pneumococcal pneumonia. Behind the advancing edge, there is massive migration of polymorphonuclear leukocytes and a few mononuclear phagocytes from the congested alveolar septa (*arrows*) into the alveolar spaces. The alveolar septa remain intact.

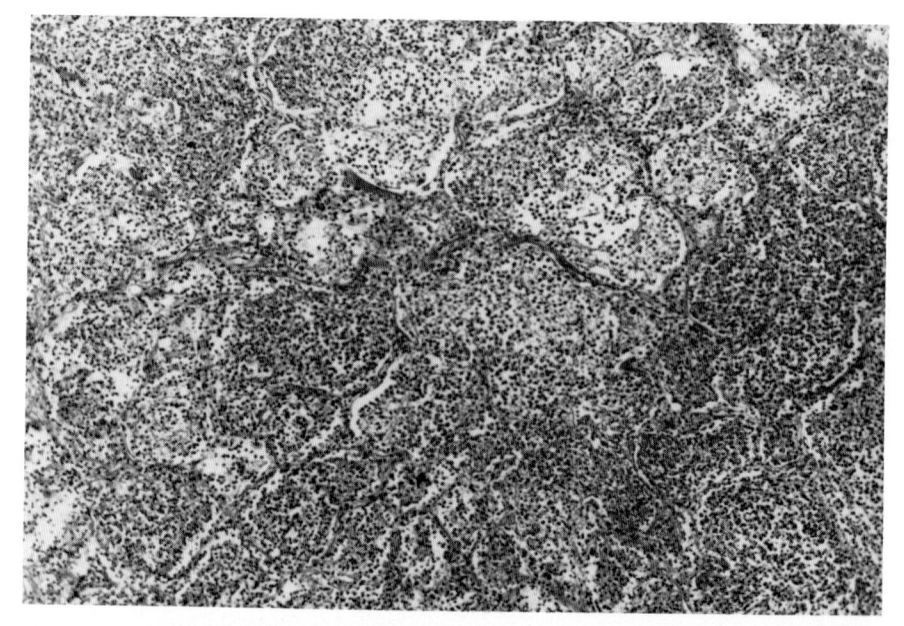

Figure 4.3. Pneumococcal pneumonia. There is marked consolidation of the lung, with the alveolar spaces packed with polymorphonuclear leukocytes, some of which are degenerating, and variable amounts of fibrin. Note that the normal pulmonary architecture is still visible. In most instances, pneumococcal pneumonia does not injure the basic structure of the lung.

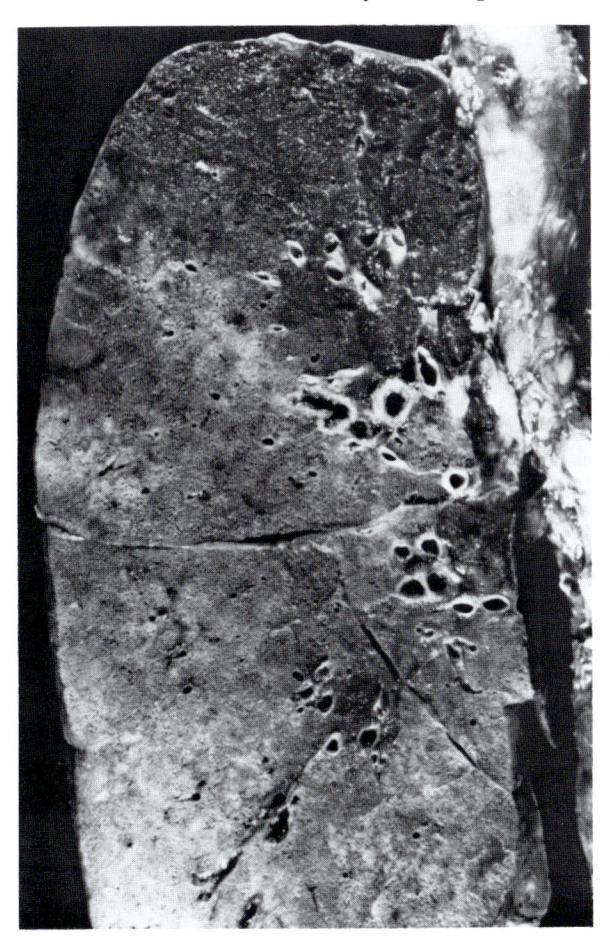

Figure 4.4. Pneumococcal pneumonia. The upper portion of the upper lobe of this lung appears normal and is normally aerated. The entire lower portion of the lung is massively consolidated, being pale gray in color, firm in consistency, and containing very little air.

The Staphylococcus

Staphylococcus aureus is unlikely to produce pulmonary disease in the normal host. In infants, children with cystic fibrosis, adults with influenzal pulmonary infections, or those with compromised resistance, staphylococci can reach the lung through the respiratory passages. Staphylococci produce a variety of exotoxins, among them hemolytic, necrotizing, and leukocidal toxins. They also produce lysozyme, fibrinolysins, coagulase, and a thermonuclease. In the lung, there is extensive destruction of bronchiolar and alveolar walls, and an intensive reaction characterized by massive numbers of polymorphonuclear leukocytes and fibrin deposition. Staphylococci are phagocytized, but they are not readily digested, and many leukocytes are destroyed. There is progressive enzymatic digestion, and an abscess forms. It is characterized by a necrotic, liquefied center containing cellular debris derived from the destroyed pulmonary architecture and polymorphonuclear leukocytes, active polymorphonuclear leukocytes, and numbers of living and dead microorganisms (Fig. 4.6). The area of destruction tends to be walled off

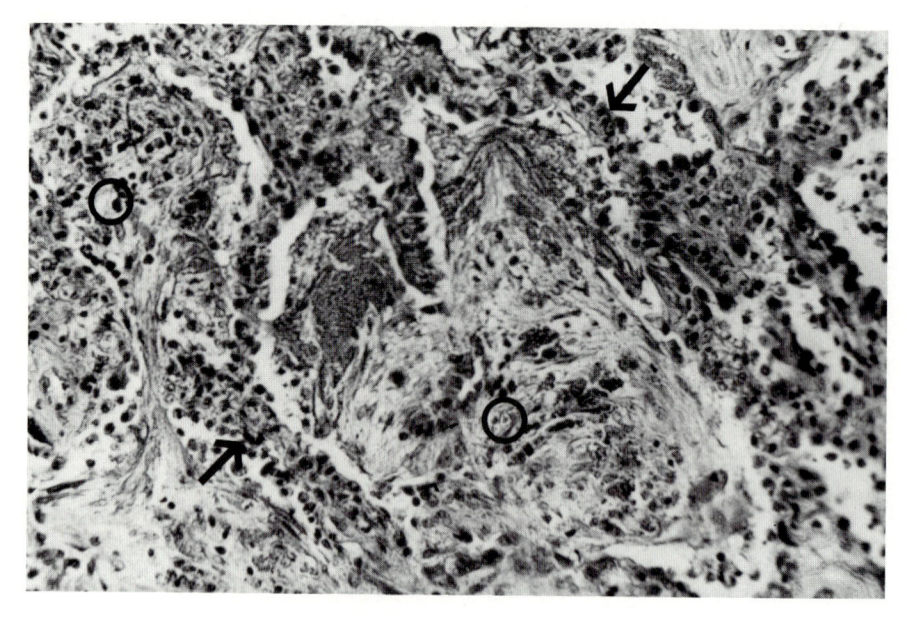

Figure 4.5. Organizing pneumococcal pneumonia. The alveolar exudate has failed to heal by resolution, and is being replaced by proliferating fibroblasts and capillaries (*circles*). The alveolar septa (*arrows*) are thickened, and their lining cells are prominent.

effectively by a zone of intense polymorphonuclear leukocytic infiltration and fibrin deposition (Fig. 4.7), although some fibroblastic and vascular proliferation may be seen quite early. As is true of abscesses elsewhere in the body, healing can be rapid, if the abscess drains itself effectively, by ingrowth of granulation tissue and scar formation.

A staphylococcal abscess is again an example of acute inflammation, even though, because of extensive tissue destruction, healing has required organization and scar formation. A highly pathogenic organism has produced rapid tissue destruction, but the area of injury has been effectively walled off, and if drainage is achieved healing is rapid. The early phases of the inflammatory response, especially polymorphonuclear leukocytic migration and fibrin deposition, have dominated the reaction to an injury produced by the *Staphylococcus*.

Tubercle Bacillus

The tubercle bacillus produces no toxins of significance in tuberculous infection. Its pathogenicity rather lies in its ability to survive and grow slowly within host cells, and its ability to induce cell-mediated immunity, or delayed type hypersensitivity, to its proteins. When tubercle bacilli are introduced into the lung of a susceptible but previously unexposed host, they are ingested by mononuclear phagocytes. They do not destroy the cells, and the cells do not interfere with their slow growth. After several weeks, when cell-mediated immunity is demonstrable, there is rapid change. The cells containing the organisms become necrotic, and there is a brief appearance of polymorphonuclear leukocytes (Fig. 4.8). These

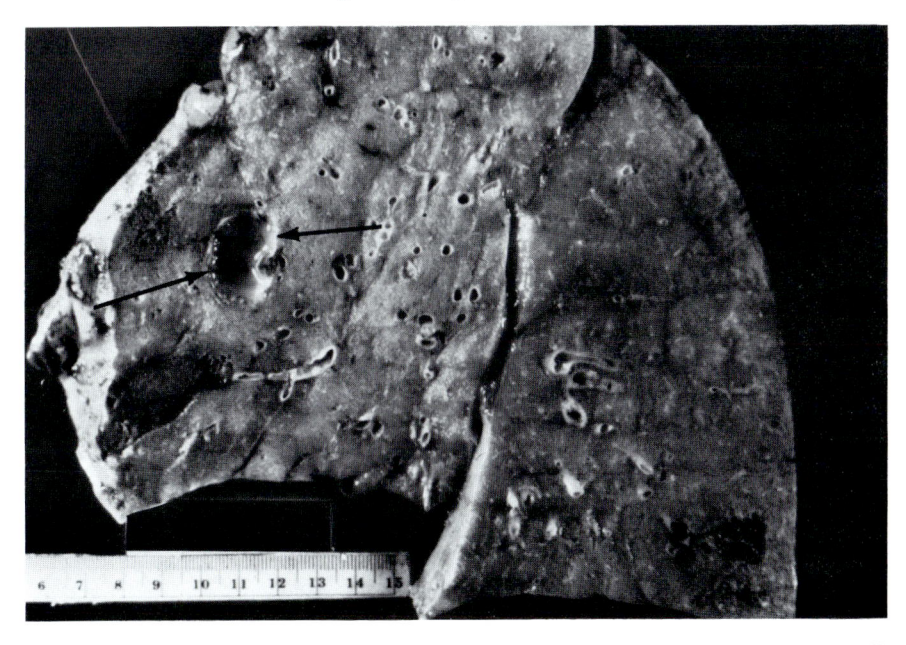

Figure 4.6. Lung abscess. The abscess cavity, which has been evacuated, is lined by a delicate membrane composed of masses of polymorphonuclear leukocytes in a fibrin network.

are replaced by a new migration of mononuclear phagocytes. Cellular and tissue necrosis occurs, and is only partially digested (caseation necrosis), and there is gradual evolution of a lesion called a *granuloma* (Fig. 4.9). This lesion is circumscribed. It has a center of caseation necrosis, containing remnants of tissue and phagocytic cells, living and dead organisms, and products of the tubercle bacillus. This is surrounded by many mononuclear phagocytes. Some of them have assumed a superficial resemblance to epithelial cells, and are called *epithelioid cells*. Others have fused to form multinucleated giant cells. Lymphocytes are usually present. The lesion is surrounded by a zone of fibroblastic proliferation containing numbers of lymphocytes (Fig. 4.10). A fibrous wall gradually forms, and the lesion may appear to remain quiescent for a prolonged period of time.

The tubercle bacillus and the host lived in harmony up to the moment that cell-mediated immunity was demonstrable. From then on, the bacillus had some ability to injury host tissue, but there was also an enhanced capacity of host cells to destroy the organism. A relationship of relative stalemate was achieved in which host and parasite had only limited ability to destroy each other. This is characteristic of *chronic inflammation*. The later phases of the inflammatory response, mononuclear phagocytes and reparative fibrosis, dominated the morphologic expression of the relationship.

ACUTE, CHRONIC, AND GRANULOMATOUS INFLAMMATION

Inflammatory reactions are subclassified as acute or chronic. Acute inflammatory lesions result from a host-injurious agent relationship in which tissue injury

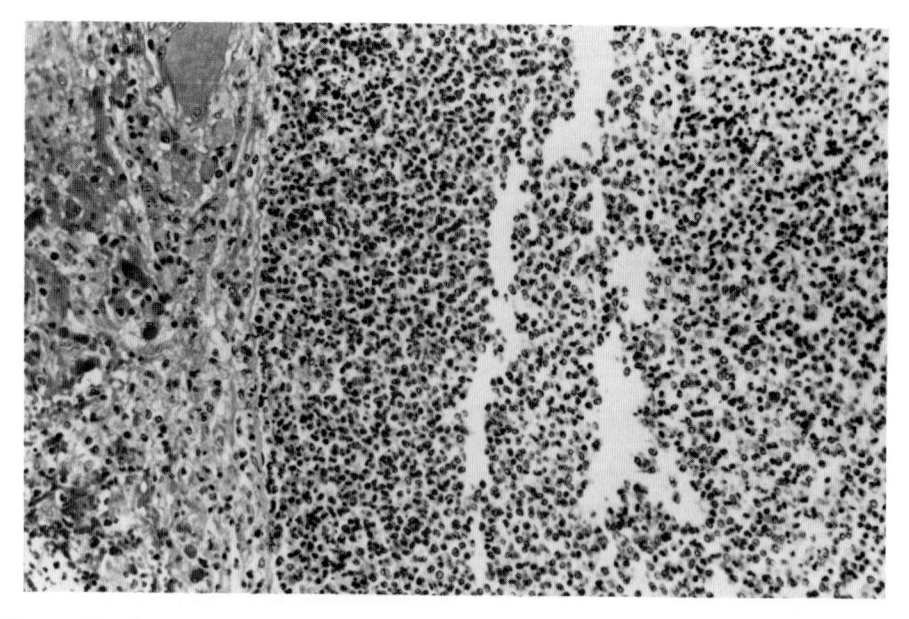

Figure 4.7. Lung abscess. The abscess wall is shown to the *left*, and consists of tightly packed polymorphonuclear leukocytes surrounded by a few strands of collagen. To the *right*, many of the leukocytes are becoming necrotic and fragmented, and this area is becoming liquefied.

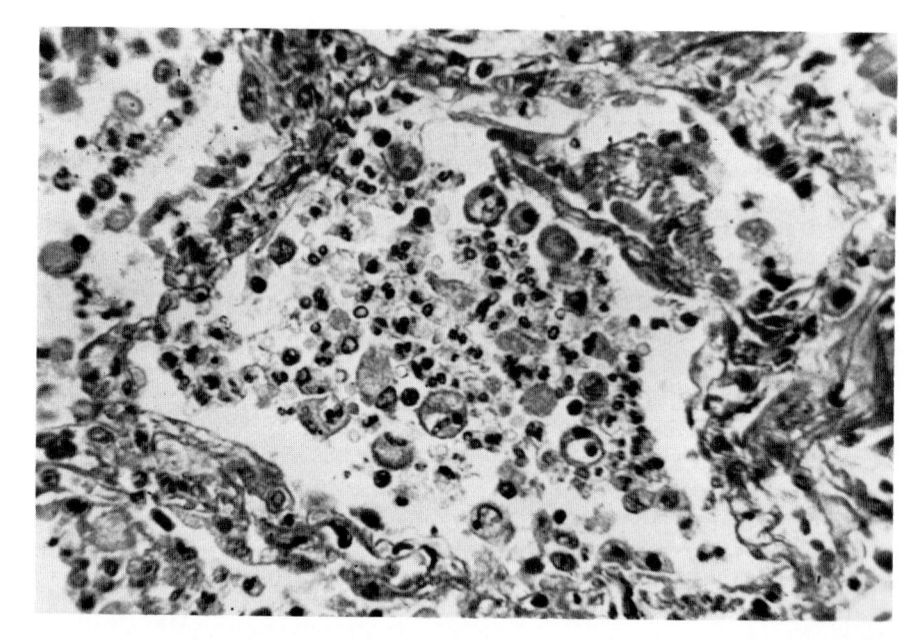

Figure 4.8. Pulmonary tuberculosis. This field shows an alveolar space with an early lesion of tuberculosis. Mononuclear phagocytes containing tubercle bacilli have become necrotic, and there is a transient polymorphonuclear leukocytic reaction.

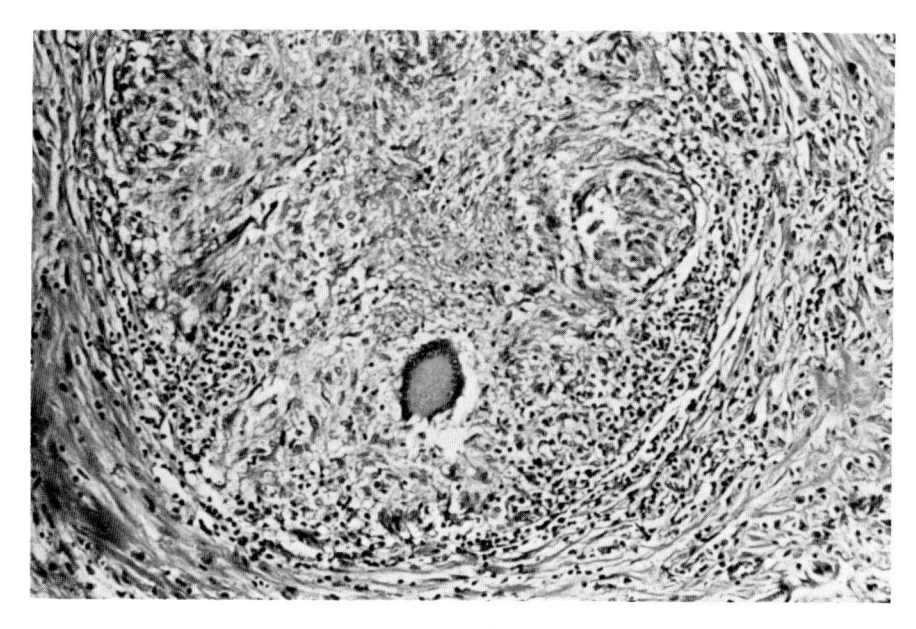

Figure 4.9. Pulmonary tuberculosis. There is early granuloma formation, with a central area of caseation necrosis and surrounding mononuclear phagocytic reaction. A multinucleated giant cell is seen *below* the area of necrosis.

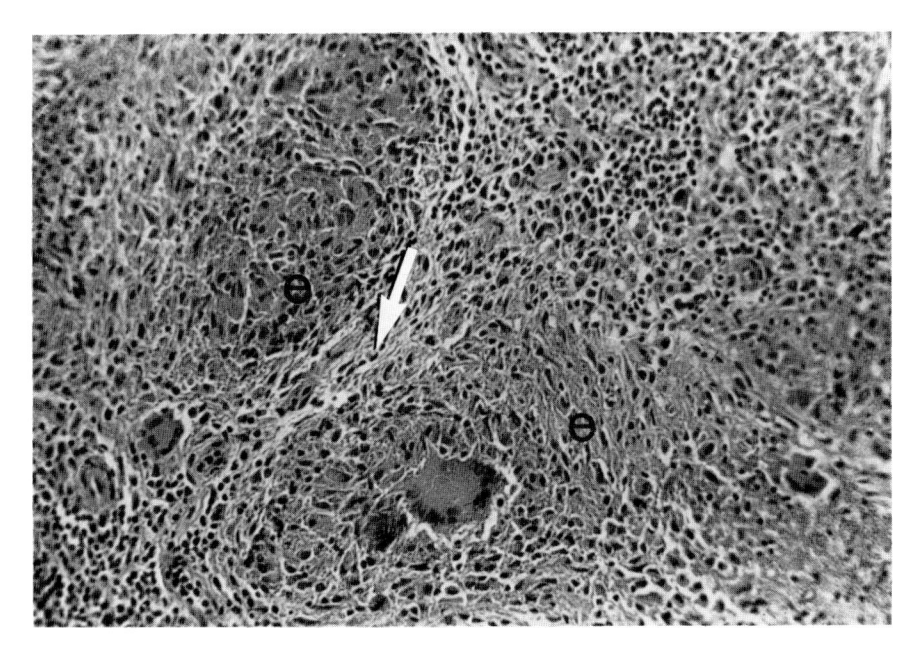

Figure 4.10. Granulomatous inflammation in tuberculosis. Several groups of epithelioid cells are seen (*e*), and multinucleated giant cells are noted in the *lower portion* of the photograph. Elsewhere, there is fibroblastic proliferation (*arrow*) and groups of small lymphocytes.

may be extensive, but, assuming survival, the host gains mastery over the injurious agent and heals the injury. Chronic inflammation results from a relationship in which host and injurious agent have limited capacity to injure each other, so that continuing low grade injury is accompanied by constant attempts at healing. Acute inflammation is usually of brief duration, lasting days or, at most, a few weeks, and the dominant cell is the polymorphonuclear leukocyte. Chronic inflammation generally lasts months or years, and mononuclear phagocytes and fibroblasts are the cells most seen. There are many exceptions to the temporal and cytologic aspects of acute and chronic inflammation, and it is important to recognize the interaction of host and injurious agent as the fundamental basis for classification.

A *granuloma* is a localized area of chronic inflammation. The etiologic agent, when known, is generally found near its center. Most granulomas have necrotic centers; others do not. The most characteristic aspect of the lesion is the accumulation of mononuclear phagocytes, some of which fuse to form multinucleated giant cells. The area of mononuclear phagocytic infiltration is surrounded by a zone of fibroblastic proliferation and collagen production, often with an intermingling of lymphocytes (Figs. 4.11, 4.12, and 4.13). The mononuclear phagocytes observed in granulomas are activated cells; *i.e.*, they have been stimulated, often by lymphokines, to increase their phagocytic functions. Activated mononuclear phagocytes are nonspecific in these reactions, responding to many types of organisms and particulate matter. Many granulomas demonstrate a change of mononuclear phagocytes to epithelioid cells. These cells have lost

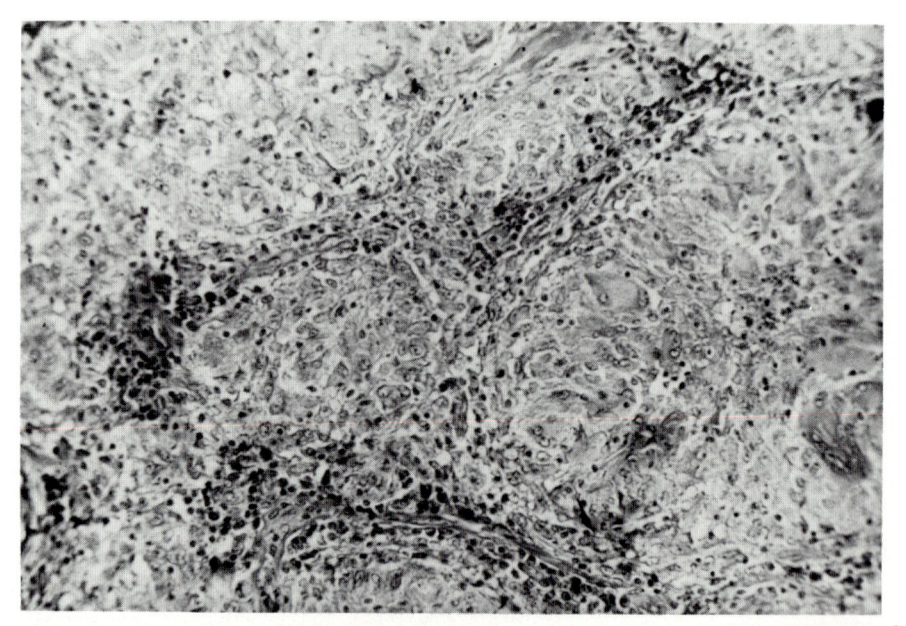

Figure 4.11. Granulomatous lymphadenitis in sarcoidosis. There are nodular accumulations of epithelioid cells and a few small giant cells. These nodules are surrounded by delicate fibrous tissue and numbers of small lymphocytes. No necrosis is seen.

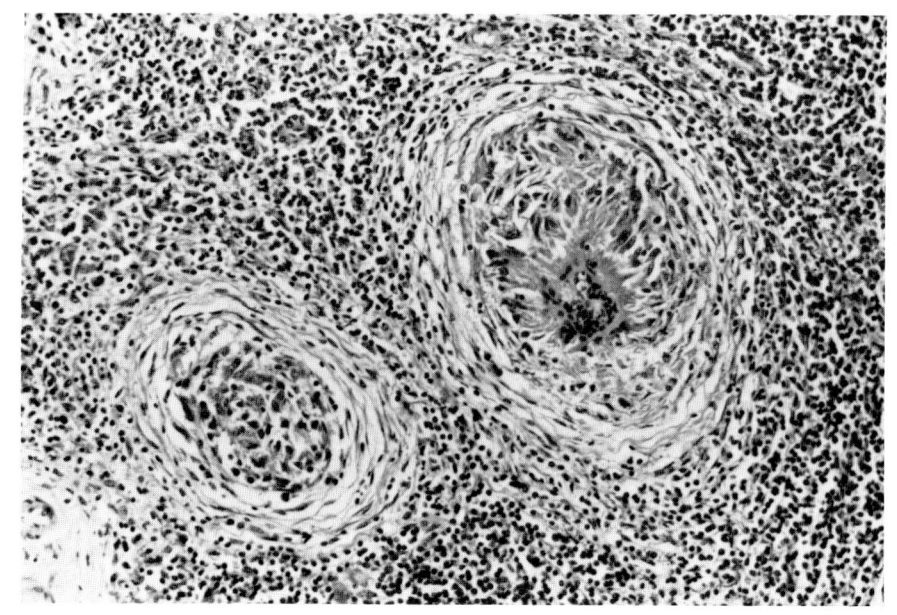

Figure 4.12. Granulomatous lymphadenitis in sarcoidosis. Two well demarcated granulomatous lesions are seen. The central area is composed of large numbers of epithelioid cells, and one granuloma contains a large multinucleated giant cell. There is no necrosis. The granulomas are well circumscribed by fibrous tissue.

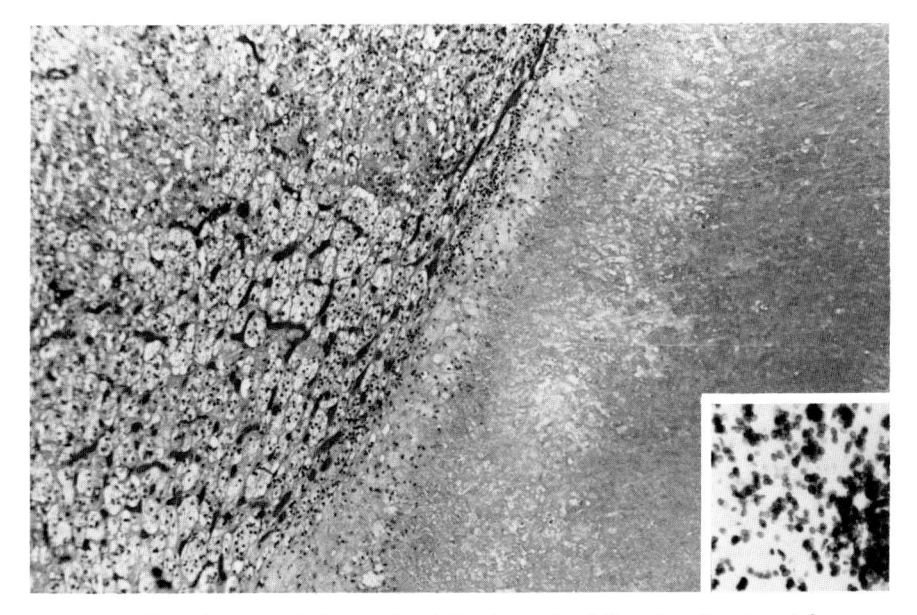

Figure 4.13. Granulomatous inflammation: histoplasmosis of the adrenal cortex. A large area of necrosis is seen to the *right*, separated from the adrenal cortex by a narrow band of mononuclear phagocytes and proliferating fibroblasts. The *inset*, at higher magnification, shows large numbers of *Histoplasma* organisms stained with silver.

some of their capacity to phagocytize, but they have markedly enhanced ability to kill microorganisms.

Granulomatous inflammation is characteristic of many disorders in which cell-mediated immunity is demonstrable, but granulomas are also prominent in the response to many foreign materials to which there is no immunologic reaction. In general, it is thought that those granulomas containing epithelioid cells and lymphocytes represent a manifestation of cell-mediated immunity.

Many human diseases manifest granulomatous inflammation, among them tuberculosis, many fungus diseases, brucellosis, and the late stages of syphilis. Granulomatous inflammation is also the rule in disorders resulting from incorporation of such foreign materials as silica, asbestos, and beryllium. In the disease *sarcoidosis*, there is extensive granulomatous inflammation with many epithelioid cells in response to an unknown etiologic agent.

THE PATHOGENICITY OF MICROORGANISMS

The pathogenicity of microorganisms lies in their ability to survive and grow in the human body and to produce injury to its cells and tissues. There are many mechanisms to explain pathogenicity.

Many organisms are able to resist phagocytosis by virtue of their component structures. These include the thick polysaccharide capsule of the pneumococcus, the M-protein of the cell wall of streptococci, and the waxy capsule of the tubercle bacillus. Organisms vary in their ability to spread in tissue. Some are motile. Many Gram-positive bacteria produce a hyaluronidase that loosens interstitital structures. Some, such as staphylococci and streptococci, produce kinins that activate fibrinolytic enzymes. The clostridia that cause gas gangrene are thought to spread because of their production of powerful collagenases.

Powerful exotoxins are secreted by many organisms, often, as in the case of diphtheria, tetanus, and botulism, acting at distances from the site of infection or portal of entry. Others act locally, and are responsible for producing tissue injury. Most, but not all, exotoxins are produced by Gram-positive organisms. A strong exotoxin elaborated by *Pseudomonas aeruginosa* is an important aspect of its pathogenicity. Gram-negative organisms are likely to release endotoxins when they are lysed. Endotoxins are components of the bacterial cell wall, and contain phospholipids and polysaccharides. Endotoxins are associated with fever production and cardiovascular shock, and, most important, they may produce diffuse injury to vascular endothelium leading to the syndrome of disseminated intravascular coagulation, with consumption of various clotting factors. The ability to induce immunologic reactions can be an important mechanism of pathogenicity. Cell-mediated immunity is the major element of the pathogenesis of tuberculosis. Some organisms produce disease by altering host tissues so that they behave as antigens and evoke autoimmune responses. Still others may produce antigens closely related to host proteins, so that antibodies to the exogenous antigen react also with normal body structures.

The pathogenicity of viruses resides in their ability to be incorporated in the genome of host cells. The cell may be destroyed, or its growth pattern may be seriously altered, but a long period of latency may precede these events.

A newly recognized basis of pathogenicity is the ability to bind to cell receptor sites for normal substances. For example, the microorganism causing cholera does not invade tissue or produce recognizable injury to the small intestine. Disease is produced because a product of the organism binds to mucosal receptor sites, and, through stimulation of adenylate cyclase, leads to the outpouring of massive quantities of water and electrolytes into the intestinal lumen.

HOST RESISTANCE

Host resistance consists of the ability to destroy or inactivate injurious influences, and to repair the injury they have produced. Normal resistance implies good general health and nutrition, a normal vascular system, integrity of the inflammatory response, and an intact capacity for immunologic reactions.

There are variations in natural resistance to certain infections among the races and peoples of the world. These are based on the cumulative experience of a population over a prolonged period of time. Thus, white Americans have a greater natural resistance to tuberculosis than do American Indians or Eskimos. Introduction of diseases not previously experienced by isolated population groups can have devastating effects.

Some differences in resistance are age-related. Infections with *Haemophilus influenzae* are common before the age of 8, but uncommon in normal adults. Resistance to tuberculosis is impaired in infancy and old age.

Variations in resistance to injury are also dictated by characteristics peculiar to certain tissues and organs, including their ability to regenerate normal tissue, their susceptibility to the injurious effects of certain immunologic phenomena, and such constraints as limited blood supply, a rigid or nonexpandable architecture, or a tissue structure resistant to phagocytosis and enzymatic digestion. Liver and renal tubules have a great capacity for regeneration and reconstitution of normal architecture following acute injury, but muscle has at most very limited capacity, and most muscle injuries are followed by scar formation. Glomeruli, small blood vessels, and joint tissues are particularly subject to immunologically mediated injury. The rigid structure of bone resists expansion due to edema during the early inflammatory response; this may result in vascular compression and extensive ischemic necrosis of bone and bone marrow. Necrotic bone may require months or years to be removed by enzymatic digestion.

Resistance is impaired in patients suffering from a multitude of inherited and acquired deficiencies of the inflammatory and immune responses. These can be given but cursory consideration.

Altered leukocytic function, particularly of chemotactic behavior and phagocytosis, is observed in patients with diabetes mellitus, malnutrition, and certain tumors. These functions are also abnormal in patients with inadequate numbers of leukocytes (leukopenia or agranulocytosis) and in those with leukemia. Patients with sickle cell disease are deficient in certain opsonins, and particularly prone to pneumococcal infection. Deficiencies in the various components of complement are also reflected in altered response to injury.

There are many inborn immunodeficiency states. In *Swiss type agammaglobulinemia*, there is a deficiency of both T and B lymphocytes, and impaired humoral and cell-mediated immunity. Those afflicted suffer repeated infections by bacterial agents, fungi, protozoa, and viruses. In the *Di George syndrome*, there is absence of the thymus and other third and fourth pharyngeal pouch derivates. B cell function is normal, but death is usually due to viral or fungal infections in infancy. In *Bruton type agammaglobulinemia*, there is sex-linked failure of B cell differentiation, and inability to produce humoral antibodies. Cell-mediated immunity and resistance to virus and fungus disease are normal. The *Wiskott-Aldrich syndrome* is transmitted as a sex-linked recessive. Patients suffer recurrent infections due to many organisms, although levels of IgG, IgE, and IgA are normal or elevated. IgM is present but decreased. This disorder is poorly understood, but it is thought that there is deficient production of antibodies to the carbohydrate components of bacteria that grant antigenic specificity. Defects of T cell function may be noted, and there is also a striking thrombocytopenia. *Ataxia telangiectasia* is a syndrome composed of disturbances of motor function, abnormal dilatation of postarteriolar capillaries (telangiectases), and increased susceptibility to infection. There is disturbed T cell function and poor synthesis of IgA and IgE immunoglobulins.

Immunodeficiencies may also result from disease. Patients with Hodgkin's disease characteristically have disturbances of cell-mediated immunity due to altered T cell function. Certain leukemias and multiple myeloma are associated with poor immunoglobulin synthesis.

The ability to repair injury can be affected by disorders such as scurvy, where fibroblasts do not proliferate normally or produce collagen.

Some of the most serious disturbances of host resistance are related to the administration of therapeutic agents. Broad spectrum antibiotics may change the natural flora in various parts of the body, with the result that there is massive overgrowth of unaffected organisms. Successful treatment of certain infections may open the way for infection by antibiotic-resistant organisms. Adrenal steroid preparations affect many aspects of host resistance. Most phases of the inflammatory response are depressed, including changes in vascular permeability and the migration of leukocytes. Large doses suppress both cell-mediated and humoral immunologic mechanisms. Fibroblastic repair is also inhibited. All antineoplastic chemotherapeutic drugs suppress leukocyte function and immune reactions.

The resistance to infection of many patients is severely compromised by the combined administration of broad spectrum antibiotics, adrenal steriods, and cytotoxic agents in the treatment of neoplastic diseases, in certain autoimmune diseases, and in the prevention of rejection reactions following organ transplantation. The result has been the emergence of *nosocomial* or hospital-acquired infections caused by organisms that do not ordinarily produce disease in the normal host. Among these have been bacterial infections due to *Pseudomonas aeruginosa*, enteric streptococci, and certain Gram-negative organisms; many fungus infections, including aspergillosis and mucormycosis; systemic dissemination of infections with cytomegalovirus, herpes simplex, and herpes zoster viruses; infection with the protozoan *Pneumocystis carinii*, and pulmonary and cerebral dissemination of the intestinal parasite strongyloides. Legionnaire's disease has forced temporary closing of a large transplantation service in Los Angeles.

Patients with compromised resistance are also likely to suffer recrudescence of apparently arrested infections, particularly those due to tuberculosis.

CONCLUSION

It is apparent that a great many factors affect the interplay between the injury-producing capacity of injurious agents and the healing powers of the host. All of these factors have modifying effects on the morphologic sequence of events that constitutes inflammation. They become signally important in such disorders as tuberculosis, where the delicate balance between host and injurious agent is readily upset and the outlook for recovery profoundly altered.

Suggested Reading

Adams DO. The granulomatous inflammatory response. Am. J. Pathol. *84:* 163, 1976.
Cohen S. The role of cell-mediated immunity in the induction of inflammatory responses. Am. J. Pathol. *88:* 501, 1977.
Nathan CF, Murray HW, Cohn ZA. The macrophage as an effector cell. N. Engl. J. Med. *303:* 622, 1980.
Unanue ER. Secretory function of mononuclear phagocytes. Am. J. Pathol. *83:* 395, 1976.

Chapter 5

Patterns of Infection

In Chapter 4, consideration was given to many of the factors that contribute to pathogenicity and resistance, and to how they interact to determine the pathogenesis, extent, character, and ultimate fate of injury. An understanding of these factors and their interplay is central to the study of infections.

There are many hundreds of human diseases caused by microbial agents, and even a sketchy overview would be far beyond the scope of this book. Instead, a small group of selected disorders is discussed in some detail. They have been chosen because of their contemporary importance or because they illustrate certain pathogenetic mechanisms. Pneumococcal pneumonia was described in Chapter 4. The infections considered here are *Escherichia coli* pyelonephritis, gonorrhea, tuberculosis, Rocky Mountain spotted fever, cytomegalic inclusion disease, candidiasis, and pneumocystis pneumonia.

ESCHERICHIA COLI PYELONEPHRITIS

Pyelonephritis is an infection of the kidney. It is particularly likely to occur in individuals with obstructive lesions of the urinary tract. It may be unilateral or bilateral, and usually has a focal distribution within the kidney. Infection starts in the interstitium of the kidney, but extends to involve the tubules and, at times, the glomeruli. It often occurs as a very acute disease, with fever, prostration, costovertebral angle pain, and dysuria. Acute episodes usually subside, particularly with effective antibiotic therapy, but there is a marked tendency to relapse or recurrence. Pyelonephritis may occasionally follow a more chronic course, with progressive destruction of the renal parenchyma and renal failure.

E. coli, the most common cause of urinary tract infections, is the causative agent in some 85% of kidney infections, particularly in an initial episode of disease. It is a normal inhabitant of the gastrointestinal tract and, in general, an organism of very low pathogenicity. It releases endotoxins upon lysis of the bacterial wall, and a very few strains, those that may be associated with acute enteritis, produce an enterotoxin. When *E. coli* gains access to a location not normally inhabited, it can produce destructive disease. Infections may be associated with bacteremia, shock, and the syndrome of disseminated intravascular coagulation.

Obstructive lesions of the urinary tract play an important role in the pathogenesis of pyelonephritis; they are demonstrable in more than half of patients. Obstruction may be located at any point in the urinary tract, the most frequent sites being the outflow tract of the bladder, the ureterocystic junctions, and the

Patterns of Infection

renal pelves. It is not surprising that pyelonephritis is most likely to occur in children with congenital anomalies of the urinary tract, during pregnancy, and in elderly men with enlarged prostate glands.

Coliform organisms frequently gain transient access to the lower urinary tract, particularly in women because of the short length of the urethra. Organisms may also be introduced through instrumentation of the lower tract. Any obstruction may result in pooling and incomplete evacuation of urine and the opportunity for bacterial growth. Organisms reach the kidney in most instances through the urinary column itself. Within the kidney, particularly in the renal medulla, the ability of coliform organisms to produce injury relates to two local conditions. The normal hypertonicity of the medulla interferes with phagocytosis by both polymorphonuclear leukocytes and mononuclear phagocytes. Hypertonicity, furthermore, may induce the formation of protoplast forms, microorganisms that have lost their capsules, are resistant to antibiotics, and can persist for long periods in hypertonic media. The high ammonia content of the medulla inhibits the C4 component of complement, and interferes with bactericidal mechanisms.

Pyelonephritis is a destructive lesion of the renal parenchyma. Although inflammation may at times be confined to the interstitium, injury usually extends to involve tubules and, at times, glomeruli (Fig. 5.1), and abscess formation is common (Fig. 5.2). The lesions heal with scarring, and these scars can add a new

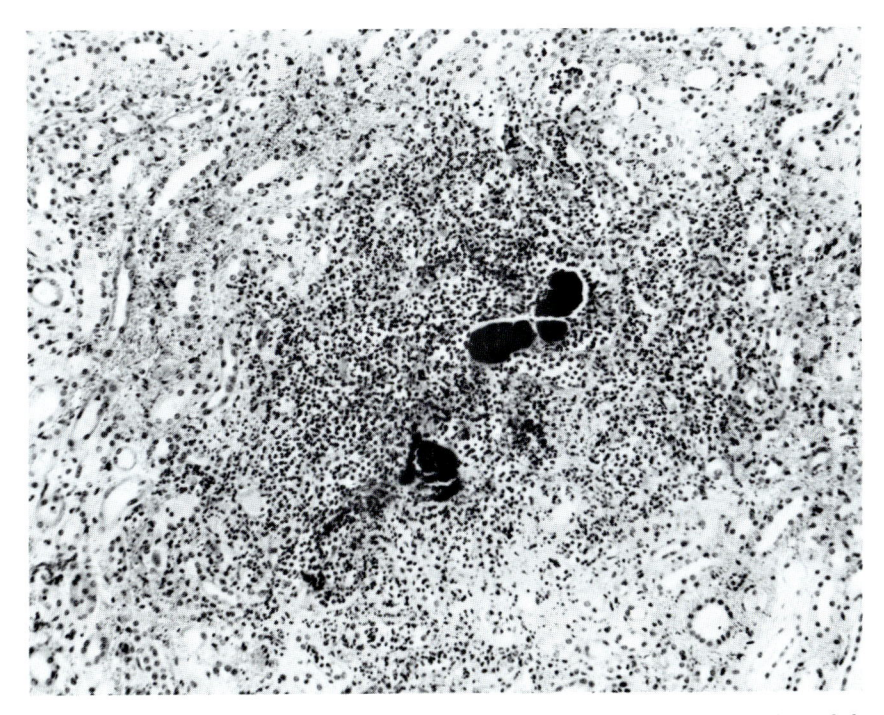

Figure 5.1. Acute pyelonephritis. Infection started in the interstitum of the medulla, and there is marked infiltration of polymorphonuclear leukocytes. The tubules in the central area have been destroyed, and there is early abscess formation. The dark-staining masses are conglomerations of bacteria, in this instance, staphylococci.

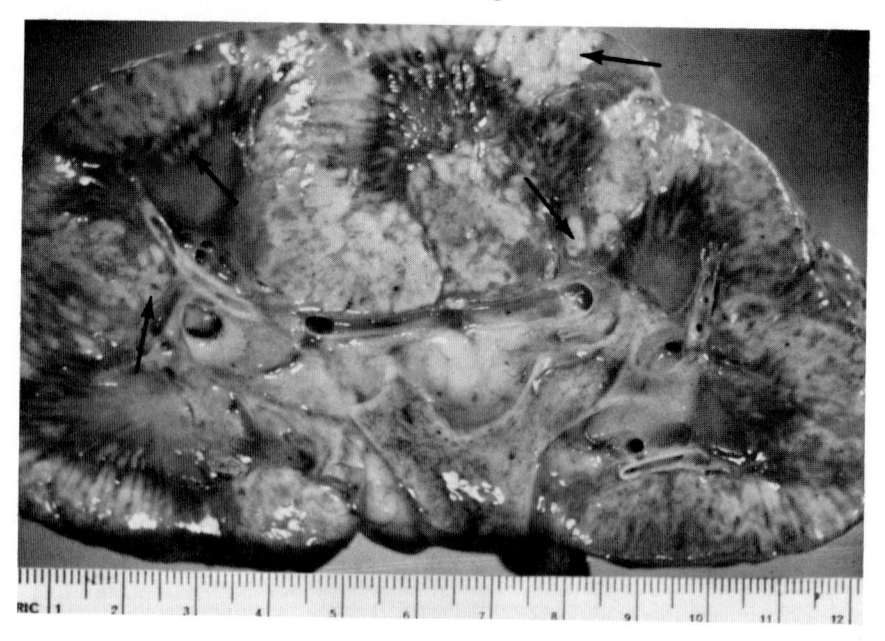

Figure 5.2. Acute pyelonephritis. Myriads of abscesses are seen, predominately involving the cortex, but some medullary lesions are seen as well.

obstructive element within the kidney that adds to the proclivity for recurrent infection.

GONORRHEA

Gonorrhea is a disease of epidemic proportion in the United States. The introduction of penicillin therapy resulted in a drop in reported cases from approximately 300 to 130 per 100,000 population between 1945 and 1957. Since 1957, however, there has been a steady increase in cases, reaching 468 per 100,000 population in 1978. This rise may in part reflect improved reporting, but the emergence of antibiotic-resistant and penicillinase-producing strains of gonococci is probably the most important explanation.

Several factors other than antibiotic resistance contribute to the high incidence of gonorrhea. It is a highly transmissible disease. There is a large reservoir in asymptomatic patients, mostly women, but including 10% of men with the disease. Over 60% of infections are in the young, aged 15 to 24, where changes in sexual mores, activity, and practices have been greatest. Finally the immune response to gonorrheal infection is poor, and does little to protect from new infection.

The pathogenicity of the organism, *Neisseria gonorrhoeae*, is poorly understood. The organism contains a rather weak endotoxin. Virulent organisms have hair-like projections, or *pili*, that may aid in attachment to mucosal epithelial cells. They also produce a protease that inactivates IgA and may open the way to mucosal surface infection.

Infection is virtually always the result of sexual contact. The initial sites of infection are usually the anterior urethra in men and the urethra, vulvovaginal glands, and endocervical glands in women. Other portals of entry include the anus and pharynx. The incubation period is between 2 and 7 days. In men, the disease most often starts as a very acute purulent urethritis, with dysuria and an inflamed meatus. The urethral discharge includes large numbers of polymorphonuclear leukocytes, most of them containing the organisms in their cytoplasm. There is frequent extension to involve the prostate, seminal vesicles, and the epididymis. If infection persists, abscesses may form in the prostate and seminal vesicles, and the epididymitis can result in sterility. Urethral stricture, formerly a frequent complication, is uncommon.

In women, the onset of disease is usually less dramatic, and symptoms may be ignored. Vaginal discharge and dysuria are frequent. Painful swelling and inflammation of Bartholin's and Skene's glands may occur. The endocervix is often inflamed. The most serious complications are extension to the Fallopian tubes and pelvic peritoneum. This is most likely to occur at the time of menses. Adhesions form between the fimbria and ovary, leading to tubo-ovarian abscess formation. Gonorrheal salpingitis frequently results in sterility or a high incidence of ectopic pregnancy. Pelvic peritonitis, with extensive adhesion formation, can be extremely painful and disabling.

Anal gonorrhea is observed in women and homosexual men. In women it may result from anal sex or from contamination from the genital tract. It is usually manifested by a purulent proctitis, often painful. Active pharyngitis is found in 20% of men and women with gonorrhea.

Dissemination of disease is more likely in women and homosexual men; in heterosexual men, the severity of urethritis leads to earlier therapy. Occasional patients manifest a syndrome similar to that observed in low grade meningococcal bacteremia, consisting of fever, skin rash, arthralgias, and tenosynovitis. Septic arthritis, involving one or several joints, may occur some weeks after infection. There is fever and leukocytosis, and organisms are usually demonstrable in the purulent joint fluid.

Gonorrhea is likely to remain a major health problem for some time to come. The introduction of each new antibiotic is followed by the emergence of resistant strains of gonococci. The possibility of effective immunization against the disease perhaps holds the greatest promise.

TUBERCULOSIS

The pathogenicity of the tubercle bacillus and the formation of an epithelioid granuloma were discussed in Chapter 4. Tuberculosis is considered here because it remains an important disease, and because it is a prototype of disease in which cell-mediated immunity is the key to pathogenesis.

The granuloma of tuberculosis is called the *tubercle*. It is the basic and characteristic lesion of tuberculosis, regardless of site of infection, age of patient, or stage of disease. The tubercle consists of a central zone of caseation necrosis, containing partially digested necrotic debris, tubercle bacilli, and protein and lipid residues of destroyed organisms. The necrotic area is surrounded by mononuclear phagocytes, many of them having the appearance of epithelioid cells, and varying numbers of multinucleated giant cells (Fig. 4.10). The giant cells often show a peripheral arrangement of nuclei, and are called *Langhans* cells. The tubercle is circumscribed by a zone of active fibroblasts, often including groups of T lymphocytes. Lesions of tuberculosis do not appear until cell-mediated immunity can be demonstrated in the host. Except in patients with overwhelming infection or with altered immune responses, the presence of tuberculous lesions signals demonstrable cell-mediated immunity. Were it not for cell-mediated immunity, tuberculosis as we know it would not exist.

Cell-mediated immunity results in an enhancement of the ability of mononuclear phagocytes, especially epithelioid cells, to kill the tubercle bacillus. It is also responsible for tissue necrosis. In general, when few organisms are present, cell-mediated immunity results in increased function of mononuclear phagocytes, destruction of the organisms, and healing (*proliferative* lesions). When there are large numbers of organisms, cell-mediated immunity leads to tissue necrosis and spread of infection (*exudative* lesions). The fate of the tubercle depends on the degree of success in killing the tubercle bacilli. The more caseation, the more difficult to heal the tubercle. The lesions enlarge, but may become encapsulated, isolating the organisms. Such a lesion is arrested, but can be reactivated at some future time if host resistance is changed (Fig. 5.3).

The pattern of tuberculosis differs in children and adults. The characteristic pattern in childhood is the *Ghon complex*. In pulmonary disease, it consists of a small subpleural focus of tuberculous infection, with involvement of lymphatics, and striking caseation necrosis of hilar lymph nodes (Fig. 5.4). Healing takes place in the vast majority of children, leaving calcified scars in the lung and hilar nodes. Tubercle bacilli may be eliminated, but some may persist in apparently healed tubercles for many years.

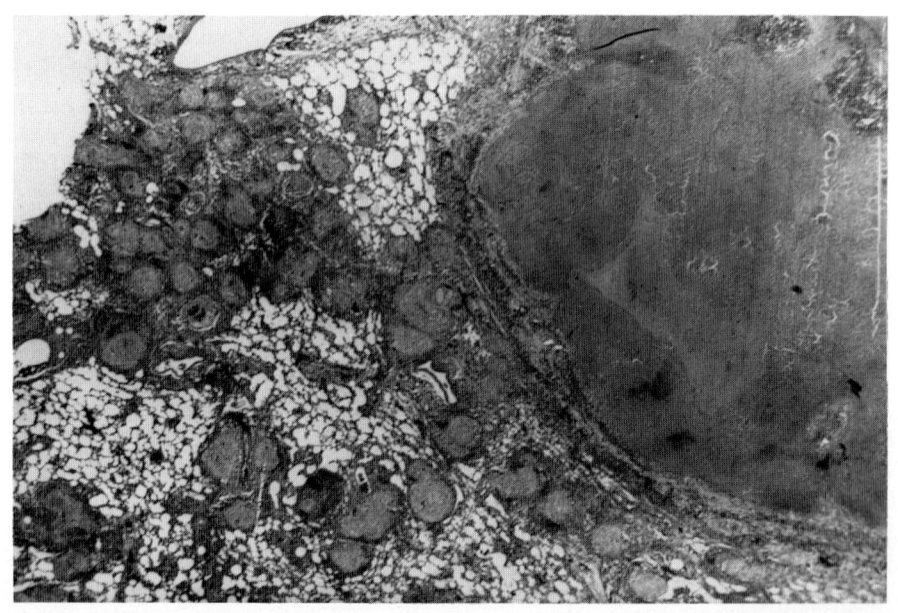

Figure 5.3. Pulmonary tuberculosis. A large tubercle is seen to the *right*. It consists of a mass of caseation necrosis surrounded by a thin wall of fibrous tissue. There has been dissemination, apparently through the bronchial tree, and many small tubercles are seen to the *left* and *below*.

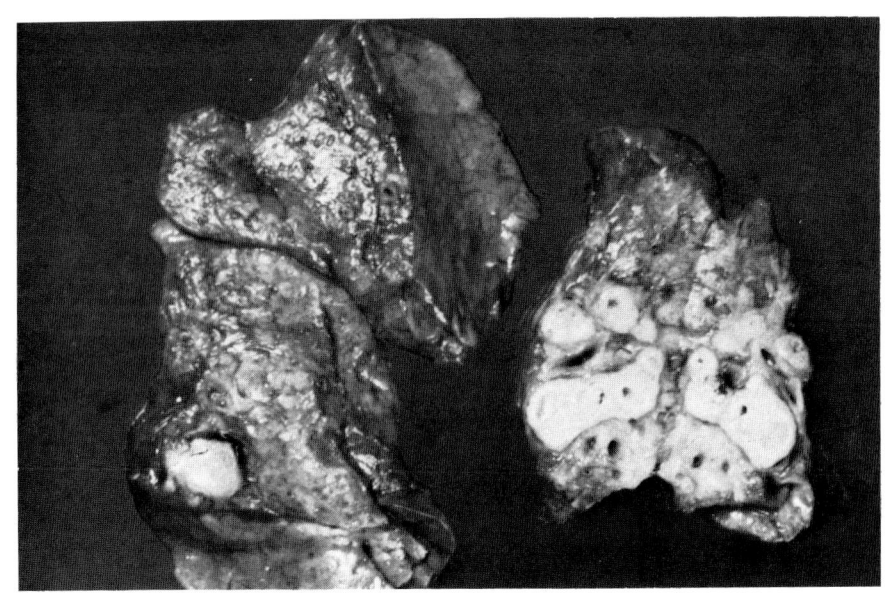

Figure 5.4. Ghon complex of childhood tuberculosis. A subpleural lesion of tuberculosis is seen at the *left*. The bisected hilar lymph nodes are shown at the *right*; there is massive caseation necrosis of these structures.

Pulmonary involvement in the adult is called *fibrocavitary tuberculosis*. There is spreading infection, usually starting in the subapical regions, characterized by progressive destruction of pulmonary architecture together with fibrous scarring. Emptying of necrotic material into bronchi results in cavity formation, often with rapid growth of tubercle bacilli and dissemination of disease (Fig. 5.5). Fibrocavitary tuberculosis may spread through the lungs, or may be arrested at any point. Tubercle bacilli generally remain viable in the arrested lesions.

Tuberculous infection can spread locally through structures such as bronchi, through lymphatics, and through the bloodstream. Hematogenous dissemination of tuberculosis is almost the rule in every infection, but most hematogenous lesions heal completely, leaving only tiny calcified nodules. When hematogenous dissemination is massive, *miliary tuberculosis* results, with myriads of tubercles in many organs of the body. Complications of tuberculosis are more frequent in adults, but they tend to be more severe in children. In children, tuberculous pneumonia resulting from dissemination of a large amount of caseous material through the bronchial tree is a potentially fatal complication of hilar node involvement. Hematogenous spread to bones and joints also occurs. In adults, hematogenous spread to kidneys, epididymides, or Fallopian tubes is frequent. Tuberculous destruction of the adrenal glands used to be the principal cause of Addison's disease. Extensive ulceration of the intestinal tract can follow swallowing large amounts of infected sputum. Tuberculous meningitis is a serious complication of both childhood and adult tuberculosis. It results most often from rupture of a hematogenous focus in the brain into the ventricles or subarachnoid space, with dissemination of caseous material in the cerebrospinal fluid.

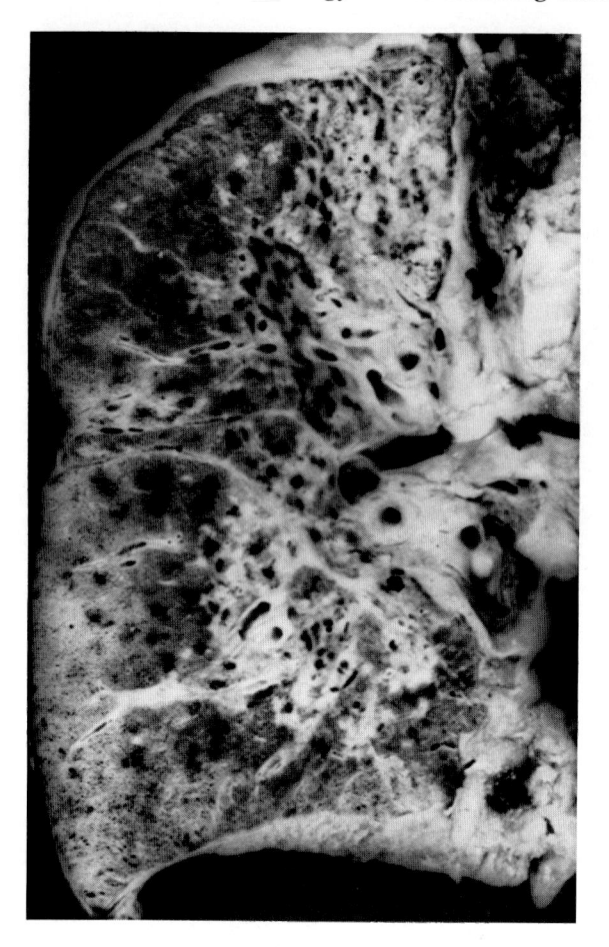

Figure 5.5. Tuberculosis in the adult. There is extensive caseation necrosis and fibrosis extending from the apical portion of the lung to the hilar region. Some involvement is noted also around the larger bronchi of the lower lobe. No involvement of hilar lymph nodes is seen.

Tuberculosis has afflicted man since the dawn of history. It has been epidemic during times of widespread malnutrition and debilitation. Modern chemotherapy permits cure of virtually all patients with this disease, but it remains a serious problem among economically and socially deprived persons, and in those whose resistance has been impaired by such concomitant disorders as diabetes mellitus, alcoholism, uremia, and silicosis, and by the administration of adrenal cortical steroids and immunosuppressive agents.

Much that has been said in this section is applicable to other diseases characterized by cell-mediated immunity and granulomatous lesions. They include systemic fungus diseases, particularly histoplasmosis and coccidioidomycosis, leprosy, some of the lesions of syphilis, and cat-scratch disease.

ROCKY MOUNTAIN SPOTTED FEVER

Rocky Mountain spotted fever, or tick-borne typhus fever, a disease of the rickettsial group, has been increasing in incidence since 1960. Over 1100 cases were reported nationally in 1977. Although first described in the Rocky Mountain

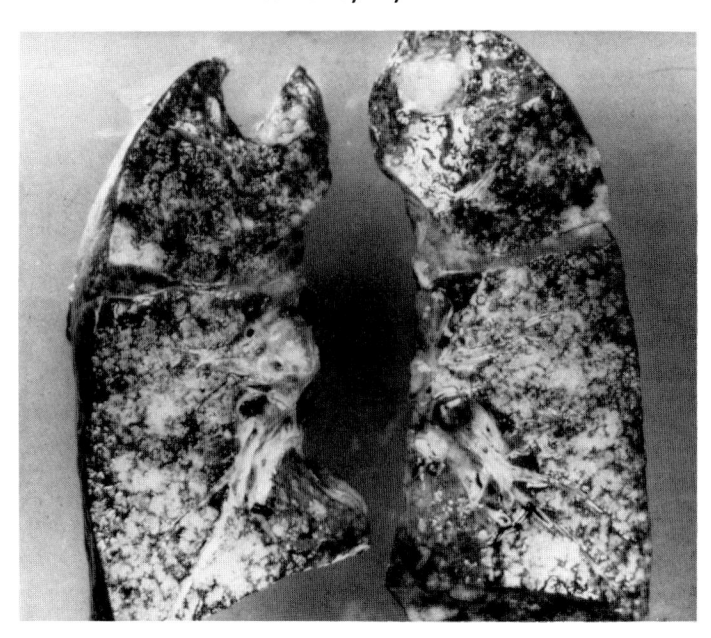

Figure 5.6. Bilateral pulmonary tuberculosis in the adult. Both lungs show massive numbers of tuberculous lesions, largely concentrated about the bronchi. Large cavities are noted at both apices. The hilar lymph nodes are not enlarged, and there is at most minimal tuberculous involvement.

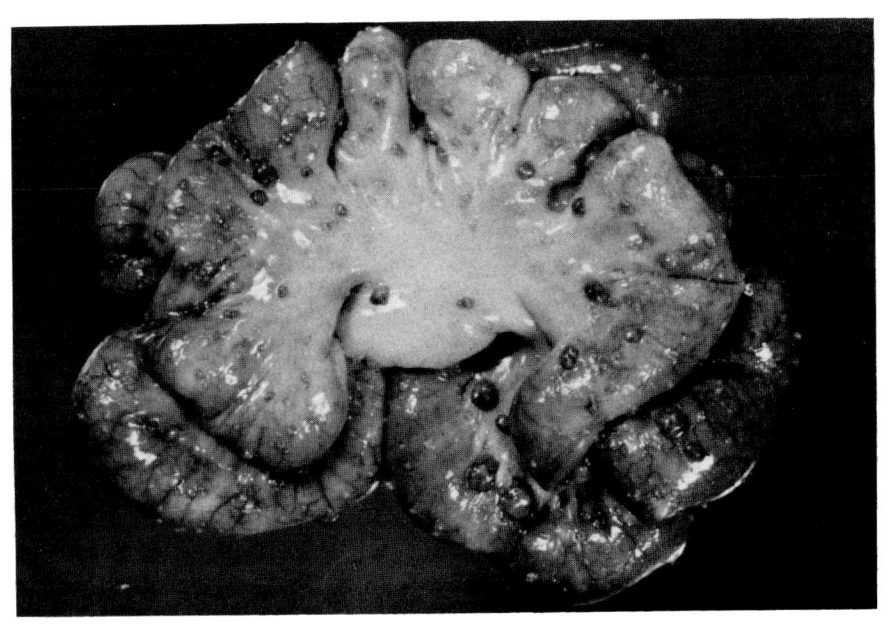

Figure 5.7. Tuberculous peritonitis. The mesentery and intestine are studded with tuberculous lesions. This complication of tuberculosis, in all likelihood, resulted from rupture of a caseous lymph node into the peritoneal cavity.

states, the greatest number of cases occurs east of the Mississippi, and particularly along the Atlantic seaboard.

The causative organism, *Rickettsia rickettsii* is a Gram-negative bacterium that is an obligate intracellular parasite, with capacity to invade and live in endothelial cells. It is transmitted by several species of ticks, among them *Dermacentor andersoni*. The ticks and several species of wild rodents constitute a reservoir of the organisms. Following inoculation, the organism colonizes the vascular endothelium of the microcirculation, particularly in arterioles (Fig. 5.8). After an incubation period of 4 to 12 days, patients manifest chills and high fever, often with stupor. Several days later, there is a rash, at first maculopapular, then petechial, and finally hemorrhagic or purpuric. The morphologic findings consist of widespread vascular necrosis and thrombosis with infiltration of polymorphonuclear leukocytes and some mononuclear phagocytes. Lesions are most prominent in the brain where they consist of microinfarcts and proliferation of glial cells (*glial nodules*), in the myocardium (interstitial myocarditis), the lungs (interstitial pneumonitis), and in skeletal muscle, kidneys, and testes (Fig. 5.9). The widespread vascular injury and thrombosis constitute a form of disseminated intravascular coagulation, and many of the hemorrhagic phenomena may relate to consumption of coagulation factors (Chapter 7). The mortality rate among untreated patients may be quite high.

Most of the rickettsial diseases have many clinical and morphologic findings in common. All but Q fever are transmitted by insects. All produce injury by invasion of vascular endothelium. In the rickettsial diseases, both humoral and cell-mediated immunity are demonstrable.

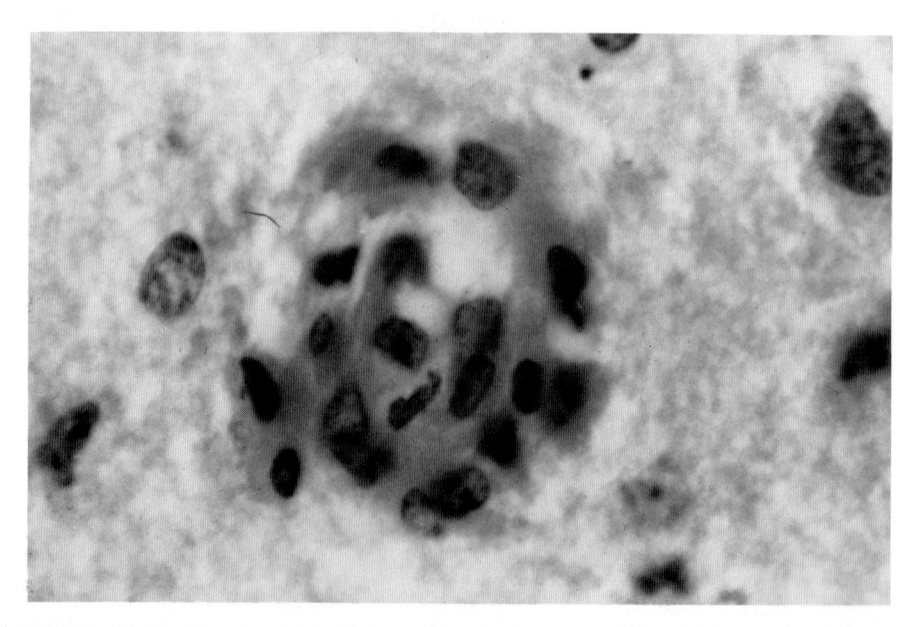

Figure 5.8. Rocky Mountain spotted fever. Early in disease, the rickettsial organisms parasitize endothelial cells, particularly of small blood vessels. There is striking proliferation of endothelium, as shown here, prior to vascular necrosis and thrombosis.

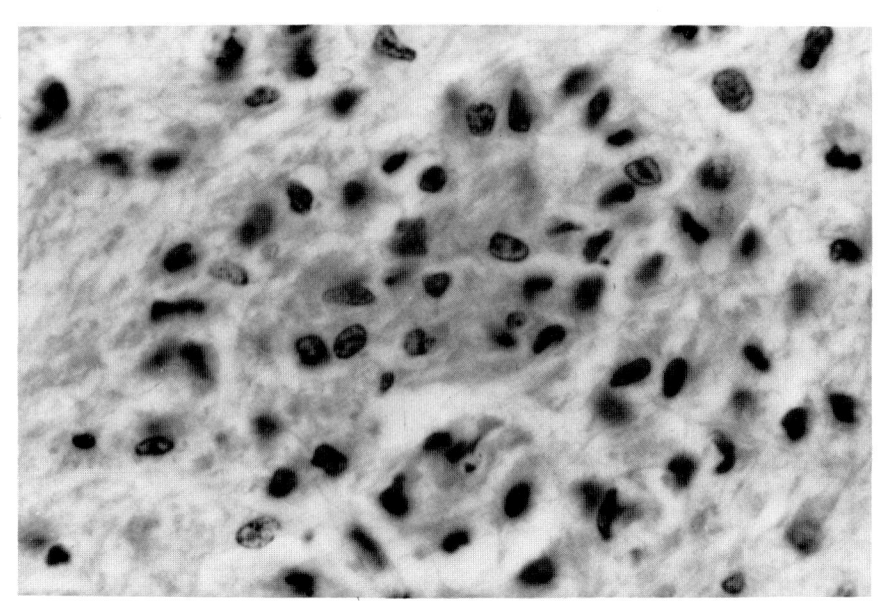

Figure 5.9. Rocky Mountain spotted fever: a *glial nodule*. This lesion is the response to a small area of necrosis of brain tissue secondary to vascular thrombosis. There is a proliferation of glial cells, chiefly astrocytes.

CYTOMEGALIC INCLUSION DISEASE

Cytomegalic inclusion disease is caused by a DNA virus of the herpes group. The virus causes severe disease when infection is congenital, and milder disease when contracted in infancy. It is observed in adults primarily as an opportunistic infection in the immunologically compromised host. All lesions of cytomegalic inclusion disease show markedly enlarged cells, with large nuclear inclusion bodies composed of virions and chromatin material, and at times smaller cytoplasmic inclusions.

The congenital form of disease resembles erythroblastosis fetalis, and is associated with prematurity, hemolytic anemia, jaundice, thrombocytopenia, pneumonitis, and enlargement of liver and spleen, together with evidence of severe brain injury. There is a 50% mortality. Those who survive tend to be mentally retarded, but some appear to be normal. Milder and latent forms of disease are seen, sometimes followed by delayed evidence of brain damage. In severe cases, the brain lesions show focal necrosis of neural elements, with polymorphonuclear leukocytic infiltration, and many giant cells with inclusions. They are distributed in laminar fashion in subpial and subependymal areas, especially around the cerebral aqueduct. Calcification may be seen in the necrotic areas. Cytomegalic lesions are widespread; they are seen in the liver, kidneys, lungs, gastrointestinal tract, pancreas, and adrenals. Renal tubular cells are prominently involved and are sloughed into the urine. The pulmonary lesion is an interstitial pneumonitis, with inclusions seen in lining cells and alveolar capillaries (Fig. 5.10).

A milder disease occurs in infancy after maternal antibodies have disappeared.

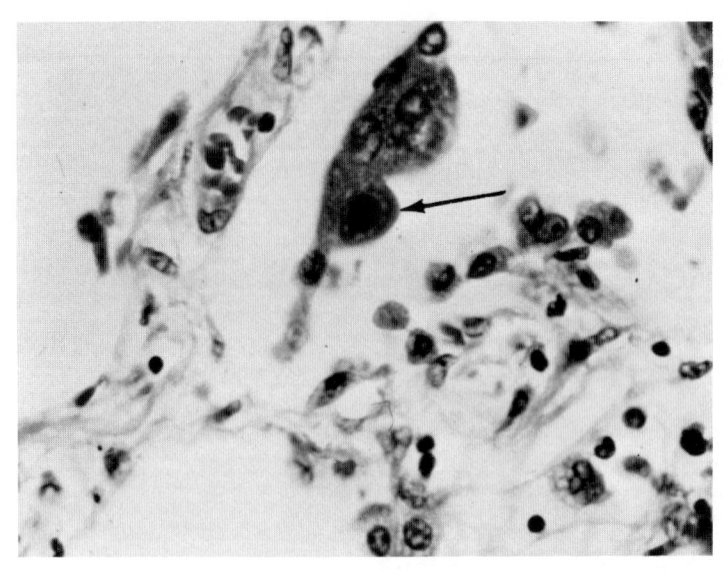

Figure 5.10. Cytomegalic inclusion disease. A greatly enlarged nuclear mass is seen in an alveolar lining cell in an area of pneumonitis.

There may be enlargement of liver and spleen, interstitial pneumonitis, and occasionally an enterocolitis. Some 5 to 15% of infants develop complement-fixing antibodies to cytomegalic virus during the first year of life.

Infection in adult life is probably common, but usually latent and asymptomatic. Fifty per cent of pregnant women have complement-fixing or IgM antibodies to cytomegalic virus, and virus may be excreted in urine and breast milk for prolonged periods. In the severely compromised or debilitated host, however, cytomegalic inclusion disease may be life-threatening, with severe and progressive pneumonitis, hemolytic anemia, purpura, pericarditis, and hepatitis. Encephalitis occurs only occasionally. An infectious mononucleosis-like syndrome due to cytomegalic virus may occur following administration of transfusions to young adults.

CANDIDIASIS

Candida albicans is an opportunistic fungus, having very low pathogenicity in the normal host. It is a frequent commensal in the mouth and vagina. Disease occurs when colonized patients become more vulnerable to tissue invasion by the organisms. Predisposing factors include diabetes mellitus, pregnancy, and administration of penicillin and broad spectrum antibiotics, adrenal cortical steroids, and oral contraceptives. Chronic maceration of skin, as occurs in obese individuals, may also set the stage for tissue invasion.

Candida organisms are usually confined to epithelial surfaces. Invasion and dissemination may result in extensive growth of organisms and tissue injury, but there is usually little if any inflammatory reaction (Fig. 5.11), since this occurs almost exclusively in patients with impaired resistance and reaction to injury.

Superficial lesions of the oral mucous membranes, or *thrush*, are common in children with infectious diseases. Candida vaginitis, often associated with anti-

Patterns of Infection 53

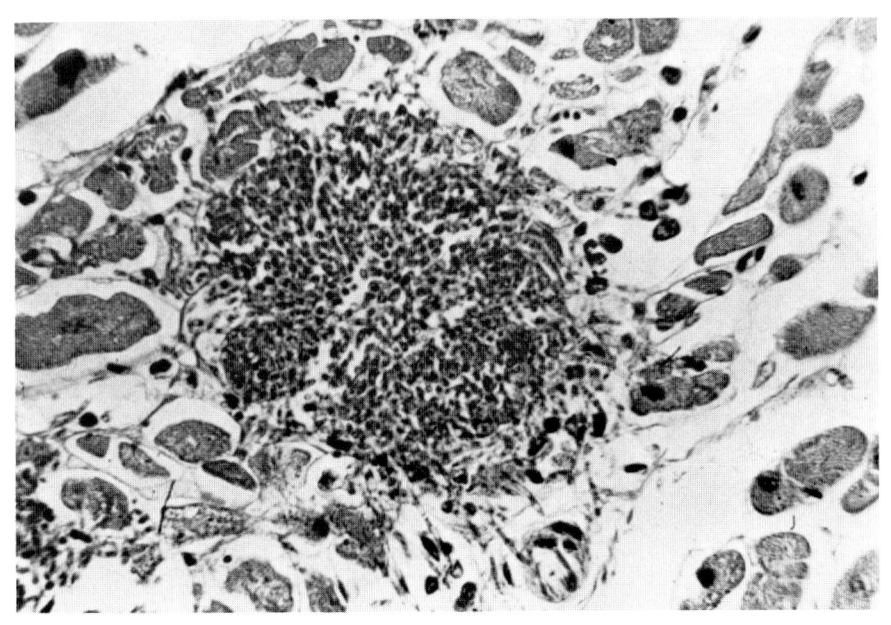

Figure 5.11. Systemic candidiasis. A large mass of candida organisms is seen in the myocardium of a patient with disseminated disease. Although myocardial fibers have been destroyed, there is little inflammatory response.

biotics or oral contraceptives, is also a common disorder, with a curd-like discharge and burning pain, and diffuse inflammation of the vaginal mucosa. Superficial ulceration of the lower esophagus with overgrowth of the organisms is frequent in debilitated patients. *Candida* endocarditis can occur on normal or diseased cardiac valves, is characterized by large bulky vegetations, and frequent embolic phenomena. It is almost always fatal. Infection also may occur in relation to insertion of central venous lines and in recipients of prosthetic cardiac valves. Widespread dissemination of candidiasis may occur in the compromised host, particularly in leukemic patients receiving antimetabolites.

The syndrome of *familial candidiasis endocrinopathy* is the association of mucocutaneous candida infection with decreased function of one or more endocrine organs. It probably represents an immunologic disorder, with a defect of suppressor T cell function. It appears to be inherited as an autosomal recessive. IgG levels are high, but IgA is deficient. The patients may suffer from chronic active hepatitis, autoimmune endocrine lesions of several endocrine glands, pernicious anemia, myasthenia gravis, and diabetes mellitus.

PNEUMOCYSTIS PNEUMONIA

Pneumocystis carinii is an opportunistic protozoan of wide distribution. It causes an important and often fatal acute pulmonary disease in immunodeficient patients, particularly those receiving antimetabolites and adrenal cortical steroids. Pneumocystis pneumonia also occurs, primarily in European countries, in malnourished and premature infants 3 to 4 months of age.

Pulmonary lesions are grossly firm and pale, either nodular or diffuse. Micro-

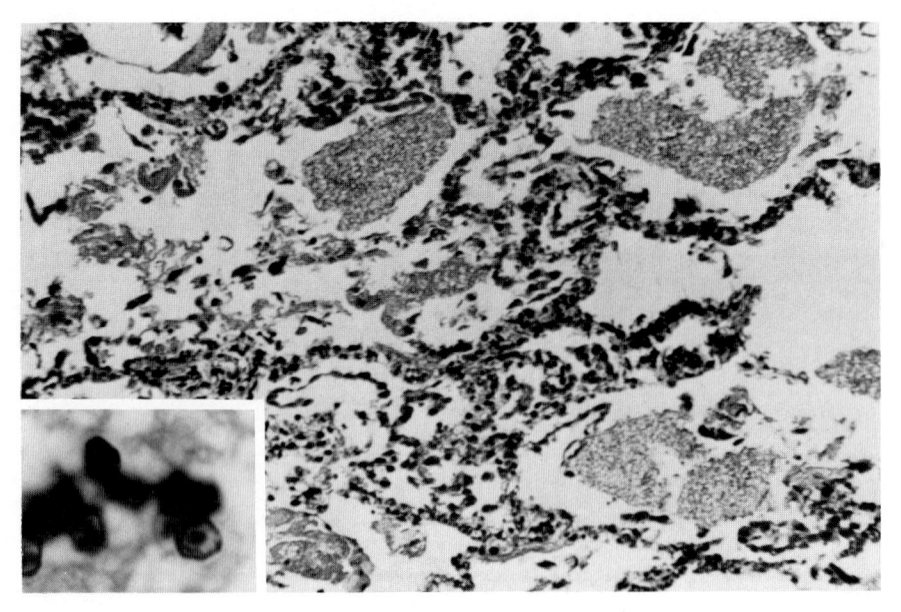

Figure 5.12. Pneumocystis pneumonia. The alveoli are filled with a foamy proteinaceous fluid. There is patchy mononuclear inflammatory cell infiltration. The *inset* shows pneumocystis organisms, seen at much higher magnification.

scopically, the alveoli are filled with foamy honeycombed appearing eosinophilic fluid, containing pneumocystis cysts and trophozoites (Fig. 5.12). Few inflammatory cells are seen, mostly mononuclear phagocytes, lymphocytes, and occasional eosinophils.

Pneumocystis pneumonia may occur together with other opportunistic infections. Some 10 to 25% of patients with pneumocystis pneumonia also have cytomegalic inclusion disease or fungus disease.

Suggested Reading

Cassell GH, Cole BC. Mycoplasmas as agents of human disease. N. Engl. J. Med. *304:* 80, 1981.
Craighead JE, et al. Chronic and persistent viral infections. Fed. Proc. *38:* 2659, 1979.
Dannenberg AM Jr. Pathogenesis of tuberculosis. In: Fishman AP, ed. Pulmonary diseases and disorders. New York, McGraw-Hill Book Co, 1980.
Glassroth J, Robins AG, Snider DE Jr. Tuberculosis in the 1980s. N. Engl. J. Med. *302:* 1441, 1980.

Chapter 6

Disturbances of Fluid, Electrolyte, and Acid-Base Balance

Disorders of fluid, electrolyte, and acid-base balance are some of the most important and frequently life-threatening manifestations of disease. The functional changes are dramatic, and there may, at times, be structural changes that are equally severe. At other times, however, the morphologic alterations are minimal and difficult to define. This chapter includes discussions of shock, congestion and edema, alterations of sodium and potassium metabolism, and the important abnormalities of acid-base balance.

SHOCK

Shock exists when the cardiovascular system fails to maintain sufficient perfusion of body tissues to meet their metabolic needs. It can result from a drop in cardiac output or from a decrease in peripheral vascular resistance. It leads to altered membrane function and cell metabolism, and, when severe, to cell death.

The principal manifestations of shock are hypotension, with the systolic pressure usually less than 90 mm mercury, tachycardia, with a weak thready pulse, and extremities that are cold, clammy, and cyanotic. Mental confusion and combativeness signal inadequate cerebral perfusion. Oliguria results from decreased glomerular filtration.

Shock can result from changes in cardiovascular function induced by hemorrhage, hypovolemia (*e.g.*, following severe vomiting or diarrhea), and failure of the myocardium to maintain cardiac output. It may also be initiated by extensive cellular injury due to trauma and burns. Shock is part of anaphylactic hypersensitivity reactions. Bacterial sepsis is often accompanied by shock due to widespread endothelial injury that causes severe vascular dilatation and altered permeability.

Early in shock due to decreased cardiac output, the blood pressure is maintained by reducing the peripheral vascular bed and shunting blood so as to maintain circulation to the vital organs, including brain and heart. After a time, this compensatory mechanism fails, and there is reduced perfusion of all organs. This results in altered cerebral function, decreased urine output, and impaired coronary blood flow. The skin is cyanotic, cold, and clammy, evidence of marked sympathetic activity. In the late stages of shock, there is marked alteration of the microcirculation and evidence of severe cell injury. There is inadequate perfusion of vital organs. One result may be dilatation and evidence of injury to the renal tubules, with the clinical syndrome of *acute tubular necrosis* (p. 199). *Shock lung* consists of the accumulation of fluid of high protein content in the pulmonary alveoli, often with hyaline membrane formation (p. 221). Aggregation of polymorphonuclear leukocytes, platelets, and red blood cells is noted in the alveolar capillaries, and release of enzymes from polymorphonuclear leukocytes is probably responsible for the greatly increased capillary permeability. Mucosal necrosis may occur in the gastrointestinal tract, permitting the entrance of many coliform organisms into the circulation, and exacerbating the shock. Myocardial contractility is depressed, further lowering cardiac output and arterial pressure. Diffuse endothelial injury results in severe loss of intravascular fluid, with further hypovolemia and hypotension. Sludging of blood (clumping and rouleaux formation) may be seen seen in capillaries throughout the body. Disseminated intravascular coagulation (p. 72) often results from the diffuse injury to vascular endothelium, and can cause such further tissue injury as bilateral cortical necrosis of the kidneys (Fig. 6.1). Individuals whose circulation to various organs is already compromised by atherosclerosis may suffer infarction of the myocardium, brain, or kidneys.

Many of the changes in cellular metabolism that result from shock tend to exacerbate and perpetuate it. The affinity of red cell hemoglobin for oxygen may

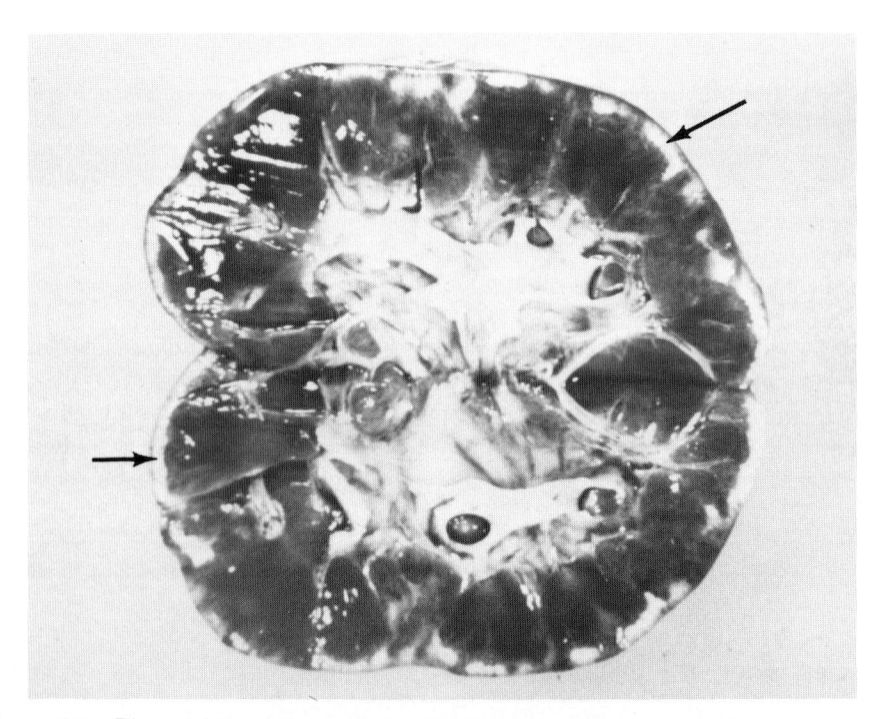

Figure 6.1. Bisected kidney from patient with bilateral cortical necrosis. There is an almost continuous zone of infarction of the superficial portion of the cortex. This event, usually followed by cessation of renal function, may occur in patients with severe hemorrhage and shock, sometimes in the syndrome of disseminated intravascular coagulation.

Disturbances of Fluid, Electrolyte, and Acid-Base Balance

be decreased, further altering the delivery of oxygen to the tissues. Ischemia results in severe mitochondrial injury and then cell death, with release of lysosomal hydrolases. Pancreatic hydrolases release peptides that depress myocardial contractility. Complement may be activated in shock, attracting polymorphonuclear leukocytes which then release their lysosomal enzymes. Finally, the shift to anaerobic cellular metabolism increases production of lactic acid, still further increasing vascular permeability and volume depletion.

CONGESTION AND EDEMA

Congestion is defined as an increased blood content of an organ, particularly within its capillaries. Congestion can be *active*, due to arteriolar dilatation, or *passive* due to interference with venous blood flow.

Passive congestion occurs whenever there is an increase in venous pressure, most notably in congestive heart failure. It is a frequent consequence of obstructive lesions of large veins, such as thromboses or tumor invasion, and external compression of veins by tumors and other masses. The congested tissue will demonstrate a dilated microvasculature packed with blood cells. Decreased blood flow through an organ results in impairment of its cellular metabolism. There may be accumulation of acid products and decreased oxygen tension, although extraction of oxygen from hemoglobin is more complete. There is increased passage of fluid into the extravascular compartment. Reversible or irreversible cellular injury may be observed. Passive congestion of the liver is often manifested by hypoxic injury to cells in the central lobular areas (Fig. 6.2). Fatty change may be followed by cell necrosis and an inflammatory reaction. Repeated episodes of

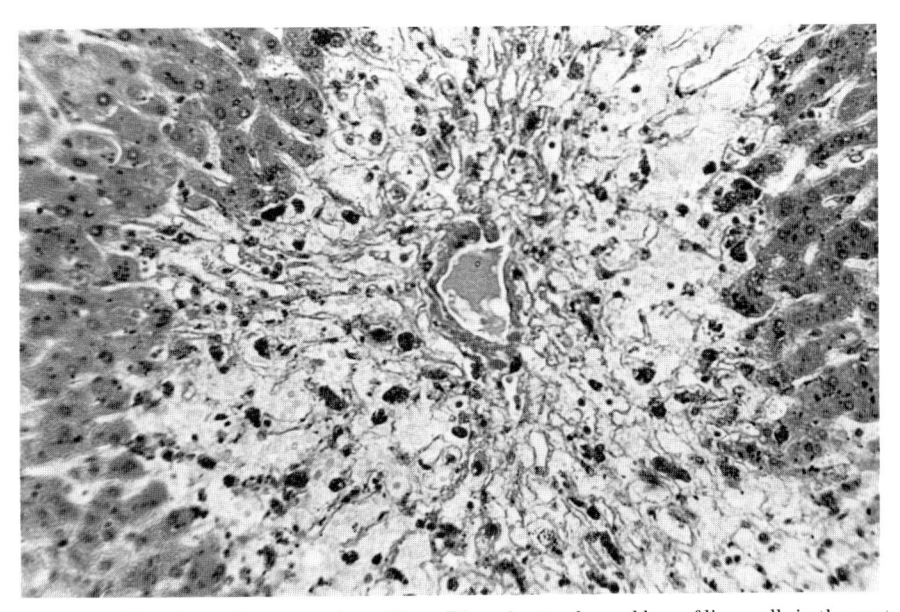

Figure 6.2. Chronic passive congestion of liver. There is atrophy and loss of liver cells in the central lobular region, and some fibrosis around the central vein. The sinusoids are congested. This picture can follow the more acute changes shown in Figure 2.4.

congestion can lead to atrophy of the central lobular hepatocytes and increased fibrous tissue around the central veins. Chronic passive congestion of the lungs is associated with fibrous thickening of alveolar septa and interference with gas exchange. The passively congested spleen is enlarged and in time fibrotic, with dilated sinusoids and, often, evidence of increased destruction of blood elements. The effects of visceral congestion in congestive heart failure are discussed in greater detail in Chapter 15.

Edema is the accumulation of excessive fluid in tissue spaces. It can be localized, as in inflammatory reactions, or generalized (*anasarca*). Fluid normally enters the extravascular space because postarteriolar capillary hydrostatic pressure exceeds blood osmotic pressure. Some resorption takes place at the venous end of the capillary, and the remaining portion is removed by lymphatics. Excessive accumulation of tissue fluid can result from increased capillary hydrostatic pressure, reduced blood osmotic pressure, or lymphatic obstruction. Increased capillary permeability from endothelial damage due to bacterial products, burns, chemical irritants, or immunologic reactions can cause leakage of plasma.

Generalized edema occurs most frequently in patients with congestive heart failure, cirrhosis of the liver, and certain forms of renal disease. The mechanisms responsible for edema in each of these circumstances are discussed in Chapters 15, 17, and 21. Generalized edema is likely to be most prominent in dependent portions of the body, as a result of the gravitational effects on hydrostatic pressure, and where tissue pressure offers least resistance to the accumulation of fluid. Ambulant patients tend to accumulate fluid in tissues around the ankles and anterior tibias. When recumbent, edema shifts to the back and sacral area, to loose periorbital tissues, or to the lung. Fluid also accumulates in serous cavities, *i.e.*, pleural and pericardial *effusions* and peritoneal *ascites*.

Most edema fluid contains solutes of less than 10,000 molecular weight. Very little protein is present, and the specific gravity of edema fluid is low. With injury to the microvasculature, there is leakage of protein and a higher specific gravity.

Edema produces remarkably little functional disturbance when located in subcutaneous tissues. Large pericardial effusions may interfere with venous return to the heart and with diastolic filling. Large pleural effusions may interfere with normal lung expansion. Ascites, however, has relatively little effect on abdominal organ function.

The osmotic pressure in pulmonary capillaries normally exceeds hydrostatic pressure, and no fluid escapes to the alveoli. Pulmonary edema results from increased capillary hydrostatic pressure in left ventricular failure or hypervolemia, or from increased permeability due to hypoxia or inhaled irritants. It may be moderately high in protein content. Pulmonary edema often starts in the loose alveolar interstitium before spilling over into the alveolar spaces. In either location, it interferes with alveolar gas exchange.

The brain cannot accommodate much edema because of ridigity of the skull. Edematous expansion of the cerebrum may result in herniation of uncal gyri through the tentorium or of cerebellar tonsils into the foramen magnum, with disturbed function of vital control centers.

Recurrent or long standing edema may have permanent effects. Subcutaneous tissues tend to become brawny because of an increase in fibrous tissue. The serosal surfaces of pericardium, pleura, and peritoneum may become thickened and fibrotic. Pulmonary edema, together with passive congestion, is responsible for the fibrous thickening of alveolar septa observed in chronic congestive heart failure.

VOLUME DEPLETION

Volume depletion can follow loss of water alone, as in simple dehydration, but more often results from loss of water and electrolytes. The major sites of loss are the skin, the gastrointestinal tract, and the kidneys. Skin loss results from excessive sweating, including that in normal individuals and in children with cystic fibrosis. Massive loss may accompany burns. Vomiting, diarrhea, and enterostomies are causes of loss through the gastrointestinal tract. Excessive fluid loss through the kidneys can occur during an osmotic diuresis, during the diuretic phase of acute tubular necrosis, and in renal lesions characterized by sodium (and water) wasting.

Volume depletion is manifested by thirst, nausea, and weakness. If severe, hypotension, tachycardia, oliguria, and other signs of shock follow.

HYPONATREMIA AND HYPERNATREMIA

Sodium, as the most plentiful extracellular ion, is an important determinant of plasma osmolality. Changes in sodium concentration can profoundly affect the distribution of water among vascular, interstitial, and cellular compartments.

In hyponatremia, water passes from plasma and interstitium into cells, producing manifestiations of water intoxication: irritability, confusion, lethargy, and convulsions. Hyponatremia is seen in untreated adrenal cortical insufficiency (Addison's disease), in the syndrome of inappropriate antidiuretic hormone secretion, where there is sodium loss together with water retention, with excessive use of diuretics, and administration of drugs such as chlorpropamide and cyclophosphamide. It occurs in acute and chronic renal failure if water intake is greater than can be excreted. It can also occur with tremendous water intake in patients with psychogenic polydipsia. Dilutional hyponatremia is seen in the presence of severe hyperglycemia, where cellular water passes to the extracellular fluid.

Hypernatremia is a reflection of water loss, as with excessive sweating or vomiting. Severe hypernatremia occurs in the absence of fluid intake, in patients with diabetes insipidus, and during an osmotic diuresis. This can occur in patients immediately following renal transplantation and when a very high protein diet presents the kidney with a heavy urea load.

Hypernatremia leads to cellular dehydration. Patients with hypernatremia generally have serious predisposing illnesses, and it is difficult to ascribe clinical manifestations to the hypernatremia *per se*.

DISORDERS OF POTASSIUM METABOLISM

Potassium plays a major role in cellular osmotic control; its concentration in body fluids affects cardiac and striated muscle contractility. Extracellular potas-

Pathology: Understanding Human Disease

sium is a very small proportion of total body potassium. At times, plasma potassium is a good reflection of cellular potassium; at other times, as in chronic renal failure, it may be deceiving. The plasma level is controlled by distal tubular exchange in the kidney.

Hypokalemia and Potassium Deficiency

Hypokalemia and potassium deficiency result from renal loss or loss through the gastrointestinal tract. Increased sodium-potassium exchange in the renal distal tubule occurs with many diuretics and in primary hyperaldosteronism, in Cushing's syndrome, and with administration of adrenal steroids. Prolonged vomiting and diarrhea account for most gastrointestinal loss, but villous adenomas of the rectum characteristically secrete large quantities of potassium.

Musclar weakness and paralysis, at times with myoglobinemia, may be manifestations of hypokalemia. Although striking electrocardiographic changes are seen, and digitalized patients may suffer arrhythmias, cardiac function is usually not disturbed. The myocardium may show focal fiber degeneration and necrosis, with interstitial edema containing mononuclear phagocytes. *Hypokalemic nephropathy* is seen with prolonged or severe hypokalemia, and consists of a defect in renal concentration ability with polydipsia and polyuria. Both proximal and distal convoluted tubules show striking vacuolar degeneration (Fig. 6.3).

Hyperkalemia and Potassium Intoxication

Hyperkalemia and potassium intoxication are manifested by disordered intraventricular cardiac conduction, sometimes with cardiac arrest, although no mor-

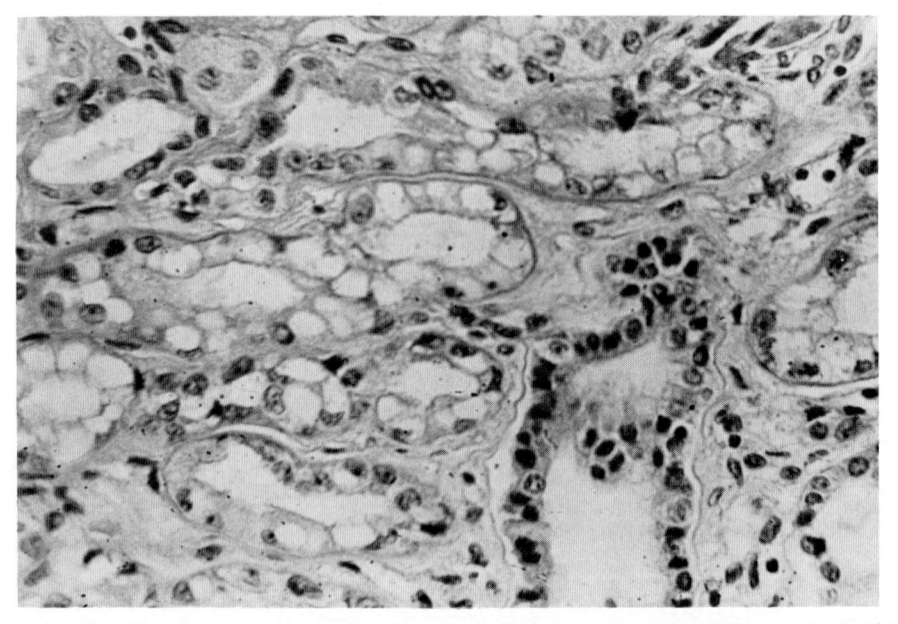

Figure 6.3. Hypokalemic nephropathy. There is striking vacuolar degeneration of the tubular epithelial cells.

phologic changes in the myocardium have been defined. The electrocardiogram shows tall peaked T waves and widened QRS complexes. Patients may also suffer generalized muscle weakness and flaccid paralysis.

Decreased renal potassium excretion is the usual mechanism of hyperkalemia. This occurs in both acute tubular necrosis and chronic renal failure. It also characterizes severe adrenal cortical insufficiency and may follow administration of spironolactones that interfere with sodium-potassium exchange in the distal nephron.

DISTURBANCES OF ACID-BASE BALANCE

Body metabolism yields an excess of acids. Carbonic acid is excreted by the lung, but nonvolatile or "fixed" acids, including sulfuric, phosphoric, lactic, and β-hydroxybutyric acids can be excreted only by the kidney. A 70-kg man excretes some 20 moles of acid through the lungs as carbon dioxide and some 70 millimoles through the kidneys. This is accomplished without change of the pH of the plasma or extracellular fluid; it reflects effective buffer systems and intact renal and respiratory function. Hydrogen ions from fixed acids must react with phosphate buffer or ammonia before they can be excreted. The sodium-hydrogen (and potassium) exchange mechanism in the distal nephron plays a key role in the renal handling of acids.

The carbonic acid-bicarbonate system is the major buffer of the extracellular fluid. Its critical role in determining pH is indicated by the Henderson-Hasselbalch equation:

$$pH = pK + \log \frac{(HCO_3^-)}{(H_2CO_3)}$$

In normal man, this is:

$$7.4 = 6.1 + \log \frac{24 \text{ mM/l}}{1.2 \text{ mM/l}}$$

The normal ratio of bicarbonate to carbonic acid (dissolved CO_2—see below) is approximately 24:1.2, or 20:1.

In evaluating acid-base status, several measurements are made. The $PaCO_2$ is the partial pressure of carbon dioxide. It averages 36 mm mercury in alveolar air and 40 mm in arterial blood. The $PaCO_2$ is normally in equilibrium with and a reflection of the "dissolved CO_2" of plasma, which includes dissolved CO_2 and a tiny fraction of undissociated carbonic acid. The plasma "bicarbonate" includes bicarconate and carbonate ions and carbamino compounds (proteins and amino acids that do not affect pH). In other words, it represents the total plasma CO_2 minus the "dissolved CO_2." The pH, of course, is also measured.

Normal acid-base balance can be disturbed by disordered metabolic function or by changes in respiratory function. A primary reduction in plasma bicarbonate is indicative of *metabolic acidosis*, a primary increase of bicarbonate of *metabolic alkalosis*. A primary elevation of arterial $PaCO_2$ reflects *respiratory acidosis*, while a low $PaCO_2$ is indicative of *respiratory alkalosis*.

Metabolic Acidosis

Metabolic acidosis can result from increased acid production, loss of base, as in diarrhea, or failure of the kidney to handle an acid load. The latter can be related to inability to produce ammonia or loss of capacity to resorb bicarbonate. Some of the principal causes of metabolic acidosis are shown in Table 6.1. The metabolic acidosis of diabetes mellitus results from increased production of β-hydroxybutyric and acetoacetic acids. Lactic acidosis is most often related to shock or cardiovascular disease, and is the product of anaerobic glycolysis. In metabolic acidosis due to those factors in the left-hand column of Table 6.1, there is an increased *anion gap*. The anion gap is a useful clinical concept, and is defined as the difference, in millimoles per liter between the sum of plasma bicarbonate and chloride and the level of sodium. It is composed of anions not usually measured: phosphate, sulfate, organic anions, and protein. The normal anion gap is about 12 mM per l, and it may be higher than 30 in severe diabetic or lactic acidosis.

In metabolic acidosis, the ratio of plasma bicarbonate to dissolved CO_2 may be 12.5:1, with a pH of 7.20. Increased respiratory activity will increase the ratio to perhaps 15:0.95 (16:1), increasing the pH to 7.30. Renal excretion of hydrogen ion with phosphate, production of ammonia, sodium-hydrogen exchange, and bicarbonate resorption may return the ration to 20:1 with a pH of 7.40. Then the acidosis is completely compensated, although the basic defect, a bicarbonate deficit, has not been corrected.

Metabolic Alkalosis

Metabolic alkalosis results from retention of base, or an abnormal loss of acid. It occurs with vomiting and use of chlorothiazide diuretics, in some patients with Cushing's syndrome, in primary hyperaldosteronism, in patients receiving glucocorticoids (through potassium loss), and with administration of alkali. With vomiting, there is loss of hydrochloric acid. The kidneys now filter sodium with bicarbonate, rather than chloride, and there is decreased sodium resorption in the proximal tubules. There is loss of sodium in the urine, since the distal tubular exchange cannot fully compensate, and there is depletion of extracellular fluid volume. This leads to conservation of all sodium and bicarbonate, and persistence of a high plasma bicarbonate. The ratio of bicarbonate to dissolved CO_2 might be 40:1.25 (32:1), and the pH 7.60. Decreased respiratory function can retain carbon dioxide and could change the ratio to something like 40:1.57 (25.5:1), and the pH to 7.51. Decreased renal sodium-hydrogen exchange and ammonia formation could complete the compensation. The ratio might be 31:1.57 (20:1), and the pH 7.40. There would still be, however, a primary bicarbonate excess.

Table 6.1
Some Causes of Metabolic Acidosis

Renal failure	Diarrhea
Diabetic acidosis	Ammonium chloride intake
Lactic acidosis	Renal tubular acidosis
Salicylate toxicity	Carbonic anhydrase inhibitors
Ethylene glycol poisoning	Pancreatic fistula
Methanol poisoning	

Disturbances of Fluid, Electrolyte, and Acid-Base Balance

Respiratory Acidosis

Respiratory acidosis represents a failure to eliminate carbon dioxide because of pulmonary disease or depressed function. It is prominent in chronic obstructive pulmonary disease and pneumonia, in patients with morphine narcosis, and in patients with pulmonary vascular obstruction. There is elevation of $PaCO_2$ and dissolved CO_2. The bicarbonate-dissolved CO_2 ratio might be 27:1.8 (15:1), with a pH of 7.28.

Respiratory Alkalosis

Respiratory alkalosis results from an increased rate or depth of respiration. It occurs with fever, hysteria, and salicylate toxicity and as a response to hypoxia. It is usually observed as a compensatory mechanism in the presence of metabolic acidosis. $PaCO_2$ and dissolved CO_2 are reduced. The bicarbonate-dissolved CO_2 ratio might be 27:1, and the pH 7.53. Respiratory alkalosis cannot usually elevate the pH above 7.60, unless an element of metabolic alkalosis is also present.

It is apparent that various compensatory mechanisms help mollify the effects of acidosis and alkalosis: they do not, however, correct the initial defect responsible for disturbed acid-base balance. When that is accomplished, all parameters return to normal.

Suggested Reading

Bave AE, Metabolic abnormalities of shock. Surg. Clin. North Am. *56:* 1059, 1976.
Tietz NW, Siggaard-Andersen O. Acid-base and electrolyte balance. In: Tietz NW, ed. Fundamentals of clinical chemistry. Philadelphia, WB Saunders Co, 1976.

Chapter 7

Hemostasis and Blood Coagulation

Hemostasis plays a critical role in preserving the internal environment, permitting healing of injury to blood vessels and preventing or limiting the severity of hemorrhage. There are two aspects to this reaction to injury, one reflecting the function of circulating platelets and the other the coagulation of blood. Disorders of the hemostatic mechanism include both pathologic clotting of blood and a large group of bleeding disorders resulting from deficiencies of platelet function or factors essential to the coagulation of blood. The disorder *disseminated intravascular coagulation* consists of abnormal coagulability followed by failure of hemostasis and hemorrhage. Thrombotic disorders are an important cause of morbidity and mortality, responsible for some 200,000 hospital admissions and 50,000 deaths each year. Bleeding disorders are considerably less frequent, but at least one, hemophilia, has had an important influence on history.

PLATELETS

Injury to vascular endothelium exposes underlying collagen. Possibly because of a change in electric potential, platelets, which have receptor sites for collagen, adhere at the site of injury, bound to collagen fibrils and to each other. Normally appearing as convex discs, they become spherical, and projecting pseudopods facilitate their adherence and aggregation. They release factors included in their cytoplasmic dense bodies: adenosine diphosphate (ADP), calcium, and serotonin. ADP release, controlled by cyclic adenosine monophosphate (AMP), itself promotes further aggregation of platelets.

Prostaglandins play a key part in the mediation of platelet function. Two prostaglandins are derived from arachidonic acid contained in platelets and vascular endothelium. Thromboxane A_2 promotes platelet aggregation and release of platelet factors. These serve to generate more thromboxane A_2. It is very unstable, having a half-life of some 30 sec. Prostacyclin, PGI_2, antagonizes the action of thromboxane A_2, interfering with adherence to endothelium and platelet aggregation.

As platelets aggregate, changes in their membranes expose an important phospholipid, *Platelet Factor 3*, necessary for the conversion of prothrombin to thrombin in the intrinsic coagulation pathway. Thrombin, in turn, has a positive feedback effect on platelets, stimulating further aggregation, release, and exposure of Platelet Factor 3.

The platelet aggregate constitutes a "white thrombus." It can serve as a

Hemostasis and Blood Coagulation

temporary plug to maintain vascular integrity, but most injuries require coagulation of blood to prevent leakage more effectively and to promote healing.

COAGULATION

Blood coagulation consists of a series of reactions culminating in the conversion of the globulin dimer *fibrinogen* to *fibrin*. This is accomplished by the protease *thrombin* which splits off two peptide fragments from each fibrinogen chain, yielding a fibrin monomer. Unstable fibrin polymers, together with formed elements of the blood, constitute a gel. Activated *fibrin stabilizing factor* (Factor XIIIa) promotes the formation of stable covalent linkages between fibrin monomers.

The coagulation system consists of 10 proteins, calcium, and tissue thromboplastin. These factors are listed in Table 7.1, with their international nomenclature and synonyms.

The sequence of coagulation can be viewed as an example of biologic amplification, similar in many respects to the complement cascade. The 10 coagulation proteins are enzymes or enzyme cofactors. Each is activated by a previous reaction and activates the next enzyme. Two of the activations are greatly facilitated and accelerated by phospholipids: the conversion of prothrombin to thrombin (II to IIa), and factor X to Xa.

There are two coagulation pathways. In the *intrinsic pathway*, all factors necessary for coagulation are present in the blood. The *extrinsic pathway* is dependent upon the release of phospholipid and a lipoprotein from injured tissue.

The intrinsic pathway is outlined in Figure 7.1. It starts with activation of Hageman factor (Factor XII) by surface contact at the site of endothelial injury and platelet aggregation. There is sequential activation of Factors XI and IX. Activated Factor IX (IXa) forms a complex with Factor VIII, Platelet Factor 3 and calcium, which, in turn, activates Factor X. Factor Xa, Factor V, and Platelet Factor 3 constitute *plasma thromboplastin,* or prothrombin converting factor, which in the presence of calcium, converts prothrombin to thrombin (II to IIa).

Table 7.1
Blood Coagulation Factors

International Nomenclature	Synonyms
Factor I	Fibrinogen
Factor II	Prothrombin
Factor III	Tissue thromboplastin
Factor IV	Calcium
Factor V	Prothrombin accelerator
Factor VII	Stable factor, convertin
Factor VIII	Antihemophilic globulin
Factor IX	Christmas factor
Factor X	Stuart-Prower factor
Factor XI	Plasma thromboplastin antecedent
Factor XII	Hageman factor
Factor XIII	Fibrin-stabilizing factor

```
                Surface contact
                      ↓
           XII ——→ XIIa
                      ↓
              XI ——→ XIa
                      ↓
                 IX ——→ IXa
                      ↓
       VIII + Platelet Factor 3 + IXa + Ca⁺⁺
                      ↓
                  X ——→ Xa
                      ↓
        V + Platelet Factor 3 + Xa + Ca⁺⁺
                      ↓
         Prothrombin ——→ thrombin ——┐
                      │             │
                      │         XIII ——→ XIIIa
                      │             ↓
         Fibrinogen ——→ fibrin gel ——→ cross-linked fibrin
```

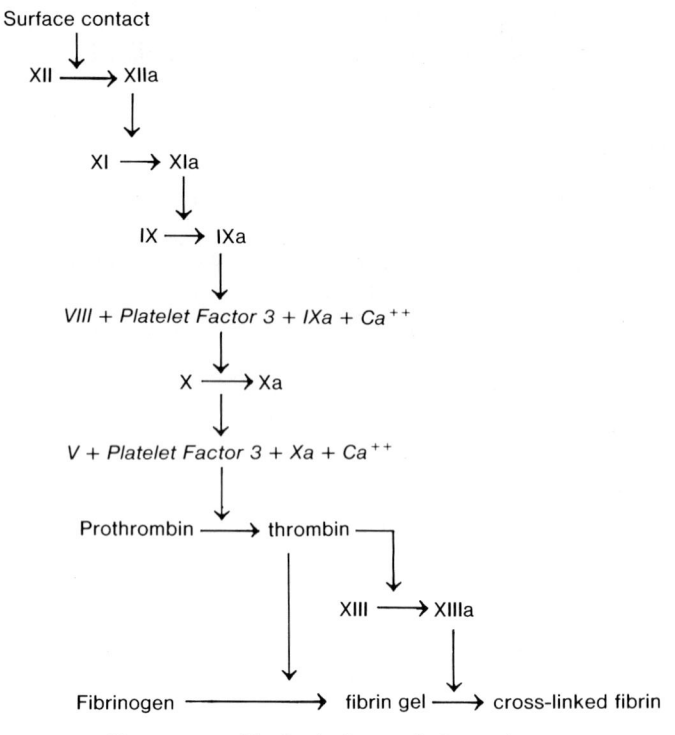

Figure 7.1. The intrinsic coagulation pathway.

In the extrinsic pathway (Fig. 7.2), tissue thromboplastin in the presence of Factor VII activates Factor X. Tissue thromboplastin contains phospholipid and a protein moiety which activates Factor VII. This phospholipid also serves to promote thrombin generation.

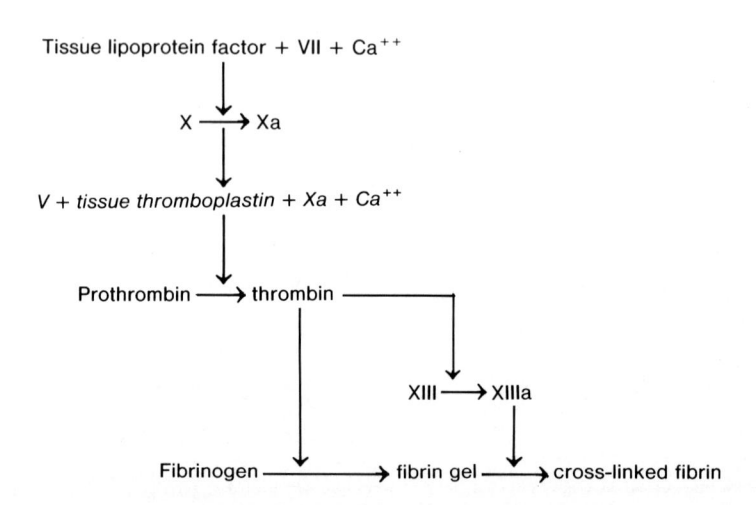

```
          Tissue lipoprotein factor + VII + Ca⁺⁺
                      ↓
                  X ——→ Xa
                      ↓
       V + tissue thromboplastin + Xa + Ca⁺⁺
                      ↓
         Prothrombin ——→ thrombin ——┐
                      │             │
                      │         XIII ——→ XIIIa
                      │             ↓
         Fibrinogen ——→ fibrin gel ——→ cross-linked fibrin
```

Figure 7.2. The extrinsic coagulation pathway.

Hemostasis and Blood Coagulation

The activation of Factor X is central to both pathways. The difference between them is the means of activating Factor X and the source of phospholipid necessary for prothrombin activation.

The events of coagulation take place on the surfaces of platelet aggregates. The generation of thrombin induces further platelet aggregation and exposure of Platelet Factor 3, which, in turn, stimulates further coagulation. The resulting *thrombus* which forms is composed of alternating layers of platelets and fibrin, recognizable as the *lines of Zahn* (Fig. 7.4).

Control of Coagulation

It is obvious that platelet activation and blood coagulation must be confined to a local area rather than being permitted to spread throughout the vascular system. There are various factors that serve this purpose. Activated coagulation factors are unstable, and tend to be washed away rapidly by the circulation. Consumption of available coagulation factors also limits the spread of intravascular coagulation. An antithrombin is present in the $\alpha 2$-globulin fraction of plasma; antithrombin III is a cofactor of heparin, and an inhibitor of the action

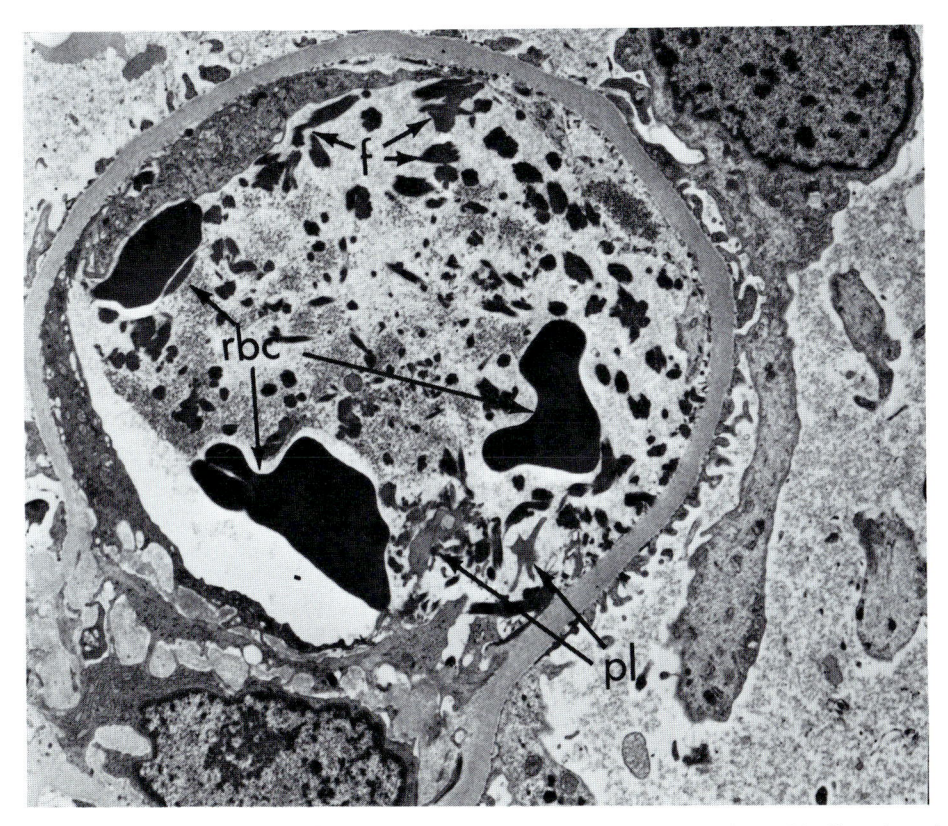

Figure 7.3. Electron micrograph of early thrombus formation from a patient with disseminated intravascular coagulation. A glomerular capillary is almost occluded by a forming thrombus. Three dark staining red blood cells are seen (*rbc*). There are many strands of fibrin (*f*) and several platelets (*pl*).

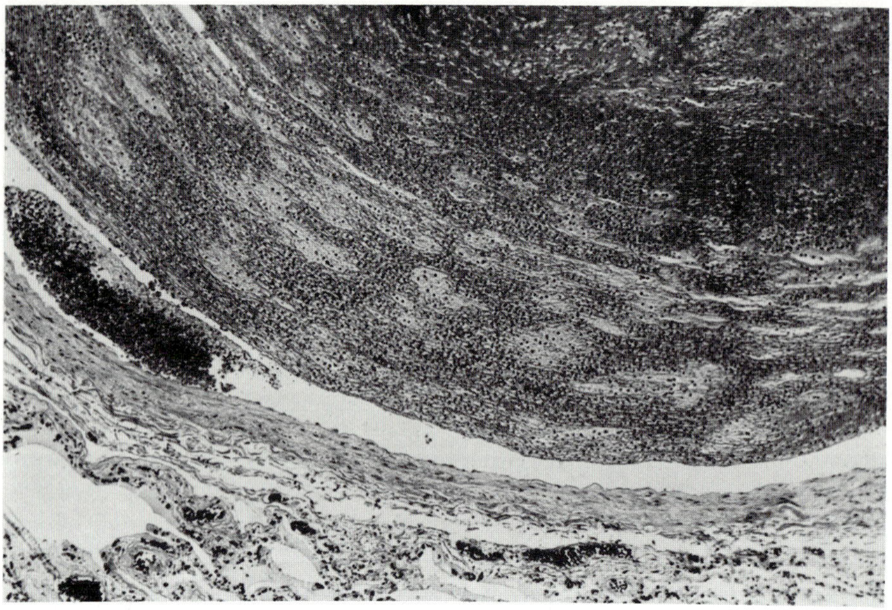

Figure 7.4. Thrombus forming in large vessel. The alternating layers of fibrin and platelets are recognized as prominent lines of Zahn. These help distinguish between an antemortem thrombus and a postmortem clot.

of thrombin on fibrinogen. A fibrinolytic system is activated by Factor XIIa: plasminogen is converted to plasmin, which degrades fibrin by splitting arginine-lysine bonds.

Hageman Factor

Hageman factor plays an important role both in the intrinsic coagulation pathway and in the fibrinolytic system. This substance is also key to the generation of kinins in the early phases of the inflammatory response (see Chapter 3) and it may also be related to activation of complement. Through Hageman factor, the inflammatory reaction, coagulation of the blood, and certain immunologic reactions are closely interrelated.

BLEEDING DISORDERS

Bleeding may be due to such anatomic lesions as esophageal varices, hemorrhoids, or ruptured arterial aneurysms, or it may reflect a congenital or acquired bleeding tendency. In determining the cause of bleeding, it is often necessary to evaluate both platelet function and the coagulation system. Defects or deficiencies occur virtually at every point in the mechanisms described in this chapter. Disturbances of platelet numbers or function are most frequently manifested by petechial and purpuric hemorrhage of the skin and oozing from the mucous membranes. Bleeding in patients with coagulation defects often follows trauma, or occurs in deeper structures such as joints.

Platelet Abnormalities

Platelet function is evaluated by the *bleeding time* test, which measures the duration of bleeding following a standardized superficial incision. A normal test depends on platelet aggregation and formation of a plug. The test will be abnormal in the absence of adequate numbers of platelets, or *thrombocytopenia*. This occurs in association with leukemias, aplastic anemia, and the administration of agents that depress the bone marrow. In *autoimmune* thrombocytopenia, antiplatelet antibodies coat the platelets, and there is accelerated platelet destruction in the spleen. Drugs such as Sedormid and sulfonamides may lead to platelet destruction by acting as haptens attached to platelet membranes.

Platelets may be normal in number, but abnormal in function. In *thrombasthenia*, platelets do not form normal aggregates. In von Willebrand's disease (see below), they fail to adhere to sites of endothelial injury. Aspirin interferes with platelet aggregation and release by inhibiting thromboxane A_2 synthesis and ADP release. It acetylates cyclo-oxygenase, permanently injuring formed platelets.

Disturbances of Coagulation

Congenital deficiencies of each of the coagulation proteins have been described. Most are rare, transmitted as autosomal recessives, requiring the homozygous state for expression. Less rare are the sex-linked hemophilias A and B, and von Willebrand's disease, transmitted as an autosomal dominant. Acquired defects in coagulation may result from failure to produce certain coagulation factors, as in severe liver disease, or increased consumption of factors, as in disseminated intravascular coagulation. There may be selective loss of coagulation factors in the urine of patients with the nephrotic syndrome. Autoimmune reactions may inhibit the function of individual factors; this is particularly true of antibodies to Factor VIII, which may occur in patients with hemophilia or in otherwise normal individuals.

The extrinsic coagulation pathway is evaluated by the *prothrombin time,* where tissue thromboplastin and calcium are added to a patient's plasma. Clotting is normally rapid, occurring in 11 or 12 sec. The test is thus very useful in monitoring anticoagulant therapy. The test is also abnormal in the presence of liver disease.

The *partial thromboplastin time* is used to evaluate the intrinsic pathway. Phospholipid (a substitute for Platelet Factor 3) and calcium are added to plasma. Clotting is slower than in the prothrombin time, taking some 30 sec. The partial thromboplastin time is abnormal in the presence of deficiencies of Factors VIII, IX, X, or XII. This test is used in monitoring heparin therapy.

The plasma *thrombin test* evaluates the last stage of coagulation by adding thrombin to plasma. It is abnormal in the absence of normal fibrinogen. This occurs in congenital afibrinogenemia, in patients with dysfibrinogenemias (where abnormal polypeptide chains produce deficient polymers of fibrin), and in disseminated intravascular coagulation. The time is markedly prolonged in the presence of a thrombin inhibitor, such as heparin.

Deficiency of Factor XII is accompanied by marked prolongation of clotting time and partial thromboplastin time. For reasons incompletely understood, patients do not bleed. In fact, the first patient recognized as having this defect,

Mr. Hageman, died of a pulmonary embolus. By contrast, in deficiency of Factor XIII, fibrin-stabilizing factor, the tests of coagulation are all normal, but since fibrin remains in unstable form, there may be severe bleeding. Deficiency of Factor X is reflected in prolongation of both prothrombin time and partial thromboplastin time.

Hemophilia

Hemophilia may be due to deficiency of Factor VIII (hemophilia A, or *classical hemophilia*) or Factor IX (hemophilia B, or *Christmas disease*). Factor VIII deficiency is the more frequent, accounting for 85% of patients with hemophilia, and occurring in one of every 3000 or 4000 American live-born males. Both Factor VIII and Factor IX deficiency are inherited as sex-linked traits. Male progeny of hemophiliac men are normal and do not transmit disease. Daughters of male patients are asymptomatic, but transmit the trait to half of their sons.

There is marked prolongation of the intrinsic coagulation pathway (partial thromboplastin time) and the time that it takes whole blood to clot in the test tube. Bleeding time is normal, indicating normal platelet function; however, the positive feedback effect of thrombin on platelets is lacking.

Bleeding is usually related to trauma, even though trivial, or surgical procedures. It is prominent in soft tissues, muscles, and joints, but can occur in any area. Repeated hemorrhages into joints can produce a chronic arthritis, with destruction of cartilage surfaces and fibrous obliteration of the joint space. Calcified hematomas may resemble bone tumors on roentgenologic examination.

There are three levels of clinical severity in classical hemophilia. In the severe form, the plasma contains <1% of the normal Factor VIII. The disease is severe throughout life, and the transmitted disease is severe. Those with moderate hemophilia have 1 to 5% of the normal Factor VIII. Bleeding is severe only after obvious trauma or surgery. In mild hemophilia, there is 5 to 25% of normal Factor VIII; bleeding is uncommon, and may first occur during surgery. Those with mild disease transmit mild disease. Similar levels of activity are observed in hemophilia due to Factor IX deficiency.

von Willebrand's Disease

In this disease, there is prolongation of both bleeding time and partial thromboplastin time. There is a marked decrease in adherence of platelets at sites of endothelial injury. This is due to a deficiency of a plasma factor, *von Willebrand's factor*, that also is expressed as decreased Factor VIII activity. The disorder is usually inherited as an autosomal dominant. It is not uncommon, and it may well be that the term "von Willebrand's disease" is being applied to a group of disorders with somewhat varying deficiencies and manifestations.

THROMBOTIC DISORDERS

The product of hemostasis and coagulation is the thrombus, composed primarily of platelet aggregates and fibrin. Pathologic thrombi have been described as "hemostasis in the wrong place." They consist of solid masses formed from elements of the blood in the heart or blood vessels. Such thrombi may be mural,

Hemostasis and Blood Coagulation

lying along the wall, or totally occluding. Occlusion of a vein may be followed by an extensive centripetal propagation of a thrombus. Propagation is less likely to follow arterial occlusion. Thrombi tend to be rather dry, granular, and friable, although a propagated tail may appear as a simple gelatinous blood clot.

Virchow stated that thrombosis is likely to occur in any of three circumstances (*Virchow's triad*): alteration of vessel walls, stasis of blood flow, and altered composition of the blood. Injury to vessel walls is most frequent in the arterial circulation, where ulceration of atherosclerotic plaques and immunologic injury is often associated with thrombus formation. Mural thrombi are frequent in the left ventricle after myocardial infarction. Stasis of blood flow is most frequent in the venous system, resulting from varicosities, from compression of veins by tumors and other masses, or as a consequence of congestive heart failure. Stasis occurs during bedrest, particularly in a postoperative patient. Thrombosis of atrial appendages is a common complication of atrial fibrillation. The blood is hypercoagulable in patients with deficiencies of antithrombin III or fibrinolytic factors and in those with thrombocytosis or polycythemia. Thrombosis is likely to occur in patients with sickle cell anemia, in patients with hyperlipidemia, and in those taking estrogens, or oral contraceptive preparations with high estrogen content.

Thrombi, once formed, may be dissolved by fibrinolysins and proteolytic enzymes from leukocytes. They may, on the other hand, be covered by endothelium and be organized by the ingrowth of capillaries and fibroblasts (Fig. 7.5). This often leads to varying degrees of recanalization with re-establishment of blood flow. Finally, thrombi may embolize (Fig. 7.6).

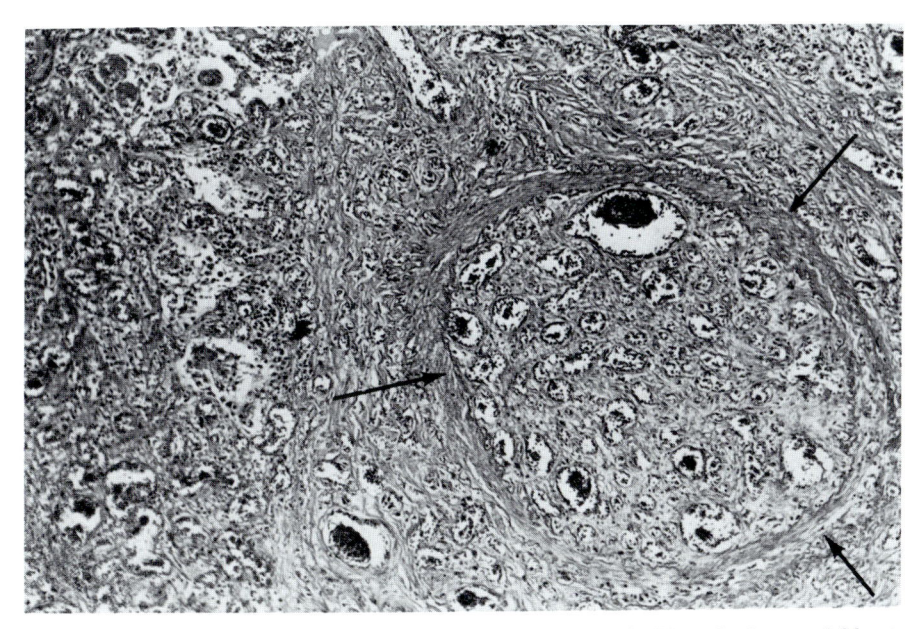

Figure 7.5. An organized thrombus in a pulmonary artery branch. Thrombotic material has been replaced by connective tissue, and many new vascular channels are seen. The *arrows* indicate the arterial wall.

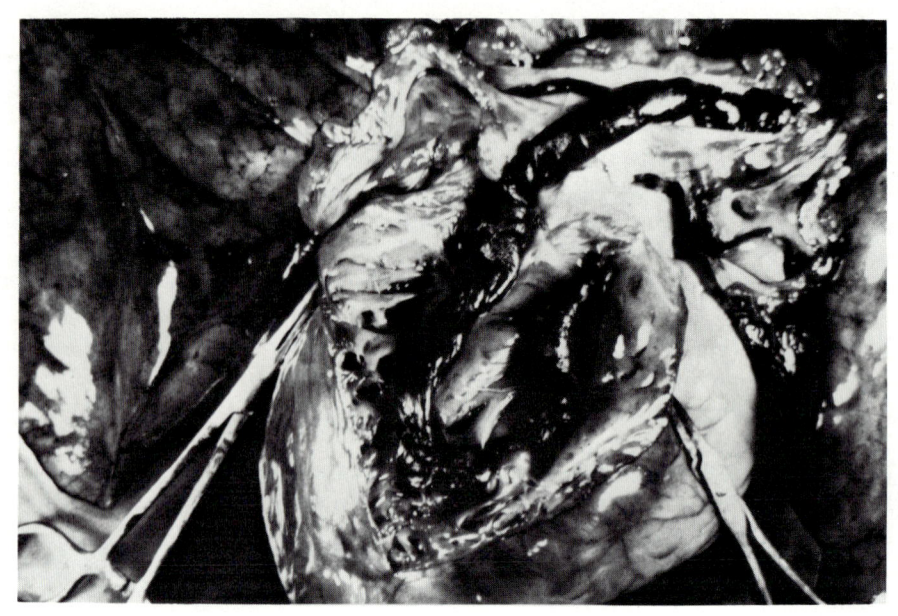

Figure 7.6. Thrombotic embolus. A long embolus from a lower extremity is seen filling the right ventricle of the heart, and extending in continuity into the pulmonary artery and its bifurcation.

EMBOLISM

Embolism is the transportation of thrombi or nonhemic substances through the circulation, until they impact in arteries. Although thrombi are by far the most frequent type of emboli, emboli may also consist of fragments of bone marrow (Fig. 7.7), neutral fat, amniotic fluid, air, material from atherosclerotic plaques, clumps of tumor cells, bits of valvular vegetations, and foreign matter introduced into veins.

DISSEMINATED INTRAVASCULAR COAGULATION

The syndrome of disseminated intravascular coagulation has assumed major importance in clinical medicine. It consists of a massive stimulus to coagulation in the microcirculation, most dramatically observed in the brain, kidneys, lungs, and skin (Figs. 7.8 and 7.9). Coagulation inhibitors and the fibrinolytic system are overpowered. There is rapid consumption of platelets, or one or more coagulation factors, particularly fibrinogen, and Factors V, VIII, or X. In effect, plasma has been converted to serum, and the depletion of clotting factors is followed by a severe and life-threatening bleeding tendency.

Disseminated intravascular coagulation is never a primary disorder, but occurs in association with widespread endothelial injury. It is seen most often in shock and bacterial sepsis, particularly due to such Gram-negative organisms as the meningococcus and *Escherichia coli*, and it is a major pathologic finding in the rickettsial diseases. Release of tissue thromboplastin in the bloodstream may also

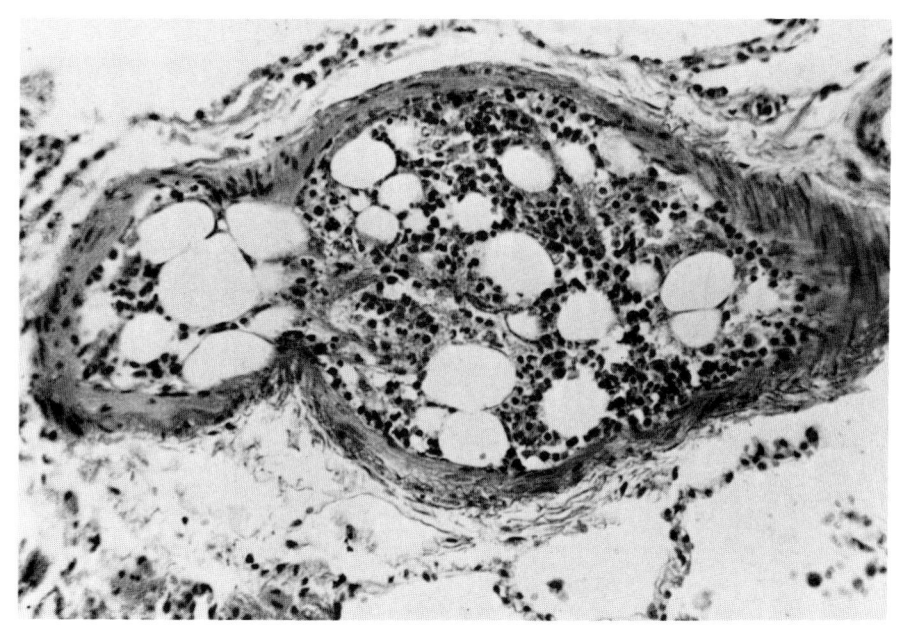

Figure 7.7. Bone marrow embolus. A branch of the pulmonary artery is occluded by a mass of bone marrow. This is a not infrequent complication of cardiopulmonary resuscitation.

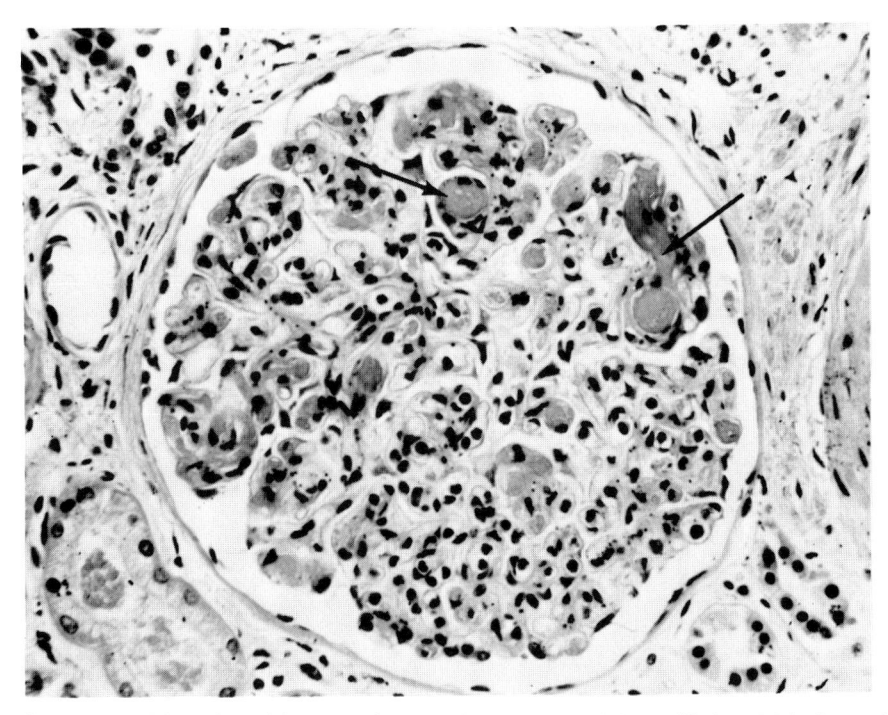

Figure 7.8. Disseminated intravascular coagulation. Many of the capillaries of this glomerulus are occluded by thrombi.

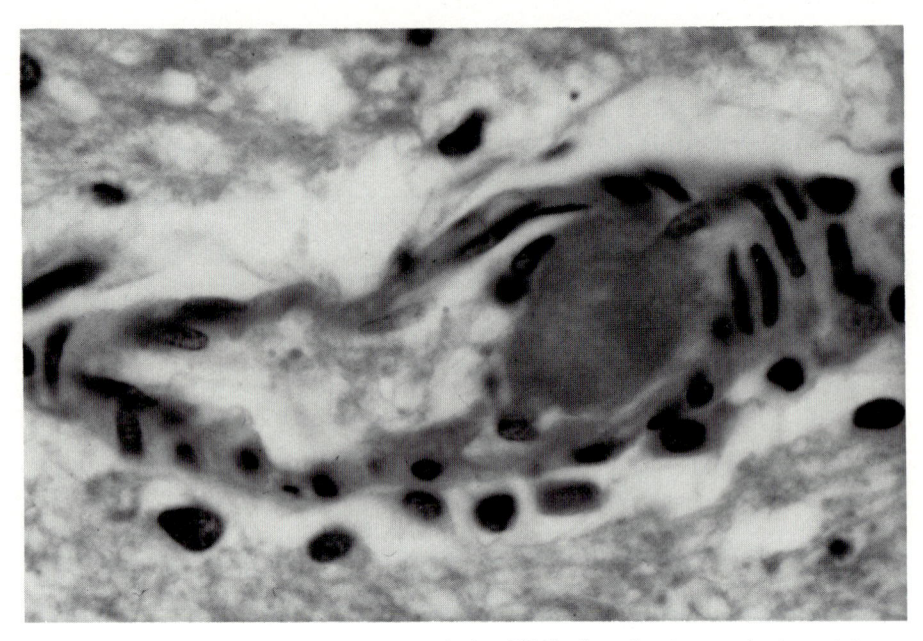

Figure 7.9. Disseminated intravascular coagulation. Fibrin thrombus in a cerebral arteriole.

trigger disseminated intravascular coagulation. This can occur with crush injuries, in many neoplastic diseases, and at the time of parturition. The disorder *thrombotic thrombocytopenic purpura* is thought to be another example of disseminated intravascular coagulation. It is an acute illness, characterized by fever, anemia, impaired renal function, altered neurologic function, and thrombocytopenia.

Suggested Reading

Mason RG, Saba HI. Normal and abnormal hemostasis—an integrated view. Am. J. Pathol. *92:* 773, 1978.
Zimmerman TS, Abildgaard CF, Meyer D. The factor VIII abnormality in severe von Willebrand's disease. N. Engl. J. Med. *301:* 1307, 1979.
Zucker MB. The functioning of blood platelets. Sci. Am. *242:* 86, 1980.

Chapter 8

Immunologic Mechanisms of Injury

The role of the immune response in host reaction to injury was emphasized in the early sections of this volume. This chapter, in contrast, considers the ways in which immunologic responses can themselves be responsible for producing injury and causing disease. Consideration is given to the classes of immunoglobulins, the four basic types of immunologic injury observed in human disease, the autoimmune disorders, and the immunologic consequences of organ transplantation.

THE IMMUNOGLOBULINS

The characteristics of the five classes of immunoglobulins are summarized in Table 8.1. While they share the capacity to bind antigens at the variable end of the Fab segment of the molecule, each class has its own specific heavy chains, and these determine its functional behavior. Many of these functions require changes in the Fc region of the molecule that occur following binding of antigen.

Immunoglobulin G

IgG is the most prevalent of the immunoglobulins. It accounts for some 80% of circulating antibody globulin. It is freely diffusable between the vascular and extravascular compartments and is unique among immunoglobulins in traversing the placenta and entering the fetal circulation. It occurs as a monomer, and its flexible hinge area permits both Fab areas to bind simultaneously with antigen. Although occasionally resulting in agglutination reactions, it usually acts as an opsonin, coating cells and particles. This action is possible because polymorphonuclear leukocytes and mononuclear phagocytes have receptor sites for the Fc portion of IgG once it has been altered by reacting with antigen. Antigen-bound IgG also activates the C1 component of complement, aiding its opsonizing function (granulocytes also have C3 receptor sites), and initiating an inflammatory response. IgG antibodies appear later than IgM following a first exposure to antigen, but IgG is the predominant immunoglobulin in response to many antigens on all subsequent exposures. Specific IgG antibody may be produced long after antigen can no longer be detected.

Immunoglobulin M

IgM is the largest of the immunoglobulin molecules, occurring as a pentamer. It is present only in the plasma, and does not cross the placenta. Since antibodies

Table 8.1
The Immunoglobulins

	IgG	IgM	IgE	IgA
Molecular weight	150,000	900,000	200,000	170,000 (monomer)
Sedimentation constant	7 S	19 S	8 S	7 S
Principal location	Serum	Serum	Attached to mast cells	Gastrointestinal and respiratory secretions, milk
Polymerization	Monomer	Pentamer	Monomer	Monomer or dimer
Placental transmission	+	–	–	–
Complement activation, classical pathway	+	+	–	–
Complement activation, alternative pathway	+	+	Slight	+

to coliform organisms are of the IgM class, neonates are particularly susceptible to infection by these organisms, notably *Escherichia coli*. IgM is the most effective immunoglobulin in agglutination reactions involving red blood cells and bacteria. By itself, it is useless as an opsonin, since granulocytes do not have IgM receptor sites. It is, however, very efficient in activating complement and, once C3 is bound, it can function as an opsonin. It is the first antibody globulin to appear after a first exposure to antigen, but its production continues only so long as antigen persists in the body.

Immunoglobulin E

IgE is unique in that it is bound by its Fc segment to mast cells and circulating basophils. When exposed to specific antigen, it signals the release of histamine from these cells. Complement is not involved in this reaction. IgE does not bind complement, although it may occasionally activate the alternative pathway. IgE antibodies are most active at sites of interface with the environment, and have specificity against such antigens as dusts, pollens, and animal products.

Immunoglobulin A

IgA is the second most prevalent immunoglobulin. Often referred to as "secretory immunoglobulin," it is found predominantly in the surface secretions of the respiratory and gastrointestinal tracts, and serves as the first line of defense against many environmental pathogens that enter through these portals. It is also present in collostrum and breast milk, carrying some passive immunity against enteric organisms. It is usually present as a dimer, and is capable of activating complement through the alternative pathway.

Immunoglobulin D

The function of immunoglobulin D is not well understood. It is present on the surface of many B lymphocytes, perhaps those that have never been in contact with specific antigen. It might serve a recognition function, perhaps as B cell receptor for antigen.

Although complement plays no role in some immunologic reactions, it is critical to many; indeed, most antigen-antibody reactions would be ineffective were they not augmented by activation of the complement cascade. The C3b fragment promotes immune adherence and conglutination and enhances phagocytosis. Anaphylotoxins C3a and C5a stimulate release of vasoactive amines from mast cells. The activated C$\overline{567}$ complex is chemotactic for polymorphonuclear leukocytes and mononuclear phagocytes, and activation of C8 and C9 often leads to cytolysis. IgM and most IgG can activate the classical pathway; IgG, IgM, IgA, and occasionally IgE can trigger the alternative pathway of complement activation.

IMMUNOLOGICALLY MEDIATED INJURY

There are four fundamental mechanisms of immunologically mediated injury, or *hypersensitivity*. They are *anaphylaxis, cytotoxicity, complex-mediated disease*, and *cell-mediated immunity*. The salient features of these basic reactions are summarized in Table 8.2.

Type I: Anaphylaxis

In anaphylaxis, the reaction of antigen with IgE antibody attached to the surface of mast cells triggers the degranulation of mast cells and the release of histamine. The immediate local effects are an increase in vascular permeability and smooth muscle contraction. Complement is not involved. Disorders resulting from localized anaphylactic reactions include hay fever, asthma, and gastrointestinal allergies. Generalized, or systemic, anaphylactic reactions are characterized by hypotension and shock, with urticaria, bronchiolar spasm, and laryngeal edema. They are the cause of acute death in patients hypersensitive, or "allergic," to the stings of bees, wasps, and other insects or to such pharmacologic preparations as penicillin and procaine. Some 100 deaths occur each year in this country as a result of insect bites.

The term *atopy* is often used in connection with Type I reactions. It implies a

Table 8.2
Immunologically Mediated Reactions

	Type I Anaphylaxis	Type II Cytotoxicity	Type III Immune Complex Disease	Type IV Cell-mediated Immunity
Mediator	IgE	IgG, IgM	IgG, IgM (IgA)	T lymphocytes
Mechanism	Histamine release	Antibodies to cell membranes	Vascular injury	Lymphokine activation of inflammatory reaction
Complement activation	−	+	+	−
Examples	Insect stings Penicillin allergy Hay fever Asthma	Hemolytic anemia Drug reactions Insulin resistance Graves' disease Myasthenia gravis	Poststreptococcal glomerulonephritis Lupus nephritis Rheumatoid arthritis	Tuberculosis Fungus disease Poison ivy Graft rejection

tendency to experience recurrent localized anaphylactic reactions, such as urticaria, hay fever, and bronchial asthma. There is a distinct genetically determined predisposition to these reactions; *e.g.*, the children of individuals with hay fever will have an increased tendency to bronchial asthma or food allergies. Eosinophilia, an increase in circulating polymorphonuclear eosinophils, is a common manifestation of many atopic disorders.

IgE-mediated anaphylaxis is totally independent of complement. It should be emphasized, however, that activation of complement, particularly C3, and the release of anaphylotoxins (C3a and C5a) can result in localized lesions with the characteristics of anaphylaxis. Thus, urticaria may be prominent in patients with serum sickness and other immune complex-mediated disease.

Type II: Immunologic Cytotoxicity

In Type II reactions the antigen is either a component of the cell or is attached to the cell wall. The cells most often affected are red blood cells, white blood cells, platelets, and vascular endothelial cells. Reaction with antibody leads to cell destruction by one of two mechanisms. The antigen-antibody reaction may trigger activation of the complement cascade, with the later components injuring the cell wall and initiating lysis of the cell. Alternatively, antibody and bound C3b may coat the cells, cause agglutination, and lead to phagocytic destruction by mononuclear phagocytes, particularly in the spleen or liver. Most of these reactions involve IgG or IgM.

Destruction of red blood cells due to transfusion of ABO-incompatible blood is an important example of immune cytotoxicity. Another is *erythroblastosis fetalis*, the hemolytic anemia of the Rh^+ newborn whose Rh^- mother has produced anti-Rh IgG antibodies. Many of the autoimmune diseases, discussed below, manifest cytotoxic reactions, and patients with these disorders often have a variety of antibodies directed against their own cells or cell components. Autoimmune hemolytic anemia, leukopenia, and thrombocytopenia are frequent findings in patients with *systemic lupus erythematosus* as well as in patients with certain neoplasms involving the lymphoreticular organs.

Many drugs are bound to the membranes of circulating cells, and may function as haptens; a few alter their antigenicity. Thus, penicillin is merely attached to red blood cells, while α-methyldopa changes red cell proteins. Sedormid is a hapten on the surface of platelets, and is associated with thrombocytopenia. Sulfapyridine and aminopyrine may cause leukopenia or agranulocytosis.

Antigen-antibody reactions that neutralize or inactivate biologically reactive molecules are often included in Type II reactions. Reactions involving insulin, Clotting Factor VIII, and gastric intrinsic factor are examples.

Type III: Complex-mediated Disease

In these reactions, injury results from circulating immune complexes. When there is an excess of antibody, large precipitates are formed and these are readily removed and digested by phagocytosis. However, if there is antigen excess, soluble antigen-antibody complexes circulate and settle out in blood vessel walls. Most immune complexes contain IgG or IgM, and IgA is encountered in a few disorders.

Immunologic Mechanisms of Injury

IgE may contribute to some reactions by aiding the entrance of complexes into vessel walls.

The vascular system is primarily affected, including blood vessels in the renal glomeruli. Within vessel walls, immune complexes activate complement, usually through the classical pathway, but at times by the alternative pathway. Anaphylotoxins are released, and granulocytes are attracted to the area. These release their lysosomal enzymes, and the vessel walls are injured, stimulating a further inflammatory response. Thrombosis is frequent. On light microscopy, the vessel wall may appear deeply eosinophilic and smudgy, and because this appears similar to fibrin has been called *fibrinoid necrosis* (Fig. 8.1). Actually, the lesions do contain large deposits of fibrin.

Immune complexes are responsible for the injuries that characterize many forms of glomerulonephritis, systemic lupus erythematosus, rheumatoid arthritis, polyarteritis nodosa, and dermatomyositis (Figs. 8.2 to 8.5). At times, complexes form by antibody reacting with normal or altered structures, such as basement membranes. One type of glomerulonephritis is due to antiglomerular basement membrane antibodies that complex with the basement membranes and activate complement (Fig. 8.6).

Type IV: Cell-mediated Immunity

Sensitized T cells, when coming in contact with specific antigen, are activated and release lymphokines. Some of these are chemotactic for granulocytes, mononuclear phagocytes, and especially other lymphocytes. Lymphokines also enhance

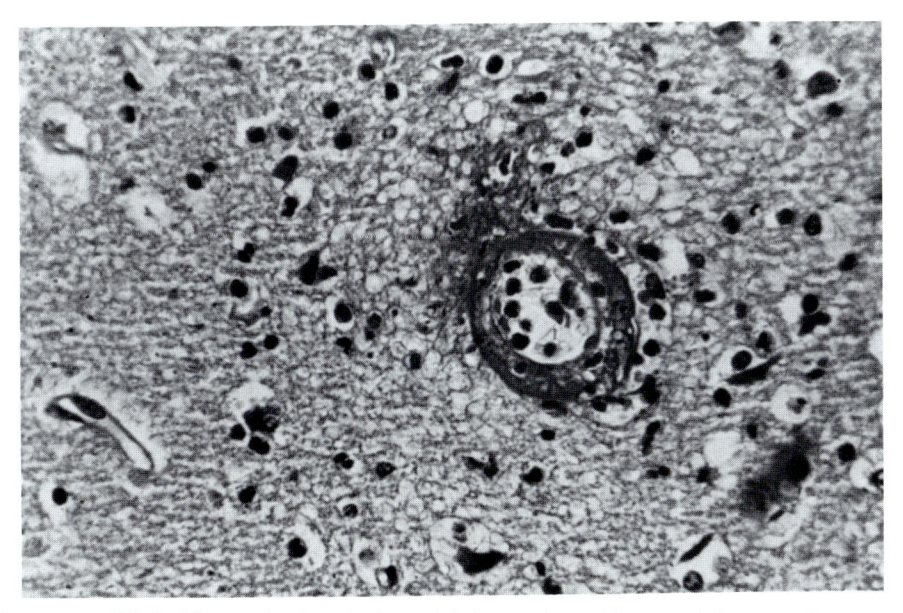

Figure 8.1. Fibrinoid necrosis of cerebral arteriole in a patient with systemic lupus erythematosus. The arteriolar wall is smudgy in appearance and disrupted. Several leukocytes are adhering to the intimal wall, and others are seen in the tissue immediately surrounding the vessel.

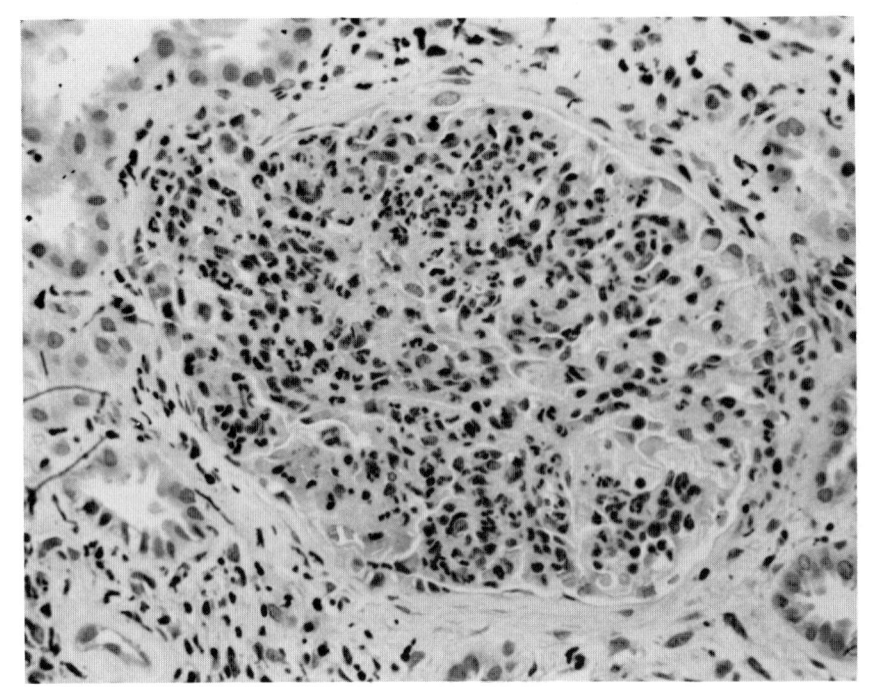

Figure 8.2. Complex-mediated acute glomerulonephritis. This glomerulus shows a striking increase in cellularity, predominantly endothelial and mesangial, although many polymorphonuclear leukocytes are present. Few patent capillaries are recognizable.

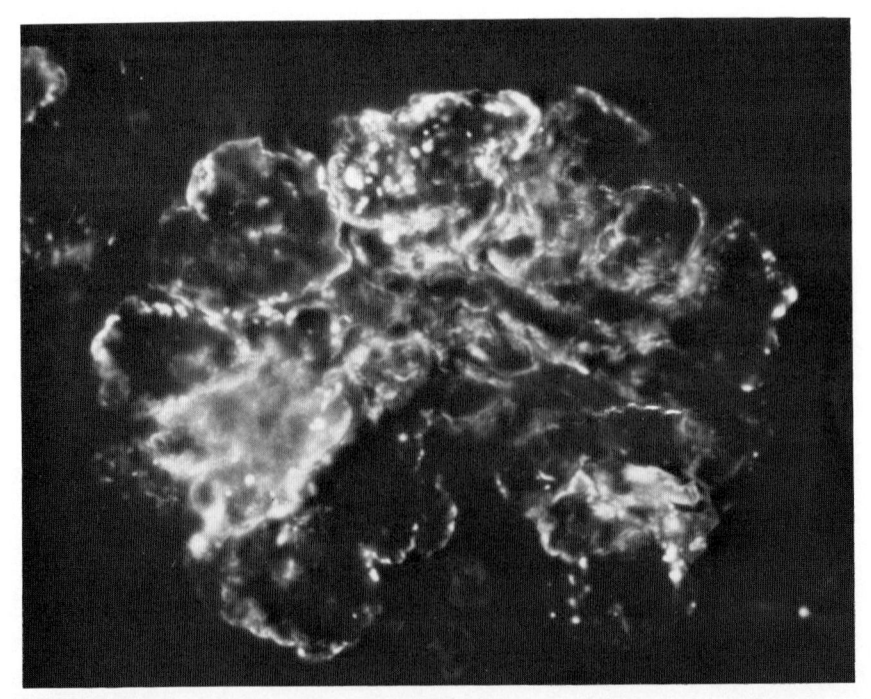

Figure 8.3. Complex-mediated glomerulonephritis. This immunofluorescent preparation, stained for IgG, shows numerous subepithelial and subendothelial granular deposits at the periphery of the glomerular lobules. Some large deposits are also seen in the mesangium.

Immunologic Mechanisms of Injury 81

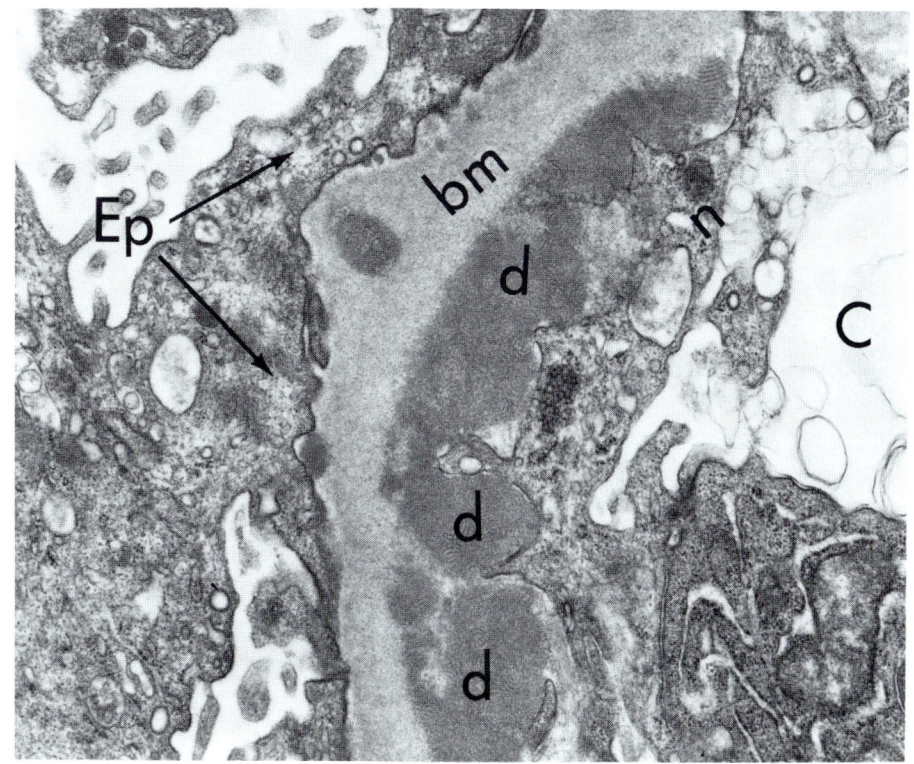

Figure 8.4. Glomerulonephritis in systemic lupus erythematosus. Electron micrograph showing extensive subendothelial immune deposits. There is prominence of the endothelial cell lining this glomerular capillary and fusion of the epithelial foot processes at the left. *d*, deposits; *C*, capillary lumen; *bm*, basement membrane; *Ep*, epithelial foot processes.

the inflammatory reaction by nonspecifically activating other lymphocytes to multiply and produce lymphokines. Mononuclear phagocytes are activated, again nonspecifically, and migration inhibitory factor keeps them in the local area. A chronic inflammatory lesion develops, often a granuloma, and the extent of tissue injury is dependent, at least in part, on the amount of antigen present and the effectiveness of the cell-mediated immune response. T lymphocytes sensitized to cell surface antigens can be cytotoxic, and K (killer) lymphocytes may be nonspecifically cytotoxic, having Fc receptors for immunoglobulin that permit attachment to antibody-coated cells. Epithelioid macrophages, also formed under stimulation by lymphokines, have lost most of their capacity for phagocytosis, but produce both intracellular and secreted enzymes that are effective in eliminating microorganisms. Epithelioid cells are characteristically seen in the granulomas mediated by sensitized T cells. Their enzymes may also be responsible for tissue injury and for the characteristics of necrosis.

Cell-mediated immunity is central to the pathogenesis of tuberculosis, leprosy, many fungus diseases, and other infections. It is also the pathogenetic mechanism of disorders such as poison ivy, where a chemical agent denatures skin proteins, and lymphocytes become sensitized to an antigen composed of altered protein

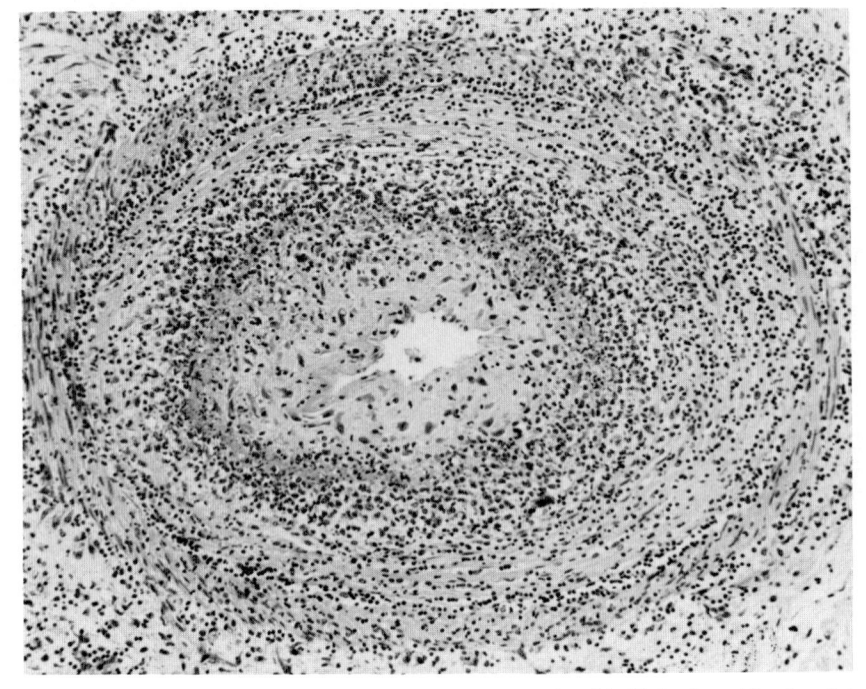

Figure 8.5. Polyarteritis nodosa. There is extensive necrosis with fibrin deposition involving the outer intima and much of the media. Many inflammatory cells, mostly polymorphonuclear leukocytes, are seen in the arterial wall and in the surrounding connective tissue.

and the chemical substance. Most noteworthy today, cell-mediated immunity is the principal component of graft and transplant rejection phenomena.

AUTOIMMUNE DISEASE

In the autoimmune diseases, an individual's immune response is directed against his own tissues. Although antibodies directed against self may be a consequence of disease and have little physiologic significance, in the autoimmune diseases they are the pathogenetic mechanism of tissue injury and altered function.

The immune response is not normally active against autologous antigens; *i.e.*, there is *immune tolerance*. The mechanisms by which autologous antigens can evoke a disease-producing immune response have been poorly understood, possible explanations including mutational development of abnormal clones of lymphocytes, reaction to normally "sequestered antigens" such as thyroglobulin and intracellular proteins, alteration of self-antigenic structure by viral and other infections, and the cross-reactivity of antibodies against exogenous agents with some normal tissue antigens. Although these mechanisms may be pertinent to the pathogenesis of certain disorders, including rheumatic fever and demyelinating diseases, it has been difficult to understand the prevalence of autoimmune disease, particularly its association with so many pharmacologic agents.

Lymphocytes with receptors for autologous antigens, including thyroglobulin,

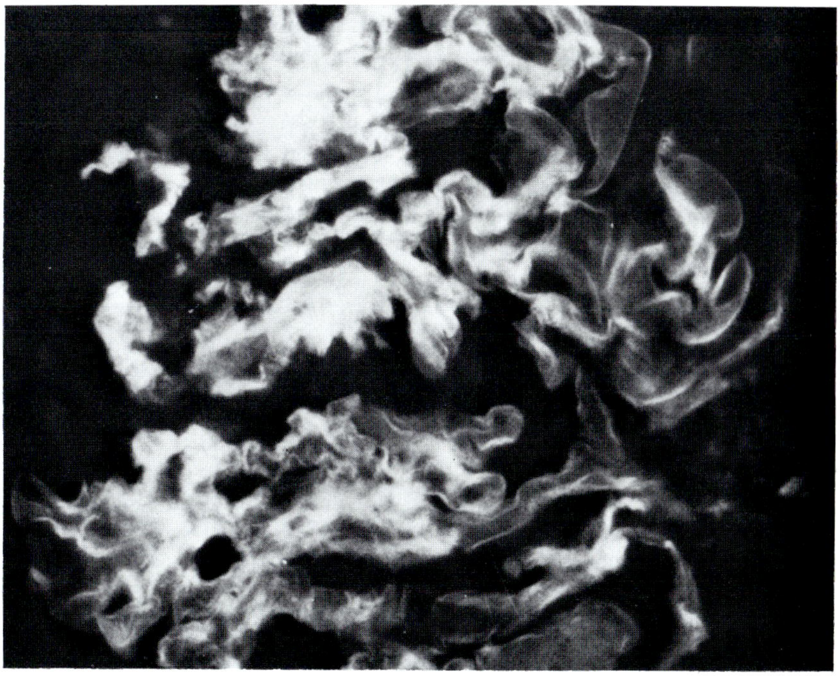

Figure 8.6. Glomerulonephritis due to antiglomerular basement membrane antibodies. Immunofluorescent preparation showing diffuse, ribbon-like deposition of IgG in the glomerular basement membrane. Specimen from a patient with Goodpasture's syndrome.

DNA, and red blood cell antigens, are normally present, although their function is quite unknown. There are substances, such as the lipopolysaccharides of bacterial cell walls, that can stimulate broad groups of B lymphocytes to produce antibodies, including autoantibodies. In other words, the potential for autoimmune reactions is always present, and the fact that they are not universal points to the influence of powerful suppressor mechanisms. Autoimmune diseases, then, can result from a failure of suppression of mechanisms that promote anti-self immune responses. Regulation of the immune system, including suppressor function, is controlled by genes located in close association with the histocompatability loci. It is not surprising, then, that so many of the autoimmune diseases show genetic linkage with HLA antigens (see Table 10.4).

It is of interest that several of the autoimmune diseases show a distinct female predominance, as great as 10:1 in systemic lupus erythematosus. This appears to be related to estrogen function and, in the case of lupus, alterations of estrogen metabolism are described. There are other interactions between endocrine organs and the immune system, and it is suggested that predisposition to autoimmune disease may be determined by both genetic and hormonal factors, and that viruses, other microbial agents, and drugs serve to initiate the autoimmune process.

Once self-tolerance is broken, injury is produced by the same mechanisms observed with exogenous antigens, namely Types I, II, III, and IV. In many autoimmune diseases, both cell-mediated and antibody-mediated reactions are observed, although one or the other is usually predominant. Type I IgE reactions are uncommon, but they may contribute to complex-mediated injury by increasing vascular permeability and enhancing the ability of immune complexes to enter vessel walls.

Many of the autoimmune diseases are listed in Table 8.3. Their division into systemic and organ-specific disorders is somewhat artificial, since most patients with these diseases have multiple autoimmune manifestations. Thus, patients with Goodpasture's syndrome, in which a severe glomerulonephritis results from antiglomerular basement membrane antibodies (antibodies that also react with pulmonary alveolar basement membranes), may also have antinuclear antibodies and antiparietal cell antibodies. There are frequent overlappings of manifestations among diseases in the systemic group, as well as among those in the organ-specific group.

Immune cytotoxicity is frequent in the autoimmune diseases, causing hemolytic anemia, and destruction of white blood cells and platelets. Type II reactive antibodies may also be directed against cell receptor sites. In *myasthenia gravis*, antibodies to acetylcholine receptors at the motor end plate interfere with the effectiveness of acetylcholine. Antibodies to insulin receptor sites account for the development of insulin resistance in the course of diabetes mellitus. Antiparietal cell antibodies and anti-intrinsic factor antibodies interfere with the absorption of vitamin B_{12} in *pernicious anemia*. In *Graves' disease*, antibodies against thyroid cell receptors for thyrotrophin have the peculiar capacity to activate the

Table 8.3
Some Autoimmune Diseases

Diseases	Antigen(s)
Systemic	
Systemic lupus erythematosus	DNA, IgG, blood cells
Rheumatoid arthritis	IgG
Polyarteritis nodosa	Hepatitis virus-related (50%)
Rheumatic fever	Cardiac tissue
Progressive systemic sclerosis	?
Sjögren's syndrome	Salivary gland ducts
Organ-specific	
Hemolytic anemia	Red blood cells
Leukopenia	Leukocytes
Thrombocytopenia	Platelets
Allergic encephalitis	Myelin
Multiple sclerosis	Myelin
Graves' disease	TSH receptor
Chronic thyroiditis	Thyroglobulin
Addison's disease	Adrenal cortical cells
Pernicious anemia	Intrinsic factor
Chronic active hepatitis	Smooth muscle, mitochondria, nuclear proteins
Goodpasture's syndrome	Glomerular basement membrane
Myasthenia gravis	Motor end plate
Sympathetic ophthalmia	Uveal tract tissues
Pemphigus	Prickle cell cement

receptors and induce uncontrolled synthesis of thyroid hormone and thyrotoxicosis.

Among the systemic disorders, systemic lupus erythematosus has been studied most extensively. It is seen predominately in young women, and is characterized by fever, skin lesions, polyarthritis, inflammation of serous membranes, diffuse vasculitis, and a life-threatening glomerulonephritis. Hemolytic anemia, leukopenia, and thrombocytopenia are frequent. Most of the manifestations are immune complex-mediated; others are cytotoxic or cell-mediated. Specific antibodies to double stranded DNA are demonstrable, as are other nonspecific antinuclear antibodies and a variety of apparently unrelated immune phenomena. Based on human observations and the study of animal models, it is thought that systemic lupus erythematosus results from a genetically determined predisposition to impaired control of the immune response, particularly suppressor T cell function, and an RNA virus infection that somehow induces the production of anti-DNA antibodies. Patients with systemic lupus have augmented reactions to many antigens. They are very prone to immune drug reactions.

Many of the disorders shown in Table 8.3 are discussed elsewhere in this volume. In *progressive systemic sclerosis* (scleroderma), an immunologic mechanism of injury is not demonstrable, although patients have antibodies to various intracellular structures. In this disease, a lymphokine of T cell origin stimulates fibroblasts to overproduce collagen in the skin, musculature, gastrointestinal tract, lungs, and heart.

TRANSPLANTATION

More than 10,000 kidney transplants are performed each year across the world. If a kidney comes from a living donor, three-fourths will be functioning 3 years after transplantation; if from a cadaver, only one-third survive. Some 500 to 1,000 heart transplants have been accomplished; half of the recipients were alive 1 year later, and one-fourth survived for 3 years. One-half of bone marrow transplant recipients are alive after 3 years. The principal reason for failure of kidney and heart transplants is immunologic rejection by the recipient. Rejection is comparatively less of a problem with liver transplants; here, technical difficulties are the major cause of failure. Bone marrow transplants may be immunologically tolerated by the recipient but, since immunocompetent cells are transplanted, *graft versus host* reactions constitute a serious complication.

Immunologic rejection is primarily the result of the introduction of foreign, *i.e.*, non-self histocompatability or cell membrane antigens. The multiple alleles described at each of the four HLA loci mean that some 300,000 genotypes occur based on these loci alone. Identical twins have identical HLA antigens, and transplants are readily tolerated. Transplants from close relatives are more likely to succeed than those from unrelated or cadaver donors. Although efforts are made to achieve as close a match as possible, the success of any individual graft tends to be unpredictable.

Rejection is predominately a cell-mediated phenomenon, although important antibody-mediated reactions also occur. An *acute rejection* can occur 2 weeks after transplantation, and at any subsequent time. In the case of the kidney, the transplant is swollen and infiltrated by large mononuclear phagocytes and lymphocytes (Fig. 8.7). There is frequent evidence of injury to vascular endothelium, and fibrinoid necrosis of arteroles is seen. Renal function is markedly depressed by ischemic injury to the nephron. Necrosis of tubular epithelial cells may be prominent.

Antibody-mediated rejection can occur immediately upon transplantation or within 1 or 2 hr. This *hyperacute rejection* occurs in the event of ABO blood group incompatability, or when antibodies to graft antigens are already present in the host. There is severe endothelial injury and diffuse intravascular clotting. The organ is swollen and deep blue in color, may be infarcted, and is without function. *Chronic rejection* may also be antibody-mediated. Repeated endothelial injury leads to progressively severe thickening and narrowing of arteries and arterioles (Fig. 8.8), and the effects of ischemia lead to a deterioration of transplant function.

Transplant rejection of varying severity can be anticipated in all but syngeneic grafts. Prolonged survival is attributable to the administration of immunosuppressive agents. Varying combinations of drugs such as azothioprine, cyclophosphamide, and adrenal steroids have been very successful but, since they all impair the immune response, patients are highly susceptible to infections, often by opportunistic microorganisms. Antilymphocyte serum, containing antibodies to lymphocytic antigens, may suppress T cells, but has not proven regularly helpful

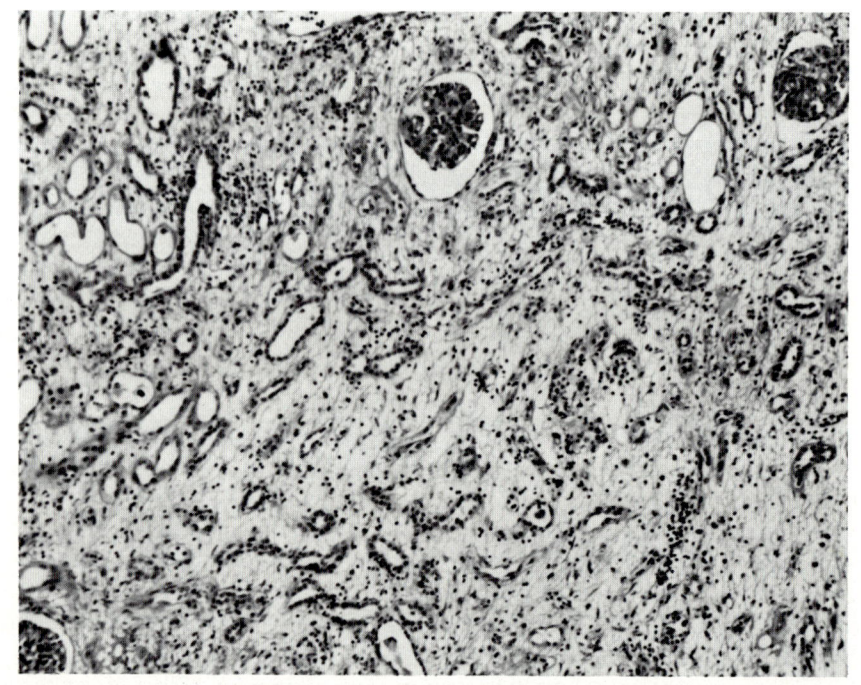

Figure 8.7. Acute kidney transplant rejection. There is striking edema of the interstitium, widely separating tubular structures. There is an extensive cellular infiltrate, composed of lymphocytes, mononuclear phagocytes, and plasma cells. The glomeruli appear shrunken.

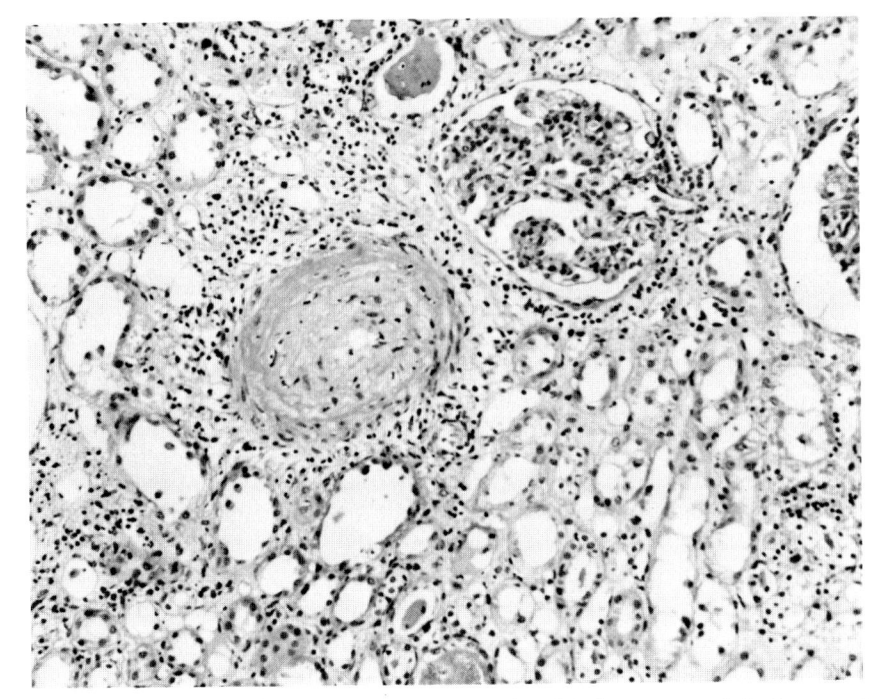

Figure 8.8. Late rejection of kidney transplant. The interlobular artery at *left of center* shows marked thickening of its intima with a mucoid appearance. Several areas of interstitial inflammatory cell infiltration are seen.

in the care of transplant patients. Of great interest is the recent observation that giving transfusions to patients prior to kidney transplantation increases by some 20% the 1-year survival rate of the grafts. This contribution is greater than that of good HLA matching for A and B loci, but matching for D-related (DR) antigens is at least equally important.

Suggested Reading

McDevitt HO. Regulation of the immune response by the major histocompatibility system. N. Engl. J.Med. *303:* 1514, 1980.

Rose NR. Autoimmune diseases. Sci. Am. *244:* 80, 1981.

Rowlands DT, Hill GS, Zmijewski CM. The pathology of renal homograft rejection. Am. J. Pathol. *85:* 773, 1976.

Russell PS, Cosimi AB. Transplantation. N. Engl. J. Med. *301:* 470, 1979.

Sell S. Immunopathology (a teaching monograph). Am. J. Pathol. *90:* 211, 1978.

Talal N. Systemic lupus erythematosus, autoimmunity, sex and inheritance. N. Engl. J. Med. *301:* 838, 1979.

Thomas ED. Current status of bone marrow transplantation for aplastic anemia and acute leukemia. Am. J. Clin. Pathol. *72:* 887, 1979.

Chapter 9

Nutrition and Disease

Except for the cataloging of vitamin deficiencies, the role of nutrition in human disease has received little attention in the medical curriculum. A change is currently taking place, however, reflecting our growing awareness of the significance of nutrition in host resistance, its importance in the pathogenesis of such major human diseases as atherosclerosis and diabetes mellitus, and the adverse effects on health of obesity, alcoholism, and other states of malnutrition.

Recent trends in the American diet have been a cause of growing concern among nutritionists. Reliance of many Americans on "fast foods" has meant that more than half of their caloric intake comes from fats, particularly saturated fats. The average American consumes over 100 pounds of refined white sugar each year, at the expense of more nutritious foods, and probably increasing susceptibility to dental caries. Large quantities of such food additives as BHA/BHT, nitrates, and monosodium glutamate are ingested, although their role in body metabolism is unclear. Finally, many pharmacologic preparations can alter the need for various nutrients; for example, oral contraceptive agents increase need for folic acid and vitamin B_6. It is possible that many who consider their diets adequate may, in reality, be subject to mild or moderate vitamin deficiencies.

NUTRITION AND INFECTION

In earlier chapters, the biologic response to injury was presented as an interplay between host and injurious or infectious agent. It was pointed out that many factors enter into this interplay, particularly in situations of relative equality between the pathogenicity of microorganisms and the reparative capacities of the host. Nutrition is one of these factors. Throughout history, devastating epidemics have occurred during periods of famine and severe malnutrition. The starvation experienced by prisoners of war in World War II was associated with rapidly spreading and frequently fatal pulmonary tuberculosis. Many infections, particularly in children, have a much higher mortality among malnourished populations.

There are many mechanisms through which malnutrition lowers host resistance to infection. Inadequate protein nutrition interferes with humoral antibody production, and cell-mediated immunity is impaired with relatively mild protein or calorie deprivation. Phagocytic activity may be abnormal. Granulation tissue proliferation and collagen synthesis, necessary for healing of any injury, are inadquate in the presence of protein deficiency and scurvy.

Infection is frequently associated with an increase in gluconeogenesis, depletion of protein, and a negative nitrogen balance. It may, at times, unmask a latent nutritional deficiency, such as beri-beri, vitamin A deficiency, and scurvy.

It is interesting to note that, very occasionally, disease may be inhibited by malnutrition in the host. Poliomyelitis was observed to have a decreased morbidity and mortality in the presence of riboflavin and thiamine deficiency. Some recent evidence suggests that mild protein deficiency may be associated with enhancement of T cell function.

NUTRITION AND ATHEROSCLEROSIS

Atherosclerosis is undoubtedly the single most important disease of man in the economically developed Western countries. It is responsible for most cardiovascular disease, including myocardial infarction and cerebral infarction. More than a million deaths each year in the United States are attributable to atherosclerosis, and half of these result from myocardial infarction. The morphology and pathogenesis of atherosclerosis are discussed in Chapter 16; consideration is given here to its relationship to nutrition and the hyperlipoproteinemias.

Many observations have linked atherosclerosis to hyperlipidemia, particularly hypercholesterolemia. Serum cholesterol levels tend to be high in patients with coronary artery disease, particularly if manifest early in life, and the risk of coronary artery disease can be correlated with serum cholesterol and triglyceride levels. High dietary intake of fat can also be related to the incidence of atherosclerosis and coronary artery disease. Diseases, such as hypothyroidism, which are associated with elevated serum cholesterol, tend to be accompanied by an increased incidence and severity of atherosclerosis. Some hyperlipoproteinemias are responsive to dietary control, and this may result in a reduction in mortality from ischemic heart disease.

Lipids are carried in the blood in the form of lipoproteins, containing cholesterol, cholesterol esters, triglycerides, and phospholipids. Five classes of lipoproteins are distinguished on the basis of density. They are *chylomicrons*, which carry exogenous triglycerides, *very low density lipoproteins* (VLDL), which carry triglycerides of hepatic origin, *intermediate density lipoproteins* (IDL), *low density lipoproteins* (LDL), which transport about 60% of serum cholesterol, and *high density lipoproteins* (HDL), which carry phospholipids and fatty acids, as well as some cholesterol.

Primary hyperlipoproteinemias may be sporadic or familial. Although there is a clear-cut pattern of genetic inheritance in several, most are thought to be predominantly related to dietary factors.

Type I hyperlipoproteinemia is rare. It is characterized by an increase in circulating chylomicrons; serum cholesterol is normal, but triglycerides are markedly elevated. This disorder, inherited as an autosomal recessive and usually evident by the age of 10, is not associated with an increased incidence or severity of atherosclerosis.

Type II hyperlipoproteinemia is increased LDL, or hypercholesterolemia. *Type IIA* includes *familial hypercholesterolemia*, inherited as a monogenic autosomal dominant. Serum triglycerides are normal. This disorder is associated with severe and premature atherosclerosis, and individuals may die of coronary artery disease in childhood. In *Type IIB*, there is hypercholesterolemia and moderate elevation of triglycerides. Hyperlipidemia is thought to be primarily dietary in origin, although *familial combined hyperlipidemia* often shows a Type IIB lipoprotein pattern. Atherosclerosis may be severe, but does not occur so early as in Type IIA.

Type III hyperlipoproteinemia consists of an increase in lipoprotein intermediates (IDL). Serum cholesterol is markedly elevated, triglycerides moderately elevated. It is uncommon, often familial, inherited as an autosomal recessive.

Type IV is by far the most common hyperlipoproteinemia, involving some 15 to 25% of adults. There is elevation of VLDL and moderate to severe hypertriglyceridemia; serum cholesterol is normal. The hyperlipidemia is thought to be diet-related, associated particularly with obesity and alcoholism, but genetic factors may also be important. Type IV hyperlipoproteinemia is associated with premature atherosclerosis, although the association is not so marked as in Type II.

Type V hyperlipoproteinemia is characterized by elevation of both VLDL and chylomicrons. Inherited as a recessive trait, it is rare, apparent in early adult life, and manifested by bouts of abdominal pain, pancreatitis, an abnormal glucose tolerance, and hepatosplenomegaly. Its relationship to atherosclerosis is uncertain.

There are many causes of secondary hyperlipoproteinemia, among them hypothyroidism, diabetes mellitus, the nephrotic syndrome, alcoholism, obstructive liver disease, and pancreatitis.

It is important to remember that not all individuals with atherosclerosis have hyperlipoproteinemia. Only one-third of patients requiring surgical intervention for coronary artery disease have abnormal lipid patterns. It should also be noted that there tends to be an inverse relationship between HDL concentration and the incidence and severity of coronary artery disease.

Although results of dietary control are neither uniform nor universally accepted as valid, they appear to demonstrate at least partial correction of hyperlipoproteinemia and a decreased mortality from coronary artery disease. Weight loss and reduction in caloric intake are effective in lowering serum triglycerides. Cholesterol levels are lowered more by increasing the ratio of polyunsaturated fats in the diet. This ratio in most American diets is 0.3:1; the recommended therapeutic ratio is 2.0:1. Reducing total dietary fat to 30 to 35% of total calories appears also to be beneficial.

DIABETES MELLITUS

Diabetes mellitus is another disease of major importance, affecting some 5% of middle-aged Americans and as many as 10% of the elderly. It is a complex metabolic disorder, with both genetic and nutritional determinants.

Juvenile onset or *insulin-dependent diabetes* is thought to result from autoimmune destruction of the β cells of the pancreatic islets, probably following a viral infection. A genetically transmitted predispostion to disease is supported by the strong association of juvenile onset diabetes with two HLA haplotypes (see Chapter 10). *Adult onset diabetes*, accounting for nearly 90% of diabetics, has a high genetically determined familial incidence, but it is profoundly influenced by nutritional factors. In fact, the environment, including economic, dietary, and cultural factors, appears at times to override genetic predisposition.

There is a close correlation of adult onset diabetes with obesity and with excessive consumption of fats. In this form of diabetes, insulin levels may be normal or near normal, but the tissues appear resistant to its action. The enlargement of fat cells in obesity is associated with a decrease in the number of receptor sites for insulin, so there is diminished effect on the entrance of glucose into these cells and on lipolysis. Striated muscle and liver cells also seem resistant to the actions of insulin.

Nutrition also affects the risk of complications of diabetes. Diabetics have a higher than normal incidence and mortality from atherosclerotic coronary artery disease, but it is interesting to note that this is an uncommon complication in underprivileged societies. There is also an increased incidence of cerebrovascular disease and of peripheral atherosclerosis and gangrene of the lower extremities. Atherosclerosis in diabetic patients correlates well with obesity and saturated fat consumption. Whether or not dietary factors influence the microangiopathy of diabetes (Chapter 26) is undetermined.

Although most diabetic patients require insulin or oral hypoglycemic agents, it is estimated that under good dietary control only 25% would require medication and that there would be a significant reduction in both mortality and morbidity.

FATS, FIBER, AND CARCINOMA

Several population studies indicate a significant relationship between the level of dietary fat and the incidence of carcinoma of the breast in women and carcinoma of the colon in both men and women. In these studies, the mortality rates of the tumors appear to be proportional to the dietary fat content.

The incidence of carcinoma of the colon is significantly higher in Americans than Japanese. American diets include more fat, more cholesterol, and more calories than Japanese diets, but less vegetables, grains, and dietary fiber. The source of fat and cholesterol in American diets is primarily animal, from meats and dairy products, although some believe that total fat, including vegetable fat, is the important factor, and stress the role of hydrogenated vegetable fat. In any event, Japanese who immigrate to this country show, by the third generation, a significant increase in colon (and breast) carcinoma. The conclusions of studies like these are difficult to confirm, and studies of other population groups reveal conflicting data.

There is also the suggestion that a decrease in dietary grain fiber is associated with a high incidence of colonic diverticulosis and carcinoma. Both conditions are comparatively rare among African natives who ingest only unrefined grains. It appears that low fiber and high fat content frequently go together, and the evidence to incriminate low fiber content as conducive to carcinogenesis is lacking.

OBESITY

Obesity is the number one nutritional problem in the United States. It is variously defined as adiposity in excess of that consistent with good health, excessive storage of fat in adipose tissue, and body weight in excess of 15 to 20% above ideal weight; but regardless of definition, it is apparent that one-fourth to one-third of all American adults are obese, and that by the sixth decade, half of all women and one-third of men fall into this category. It is particularly prevalent in lower socioeconomic groups.

Obesity may be observed with hypothalmic lesions, as well as in certain endocrine disorders. Hereditary, psychologic, and cultural factors may all play a role, but, in the end, obesity results from a caloric intake in excess of need. It is most often an acquired rather than a constitutional characteristic.

Two types of obesity are known. In life-long or *juvenile onset obesity*, there is an increased number of fat cells in adipose tissue. This disorder is very resistant to therapy, and obese children become obese adults. Adipose tissue in *adult onset obesity* shows marked enlargement of fat cells, but no increase in their number. Juvenile onset obesity tends to be evenly distributed over the body whereas in adult onset disease it is most frequently central.

Many disorders are more frequent or more severe in the obese patient; obesity is considered an important risk factor in atherosclerosis, hypertension, diabetes, fatty liver, gall bladder disease, degenerative arthritis, and endometrial carcinoma. Obese patients are more subject to the complications of anesthesia and surgery. Obesity may interfere with pulmonary function; respiratory motion is decreased, because of a large abdomen and the weight of the thorax, and there is alveolar hypoventilation and respiratory acidosis. There is a compensatory increase in red cell mass, but this contributes to pulmonary hypertension and right heart failure. In the Pickwickian syndrome, there is severe retention of carbon dioxide and narcosis.

The overall death rate in obese persons is 50% higher than in the general population. A study of morbidly obese men revealed a 12-fold increase in mortality in the 24- to 34-year-old group, and a 6-fold increase between the ages of 35 and 44. The major increase was in cardiovascular disease. There were fewer instances of malignancies, but this may only reflect a shorter life span.

ALCOHOLISM

The relationship between alcoholism and nutrition is complex. Alcohol is a source of calories, therefore, a food. Some 4.5% of the calories in the average American diet are derived from alcohol, while it supplies over 50% of the caloric intake of the heavy drinker. Alcohol often replaces other nutrients. It affects the appetite, and has severe effects on the gastrointestinal tract and liver. Alcohol remains one of the few causes of florid nutritional deficiency in this country, and 20,000 alcoholics are hospitalized each year because of disorders related to malnutrition.

Alcohol is directly toxic to liver cells, regardless of diet, and it can result in a fatty liver, alcoholic hepatitis, and cirrhosis. It can cause a severe acute gastritis, and malabsorption in the small intestine. Alcoholism is a common background for acute and chronic pancreatitis. It is associated with folate deficiency, as well as with deficiencies of nicotinic acid and vitamins B_6 and B_{12}. Alcohol can cause severe neurologic disturbances and a cardiomyopathy. It may also exacerbate other disorders, such as Type IV hyperlipoproteinemia.

STARVATION

Frank starvation is uncommon in contemporary America, except in association with severe debilitating disorders or when self-imposed, as in *anorexia nervosa.*

Various metabolic adjustments accompany starvation. Glycogen stores can supply very few calories, and endogenous fat must become the major source of energy. At first, body protein is converted to carbohydrate, but, with time, even the central nervous system becomes capable of metabolizing ketone bodies. There is an overall decrease in metabolic activity. When fat depots are exhausted, there is hypotension, lassitude, and collapse. Edema may be marked, due in part to hypoproteinemia and in part to marked reduction in tissue pressure.

Some prisoners of war during World War II manifested marked weight loss and edema. There was atrophy of adipose tissue and a marked depletion of lymphoid tissue. Decreased gonadal function was severe, with cessation of ovulation and spermatogenesis. Muscle cells, both skeletal and cardiac, decreased in size, and there was as much as a 50% reduction in the weight of the liver. Specific vitamin deficiencies were not common, since the generalized reduction in metabolic functions reduced the need for these substances.

Many types of malnutrition reflecting deficiencies of protein, amino acids, or calories may be associated with retardation of brain development in infancy and perhaps in intrauterine life.

Severe protein and caloric deprivation is observed in underprivileged populations in times of famine and war. Infants and children are most severely affected, particularly when they are further stressed by infections. *Marasmus* results from a symmetrical decrease of proteins and calories. *Kwashiorkor* is observed when severe protein deficiency occurs in a setting of relatively adequate caloric intake.

Marasmus

Marasmus is an example of severe emaciation, usually apparent during the first year of life. There is total loss of subcutaneous fat and marked muscle wasting. Most organs are atrophic. Histologic changes are few, however, aside from decreased cell size. Very often, the victims remain alert, with strong appetite, and no severe disturbances of metabolism.

Kwashiorkor

Kwashiorkor is a disease of severe malnutrition, observed almost exclusively in severely deprived populations, after children are weaned from the breast. Children with this disease are apathetic, and have a weak cry. They are severely anorectic, commonly have diarrhea, are often edematous, and have protuberant abdomens due to ascites. Skin changes may suggest pellagra; the skin is dry, thickened, and pigmented, with areas of excoriation. The hair is discolored, fine, and brittle. The liver and spleen are enlarged. The liver is fatty, may with time become cirrhotic, and may be the site of malignant tumor formation. The gastrointestinal tract, pancreas, and endocrine organs are markedly atrophic.

Anorexia Nervosa

Anorexia nervosa is a self-induced severe weight loss observed primarily in school girls at puberty. It is not rare, occurring in as many as 1% of that population group. The principal manifestations are rapid weight loss, often of 40 to 50 pounds, and early cessation of ovarian function with amenorrhea. Gonadotrophic hormones cease to be released from the anterior pituitary. Although often successfully treated, this is a serious disorder, and death may result from suicide, infections, or severe potassium depletion.

Malnutrition in Debilitating Disease

Anorexia and starvation may be observed in cancer patients. This may relate to vigorous antitumor therapy and infection, as well as to the consumption of energy by tumor. Modern care aims to prevent malnutrition in these patients by maintaining proper nutrition, if necessary by oral or parenteral hyperalimentation.

Suggested Reading

Chandra RK, et al. Nutritional deficiency, immune response, and infectious illness. Fed. Proc. *39:* 3086, 1980.

Drenick EJ, Bale GS, Seltzer F, Johnson DG. Excessive mortality and causes of death in morbidly obese men. JAMA *243:* 443, 1980.

Good RA. Nutrition and immunity. J. Clin. Immunol. *1:* 3, 1981.

Shaw S, Lieber CS. Alcoholism. In: Schneider HA, Anderson CE, Coursin DB, eds. Nutritional support of medical practice. New York, Harper and Row, 1977.

Tullis F, Tullis KF. Obesity. In: Schneider HA, Anderson CE, Coursin DB, eds. Nutritional support of medical practice. New York, Harper and Row, 1977.

Chapter 10

Genetic Determinants of Disease

Genetic determinants are responsible for a wide spectrum of human diseases, among them the many inborn errors of metabolism, the hemoglobinopathies, diseases due to gross cytogenetic abnormalities, and disorders that reflect an interaction between genetic and environmental forces. Single gene defects result in specific enzyme deficiencies or the synthesis of abnormal proteins, and their expression as disease follows Mendelian principles. Chromosomal abnormalities are observed in 20% of intrauterine fetal deaths and a significant number of infants with congenital malformations, and are responsible for some 20,000 cases of mental retardation each year. Some are heritable; others are not. Complex disorders such as diabetes mellitus and essential hypertension appear to have a multifactorial etiology, with a polygenic inherited component, and equally important environmental influences. Mendelian inheritance is difficult to recognize in these diseases.

Genetic influences are undoubtedly of importance in many disorders not usually perceived as inherited. This is indicated by associations of diseases with certain genetic traits, such as the association of peptic duodenal ulcer with blood group O. More dramatic has been the discovery that many diseases, among them autoimmune diseases, certain neoplasms, and metabolic disturbances, reveal *genetic linkage* to alleles of the major histocompatibility complex (HLA).

This chapter is devoted to a discussion of some important examples of genetic disorders, including Marfan's syndrome, Niemann-Pick disease, the adrenogenital syndromes, sickle cell anemia, cystic fibrosis, glucose-6-phosphate dehydrogenase deficiency, Turner's syndrome, Klinefelter's syndrome, and Down's syndrome, and to the contributions of HLA genetic linkage to our understanding of inherited factors in such disorders as hemochromatosis and diabetes mellitus. The essential features of many disorders are presented in tabular form.

SINGLE GENE DEFECTS

There are some 2000 single gene defects known in man. Many of these involve deficiency or abnormality of enzymes, and are usually transmitted as recessive traits, since one normal gene can code sufficient production of enzyme for normal metabolism. Dominant traits usually reflect gene defects that result in the production of abnormal proteins other than enzymes, and their clinical expression tends to be less severe. Dominant and recessive defects of autosomes are carried or expressed by both sexes, although expression may be more severe in one sex.

Recessive traits of the X chromosome produce disease in males, or very occasionally in homozygous females. Sex-linked dominant disorders are rare.

Autosomal Dominant Disorders

Some disorders with autosomal dominant transmission are summarized in Table 10.1. They occur both in males and females, and in all generations of affected families. The severity of disease (*expressivity*) may vary, however, because of environmental or other genetic influences. Most afflicted individuals are heterozygotes, since the homozygous state may be rapidly lethal. The homozygous patient with Type IIA hyperlipoproteinemia (Chapter 9) is likely to die of severe coronary atherosclerosis and myocardial infarction in childhood.

Marfan's Syndrome

Marfan's syndrome is a disorder of connective tissue, although the nature of the defect has not been defined. It may be related to failure to form normal cross-linkages in collagen and elastin fibers, or to production of an abnormal ground substance. Similarities to the lesions of experimental lathyrism suggest that the mechanism of injury may relate to deficiency of lysyl oxidase. Many patients with Marfan's syndrome resemble figures painted by El Greco; they are tall and usually thin, with long extremities, and very long fingers and toes (*arachnodactyly*). Their joints are unusually flexible, because of weak periarticular ligaments. Ocular abnormalities are frequent, particularly bilateral subluxation of the lens. The most serious defects are found in the cardiovascular system. Medial cystic necrosis of the aorta, consisting of defective elastin fibers separated by lakes of mucopolysaccharide, is most marked in the ascending aorta and predisposes to aortic dissection (p. 170); indeed, one-third to one-half of patients die of this

Table 10.1
Some Autosomal Dominant Disorders

Disorder	Defect and/or Manifestations
Ankylosing spondylitis	Arthritis of spine, predominately in males. Strong genetic linkage to HLA-B27
Familial polyposis	Massive polyposis of colon. Carcinoma of colon frequent by age 40
Hereditary angioneurotic edema	Deficiency of C1 esterase inhibitor. Repeated episodes of edema
Hereditary nephropathy	Chronic glomerulonephritis associated with nerve deafness and ocular defects. More severe in males
Hereditary spherocytosis	Spheroidal deformity of red blood cells, and hemolytic anemia
Huntington's chorea	Chorea and dementia. Onset in fourth and fifth decades
Hyperlipoproteinemia Type IIA	Hypercholesterolemia. Early and severe atherosclerosis
Marfan's syndrome	Defective collagen and/or elastin. Arachnodactyly, displacement of ocular lens, "floppy" mitral valve, dissecting aneurysm
Retinoblastoma, familial	Malignant retinal tumor, often present at birth, often bilateral
von Recklinghausen's disease	Multiple neurofibromas of skin and viscera, and patchy skin pigmentation
von Willebrand's disease	Deficiency of von Willebrand factor, with impaired platelet adherence and Factor VIII activity. Bleeding

complication. A frequent cardiac finding is a floppy, incompetent mitral valve, due to abnormal connective tissue in the valve.

Although Marfan's syndrome has a dominant inheritance, many patients suffer mild forms of the disease that may be difficult to recognize.

Autosomal Recessive Disorders

This pattern of inheritance encompasses the inborn errors of metabolism and storage diseases, abnormalities of hemoglobin synthesis, and less well defined conditions, such as cystic fibrosis and hemochromatosis. Inborn errors of metabolism are traced to single enzyme deficiencies that block normal metabolic pathways, and that may be manifested by absence of end product, buildup and storage of intermediate products prior to the block, diversion of intermediates to other metabolic pathways, or loss of feedback regulation by the normal metabolic end product.

Some autosomal recessive disorders are summarized in Table 10.2.

Niemann-Pick Disease

Niemann-Pick disease is a disorder of lipid metabolism due to a deficiency of the enzyme sphingomyelinase. This lysosomal enzyme normally initiates the

Table 10.2
Some Autosomal Recessive Disorders

Disorder	Defect and/or Manifestations
Adrenogenital syndrome	Most common form 21-hydroxylase deficiency. Female pseudohermaphroditism, male precocity
Ataxia telangiectasia	"Chromosome breakage" disorder. Defective immune mechanisms. Cerebellar ataxia and telangiectases of skin and eye
Combined, "Swiss" immunodeficiency	T and B cell deficiencies; severe infections
Cystic fibrosis	Abnormal exocrine secretions. Severe pulmonary disease, pancreatic deficiency, and electrolyte disturbances
Galactosemia	Absent galactose-1-phosphate uridyl transferase. Vomiting and diarrhea in infants given milk. Malnutrition
Hemochromatosis	Excessive iron absorption. Cirrhosis, diabetes, and skin pigmentation. Genetic linkage to HLA A3 and B14
Hurler's syndrome	Storage of mucopolysaccharides due to deficient α-L-iduronidase. Multiple deformities, dwarfism, cardiovascular disease
Niemann-Pick disease	Absent sphingomyelinase. Storage of splingomyelin in liver, spleen, and CNS
Phenylketonuria	Deficiency of phenylalanine. Severe mental retardation
Pompe's disease	α-Glucosidase deficiency. Severe glycogen storage in heart
Sickle cell disease	Hemoglobin S. Sickling of red cells and hemolytic anemia
Tay-Sachs disease	Hexosaminidase A deficiency. Storage of ganglioside G_{M2}. Mental retardation and blindness
Thalassemia	Poor synthesis of α or β chains of hemoglobin A. Severe anemia
von Gierke's disease	Absent glucose-6-phosphatase. Hepatomegaly, severe hypoglycemia and hyperlipidemia
Wilson's disease	Defective binding of copper to ceruloplasmin. Copper deposits cause cirrhosis and cerebral degeneration

digestion of sphingomyelin released in the turnover of cell membranes. Its absence leads to the accumulation of spingomyelin in large lyosomes that displace other organelles in ganglion cells, hepatocytes, and other cells. Macrophages distended by sphingomyelin-laden lyosomes are seen as large foam cells in the spleen, lymph nodes, and bone marrow. There is marked hepatosplenomegaly and anemia, but the neurologic manifestations are most severe, and death usually occurs early in childhood. Niemann-Pick disease is one of the storage diseases, characterized by the accumulation of metabolic intermediates. They include the mucopolysaccharidoses (*e.g.*, Hurler's syndrome), the glycogenoses (*e.g.*, von Gierke's disease, Pompe's disease), and the lipidoses (Tay-Sachs, Gaucher's, and Niemann-Pick disease).

Adrenogenital Syndromes

The adrenogenital syndromes result from deficiencies of any of the enzymes that catalyze the synthesis of cortisol and aldosterone (Fig. 10.1). 21-Hydroxylase deficiency is the most common of these syndromes. This deficiency blocks the synthesis of both cortisol and aldosterone. The metabolic pathway is diverted to the production of androstenedione and testosterone. The result is pseudohermaphroditism in female infants and increased pigmentation and precocious sexual maturation in males. Cortisol synthesis is normally controlled by negative feedback of this end product on the hypothalamus and anterior pituitary. Its absense or deficiency in this adrenogenital syndrome leads to uncontrolled secretion of

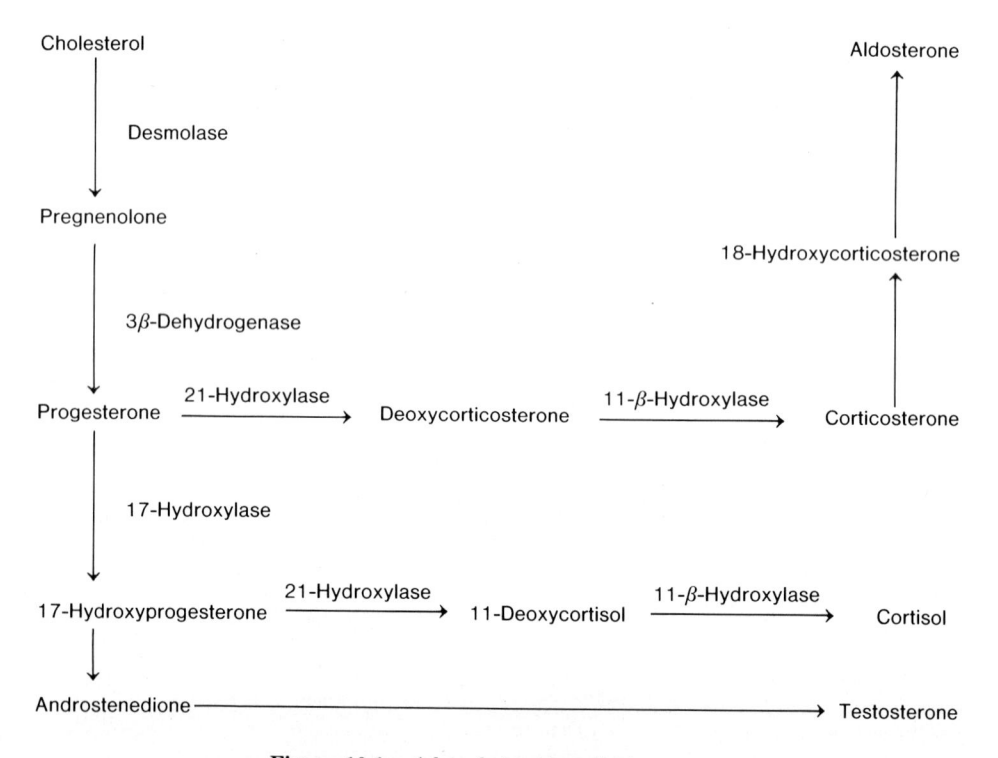

Figure 10.1. Adrenal steroid synthesis.

ACTH and, in turn, more and more androgen production. The cycle is readily broken by the administration of glucocorticoids.

Sickle Cell Disease

The hemoglobinopathies result from single substitutions in the polypeptide chain of hemoglobin, traceable to single base mutations in the DNA code. The hemoglobin of sickle cell disease, hemoglobin S, differs from normal hemoglobin A in the single substitution of a valine for glutamic acid in the β chain. This change greatly alters the solubility of reduced hemoglobin S, which tends to form a gel, changing the normal disc-shaped red blood cells to sickle cells. Intravascular sickling of red cells occurs in homozygotes, often in painfaul "crises," characterized by hemolysis and by widespread thrombosis and infarction.

Sickle cell anemia is almost entirely a disease of blacks. The heterozygous state, the *sickle cell trait*, is very common, found in some 8% of American blacks. Hemoglobin S comprises about 40% of the total hemoglobin in those with the trait, and *in vivo* sickling occurs only under conditions of severe hypoxia. The prevalence of heterozygotes in this country, and an even higher incidence in West Africa, is explained by the fact that hemoglobin S confers increased resistance to malaria, possibly because of early hemolysis of parasitized red cells. Increased resistance to malaria is also observed in those with thalassemia and with glucose-6-phosphate dehydrogenase (G6PD) deficiency.

Cystic Fibrosis

Cystic fibrosis is the most common lethal genetic disease of whites, its incidence being approximately 1 in every 1600 live births. The heterozygous carrier state is observed in 1 of every 20, or 5% of the population. Cystic fibrosis is one-tenth as common among blacks.

Although the pattern of inheritance indicates a single gene defect, the nature of the metabolic change is not known. The most striking finding is abnormality of exocrine gland function, with production of abnormally viscid secretions. These lead to severe changes in the pancreas, lungs, and other organs that are discussed in Chapter 35. Males are generally sterile, because of failure of development of the vas deferens, and females who survive to adulthood are less fertile than normal. Nasal polyposis and rectal prolapse are associated findings.

Sex-linked Disorders

Most sex-linked disorders are recessive traits. Among them are the hemophilias (Chapter 7), several immune deficiency states, and G6PD deficiency. The abnormal gene is located on the X chromosome, and disease is observed only in males and in rare instances of female homozygosity. Heterozygous females transmit the disease to half of their sons and the trait to half of their daughters. The sons of affected males are all normal, whereas all daughters are heterozygotes, or carriers. Dominant sex-linked disease is rare, one example being *vitamin D-resistant rickets*, in which there is failure to resorb phosphate from the proximal renal tubules and a defect in calcium transport from the small intestine. The disease is transmitted by male patients to all of their daughters, but none of their sons; female patients transmit disease to half of their sons and daughters.

Some of the sex-linked disorders are summarized in Table 10.3.

Table 10.3
Some Sex-linked Recessive Disorders

Disorder	Defect and/or Manifestations
Agammaglobulinemia, Bruton	B cell deficiency. Severe infections
Chronic granulomatous disease	Defect in hydrogen peroxide-halide-myeloperoxidase system. Severe infections due to impaired phagocytosis.
Glucose-6-phosphate dehydrogenase deficiency	Hemolytic anemia with certain drugs, *e.g.*, primaquine
Hemophilia A	Deficient Factor VIII. Bleeding
Hemophilia B	Deficient Factor IX. Bleeding
Lesch-Nyhan syndrome	Deficiency of hypoxanthine-guanine phosphoribosyl transferase. Hyperuricemia. Self-mutilation
Muscular dystrophy, Duchenne	Symmetrical diffuse weakness of early onset. Pseudohypertrophy. Elevated serum creatine phosphokinase
Wiskott-Aldrich syndrome	Severe infections and thrombocytopenic hemorrhage. Poor IgM response to polysaccharide antigens. Some T cell deficiency

Glucose-6-phosphate Dehydrogenase Deficiency

G6PD deficiency is of frequent occurrence, present in 10% of American blacks. Under normal circumstances, the deficiency is inapparent. G6PD is important to red blood cell carbohydrate metabolism by indirectly maintaining glutathione in the reduced state. Certain drugs, principal among them the antimalarial *primaquine*, produce a drop in reduced glutathione which in G6PD-deficient individuals results in a severe hemolytic anemia, jaundice, and hemoglobinuria.

G6PD deficiency affects as many as 25% of blacks in West Africa, and, as in the case of sickle cell trait, its frequency is relatable to the enhanced resistance of G6PD-deficient red cells to malaria.

DISORDERS WITH GROSS CHROMOSOMAL ABNORMALITIES

Chromosomal abnormalities include changes in the total number of chromosomes and abnormalities of individual chromosomes resulting from nondisjunction (trisomy) and chromosal breakage (translocations). Deletion of autosomal chromosomes is always lethal, while trisomy of chromosome 21 is the usual finding of Down's syndrome. Deletions or additions of X and Y chromosomes are tolerated quite well. Nondisjunction and chromosome breakage can occur in mitotic as well as meiotic division, as is the case in individuals whose cells show more than one chromosomal pattern (*e.g.*, patients with Down's syndrome some of whose cells are normal and others trisomic).

Chromosomal injury is at times relatable to exposure to ionizing radiation, virus infections, and immunologic reactions. The occurrence of trisomy 21 is most often relatable to maternal age.

Sex Chromosome Abnormalities

Turner's syndrome or *gonadal dysgenesis* results from deletion of an X chromosome, so that there are 44 autosomes and one X chromosome. Patients with this disorder are phenotypically female, but are short, with broad chest and webbed neck. The ovaries are thin linear structures composed only of ovarian stroma. The altered body configuration is due to loss of genes in the short arm of the X chromosome, the ovarian dysgenesis to loss of long arm genes.

The presence of more than two X chromosomes is tolerated reasonably well, although individuals with an XXX configuration tend to be mentally retarded, and severe retardation is the rule in those with XXXX or XXXXX.

Patients with *Klinefelter's syndrome* have 44 autosomes, two X chromosomes, and one Y chromosome. They are phenotypically male, but their testes do not mature normally, and spermatogenesis is rare. The seminiferous tubules are usually atrophic, and there is a real or apparent increase in interstitial Leydig cells. Enlargement of the breasts, *gynecomastia*, is not uncommon.

One in every 2000 males has an additional Y chromosome. This anomaly appears to be associated with increased height and a tendency to sociopathic behavior. The number of XYY males in maximum security prisons far exceeds chance distribution, but it is likely that only a small percentage of XYY individuals manifest criminal or sociopathic behavior.

Autosomal Abnormalities

Down's syndrome is characterized by mental retardation, short stature, hypotonic muscles and hyperflexible joints, and a characteristic facies resulting from oblique palpebral fissures and epicanthic folds. Congenital heart disease is frequent, particularly endocardial cushion defect, and there is a higher than normal incidence of acute myelogenous leukemia. By far the majority of patients with Down's syndrome have trisomy 21 from nondisjunction during meiotic division of the ovum. This event is related to maternal age, occurring in 1 in every 5000 live births from mothers 20 to 30 years old, but increasing to 1 in 30 at maternal age 45. It is a sporadic mutation, not heritable. A small percentage of patients with Down's syndrome have 46 chromosomes with two normal chromosomes 21, and a translocation combining portions of chromosomes 14 and 21. This is inherited from a parent with one normal chromosome 14, one 21, and one 14/21 translocation.

The *cri-du-chat syndrome* is due to a deletion of part of chromosome 5, usually a sporadic mutation. There is severe mental retardation and a characteristic high pitched cry.

Several neoplasms are associated with chromosomal abnormalities. The malignant tumor of the retina, *retinoblastoma*, occurs in familial and nonfamilial patterns, the latter in association with deletion of a segment of the long arm of chromosome 13. The embryonal tumor of the kidney, *Wilms' tumor*, also occurs in familial and sporadic forms, and deletion of the short arm of chromosome 11 is observed in the noninherited cases. A balanced translocation of chromosomes 3 and 8 has been observed in members of a family with a very high incidence of renal cell carcinoma. The *Philadelphia chromosome*, derived from a translocation between chromosomes 9 and 22, is found in the majority of patients with chronic myelogenous leukemia.

MULTIFACTORIAL DISEASES

This designation can be applied to many diseases which result from a combination of genetic and environmental influences. The genetic factors may serve to predispose the individual to illness, and involve multiple genes, so that Mendelian inheritance cannot be recognized. A genetic role in these diseases may be suggested by a high familial incidence, particularly in identical twins, and by associations with other genetic traits. Multifactorial diseases include diabetes mellitus, gout, essential hypertension, atherosclerosis, duodenal peptic ulcer, many neoplasms, and schizophrenia. Most of these disorders are discussed elsewhere in this volume.

Genetic Linkage to HLA Alleles

The study of HLA antigens has yielded a great deal of new information that has helped clarify genetic patterns in various complex disorders. The major histocompatibility gene complex consists of four loci on the short arm of chromosome 6, designated A, B, C, and D. Each locus may be occupied by any one of many alleles, detectable by serologic methods. Since each individual has two sets of A, B, C, and D alleles, these four loci alone account for tremendous heterogeneity in the population, perhaps exceeding 300,000 genotypes.

HLA typing has revealed many examples of genetic linkage, *i.e.*, the close physical proximity of disease-related genes with HLA alleles. Some associations of disease with HLA antigens are shown in Table 10.4. In the case of ankylosing spondylitis, the association is almost constant, suggesting that the HLA antigen itself might have a direct etiologic role.

Hemochromatosis provides an example of the contribution of HLA typing to understanding a multifactorial disease. Hemochromatosis is characterized by the triad of diabetes mellitus, cirrhosis of the liver, and increased skin pigmentation. Patients with this disorder have high serum iron levels, and increased saturation of iron binding capacity. It is predominantly a disease of men, with onset usually between ages 40 and 60. The morphologic findings include massive deposition of iron in the form of hemosiderin in the liver, pancreas, skin, adrenals, and myocardium. Normal total body iron varies between 2 and 5 g; in patients with hemochromatosis, it is often 50 to 75 g. The term hemochromatosis may well encompass a group of disorders. It is usually familial, most often relatable to high iron absorption from the gastrointestinal tract, but it can also be related to high dietary intake of iron, especially in patients with underlying cirrhosis. Excessive alcohol intake is also associated with increased iron absorption. Hemochromatosis can occur with transferrin deficiency, and occasionally, in recipients of large

Table 10.4
Some Disease with Genetic Linkage to HLA Alleles

Acute lymphocytic leukemia	Hodgkin's disease
Addison's disease	Hypertrophic cardiomyopathy
Adrenogenital syndrome (21-hydroxylase deficiency)	Juvenile onset diabetes mellitus
Ankylosing spondylitis	Multiple sclerosis
Cerebellar ataxia	Myasthenia gravis
Chronic active hepatitis	Rheumatoid arthritis
Gluten-sensitive enteropathy	Sjögren's syndrome
Hashimoto's thyroiditis	Systemic lupus erythematosus
Hemochromatosis	Thyrotoxicosis

numbers of transfusions. The heterogeneity of associated findings, the comparatively late onset of disease, and uncertainty as to the precise criteria for diagnosis made the evaluation of genetic influences virtually impossible. HLA typing of patients with a familial background for this disease reveals a close association with A3 and B14 haplotypes, *i.e.*, a tight genetic linkage of a hemochromatosis susceptibility locus to HLA antigens. Susceptibility is inherited as an autosomal recessive; homozygotes show severe iron overload, but some heterozygotes also manifest mild overload. An important benefit of HLA typing is the ability to identify family members at risk for hemochromatosis, before the onset of overt clinical manifestations.

The absence of an HLA association in no way excludes a genetic role in disease pathogenesis. Juvenile onset diabetes mellitus shows a genetic linkage to B8 and BW15 alleles, whereas there is no HLA association of adult onset diabetes. We know that inheritance is important in both forms of diabetes, and its role is actually stronger in the adult onset disease.

Suggested Reading

Gerald PS. Sex chromosome disorders. N. Engl. J. Med. *294:* 706, 1976.
Kidd KK. Genetic linkage and hemochromatosis. N. Engl. J. Med. *301:* 209, 1979.
McDonald JC. The biologic implications of HLA. Arch. Intern. Med. *141:* 100, 1981.
Motulsky AG. The HLA complex and disease. N. Engl. J. Med. *300:* 918, 1979.

Chapter 11

Aging

The maximum life span of humans lies between 90 and 100 years. To the best of our knowledge, it has not changed during recorded history. In contrast, mean survival time, or life expectancy, has grown progressively longer. Survival curves are determined by environmental factors, nutrition, sanitation, population density, and levels of preventive and therapeutic medicine. In primitive societies, many deaths occur in infancy and early years, and few individuals attain the maximum life span. In more advanced societies, most deaths are due to aging and age-related disease. The probability of dying while young has been reduced, but the maximum life span has not changed; it appears to be an intrinsic characteristic, and will not change until we understand and can alter the aging process.

Since 1900, the number of Americans 65 and over has increased from 3 million to more than 23 million. By the year 2000, the number should increase to 32 million, and by 2020, to 45 million. One-fourth of those born today will live to 85.

It was calculated over 150 years ago that the probability of dying doubles every 8 years after maturity, and that observation is still valid today. Our major causes of death are the consequences of atherosclerosis and hypertension (coronary artery disease, cerebrovascular disease, renal failure) and neoplastic disease. Atherosclerosis and hypertension are age-dependent disorders; *i.e.*, their age-specific death rates parallel death rates from all causes. The probability of death from neoplastic disease does not parallel the probability of death from any cause, at least at more advanced ages. It is estimated that elimination of neoplastic disease as a cause of death would increase life expectancy at birth no more than 2 years, and elimination of atherosclerosis and hypertension would add another 7 or 8 years. Maximum life span would not change, nor would the geometric increase in age-determined probability of death.

Increasing age greatly enhances the risk of certain diseases, among them atherosclerosis, hypertension, diabetes mellitus, osteoarthritis, dementia, and neoplastic disease. Disorders that are universal can be considered as part of the aging process, whereas those that affect fewer than 100% of the aging population are diseases. Many diseases causing death are age-related; their incidences increase with age as do their age-specific death rates. Atherosclerosis and its complications are almost universal, and many consider it an inherent part of aging. Increasing vascular rigidity and peripheral resistance make systolic and diastolic hypertension commonplace, and hypertension may be universal in women. Some neoplasms, most notably carcinoma of the colon, prostate, stomach, and skin, show a steadily increasing incidence with age.

There are other conditions that are not age-related, but which are more serious in older persons, among them accidents, influenza, and bronchopneumonia. These are responsible for more and more deaths as people approach the maximum life span. An important aspect or consequence of aging, then, is an increased susceptibility and poor resistance to infection and trauma. What is striking is that the tissue injury observed at autopsy of older patients often appears almost trivial, and would be readily tolerated by the young.

MECHANISMS OF AGING

The mechanisms of aging are poorly understood. Many observations have been recorded of altered physiologic functions, but it is difficult to distinguish causes from manifestations. This is particularly true since there is no clear biologic definition of senescence, and its expression involves such imprecise modalities as susceptibility and resistance.

The changes of aging are not inherently related to environment, nutrition, or activity. They are observable at all levels of structure and function: cells, tissues, and organs.

There is a progressive decline in many bodily functions, starting soon after maturity. Thus, with advancing age, there is a progressive decrease in cardiac output and stroke volume, glomerular filtration rate, cerebral blood flow and oxygen consumption, and pulmonary vital capacity and maximum breathing capacity. There is loss of muscle strength, a decrease in many secretions, and impaired carbohydrate tolerance. Increasing thickness of the optic lens is associated with inability to accommodate, and there is progressive hearing loss, particularly at higher frequencies. The function of virtually every organ is affected by the aging process.

Special attention has been paid to altered immune responses. Many immunologically mediated reactions are quantitatively reduced, including the primary response to foreign antigens, anaphylaxis, and cell-mediated immunity. T cell functions are particularly impaired, and there is a decrement in cell proliferation in spleen and lymph nodes as well as germinal center formation, decreased T cell response to antigens and mitogens, and decreased cell-mediated cytotoxic reactions. On the other hand, there appears to be an increase in the formation of autoimmune antibodies. The role that these widespread changes play in altered susceptibility to infection and impaired immune surveillance against neoplastic disease has not been clarified. They are, in all probability, consequences of aging rather than causes.

Aging may be an inborn or genetically determined property of normal cells. Human fetal fibroblasts in cell culture will show population doubling some 50 times, after which they die. Cells harvested from adults and older individuals go through fewer population doublings, but cultures of malignant neoplastic cells do not appear to have a finite limit to reproduction. Information controlling the reproductive behavior of cells in culture is contained in the nucleus. Aging may be related to cell-reproductive capacity; senescence may be a characteristic of cells that do not divide or divide little after maturity.

Cellular aging may reflect an accumulation of injurious events. Targets of injury include DNA, RNA, cell proteins, and membranes. DNA is particularly prone to injuries such as breaks, distortions, and additions. Cross-linkages form between DNA molecules, between DNA and RNA, and between DNA and proteins. Such injuries are inherent in normal metabolism, but are also relatable to ultraviolet and ionizing radiation, to mutagens and carcinogens, and to viruses. Most injuries to DNA and other cell components are repaired, but, with time, the cell's capacity to heal its wounds diminishes. It is thought that any one cell uses but a very small proportion of its DNA, and that many identical coding sequences permit replacement of injured DNA. With time, these replacements may be exhausted.

Injuries to collagen fibers and elastin are also a regular occurrence, and the cross-linkages that form are reflected in decreased function and the changes of senescence in connective tissue.

ANATOMIC CHANGES WITH AGING

Many morphometric measurements have been made to define the gross changes of aging. In general, aging is accompanied by a decrease in height, particularly sitting height, reduction in the circumference of the neck, thighs, and arms, narrowing of the anterior aspect of the chest, but deepening of the thoracic cage, widening of the pelvis, and such other changes as lengthening of the nose and ears. Decreased bone mass due to osteoporosis and osteoarthritic changes is almost universal. The cranial vault, however, is thickened, while the brain is reduced in weight and has dilated ventricles.

Changes in body weight largely represent body fat. Men tend to gain weight until about age 50, then gradually lose. Women are likely to gain until 70 before starting to lose.

Total body water decreases from about 61 to 54% of body weight. This reflects an increase in body fat together with a decreased lean body mass. A drop in body specific gravity also represents fat. Body potassium is reduced, indicating a decreased cell mass, and an elevated sodium to potassium ratio suggests that the decrease in cell mass is accompanied by an expanded extracellular compartment. Total muscle mass is reduced, partially concealed by increased muscle fat.

The heart may be mildly increased in weight, and there is an increase in fibrous tissue and, at times, a dramatic replacement of muscle fibers by fat. The myocardial fibers are often decreased in size, and contain lipofuscin pigment derived from peroxidation of lipids. Large vessels have an increased collagen content and altered elastin. Their walls are rigid and the vessels tortuous. Capillary basement membranes are diffusely thickened.

The kidneys may show a 40% reduction in nephron mass, accounting for decreased glomerular filtration rate, renal blood flow, and tubular function.

The lungs lose some of their elasticity, reducing their recoil. Mild senile emphysema is common. Although older people are less susceptible to common upper respiratory infections, they are prone to influenzal and other pneumonias and to pulmonary complications of other diseases and surgical procedures.

Atrophic gastritis, hiatus hernia, and colonic diverticulosis are often noted, as is an increasing incidence of gall stones.

The skin is wrinkled and contains less melanin pigment, and there is a loss of skin adnexa and subcutaneous fat. The loss of sweat glands is reflected in an impairment of heat regulation. Collagen is increased, and elastic fibrils are fragmented.

Skeletal changes of aging are discussed in Chapter 31.

Some of the findings noted in this section, particularly those relatable to changes in collagen and elastic fibers, and to loss of cellular functions following death of such nonmitotic cells as neurons and striated muscle, are probably inherent to senescence. Many of the others represent consequences or phenomena secondary to the still elusive basic mechanisms of aging.

Suggested Reading

Fries JF. Aging, natural death, and the compression of morbidity. N. Engl. J. Med. *303:* 130, 1980.
Hayflick L. The cell biology of human aging. Sci. Am. *242:* 58, 1980.
Masoro EJ, et al. Biology of aging. Fed. Proc. *39:* 3162, 1980.
Rossman I. The anatomy of aging. In: Rossman I, ed. Clinical geriatrics. Philadelphia, JB Lippincott Co, 1979.
Walford R Jr. Immunology and aging. Am. J. Clin. Pathol. *74:* 247, 1980.

Chapter 12

The Environment and Health

A diversity of environmental factors can affect human health, among them air and water pollution, synthetic chemicals and drugs, tobacco and alcohol, heavy metals, microwaves, ionizing radiation, and noise. At times, an environmental influence will be directly toxic, and cause and effect are clearly defined, but, more often, it is only one of many factors in the causation of disease; it may only increase the risk of various disorders by mechanisms that are obscure. Substances in the environment may induce mutations, birth defects, or malignant neoplasms, the manifestations of injury appearing a considerable time after exposure. Mutagenesis, teratogenesis, and carcinogenesis are separate phenomena, but many environmental factors, such as ionizing radiation, can result in all three.

Some 50,000 new synthetic compounds are introduced each year, and the environmental impact of relatively few can be adequately tested. It is difficult to test new chemicals on human population groups, and reliance must be placed on laboratory animals and other biologic systems. There is, however, considerable species variation in toxic manifestations, often determined by disparate metabolic pathways. Substances that are toxic to animals, particularly in the large doses generally administered, may be quite acceptable for man. Thus, saccharin causes bladder tumors in mice, but only when it constitutes 5% of the diet. It has not been shown to increase the incidence of these tumors in man. On the other hand, thalidomide was a safe drug in animals.

The effects of environmental contamination are evaluated in terms of the individual and his health, while the causes of contamination are likely to be technologic, economic, or political. Even when the danger and toxicity of an environmental pollutant are clearly established, it may take years before corrective measures are even initiated. Although serious exposure to toxic chemicals over the infamous Love Canal was documented in 1978, it was mid-1980 before the Federal government could be coerced into moving the endangered and injured population group. Unfortunately, too many members of government regulatory bodies are representatives of the very industries they are charged with regulating. The prolonged and bitter debate over nuclear power plants triggered by the near catastrophe at Three Mile Island has not created confidence that the public welfare is given highest priority. It is also ironic that while the Department of Health and Human Services has conducted a major campaign to get Americans to stop smoking, the Department of Agriculture encourages tobacco growing by supporting tobacco prices.

As emphasized earlier in this volume, most diseases result from an interplay between environmental and genetic determinants, albeit one or the other is usually predominant. Environmental medicine could thus be a very broad discipline, and it is not surprising that chapters on the subject in major texts vary so greatly in content. This chapter considers only a few examples of environmental influence on health: air pollution, alcohol and tobacco, asbestos, drug-related disease, chemical carcinogens, metals, and ionizing radiation.

AIR POLLUTION

There are two general types of air pollution in our cities. One results from burning coal and consists predominantly of sulfur oxides and particulate matter. The other derives from gasoline combustion, and includes incompletely burned hydrocarbons, carbon monoxide, carbon dioxide, and nitric oxide. Both types of pollution frequently occur together. The magnitude of the air pollution problem is illustrated in Table 12.1.

Air pollution does not directly cause disease; rather, it aggravates existing cardiovascular and pulmonary diseases. The death rates from these disorders often rise dramatically during periods of severe air pollution.

Sulfur Dioxide

Sulfur dioxide pollution causes an increase in pulmonary airway resistance, and an increase in bronchial mucus secretion. Ciliary action is impaired, and particulate matter is not transported normally from the lung. Sulfur dioxide is thought to contribute to the pathogenesis of chronic bronchitis, and adds to the pollution-related increase in death rates.

Sulfur dioxide is quite water-soluble, but reaches the distal respiratory unit (respiratory bronchiole with its alveolar ducts and alveolar sacs) by being adsorbed to particulate matter.

Nitrogen Oxides

Nitrogen oxides are mostly derived from automobile combustion and burning of natural gas. Ultraviolet light converts nitrogen oxide to nitrogen dioxide which is highly injurious to the lung. Severe exposure can cause acute death due to pulmonary edema; lesser exposures are associated with an obliterative bronchiol-

Table 12.1
Air Pollution, United States, 1977[a]

	All Sources	Transportation	Stationary Fuel Combustion	Industrial Processes	Solid Waste	Other
		emission in 10^6 metric tons per year				
Particulate matter	12.4	1.1	4.8	5.4	0.4	0.7
Sulfur oxides	27.4	0.8	22.4	4.2	<0.05	<0.05
Nitrogen oxides	23.1	9.2	13.0	0.7	0.1	0.1
Hydrocarbons	28.3	11.5	1.5	10.1	0.7	4.5
Carbon monoxide	102.7	85.7	1.2	8.3	2.6	4.9

[a] Data from *Health, United States.* U. S. Department of Health, Education, and Welfare, 1979.

itis and a diffuse interstitial fibrosis of the alveolar septa. Nitrogen dioxide may also arise from silage, causing "silo filler's disease."

Ozone

Ozone is a powerful oxidizing agent, released by the action of ultraviolet light on nitrogen dioxide. In the lung, it causes alveolar edema, necrosis of bronchiolar epithelium and alveolar lining cells, an inflammatory reaction, and alveolar scarring. Its injurious capacity lies in altering membrane lipids and the oxidation of sulfhydryl groups. The lung changes predispose to infection.

Carbon Monoxide

Carbon monoxide pollution results from incomplete combustion of hydrocarbons. It is an important constituent of automobile exhaust (7%) and of tobacco smoke (2%). It is toxic by virtue of its affinity for hemoglobin, forming carboxyhemoglobin, and interfering with oxygen transport. Tissue hypoxia is most apparent in the central nervous system. There is cerebral edema with minute areas of hemorrhage, and necrosis of neurons. Manifestations include confusion, loss of coordination, visual disturbances, coma, and death.

Asbestos

Asbestos is an air pollutant. It is primarily an occupational hazard of workers in the insulation industry, shipyard workers, miners, and millers, but traces of asbestos are widespread, and evidence of some exposure is found in virtually all who live or work in cities.

Asbestos is a group of highly inert fibrous silicates. Inhaled into the lung, crystals of asbestos are coated by a protein-iron complex, forming characteristic ferruginous bodies (Fig. 12.1). These cannot be removed or digested, and evoke a chronic inflammatory reaction leading to extensive pulmonary fibrosis. Asbestos has been clearly implicated as a cause of carcinoma of the lung, and as the major cause of mesothelioma, a malignant tumor arising in the pleura or other serous cavities. It is also associated with an increased incidence of carcinoma of the esophagus, colon, and rectum. The risk of lung cancer is increased 10-fold in those with pulmonary asbestosis, and the risk is much greater if cigarette smoking is added. Neoplasms are likely to occur many years after exposure, as many as 20 to 40 years in the case of shipyard workers.

ALCOHOL AND TOBACCO

Alcohol and tobacco are not occupational hazards; they are, rather, threats to health from the personal or individual environment.

Alcohol

The effects of alcohol on nutrition were discussed in Chapter 9, and its role in the causation of diseases of various systems is considered in subsequent chapters. Here, it is pointed out that alcohol is a powerful co-carcinogen, *i.e.*, a promotor rather than an initiator of neoplastic transformation (p. 131). Together with tobacco, it is important in the genesis of carcinomas of the mouth and oral pharynx, the larynx, and the esophagus.

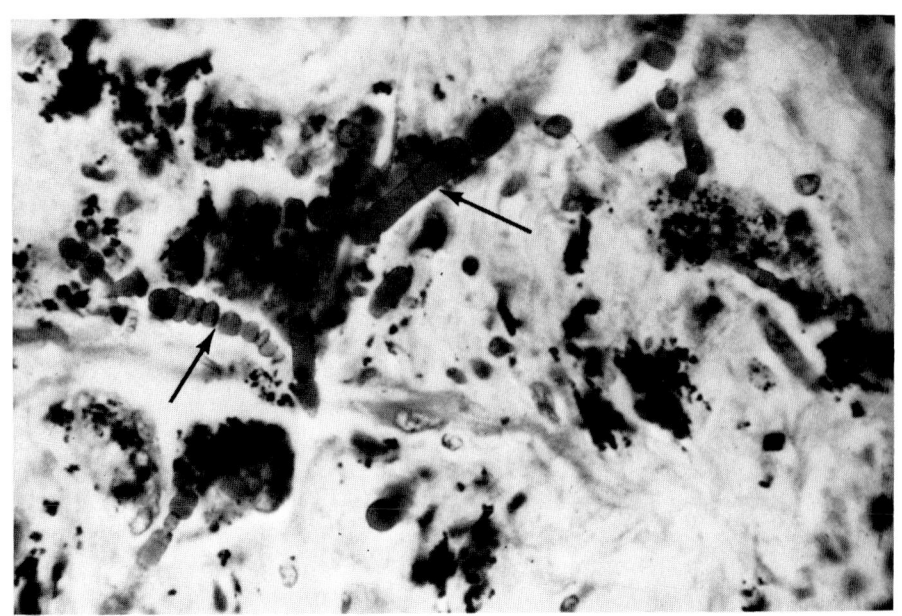

Figure 12.1. Pulmonary asbestosis. Several ferruginous bodies are seen in an area of pulmonary fibrosis. They are composed of crystals of asbestos coated with a protein-iron complex.

Maternal alcoholism poses a threat to the fetus. The *fetal alcohol syndrome* occurs once in every 500 to 1000 live births, and some manifestations are noted in perhaps 1 of every 200 neonates. The syndrome is marked by a characteristic facial appearance, retardation of growth and mental development, hyperactivity, and poor physical coordination. It is generally associated with maternal intake equivalent to about 90 ml of absolute alcohol per day.

Some 20% of alcohol-related deaths are violent.

Cigarette Smoke

Cigarette smoke may well be our worst environmental hazard. The gas phase constitutes 90% of the smoke, and contains over 200 compounds, including dimethyl ether, vinyl chloride, formaldehyde, hydrogen cyanide, and carbon monoxide. The particulate phase consists of nicotine and tars, and more than 3000 other constituents, including polycyclic hydrocarbons and phenols. Nicotine is thought responsible for addiction and for ganglionic stimulation, releasing catecholamines, elevating pulse and blood pressure, and promoting platelet adherence. There is elevation of blood cholesterol and a decrease in high density lipoproteins.

Various studies have indicated that cigarette smoking increases death rates 54 to 86%. It is a major factor in the etiology of chronic obstructive pulmonary disease (COPD), including centrilobular emphysema and chronic bronchitis. Smokers have impaired ability to force air from the lungs, and have ventilation-perfusion disturbances. There is altered ciliary action, disturbed macrophage function, and an increased susceptibility to infections. The risk of death from COPD is increased some 35-fold.

Cigarette smoking is one of the cardinal risk factors for coronary artery and peripheral vascular disease. This may reflect the action of nicotine on blood pressure, pulse, lipids, and platelets. Coronary artery disease alone accounts for half of the increased death rates of cigarette smokers. The combination of oral contraceptive agents and cigarette smoking greatly increases the risk of myocardial infarction in women, particularly after the age of 40.

Men who smoke one pack of cigarettes per day have a 40-fold increase in the likelihood of developing carcinoma of the lung; the increase is 80-fold in smokers of two packs. The risk is only slightly less in women. Lung cancer accounts for one-fifth of all malignancies in men, and for 30% of all cancer deaths. Cigarette smoking greatly increases the incidence of squamous cell and small cell carcinoma; its effect on adenocarcinoma is less dramatic. Smokers are also at increased risk of developing carcinoma of the larynx, pancreas, bladder, and kidneys. Cigarette smoke may serve as a promotor of carcinogenesis; it induces an enzyme, aryl hydrocarbon hydroxylase, which is thought to activate some carcinogens.

There is no evidence that cigarette smoking has teratogenic effects, although infants of smoking mothers average 200 g less in weight than those of nonsmokers, and a difference in weight may persist for several years.

DRUG-RELATED DISORDERS

Drug-related disorders have become prominent in the spectrum of human disease. It is estimated that 5% of hospital admissions are because of drug reactions, that as many as one in every six patients admitted to the hospital will have an adverse reaction to drugs, and that these may account for as many as 3% of inpatient deaths.

Drug-related injury may be the result of direct toxicity or an immunologically mediated reaction; some reactions are idiosyncratic. Other drugs have the ability to induce neoplastic transformation. Examples of each category are given, and some of the better known drug-related disorders are summarized in Table 12.2.

Doxorubicin is an antineoplastic drug. Its usefulness is limited because of a dose-related cardiotoxicity. The myocardial fibers become vacuolated and then necrotic, and are replaced by fibrous tissue. Congestive heart failure may be the principal clinical manifestation of toxicity.

The analgesic *phenacetin* tends to accumulate in the renal medulla. It is associated with renal papillary necrosis and interstitial nephritis (Fig. 12.2), apparently causing altered cell respiration and death by its oxidizing action. Some 5% of American patients with chronic renal failure are thought to have renal disease secondary to analgesic abuse. The incidence is more than twice that high in the United Kingdom, and is 22% in South Africa.

A dose-related fatty change in the liver occurs following intravenous administration of *tetracycline*. This antibiotic interferes with mitochondrial function and protein synthesis, and triglyceride accumulates in the liver cell. The fatty change is reversible. Renal tubular function may also be altered, and renal failure may follow. Toxicity to tetracycline thus is seen where it is metabolized and where it is concentrated during excretion.

Table 12.2
Some Drug-induced Disorders

Organ/System	Drug	Toxicity
Cardiovascular	Doxorubicin	Myocardial necrosis
	Oral contraceptives	Atherosclerosis; thrombosis
Lung	Bleomycin	Interstitial pneumonitis
	Methotrexate	Alveolar necrosis
	Oxygen	Hyaline membranes
	Nitrofurantoin	Interstitial fibrosis
Kidney	Amphotericin B	Tubular injury
	Methicillin	Interstitial nephritis
	Phenacetin	Interstitial nephritis, papillary necrosis
	Gentamicin	Tubular injury
Liver	Isoniazid	Hepatocellular necrosis
	Methyl testosterone	Cholestasis
	Halothane	Hepatocellular necrosis
	Tetracycline	Fatty change
	Acetaminophen	Hepatocellular necrosis
	Oral contraceptives	Benign hepatic adenoma, cholestasis
Gastrointestinal tract	Clindamycin	Pseudomembranous enterocolitis
	Potassium chloride (enteric)	Small intestine ulcers
	Corticosteroids	Gastric ulcers
	Neomycin	Malabsorption
Blood	Chloramphenicol	Aplastic anemia
	Salicylates	Platelet dysfunction
	Cytotoxic agents	Marrow suppression; leukemia
	Primaquine	Hemolytic anemia
Female reproductive	Estrogens	Endometrial hyperplasia, carcinoma
	Diethylstilbestrol	Vaginal adenosis, clear cell carcinoma of cervix
Ear	Streptomycin	Acoustic nerve dysfunction
	Gentamicin	
Eye	Oxygen	Retrolental fibroplasia
	Corticosteroids	Cataract
Gingiva	Diphenylhydantoin	Hyperplasia

Clindamycin is effective in killing many or most intestinal bacteria. It does not, however, kill *Clostridium difficile*, and this organism may grow rapidly and injure the mucosa of the small and large intestines. There is ulceration and formation of a pseudomembrane composed of fibrin, polymorphonuclear leukocytes, and necrotic debris (Fig. 12.3).

Immunologically Mediated Drug Reactions

Most drugs are small molecules, and, if they are to induce an immunologic reaction, act as haptens. *Penicillin*, or one of its metabolites, binds to the red blood cell membrane. Antibodies and complement react at the membrane, and destroy the cell, causing a hemolytic anemia. *α-Methyldopa* alters the red blood cell membrane so as to make it antigenic. *Halothane*, one of the safest of

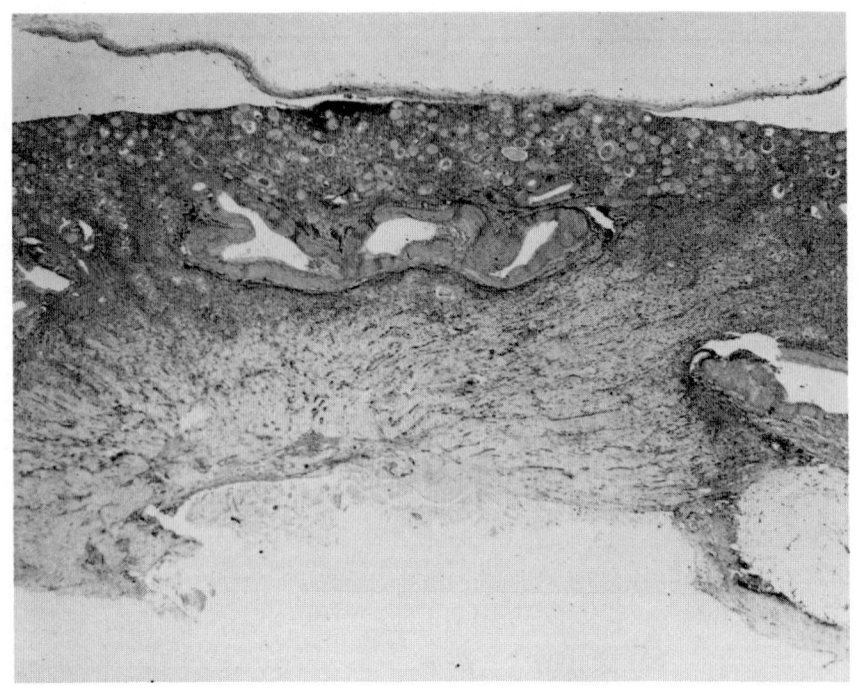

Figure 12.2. Nephropathy of phenacetin abuse. The cortex displays diffuse changes that are indistinguishable from severe chronic pyelonephritis. Necrotizing papillitis has resulted in sloughing of the papilla.

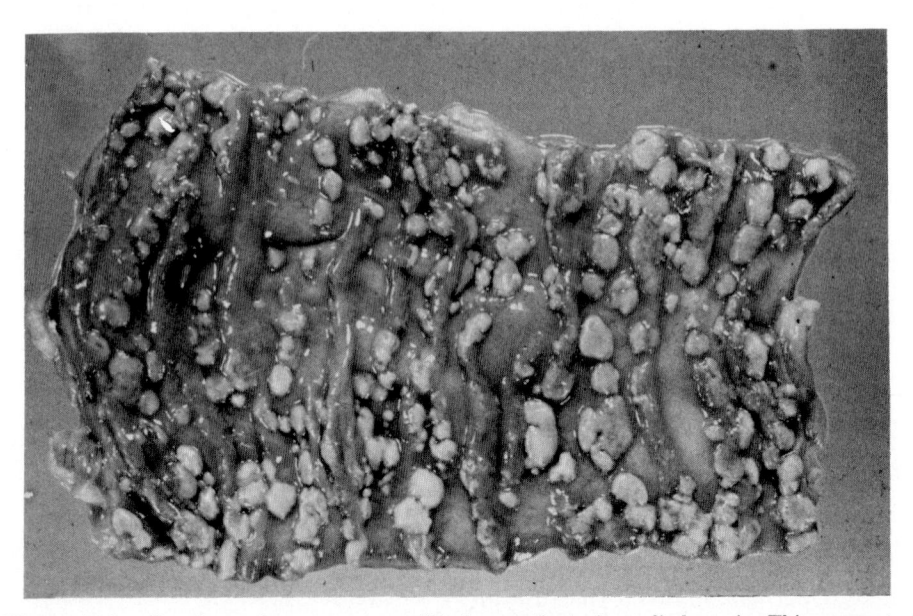

Figure 12.3. Pseudomembranous enterocolitis in a patient given clindamycin. This segment of small bowel shows multiple ulcerations covered by pseudomembrane consisting of fibrin, polymorphonuclear leukocytes, and necrotic tissue. This lesion results from overgrowth of *Clostridium difficile*.

anesthetics, can produce a severe and often fatal hepatitis in a very small number of individuals who have received it more than once. This reaction, often granulomatous, may reflect cell-mediated immunity. *Methicillin* may cause a diffuse interstitial nephritis that appears to result from both cell-mediated and antibody-mediated immune reactions.

Several drugs have the potentiality of inducing all of the serologic and clinical manifestations of systemic lupus erythematosus. Among them are phenytoin and several other anticonvulsants, chlordiazepoxide, hydralazine, α-methyldopa, and tetracycline.

Idiosyncratic Reactions

Idiosyncratic reactions are usually genetically determined. The best known is drug-induced hemolytic anemia in patients with glucose-6-phosphate dehydrogenase (G6PD) deficiency (p. 100). This deficiency, present in some 10% of American blacks, is associated with acute hemolytic anemia when patients are given primaquine, some sulfonamides, antipyretics, and analgesics. G6PD protects normal red blood cells from the oxidizing effects of these drugs. Hemolytic reactions may also occur with administration of oxidant drugs to individuals with glutathione deficiency.

Idiosyncratic reactions to drugs may also occur in acute porphyria, sickle cell anemia, and some congenital disturbances of liver metabolism.

Chloramphenicol is an excellent antibiotic, but reactions to it limit its use. There is a dose-related leukopenia and thrombocytopenia that appear to be direct toxic effects. More importantly, however, a few patients develop aplastic anemia some 2 to 4 weeks after the drug is given, and this reaction is not dose-related. It is thought to be idiosyncratic, but the mechanism is unknown.

Drug-related Neoplasms

Many chemicals employed predominately in the therapy of patients with neoplastic disease can themselves induce neoplasms. This is particularly true of the alkylating agents, such as cyclophosphamide, which injures the DNA molecule throughout the cell growth cycle. It is not unusual for a patient with Hodgkin's disease to be cured by chemotherapy and radiotherapy, only to develop acute leukemia or undifferentiated lymphoma some 3 to 5 years later. It is likely that most therapeutic agents effective in controlling neoplasms are potentially mutagenic, carcinogenic, or teratogenic.

An interesting observation has been the occurrence of benign tumors of liver cells, *hepatic adenomas*, in women taking oral contraceptive agents. These lesions are generally asymptomatic, but they may be the source of severe abdominal hemorrhage. The reason for this association is unknown. The relationship of maternal diethylstilbestrol ingestion to neoplasms in female offspring will be considered in Chapter 27.

CHEMICAL CARCINOGENS

It is estimated that between 60 and 90% of all neoplasms are related to environmental factors, including the chemical carcinogens.

Table 12.3 lists some of the chemicals known or suspected to be carcinogenic

Table 12.3
Some Carcinogenic Substances

Alkylating agents	Nitrogen mustard
	Cyclophosphamide
Aromatic amines	Benzidine
	2-Naphthylamine
Polycyclic hydrocarbons	Cigarette smoke
	Benzopyrene
	Dibenzanthracene
	Methylcholanthrene
Nitroso compounds	Nitrosamines
Natural substances	Aflatoxins
	Betel nuts
	Actinomycin D
	Asbestos
Metallic compounds	Arsenicals
	Cadmium
	Chromium
	Nickel
Miscellaneous	Vinyl chloride
	Butter yellow
	Diethylstilbestrol
	Methotrexate

in man. The mechanisms by which these chemical substances may induce neoplasms are discussed in Chapter 14. Suffice it to say here that carcinogenesis is in all likelihood a multiple step phenomenon, involving initiators and promotors. An initiator produces an irreversible change in a cell; a promotor releases that cell from normal control mechanisms. Both steps are necessary to the neoplastic process, although the promotor may follow the initiator by a period of months or years.

METALS

Table 12.4 lists the principal metals that are potentially toxic to man. All metals are toxic if sufficient quantities are ingested. Some are essential to the body, and toxicity occurs only with excessive intake or in such disturbances of metabolism as hemochromatosis (iron) and Wilson's disease (copper).

Lead

Overt lead poisoning occurs only with accidental or occupational exposure. High blood levels are not uncommon, however, and are observed in between 5 and 10% of American children.

Lead may enter the body through the gastrointestinal tract or the lungs. Only a small proportion of ingested lead is absorbed, and this is largely excreted by the kidneys. There tends to be a gradual accumulation of some 200 to 500 mg, deposited principally in bone.

Acute lead poisoning is most often seen in children and is manifested by ataxia and convulsions. Lead is toxic to neurons, and examination of the brain shows edema, focal necrosis, and proliferation of astrocytes and oligodendroglial cells.

Table 12.4
Toxic Metals

Metal	Manifestations
Mercury	Inorganic: tubular necrosis, intestinal ulceration
	Organic: CNS injury and atrophy
Lead	Anemia
	Encephalopathy
	Peripheral neuropathy
	Fanconi's syndrome
Arsenic	Lung cancer
	Acute gastroenteritis
	Weight loss, dermatitis
Cadmium	Renal tubular dysfunction
	Osteomalacia
	Pneumonitis, fibrosing lung disease
Cobalt	Cardiomyopathy
Nickel	Respiratory tract tumors
Thallium	Toxic encephalopathy
	Hair loss
Thorium	Sarcomas
Uranium	Renal tubular injury (rats)
	Lung carcinoma
Platinum	Renal tubular necrosis
	Marrow suppression

Chronic lead poisoning is associated with a microcytic, hypochromic anemia, with increased numbers of reticulocytes and basophilic stippling of many red cells. A peripheral neuropathy, manifested by wrist drop, reflects segmental demyelination and axonal degeneration. Some patients have a disturbance of proximal renal tubular function, with glycosuria, phosphaturia, aminoaciduria, and a secondary disturbance of bone metabolism (Fanconi syndrome).

Mercury

Metallic mercury is poorly absorbed from the gastrointestinal tract, although chronic low grade ingestion may lead to some injury to the central nervous system and kidneys. Mercury vapor is injurious to the lung. Bichloride of mercury is highly toxic to the proximal renal tubular epithelium and to liver cells. Its ingestion may also be associated with extensive mucosal necrosis of the colon.

Organic mercury compounds, principally methyl and ethyl mercury, are lipid-soluble, and accumulate in the central nervous system. They are most concentrated in the cerebral white matter, particularly of the occipital lobes. They result in cortical atrophy with loss of neurons, particularly in the calcarine fissure. Organic mercury compounds remain in the tissues for prolonged periods, and can cross the placenta. Seafood is the principal source of human contamination.

IONIZING RADIATION

We are all subjected to a certain amount of "background radiation" coming principally from cosmic rays, but significant additional exposure derives from the ever growing use of x-rays in medicine and dentistry, nuclear bomb testing, accidents at nuclear power plants, and inadequate disposal and storage of radioactive wastes. We know more about the effects of large exposures, less about the long term consequences of chronic low grade exposure. It is important to recognize, however, that there appears to be no threshold dosage beneath which no adverse effects occur.

Large doses of ionizing radiation applied to the total body result in the *acute radiation syndrome*. Exposures of part of the body produce localized injuries, often appearing weeks or months later. The effects of low level exposure appear gradually, often years after exposure, and involve a shortened life span, carcinogenesis, mutagenesis, and teratogenesis.

The mechanisms of cellular injury by ionizing radiation may be direct or indirect. *Direct* injury consists of alteration of the DNA molecule. Depending upon its severity, cell death may occur during the next active reproductive cycle, a permanent mutation may be produced, or the pattern of cell growth may become neoplastic. Only a few injuries to DNA are necessary to cause reproductive death. These may consist of damage to the bases, especially pyrimidines, or breaks in the chain. Such injuries can be healed by mending the breaks or excising altered nucleotides and replacing them by new DNA synthesis, but the ability to heal will be affected by the amount and duration of the exposure. A given dose is much more injurious administered in a single rapid episode than the same dose given in several fractions over a longer time frame. *Indirect* injury consists of releasing highly reactive free radicals from the ionization of cell water, which in turn can result in production of such stable molecules as hydrogen peroxide.

The injurious effects of ionizing radiation are greater in the young than in the old. Within any individual, there is striking variation in tissue susceptibility to injury. By and large, rapidly dividing cells or those with the capacity for rapid regeneration are more sensitive than those with a slow turnover rate, or in which no mitotic activity is possible. Table 12.5 groups cells by their sensitivity to ionizing radiation.

The Acute Radiation Syndrome

The acute radiation syndrome follows total body radiation. The time of onset and the principal manifestations depend on dosage. With very large doses, death can take place in hours because of extensive injury to the central nervous system. As usually seen, however, the acute radiation syndrome is an acute illness characterized by leukopenia, bleeding, diarrhea, infections, and loss of hair. These are manifestations of cessation of mitotic activity in tissues with a rapid normal turnover rate. A total body dose of 500 to 1000 rads is reflected in a few days by symptoms of gastrointestinal injury. The small intestinal mucosa is ulcerated and denuded, covered by a shaggy pseudomembrane. Necrotizing changes with thrombosis are noted in the small submucosal blood vessels. Similar changes occur a few days later in the stomach and colon. There is severe diarrhea, with extensive loss of electrolytes, and predilection to systemic infections by enteric organisms. With somewhat lower doses, the onset of symptoms is a little later, and the most striking manifestations relate to destruction of dividing cells in the bone marrow and lymphoid tissue. There is a rapid decrease or disappearance of circulating lymphocytes, polymorphonuclear leukocytes, and platelets. The decrease in red

Table 12.5
Comparative Radiosensitivity of Body Cells

	Most sensitive	Hematopoietic cells
		Short-lived lymphocytes
		Crypts of intestinal mucosa
		Spermatogonia
		Ova and granulosa cells of follicles
	Very sensitive	Basal epidermal cells
		Skin adnexa
		Gastric mucosa
	Sensitive	Vascular endothelium
		Active fibroblasts
		Growing bone and cartilage
		Glial cells
	Resistant	Liver cells
		Renal tubular epithelium
		Adrenal cortical cells
		Pancreatic acini
		Mature bone and cartilage
	Most resistant	Neurons
		Muscle cells

blood cells is more gradual. There is severe anemia, bleeding, and a striking loss of resistance to infections.

Fetal Irradiation

Fetal irradiation can cause death or retardation of growth. Severe teratogenic effects follow exposure during the period of organogenesis (2 to 6 weeks), such as a failure of normal brain development and mental retardation. Exposure of the fetus to the small dose necessary for an x-ray evaluation of the maternal pelvic outlet has led to a distinct increment in the incidence of childhood leukemia.

Delayed Effects and Carcinogenesis

Delayed effects of exposure to ionizing radiation include a shortening of life span and the induction of tumors. The mechanism of a reduction in life span is difficult to understand, although radiation-induced obliterative vascular disease may contribute. It appears to be a rather nonspecific acceleration of the aging process. Until recently, radiologists died some 5 years earlier than other physicians. Many survivors of the bombings of Hiroshima and Nagasaki showed premature aging.

Perhaps the most dramatic of the late effects is the appearance of malignant neoplasms. The incidence of leukemia in atomic bomb survivors at Hiroshima reached 140 per 100,000 population 6 years after exposure, a 35-fold increase. Other tumors, including carcinoma of the breast, lung, and thyroid, showed an increased incidence 20 to 30 years later. Patients treated with x-ray for ankylosing spondylitis have a 10-fold increase in leukemia, and twice the incidence of some other malignant tumors. Ten per cent of radium watch dial painters who tipped their brushes with their lips developed malignant bone tumors. X-ray exposure of the head and neck of children has been reported to increase the incidence of thyroid cancer, although this is now questioned. Also questioned is any adverse effect of low level diagnostic or therapeutic radiation on the incidence of leukemia. Administration of ^{131}I to hyperthyroid and euthyroid adults is not associated with an increased risk of thyroid tumors.

Suggested Reading

Hempelmann LH, Lisco H, Hoffman JG. The acute radiation syndrome. Ann. Intern. Med. *36:* 279, 1952.

Hill RB Jr, Terzian JA, eds. Topics in environmental pathology. Bethesda, Universities Associated for Research and Education in Pathology, 1980.

Linos A, et al. Low dose radiation and leukemia. N. Engl. J. Med. *302:* 1102, 1980.

Miller EC. Some current perspectives on chemical carcinogenesis in human and experimental animals. Cancer Res. *38:* 1479, 1978.

Seaton A. Asbestos. In: Morgan WKC, Seaton A, eds. Occupational lung diseases. Philadelphia, WB Saunders Co, 1975.

Chapter 13

Alterations of Cell Growth

The alterations of cell growth considered in this chapter are atrophy, hypertrophy, hyperplasia, metaplasia, and dysplasia. Changes in the number and size of cells, their differentiation, and their arrangement often appear to be adaptive and a response to a physiologic stimulus. At other times, they are pathologic, and their functional significance is difficult to evaluate.

ATROPHY

Atrophy is defined as a reduction in the size and/or number of cells in an organ or tissue, with an attendant decrease in function. It is to be distinguished from *hypoplasia* and *aplasia* in which failure of normal development accounts for small size. Atrophy is readily observed in immobilized patients, most dramatically, perhaps, when a limb is almost totally immobilized by a plaster cast. Over a period of weeks, the striated muscle cells become smaller, due to reduction in sarcoplasmic reticulum, mitochondria, and other organelles, and there is a striking reduction in muscle mass of the encased limb. The cast also removes stress and strain from the enclosed bone, so that there is no stimulus to new bone formation. Since normal bone resorption continues, there is a net loss of calcified bone, easily recognized by x-ray. There is rapid recovery from atrophy, particularly in young healthy individuals, when the cast is removed and normal function is resumed.

There are many examples throughout life of atrophy that is entirely physiologic. The neonatal adrenal cortex includes a prominent androgenic or fetal X zone. Shortly after birth, the cells of this zone become less conspicuous and begin to drop out, and, by the age of 1 to 4 months, the entire zone has disappeared, not to reappear until puberty. Some atrophy is a normal accompaniment of aging. Atrophy accounts for the loss of some secondary sexual characteristics and for the reduction or cessation of testicular and ovarian function. The heart almost always shows changes with advancing age. These consist of a loss of muscle mass, a decrease in the size of myocardial fibers, the accumulation in these cells of brownish lipofuscin pigment, and often an associated increase in interstitial fat cells. The skin tends to become thin and shiny, with loss of skin appendages and degeneration of subcutaneous elastic tissue.

Pathologic atrophy can be related to decreased use, loss of innervation, or hormonal stimulus to function, hypoxia, or decreased nutrition. The physiologic changes described in the heart and skin are greatly accentuated by the presence of occlusive vascular disease. Stenosis of a renal artery may cause striking atrophy

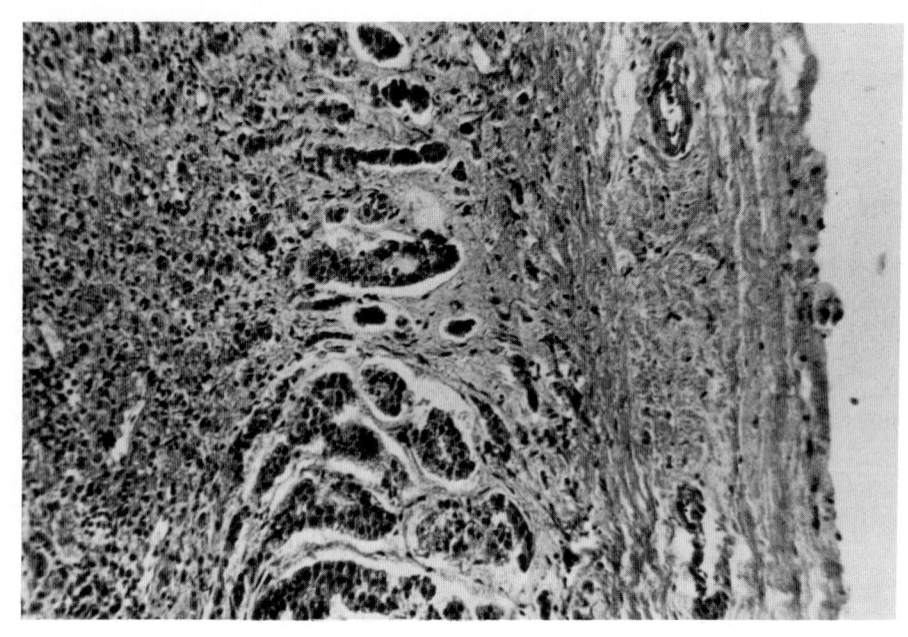

Figure 13.1. Adrenal cortical atrophy. The capsule is to the *right*. The only remaining cortical cells form a narrow band through the middle portion of the photograph. Compare with Figure 13.4. This section is from a patient with systemic lupus erythematosus who received glucocorticoids continuously for 9 years.

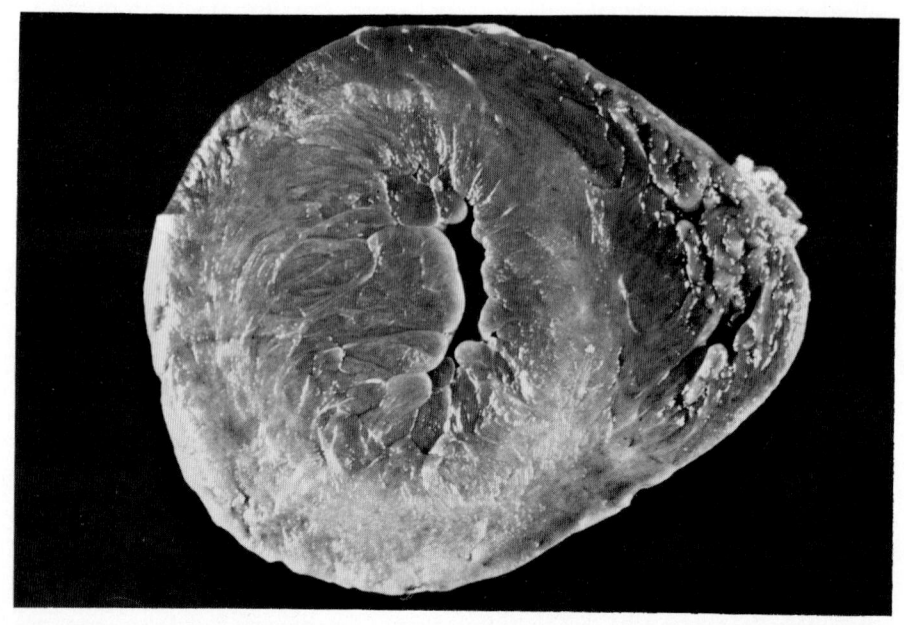

Figure 13.2. Myocardial hypertrophy. This horizontal section of heart shows striking concentric hypertrophy of the entire left ventricular wall. The right ventricle is seen at the *right*. There was a long history of systemic hypertension.

of the kidney with shrinkage of individual nephrons and loss of interstitial tissue. If adrenocorticotrophic hormone (ACTH) stimulation of the adrenal cortex is lost as a result of pituitary disease, or inhibited by the administration of glucocorticoids, the adrenal undergoes gradual atrophy, with eventual loss of the entire glucocorticoid zone, the zona fasciculata (Fig. 13.1). Similarly, the loss of thyrotrophin stimulation is followed by atrophy or involution of the thyroid gland.

HYPERTROPHY

Hypertrophy is an increase in the size of cells of a tissue or organ in response to a demand for increased function. It occurs most often in cells that cannot multiply, particularly myocardial and peripheral striated muscle fibers, but can also be observed in the pregnant uterus and in the kidney. Hypertrophied cells manifest evidence of increased synthetic and metabolic functions; their nuclei are large, with prominent chromatin material.

Myocardial hypertrophy is the means of increasing the output of the cardiac chambers, particularly the ventricles, or of maintaining output in the face of increased resistance (Fig. 13.2). Left ventricular hypertrophy is prominent in arterial hypertension and in aortic valve disease causing either stenosis or regurgitation. It may also reflect increased output in the presence of anemia or arteriovenous fistulae. The right ventricle hypertrophies as a result of pulmonary hypertension caused either by left ventricular failure or intrinsic pulmonary disease. More difficult to understand is mild hypertrophy as a response to myocardial hypoxia when diseased coronary arteries maintain a very marginal blood flow.

Loss of a normal kidney is followed by hypertrophy of the contralateral organ. Creatinine clearance is cut in half, *e.g.*, from 120 to 60 ml per minute, but in the course of several months increases to about 75. There is a concomitant 25 to 30% increase in kidney weight. The enlargement of the kidney is attributable predominantly to increased cell size, although some increase in numbers of cells is also evident.

HYPERPLASIA

Hyperplasia is defined as an increase in number of cells. It is most often physiologic, *i.e.*, a response to a stimulus for increased function. The proliferation of granulation tissue in the repair of injury is an example of hyperplasia, as is the increased cellularity of bone marrow in patients with hemolytic anemia or following a hemorrhage. Persistent hyperplasia of the bone marrow may also represent an adaptation to high altitudes, where low environmental oxygen content is compensated for by an increased red cell mass. Hyperplasia of the adrenal cortex is the response to increased ACTH secretion, hyperplasia of the thyroid to increased thyrotrophin secretion (Figs. 13.3 and 13.4). The uterine endometrium undergoes hyperplasia in the first half of every menstrual cycle, and hyperplasia becomes more marked in the presence of continuous estrogen stimulation.

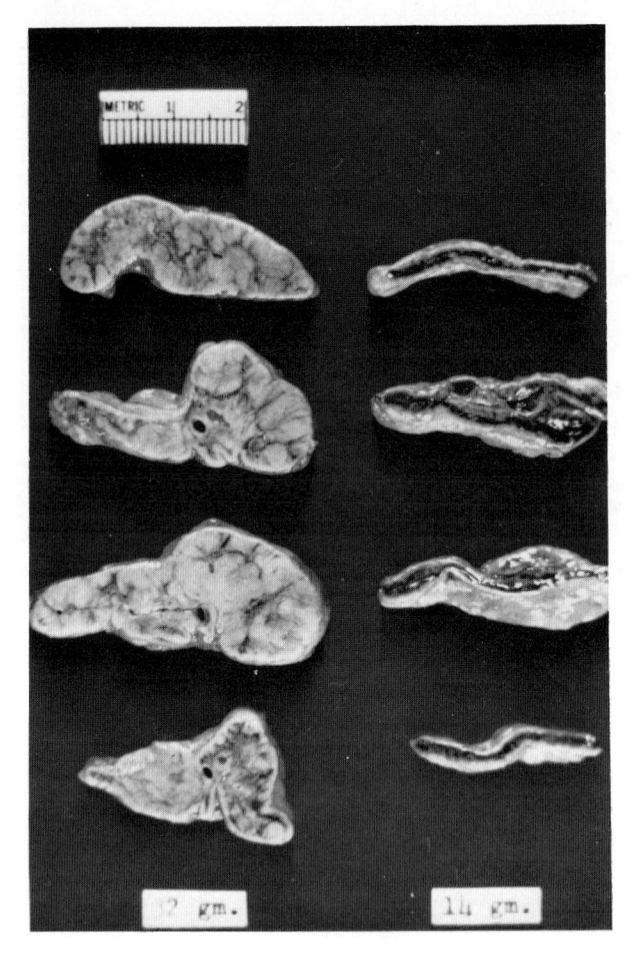

Figure 13.3. Adrenal cortical hyperplasia. Cross-sections of a normal adrenal gland are seen at the *right*. At the *left* are several cross-sections of a markedly hyperplastic gland. The cortex is greatly thickened, and the cut sections have a bright yellow color. This gland was from a patient with pituitary-dependent Cushing's disease.

Primary, Secondary, and Tertiary Hyperplasia

In many circumstances, a physiologic basis for hyperplasia may be quite difficult to define. Hyperplasia may also be clearly pathologic and indistinguishable from neoplasia.

The parathyroid glands are usually rapidly responsive to changes in the circulating level of ionized calcium. A drop in calcium is followed within minutes by an increased secretion of parathyroid hormone, and a rise in calcium rapidly cuts off further secretion. In chronic renal failure, interference with vitamin D metabolism causes a decrease in calcium absorption from the small intestine, and hypocalcemia. This is a persistent stimulus for increased parathyroid hormone secretion, and the parathyroid glands become hyperplastic. Their response tends to return ionized calcium levels toward normal. This hyperplasia is physiologic, and is called *secondary hyperplasia*.

If a patient with chronic renal failure receives a transplanted kidney, renal function may be restored to normal or near normal in hours or a few days. The physiologic need for parathyroid hormone secretion drops rapidly, but it may

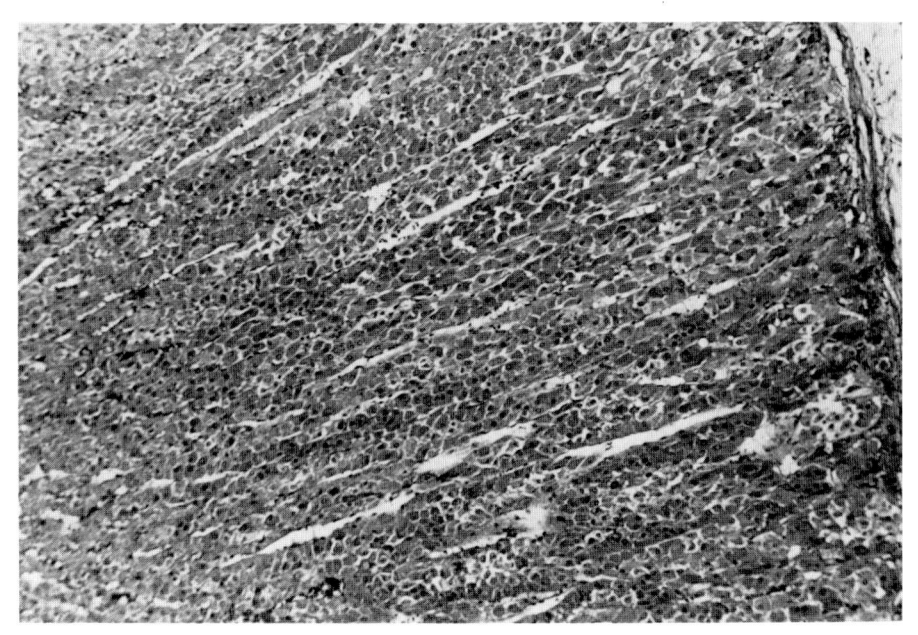

Figure 13.4. Adrenal cortical hyperplasia. This section is from the adrenal gland shown in Figure 13.3. The hyperplasia is seen to consist of extremely long columns of the zona fasciculata, the glucocorticoid-producing zone of the cortex. The capsule is at the *right*.

take months or up to 2 years to make this adjustment. With prolonged hyperplasia, there can thus be a loss of responsiveness to changes in the need for function, and the glands are at least partially autonomous of normal control mechanisms. At times, patients with long standing renal failure become hypercalcemic, again showing increased function that is autonomous. This development of autonomy in a setting of secondary hyperplasia has been called *tertiary hyperplasia* of the parathyroid glands.

Primary hyperplasia is also observed, i.e., a *de novo* hyperplasia occurring in the absence of known physiologic stimulus. This occurs in various endocrine glands. Primary hyperparathyroidism may be due to hyperplasia of all four parathyroid glands. Hyperinsulinism may be the result of diffuse hyperplasia of the islets of Langerhans, and hypercalcitoninemia may follow diffuse hyperplasia of thyroid interstitial cells. These examples of primary hyperplasia are indistinguishable in their functional behavior from neoplasms, although morphologically they do not conform to the usual concept of tumors. It is interesting that either primary hyperplasia or tumors of the parathyroid glands may be associated with tumors of the pituitary, islets of Langerhans, or adrenal medulla in the multiple endocrine syndromes.

Prolonged hyperplasia can occasionally result in the formation of clearly recognizable neoplasms. Continuous exposure of the endometrium to estrogen, as in patients with estrogen-producing ovarian tumors, leads at first to severe hyperplasia and, in some, to a malignant endometrial carcinoma.

METAPLASIA

Metaplasia is the replacement of one fully differentiated cell type by another fully differentiated cell type. It occurs most frequently in epithelial tissue, usually as an adaptation to chronic irritation. Common examples include the change from columnar respiratory epithelium to squamous epithelium in the bronchi of cigarette smokers, and the change from glandular mucus-producing endocervical epithelium to squamous epithelium in women with chronic inflammation of the uterine cervix. An example of squamous metaplasia is shown in Figure 13.5.

In many epithelia, immature undifferentiated cells are found close to the basement membrane. These *reserve cells* maintain the capacity to differentiate along different lines. In the endocervix undergoing squamous metaplasia, the reserve cells become prominent and differentiate to squamous cells, and the columnar mucus-producing cells are replaced from below. Squamous metaplasia of the endocervix or the bronchus provides a more resistant lining, but the physiologic effects of mucus secretion and ciliary action are lost.

Metaplasia may also occur in mesenchymal tissues, usually at sites of healing injury and scarring. Fibroblasts may be replaced by osteoblasts or chondrocytes, with metaplastic formation of bone and cartilage outside of the skeleton.

Although metaplasia is never considered a premalignant change, its presence

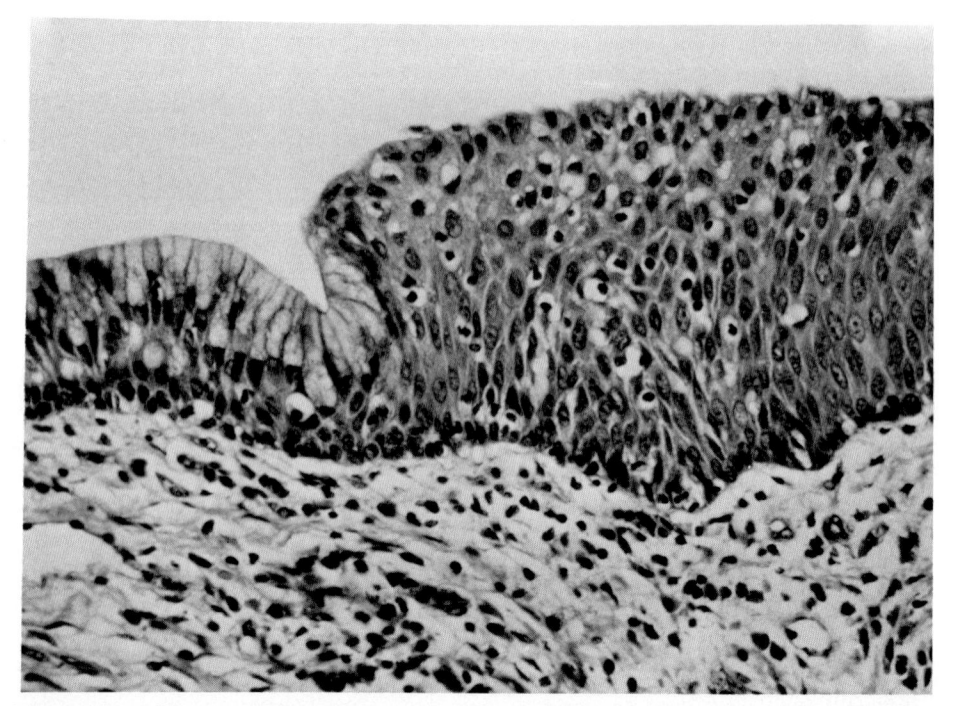

Figure 13.5. Squamous metaplasia. Normal mucus-producing epithelium is seen to the *left*. Squamous metaplasia starts at the basal layer of cells. The normal cells are at first lifted from the basement membrane and then replaced by squamous epithelial cells. The squamous epithelium at the *right* is not normal, but shows a delay in maturation.

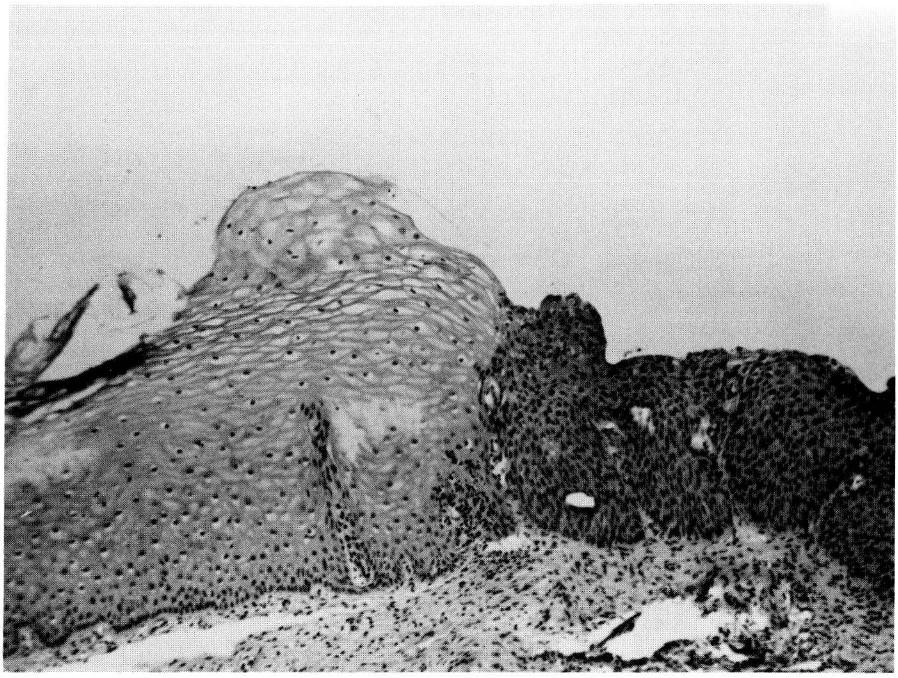

Figure 13.6. Dysplasia of squamous epithelium. Normally differentiating squamous epithelium is seen to the *left*. There is sudden transition to dysplastic epithelium, in which maturation is delayed, and the cells retain large nuclei until they are close to the surface. Very little keratinization is seen.

may signal that a patient is at increased risk for certain tumors. Thus, squamous metaplasia of bronchial mucosa suggests that there has been significant exposure to known carcinogenic agents.

DYSPLASIA

Dysplasia is a disordered and disorganized cell growth that is not an adaptive change. The maturation of individual cells and their relationships to other cells are altered. Dysplastic cells have large nuclei, dark staining because of increased DNA content, and an increased nuclear cytoplasmic ratio. There are increased numbers of mitoses. In differentiating epithelia, such as squamous epithelium, undifferentiated cells persist to the epithelial surface, and keratinization is irregular and incomplete (Fig. 13.6).

Dysplasia is best observed in epithelial cells and is usually concurrent with chronic irritation. Removal of an irritant may result in a return to normal differentiation, but often the change persists and there is evolution of a totally abnormal growth pattern that is recognizable as neoplastic. Thus, dysplasia is at least potentially premalignant, a borderline lesion that may heal or progress to cancer.

Chapter 14

Neoplastic Disease

Neoplastic disease was responsible for nearly 387,000 deaths in the United States in 1977, second only to heart disease as a cause of death. Nearly 2 of every 5 deaths were attributed to heart disease, 1 in 5 to cancer (Table 14.1). National Cancer Institute estimates of cancer deaths for 1980, including their distribution in men and women, are shown in Table 14.2.

Most age-adjusted death rates for the most prevalent neoplasms have changed relatively little during the past 45 years; some have changed dramatically. The death rate for carcinoma of the lung in men has increased from less than 5 per 100,000 population to 55, and in women from 2 per 100,000 to 15. Death rates for carcinoma of the stomach have dropped profoundly in both men and women, and uterine cancer has decreased from 27 per 100,000 to 7.

There are striking geographic differences in the incidence of many tumors. Thus, the incidence of carcinoma of the lung in men in the United States is greater than that in Japan by a factor of 3, and for prostate 10, colon 6, and rectum 3. On the other hand, the incidence of carcinoma of the stomach among men in Japan is 6 times greater than in the United States and carcinoma of the esophagus is 3 times as frequent. Among women, the incidence of carcinoma of the breast is 6 times higher in the United States than in Japan, ovarian tumors are more frequent by a factor of 6, and uterine tumors by a factor of 12.

The changes noted in age-adjusted death rates as well as geographic differences in the incidence of many tumors (differences that diminish or disappear following migration from one area to another) are interpreted as reflecting the overriding importance of environmental factors in the pathogenesis of neoplasms. Genetic predisposition plays at most a minor role in most tumors, although a very few, including the familial forms of retinoblastoma, renal cell carcinoma and Wilms' tumor, and the skin tumors associated with xeroderma pigmentosum, are clearly genetically determined.

THE NATURE OF NEOPLASMS

A neoplasm is an abnormal proliferation of cells that are relatively free of control by factors that govern the growth of normal cells. The component cells manifest a variably deranged expression of their genetic material, or altered repression or derepression of genes. The change in individual cell behavior and the interactions among groups of cells are heritable from one generation of cells to the next. Neoplasms appear to represent growths of a single clone of cells, with all cells genetically alike.

Table 14.1
Leading Causes of Death, United States, 1977[a]

Cause of Death	No. of Deaths	Death Rate per 100,000 Population	Per Cent of Deaths
Heart disease	718,850	332.3	37.8
Neoplastic disease	386,686	178.7	20.4
Cerebrovascular disease	181,934	84.1	9.6
Accidents	103,202	47.7	5.4
Influenza and pneumonia	51,193	23.7	2.7
Diabetes	32,989	15.2	1.7
Cirrhosis	30,848	14.3	1.6
Atherosclerosis	28,754	13.3	1.5
Suicide	28,681	13.3	1.5
Diseases of infancy	23,401	10.8	1.2
Homicide	19,968	9.2	1.1
All causes	1,899,597	878.1	100.0

[a] Source: *Vital Statistics of the U.S., 1977.*

Table 14.2
Estimated Cancer Deaths for 1980[a]

Site		Total	Male Cancer Deaths %	Female Cancer Deaths %
Oral		8,800	3	1
Digestive organs		106,850		
Esophagus	(7,600)		2	1
Stomach	(14,000)		4	3
Colon	(44,000)		9	13
Rectum	(8,800)		2	2
Pancreas	(20,900)		5	5
Respiratory system		106,200		
Lung	(101,300)		34	14
Bone, connective tissue, skin		9,550	2	2
Breast		35,800	—	19
Genital organs		45,300		
Uterus	(10,600)		—	6
Ovary	(11,200)		—	6
Prostate	(21,500)		10	—
Bladder and kidney		18,200	5	3
Brain and CNS		9,800	2	2
Leukemia, lymphoma		36,400	9	9
All sites		405,000		

[a] Based on rates from N.C.I. SEER Program, 1973–1976.

Despite their deviation from normal biologic behavior, an important characteristic of all tumors is that they reproduce to greater or lesser degree both the structure and function of their cells of origin. Tumors are classified as *benign* and *malignant*. Benign tumors closely resemble in structure and function their cells of origin; *i.e.*, they are well differentiated, and usually carry a favorable prognosis. Malignant tumors tend to be poorly differentiated, usually have the capacity to

130   *Pathology: Understanding Human Disease*

spread both locally and to distant parts of the body, and tend to be life-threatening. The distinction between benign and malignant may not be so simple as these sentences imply; rather, there may be a continuum of neoplasms, from those that are clearly benign to those that are patently malignant. Malignant tumors of epithelial origin are designated *carcinomas*, those arising from connective tissue *sarcomas*. Benign tumors of glandular epithelium are *adenomas*, while *papillomas* are benign lesions of covering epithelium. Benign connective tissue tumors most often carry the name of their cell of origin, such as *fibroma, lipoma*, and *chondroma*, while their malignant counterparts are *fibrosarcoma, liposarcoma*, and *chondrosarcoma*. There are many inconsistencies in the nomenclature of tumors; some are given eponymic designations, and the names of others suggest etiology. These variations, however, are best learned when considering the tumors of the various organs and systems of the body.

In order to survive, a tumor must evoke a connective tissue stroma composed of normal cells. The stroma may vary greatly from one tumor to another in terms of vascularity, degree of fibroblastic production of collagen, and presence or absence of nerves and lymphatic channels. The ability to attract a stroma is also essential to successful colonization of an area some distance from the original site of tumor formation, or *metastasis*.

Many of the features described in this section are illustrated in Figures 14.1 to 14.11.

Factors Governing Cell Growth and Proliferation

In the normal processes of repair or regeneration, cell growth results from an increase in growth promoting factors, and a release from inhibitory influences.

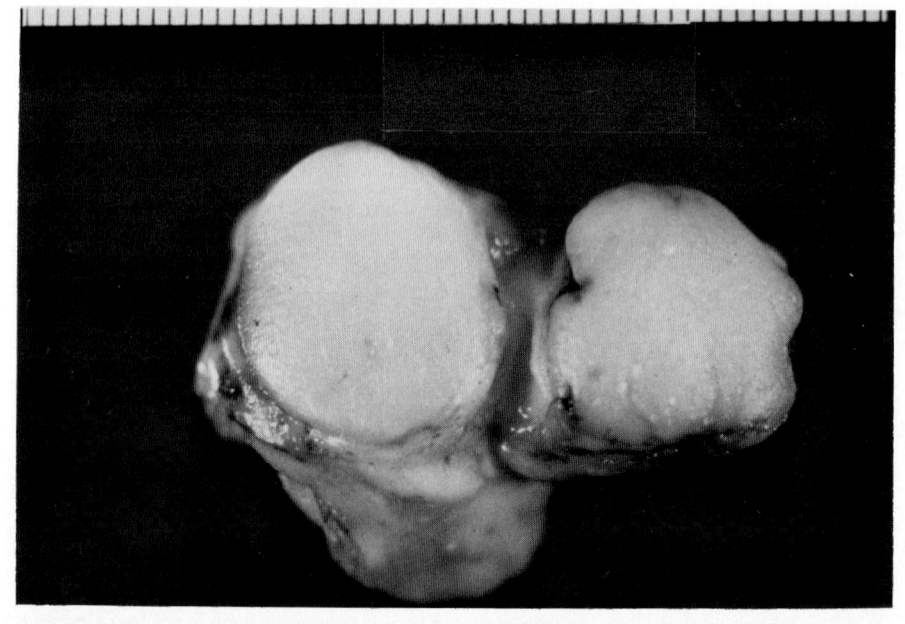

Figure 14.1. Fibroadenoma. This benign tumor of the breast is firm and homogeneous in consistency and is encapsulated and sharply demarcated from the surrounding breast tissue.

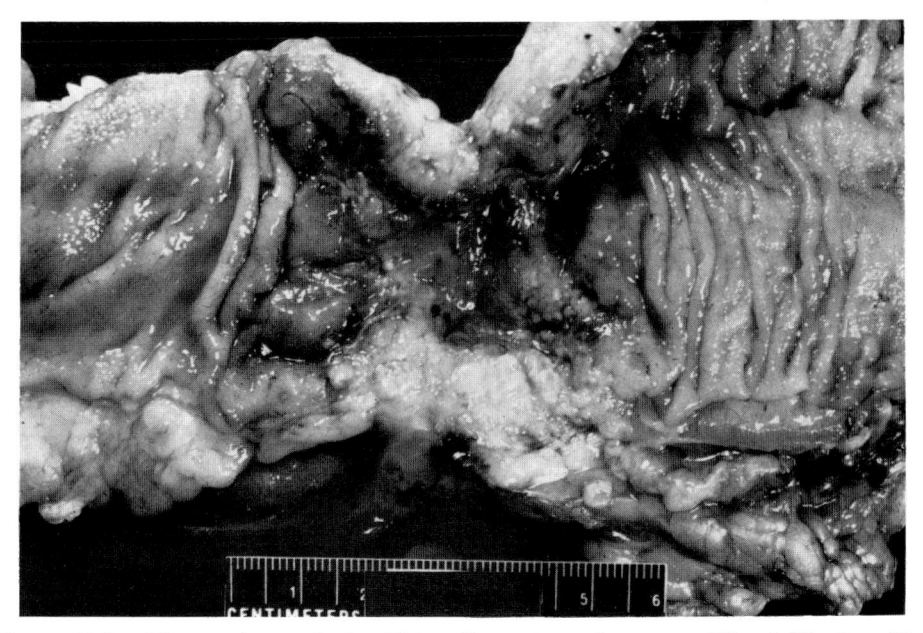

Figure 14.2. Adenocarcinoma of colon. This malignant tumor is seen as a diffuse infiltration of the wall of the intestine, with marked constriction of its lumen and ulceration of the mucosa.

Growth is stimulated by tissue hypoxia and by such hormones as somatomedin, estrogens, and androgens. There may be specific growth factors for fibroblasts and epidermal cells. *Contact inhibition* is a deterrent to growth most readily observed in tissue cultures of epithelial cells. Cell growth, migration, and mitosis are inhibited at points of contact with other cells. This may be related to modification of cell membrane receptors and to intercellular communication through cell junctions, particularly gap junctions. *Chalones* are tissue-specific intracellular growth inhibitors. With injury, these substances leak out of the cells, permitting them to grow. When injury is repaired, growth equilibrium returns through the restoration of cellular chalones. Thus, they act as effectors of an intracellular negative feedback mechanism. Malignant tumor cells in tissue culture show loss of both contact inhibition and chalones.

Neoplastic Transformation and Progression

Neoplastic transformation is a modification of a cell that permanently changes its biologic behavior, frees it at least partially from normal control mechanisms, and, in the case of malignant tumors, gives it the capacity to invade normal tissue and to *metastasize*. It is a phenomenon that occurs in immature cells, such as epithelial reserve cells, and in dysplastic cells. Transformation is usually thought of as a single cell event, creating a new and neoplastic clone, but occasionally it appears that the change occurs in many cells at the same time, or in an entire "field" of cells. Transformation may be a genetic event, or epigenetic, *i.e.*, an altered behavior and cell expression without any changes in DNA. *Progression* is a worsening, or augmentation of the changes of transformation reflected in an increasing capacity for malignant behavior.

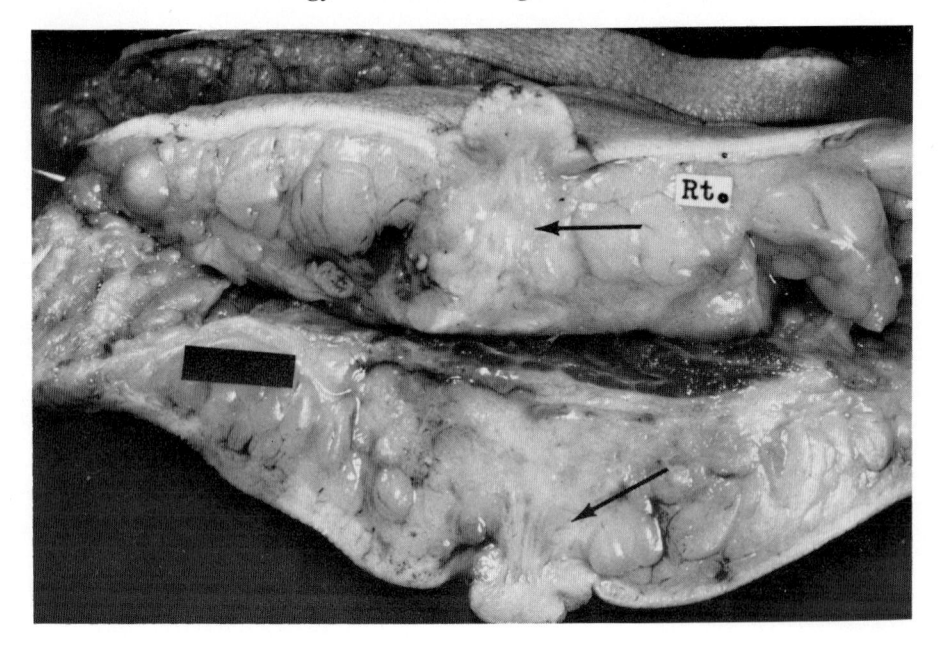

Figure 14.3. Adenocarcinoma of breast, bilateral. Firm, grayish white tumor tissue is seen infiltrating the breast beneath the nipples. The separation of tumor and normal breast tissue is poorly demarcated, and the two appear to blend.

Transformation is usually a multiple step phenomenon, involving *initiators* and *promotors*. Various carcinogens, chemical, viral, and physical, are initiators. They trigger the initial cellular event that irreversibly alters the biology of the cell. The effects of initiators are additive, and may be dormant for many years. Promotors, or *co-carcinogens*, include various growth-promoting hormones, mechanical irritants, and substances such as alcohol and coal tar phenols. The effects of promotors are not cumulative. A few chemical carcinogens are "complete" carcinogens, capable of inducing neoplasms without the help of co-carcinogens.

Characteristics of Neoplastic Cells

Although there are no features of neoplastic cells that are unique, *i.e.*, never observed in non-neoplastic cells, there are significant morphologic and functional changes that characterize and distinguish them.

The ability of tumors to spread and metastasize is relatable in part to altered cell membrane function. Tumor cells do not show contact inhibition. They form fewer junctional complexes than do normal cells, resulting in a looser architecture. They tend to have a strong negative surface charge, so that they repel each other. The spread of tumors may also be aided by the production of hyaluronidase, and by plasminogen activators promoting fibrinolysis.

It was noted in Chapter 11 that normal cells in tissue culture will stop multiplying and die after a certain number of population doublings. This does not apply to malignant tumor cells which appear able to grow indefinitely in culture.

Neoplastic Disease

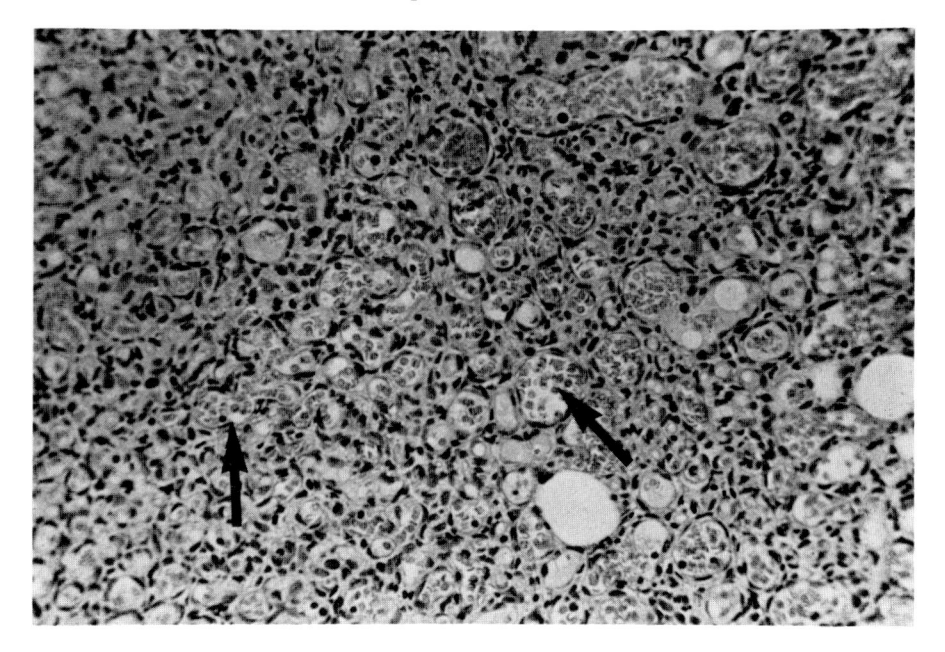

Figure 14.4. Capillary hemangioma. This benign tumor is characterized by the formation of myriads of small vascular channels, lined by endothelium, and filled with red blood cells.

There are changes in the antigenic structure of tumor cells. Many lose their HLA antigens. Tumor-specific and tumor-associated antigens are often identifiable, particularly in experimental tumors; they are generally very weak antigens.

Karyotypes of many, but not all, tumor cells are abnormal. The cells are often aneuploid, having perhaps 70 to 80 chromosomes, and the morphology of individual chromosomes may be altered. Thus far, however, only one specific chromosomal marker has been identified, the *Philadelphia chromosome* of the tumor cells in chronic myelogenous leukemia. This consists of a deletion of the long arm of chromosome 22 and its translocation to chromosome 9. Most of the chromosomal aberrations of tumor cells are thought to be late changes, the result rather than the cause of neoplastic transformation. The earliest change could be a single gene change, invisible by current techniques.

Tumor cells often show a simplification of some of the complex metabolic processes of their cells of origin. There are fewer sophisticated pathways, and loss of highly specialized enzymes. At the same time, tumor cells may assume functions not apparent in their precursor cells (see below).

The cells of malignant neoplasms show several morphologic features recognizable on light microscopy. These changes enhance the recognition of tumors in tissue sections and permit cytologic diagnosis of smears of exfoliated cells. Tumor cells are often larger than their normal counterparts. Their nuclei are larger, containing coarse and deeply staining chromatin material, and the ratio of nuclear to cytoplasmic measurements is increased. Nucleoli are large and may be multiple. Increased numbers of mitoses are often seen, as are abnormal or atypical mitotic patterns. Bizarre tumor giant cells may be prominent.

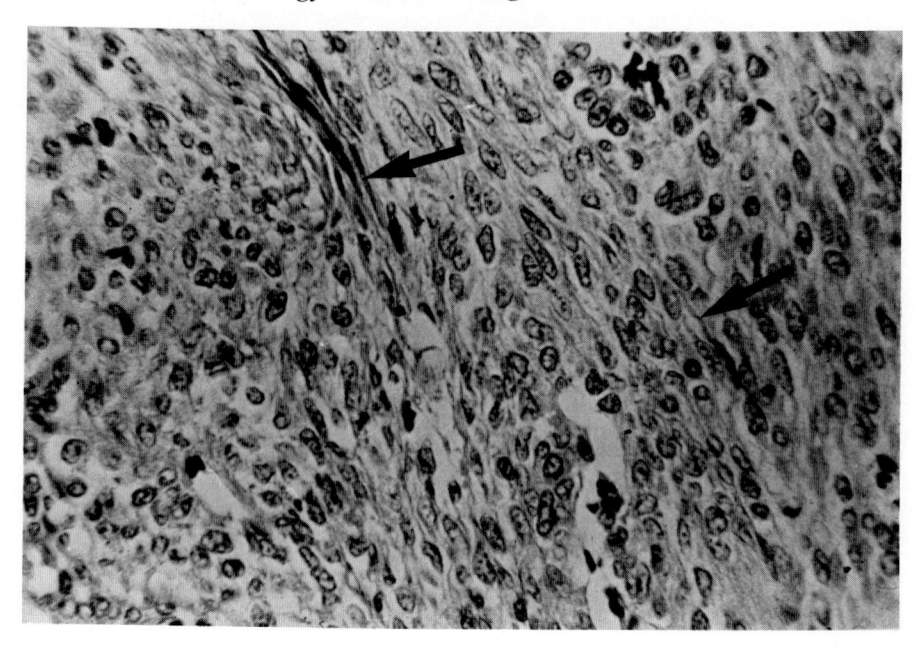

Figure 14.5. Tumor of fibroblasts. Although most of the cells comprising this tumor are not sufficiently differentiated to reveal their cell of origin, others are elongated, and are secreting collagen fibrils.

Differentiation and Anaplasia

Differentiation is the degree to which a tumor reproduces the structure and function of its cell of origin. The more closely its cells resemble their precursors, the better the differentiation. *Anaplasia* is the loss of structural and functional characteristics of the mature normal cells. It is thus inversely proportional to differentiation.

Normal differentiation involves the selective expression of some genetic information, and restriction or repression of the rest. Loss of differentiation by tumor cells results in loss of specialized function, but may also be manifested by the assumption of new functions, because of derepression of certain genes. Thus, many tumors arising from neural crest and neuroectodermal derivatives may express the capacity to produce and secrete any of the peptide hormones, including antidiuretic hormone, corticotrophin-releasing factor, adrenocorticotrophic hormone (ACTH), parathyroid hormone, calcitonin, gastrin, insulin, glucagon, and catecholamines.

Benign and Malignant Tumors

Benign tumors are characteristically well differentiated, their cells and architectural pattern resembling closely their cells of origin. Thus, the cells of a fibroma will look like fibroblasts and will secrete collagen, and those of an osteoma will look like osteoblasts and produce osteoid. A thyroid adenoma will be composed of cells arranged in follicles, usually containing colloid. Benign tumors tend to remain localized, have a round or ovoid shape, and are often

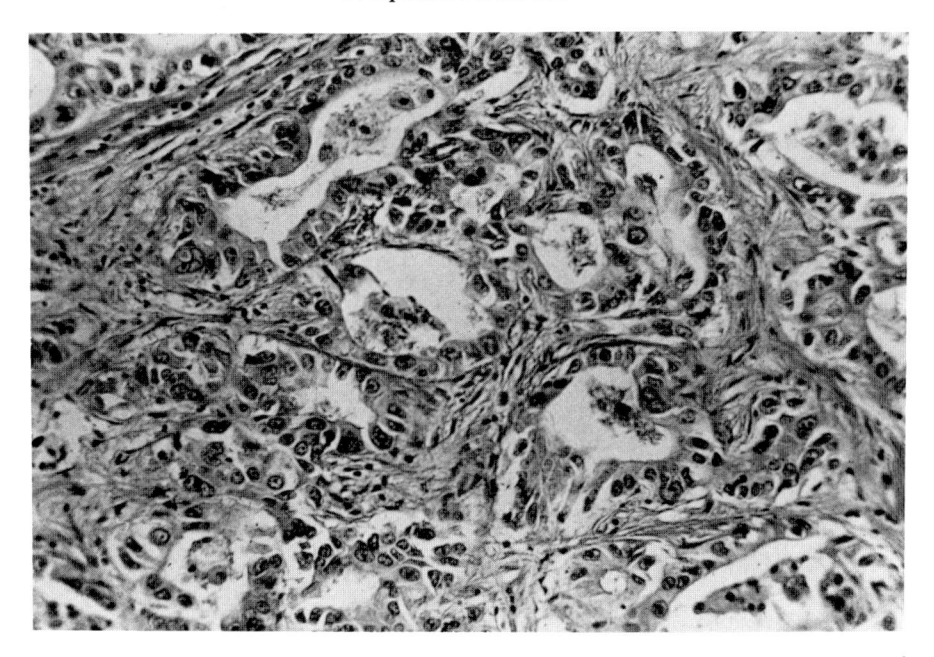

Figure 14.6. Adenocarcinoma. This tumor clearly demonstrates a ductal pattern in its growth.

encapsulated by connective tissue. They usually grow slowly and their effects are determined primarily by location and size, although in the case of endocrine adenomas there may be systemic effects of poorly controlled hormone secretion. Most benign tumors are surgically resectable, and most do not pose a threat to life.

Malignant tumors have the capacity to invade surrounding tissues and to metastasize to distant sites. They do not usually appear circumscribed or encapsulated, but have irregular borders which infiltrate and blend with surrounding tissue. They tend to be poorly differentiated, and it may be difficult to recognize their structural and functional resemblance to the normal cells of origin. A fibrosarcoma may produce little collagen, and a squamous cell carcinoma of epidermal origin may show little keratinization. An anaplastic carcinoma of the thyroid may show no follicle formation and may not secrete thyroid hormone. Malignant tumors tend to grow rapidly. They show little cohesiveness and few junctional complexes. Their increased motility permits invasion of vascular and lymphatic channels. Because of metastases, they are often incurable by surgical excision, and their progressive growth is associated with a generalized systemic cachexia.

Metastasis requires loose cells capable of gaining access to vascular and lymphatic channels, their transport to distant areas, their deposition in the microcirculation of lymph nodes, lungs, liver, or other organs, and their ability to induce a stromal response and grow at the new site. Carcinomas have a tendency, at least at first, to metastasize through lymphatic channels, sarcomas through the vascular system. Certain tumors have a predilection for metastasis to specific sites, such as bone and brain. Tumors may also metastasize by direct seeding of

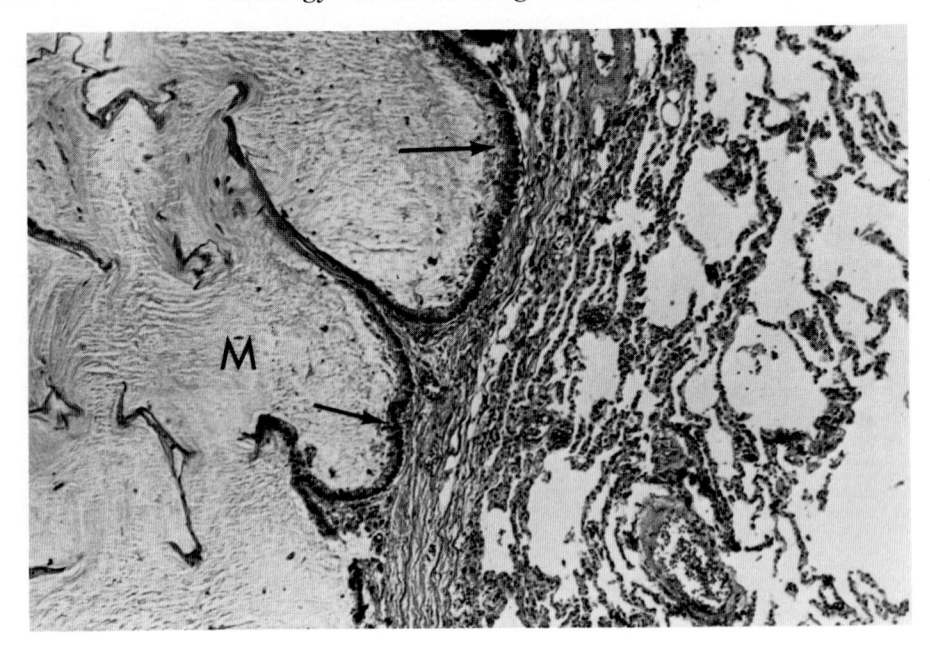

Figure 14.7. Mucin-producing adenocarcinoma, metastatic to the lung. This metastasis consists predominately of lakes of mucin (*M*). The epithelial cells of the tumor are seen at the periphery (*arrows*).

the serous cavities. Thus, carcinoma of the ovary may spread throughout the peritoneal cavity.

It must again be emphasized that the distinction between benign and malignant lesions is often hazy and many tumors are best classified as "borderline," indicating an as yet unexpressed capacity for malignant biologic behavior.

Grading and Staging

Grading of a malignant tumor is an attempt to assess its aggressiveness, or degree of malignancy. It is based on morphologic evaluation of differentiation or anaplasia. Tumors are usually graded from I to IV, the latter expressing the greatest degree of anaplasia. The grade of a tumor usually suggests its biologic behavior and may predict its responsiveness to certain therapeutic agents.

Staging is based on the extensiveness of a tumor at its primary site, and the presence or absence of metastases to lymph nodes and organs at distant sites. Staging is often critical to the selection of a therapeutic program among surgical resection, radiation, and chemotherapy.

ETIOLOGIC CONSIDERATIONS

There are three broad concepts of the etiology of neoplasms. The first, and probably the most accepted, is that neoplastic transformation is a mutation, that it results from a structural alteration of the DNA molecule. This approach is based on the fact that the great majority of oncogens, including chemicals and

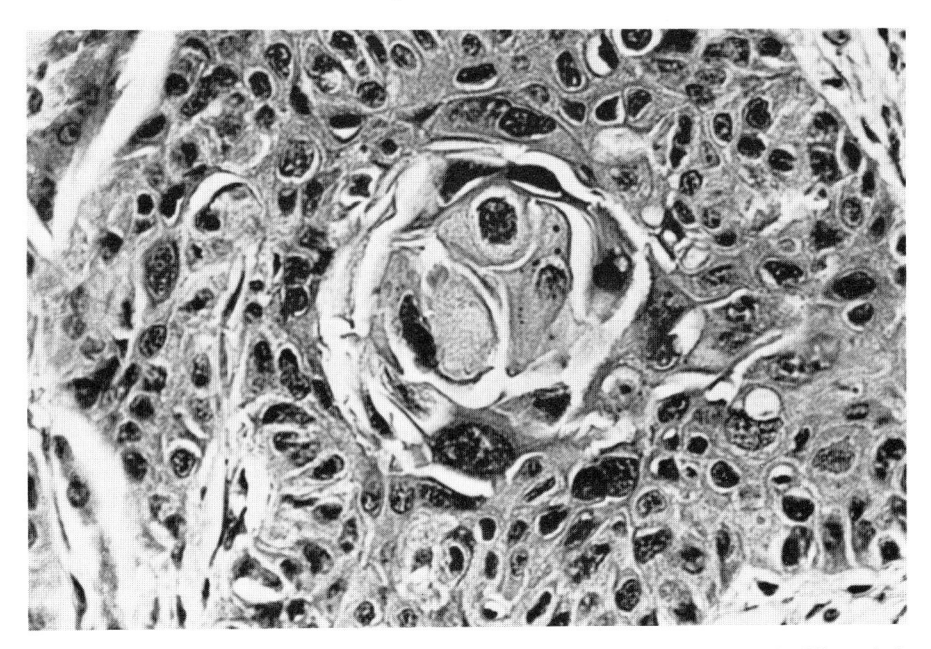

Figure 14.8. Squamous cell carcinoma. Most of the tumor cells seen here show little differentiation, but those in the center show distinct squamous differentiation and keratinization. It is this area of differentiation that permits recognition of the tumor as of squamous cell origin.

physical forces, are also mutagens, and that most neoplasms behave as clonal disorders, heritable at the cellular level. In *xeroderma pigmentosum*, there is a specific inherited defect in mechanisms of DNA repair, and those with this disorder are subject to multiple malignant skin tumors induced by exposure to ultraviolet light.

The second broad concept is that neoplastic transformation is a disturbance of cell differentiation, perhaps occurring in many cells simultaneously, and that the neoplastic cell has many disparate expressions that cannot be explained by a single gene mutation. It is pointed out that no single feature of neoplastic cells is unique, but can be identified as well in normal cells. Thus, no new genetic information is required beyond that present in all cells. Since there are no genetic differences among cell types, differentiation (either normal or abnormal) is an *epigenetic* phenomenon, a nongenetic change in the expression, repression, or derepression of various genes.

The third concept is that the genetic information of viruses becomes integrated into the host cell genome. In some respects, this would be comparable to a mutation, but there is evidence that viral genetic material may be present and awaiting activation in normal cells (an endogenous RNA virus), suggesting that viral oncogenesis is more akin to disturbed cell differentiation.

It should be emphasized that these three concepts are not mutually exclusive. They may each constitute a valid contribution to our understanding of neoplasms.

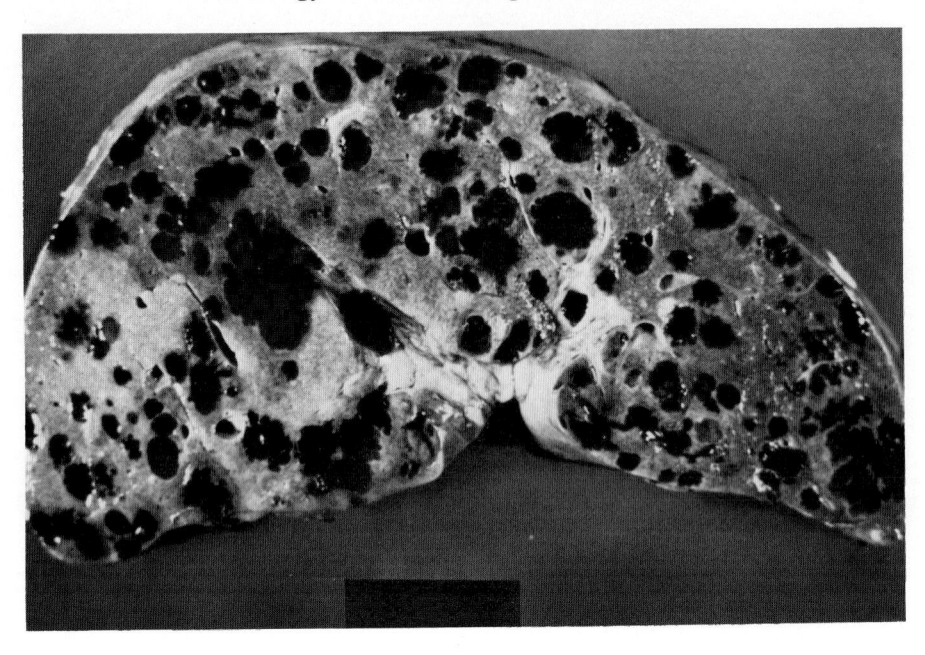

Figure 14.9. Melanoma, metastatic to liver. Multiple tumor nodules are seen. The cells comprising the tumor have not lost their ability to produce melanin, and this pigment has imparted a dark black color to the metastatic nodules.

Chemical Carcinogenesis

Many chemical carcinogens may first be activated in the body to a "proximal" form. They are electrophilic, *i.e.*, electron seekers, with a propensity to bind covalently with nucleic acids. Chemical carcinogens are initiators of neoplastic transformation, and their effects are additive and cumulative.

All chemical carcinogens are cytotoxic to target tissues if administered in sufficient dosage. Most, but not all, are mutagens, and virtually all can suppress immunologic reactions. Some can induce tumors at the site of application, others at a location distant from the exposure. Thus, 2-naphthylamine, inhaled or absorbed through the skin, causes tumors of the urinary bladder.

Chemical carcinogens were discussed in Chapter 12. Aromatic hydrocarbons are common air pollutants, and are important components of tobacco smoke. They are particularly potent carcinogens if there is also exposure to asbestos. Thus, cigarette smokers exposed to asbestos have a 90-fold increase in the incidence of carcinoma of the lung. Aromatic amines are most associated with bladder tumors. Workers in dye and rubber industries are at risk, but these carcinogens are also present in tobacco smoke. Carcinogenic nitrosamines can be formed in the stomach by interaction with nitrites used in the preservation of many meat products. Aflatoxins, produced by the fungus *Aspergillus flavus*, appear responsible for the very high incidence of liver cell carcinoma in Hawaii, Singapore, and some parts of Africa.

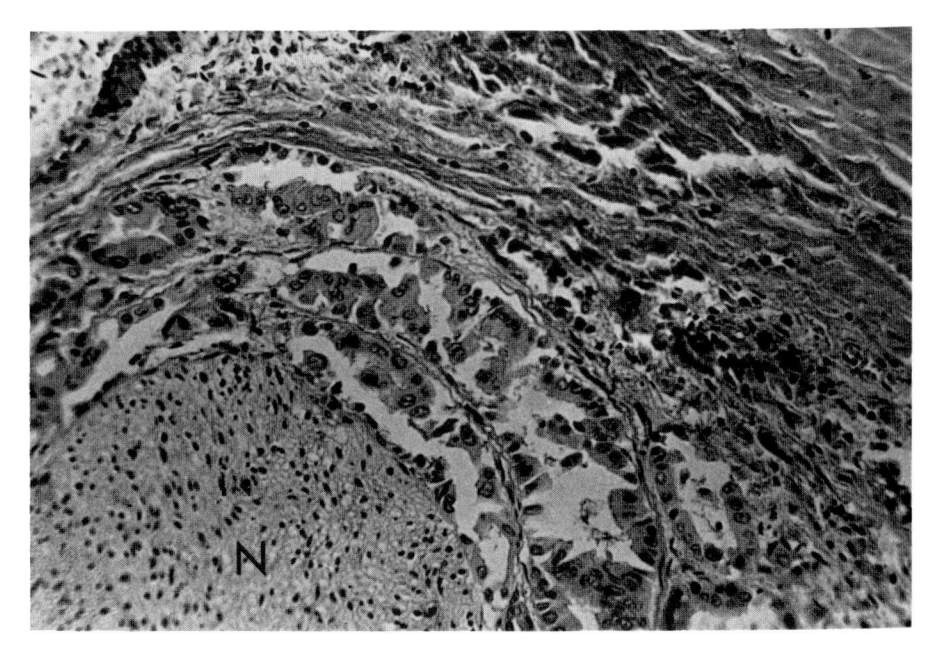

Figure 14.10. Perineural invasion. A nerve trunk is seen at the *lower left*. Tumor cells, arranged in a glandular pattern (adenocarcinoma), have filled the perineural spaces. This is an important pathway of metastasis in carcinomas of the pancreas and prostate.

Viral Oncogenesis

The study of experimental animal tumors leaves no doubt that neoplastic transformation can be induced by DNA and RNA viruses. Virus-specific genetic information is permanently integrated into the DNA of transformed cells. DNA viruses do not replicate in the cells they transform, or the end result would be cell lysis. Instead, they alter the genome. With RNA viruses transformation and replication can be concurrent. DNA derived from the reverse transcription of RNA becomes a part of the host cell DNA. As indicated earlier, viral genetic material, in the form of endogenous RNA, may already be present in the cell prior to neoplastic transformation.

Proof of the viral etiology of human neoplasms is extremely difficult to establish. Nevertheless, there is growing evidence that certain DNA viruses, specifically herpes viruses, are intimately related to some human tumors. The Epstein-Barr (E-B) virus appears to be the cause of Burkitt's lymphoma in the malaria belt of Africa and of nasopharyngeal carcinoma among Cantonese Chinese. The E-B virus is present in these tumors, and has been shown capable of transforming normal human cells *in vitro*. Although rare examples of Burkitt's lymphoma occur in the continental United States, the virus is best known here as the cause of infectious mononucleosis in adolescents and young adults. Herpes simplex virus, Type 2, has been strongly implicated in the etiology of carcinoma of the uterine cervix and of squamous cell carcinoma of the head and neck. Viral

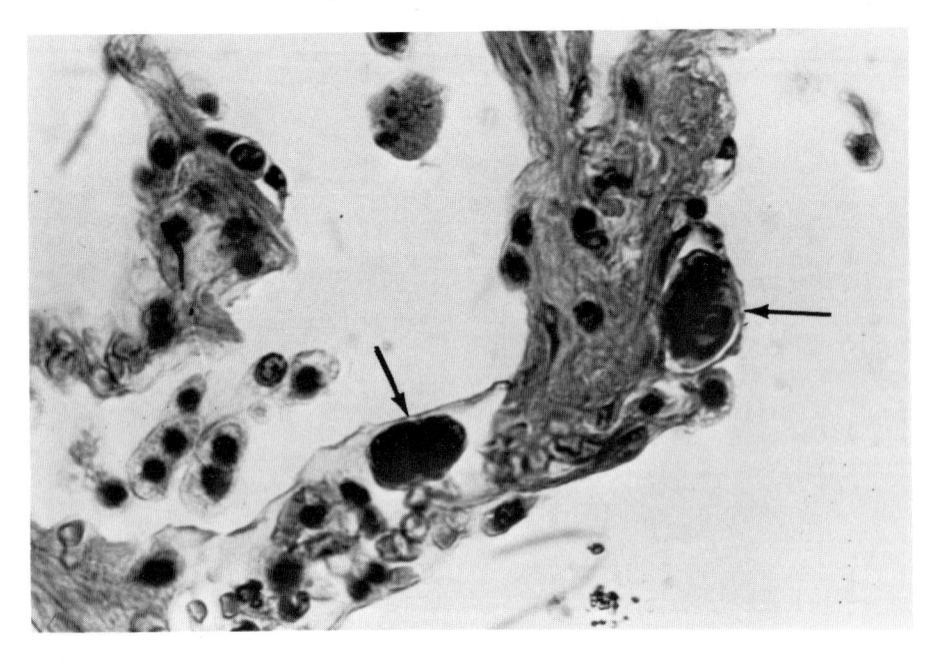

Figure 14.11. Dissemination through the bloodstream. Two large tumor cells are seen in pulmonary alveolar capillaries.

tumor-associated antigens are demonstrable in some 90% of patients with these tumors and in less than 5% of cancer-free individuals. Most recently, it appears that carcinoma of the liver (hepatocellular carcinoma) is closely related to chronic active hepatitis due to the hepatitis B virus, and that, at least in this country, it does not occur in the absence of the hepatitis B surface antigen carrier state.

Physical Carcinogens

The oncogenicity of ionizing radiation was considered in Chapter 12. Ultraviolet radiation is associated with the induction of skin tumors. It is both toxic and mutagenic, and acts by dimerization of DNA bases, particularly thymine.

TUMOR IMMUNOLOGY AND IMMUNE SURVEILLANCE

One of the characteristics of neoplastic transformation is a change in the antigenic structure of the cell membrane to one that is no longer recognizable as self. Many malignant tumor cells may activate the host's immune mechanisms, but the new antigens are generally very weak and the immunologic reaction is probably an ineffective means of destroying the altered cells. Whatever effectiveness does exist resides much more in cell-mediated immunity than in humoral mechanisms. It is likely that the immune response is ineffective because cytotoxic lymphocytes are "blocked" from reaching their target cells. This blocking effect is attributed to the tumor cell antigens themselves, possibly by their release as free antigens which react with sensitized T lymphocytes.

Some tumors manifest a re-expression of proteins normally produced predom-

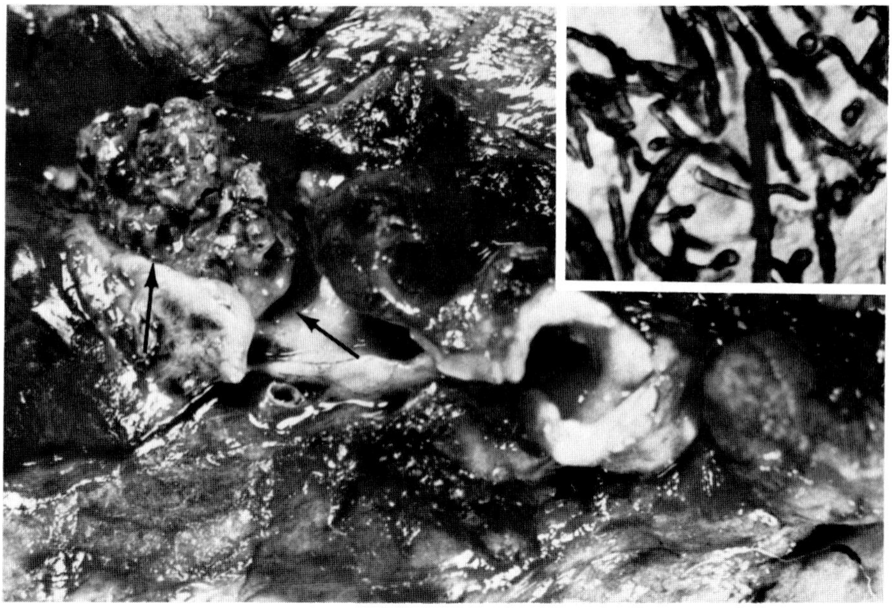

Neoplastic Disease 141

Figure 14.12. Aspergillus infection in a patient being treated for neoplastic disease. The *arrows* point to a pulmonary "fungus ball," composed of massive numbers of fungus organisms. The *inset* shows branching, septate hyphae characteristic of this organism.

inantly in fetal tissue. These antigens, called oncofetal antigens, are difficult to demonstrate in normal cells, including the normal counterparts of certain malignant tumor cells. Carcinoembryonic antigen (CEA) is a glycoprotein on the cell membranes of embryonal gut cells. High serum levels of CEA are observed in many patients with carcinoma of the colon, stomach, pancreas, or lung, as well as in many with malignant bone tumors and immature neuroblastic lesions. High serum levels of α-fetoprotein, a product of fetal liver cells, have proven useful in the diagnosis of hepatocellular carcinoma and some testicular and ovarian germ cell tumors, but may also occur in patients with hepatitis.

Virtually all experimental tumors in inbred animals have tumor-specific antigens demonstrable by transplantation to syngeneic hosts, and it is assumed that similar specific antigens are present in man. The immune response of animals to these antigens varies greatly; the longer the time interval between administration of a carcinogen and the appearance of a tumor, the weaker the immune response. Both latent period and the induction of an immune response are thought to be related to the concentration of carcinogenic agent.

The concept that immune mechanisms, designated immune surveillance, offer a defense against the development of neoplasms is currently being questioned. Although immunosuppressed transplant recipients and patients with such immunodeficiency disorders as the Wiskott-Aldrich syndrome have a greatly increased incidence of neoplastic disease, almost all of the tumors involve the lymphoreticular system; *i.e.*, they are tumors of the immune system itself. There is little if any increase in tumors of other systems or organs. Immune surveillance as a protective mechanism may be nonexistent, or of very limited importance, and there is some evidence that an early immune response may actually stimulate and enhance tumor growth.

CAUSES OF DEATH IN PATIENTS WITH NEOPLASTIC DISEASE

There is no single major cause of death in patients with neoplastic disease. *Cancer cachexia*, referred to earlier, is manifested by anorexia, early satiety, weight loss, anemia, and marked weakness, and can progress to severe emaciation and death. It can occur with any type of neoplasm. It is a metabolic disturbance, perhaps related to release of peptides produced by tumors, and not a simple starvation. It responds only to complete removal of all tumor tissue.

Death may be directly related to physical effects of the primary tumor mass or its metastases, such as destruction of respiratory and circulatory control centers in the pontine medulla, or obstruction of vital channels: the trachea, intestines, or ureters.

Hemorrhage is a less common cause of death than a few years ago. Bleeding, however, may result from the consumption of coagulation factors in a tumor-induced disseminated intravascular coagulation, from destruction or replacement of the bone marrow, and from direct invasion and disruption of blood vessels.

Death is not infrequently attributable to direct toxic effects of radiation and chemotherapeutic agents. Examples include *radiation enterocolitis*, a result of obliterative vascular lesions of the intestines, and adynamic obstruction or perforation, bone marrow depression by nitrogen mustards, and severe pneumonitis due to bleomycin or Myleran.

Infections are an important and increasing cause of death. Most cancer patients are immunologically compromised. This may in part be due to neoplasms such as Hodgkin's disease which manifest T cell deficiencies, but more often results from the immunosuppressive effects of cytotoxic drugs, the use of adrenal cortical steroids, and the effects of radiation on the immune system. In addition to immunosuppression, the normal bacterial flora of cancer patients is often dramatically altered by the administration of one or more broad spectrum antibiotics, with the result that severe and fatal infections may be due to organisms normally of very low pathogenicity. Bacterial infections due to *Escherichia coli*, *Pseudomonas aeruginosa*, and *Klebsiella pneumoniae* are common. Systemic candidiasis, cryptococcosis, and aspergillosis (Fig. 14.12) are diseases frequently encountered in cancer patients, as are such unusual infections as pneumocystis pneumonia, systemic dissemination of cytomegalovirus, and even fatal infections by the roundworm *Strongyloides stercoralis*.

Suggested Reading

Baserga R. The cell cycle. N. Engl. J. Med. *304:* 453, 1981.
Becker, FF. Recent concepts of initiation and promotion in carcinogenesis. Am. J. Pathol. *105:* 3, 1981.
Bishop JM. The molecular biology of RNA tumor viruses: a physician's guide. N. Engl. J. Med. *303:* 675, 1980.
Cancer statistics, 1980. CA *30:* 23, 1980.
Harris CC, et al. Individual differences in cancer susceptibility. Ann. Intern. Med. *92:* 809, 1980.
Prehn RT, Prehn LM. Pathobiology of neoplasia (a teaching monograph). Am. J. Pathol. *80:* 527, 1975.

Chapter 15

The Heart

This chapter includes discussions of the pathology and pathophysiology of congestive heart failure, ischemic heart disease, disorders of the valves, the various forms of cardiomyopathy, and the more important congenital cardiac anomalies. The effects of hypertension on the heart are discussed in Chapter 18.

CONGESTIVE HEART FAILURE

The heart is a pump. Heart failure exists when the heart is unable to pump sufficient blood to meet the metabolic needs of body tissues. It can be due to alterations of the pump, to changes in the body's metabolic requirements, or to alterations in the volume or composition of the blood. Heart failure can be acute or chronic. Attention here is paid primarily to chronic failure, or congestive heart failure.

Structural changes may impair the ability of the heart to contract or dilate. Thus, in constrictive pericarditis due to tuberculosis or healed rheumatic pericarditis, the heart is prevented from dilating by an inelastic fibrous envelope, and diastolic filling of the ventricles may be insufficient to maintain cardiac output. Diseases of the myocardium, such as hypertrophic cardiomyopathy, amyloid infiltration, or diffuse scarring due to coronary artery atherosclerosis (ischemic cardiomyopathy), result in both poor ventricular contraction and diastolic filling. The nutritional requirements of the myocardial musculature may not be met because of obstructive coronary artery disease, severe anemia, or such metabolic disturbances as thyrotoxicosis and beri-beri. In disturbances of rhythm, particularly tachycardias, there may be inadequate diastolic filling to maintain a normal cardiac output. The most frequent cause of failure is an increased cardiac workload. In systemic hypertension, the heart must pump against a markedly increased peripheral vascular resistance. In the presence of arteriovenous fistulae, or a patent ductus arteriosus, peripheral resistance is decreased, but the cardiac output must increase tremendously in order to maintain adequate tissue perfusion. A high output must also be maintained in severe anemia. Abnormal cardiac valve function, either stenosis or insufficiency, greatly increases the work required of the myocardium. In all situations in which cardiac work load is increased, the heart at first adjusts to the increased demand by undergoing hypertrophy; the weight of the heart may double or even treble, and the ventricular muscle mass is greatly thickened. When hypertrophy can no longer compensate for the increased load, the chambers tend to dilate and muscular contraction, or stroke volume, becomes inadequate.

Recent successes in the treatment of intractable congestive heart failure by vasodilator therapy have emphasized the importance of aortic impedence in depressing left ventricular stroke volume and output. Systemic vascular resistance is often elevated in heart failure, most likely because of activation of the sympathetic nervous system or the renin-angiotensin system. Dramatic improvement in left ventricular function may follow blockade of the formation of angiotensin II.

Manifestations of Congestive Heart Failure

The manifestations of congestive heart failure are primarily extracardiac and relate to inadequate oxygenation of body tissues and the hemodynamic effects of altered fluid balance. Fatigue, weakness, and loss of muscle mass are often the first symptoms of failure, and reflect tissue hypoxia. With time, there is altered function of virtually all organs. The hemodynamic changes include an increase in blood volume, an increased blood content of the venous system and visceral organs, and the collection of fluid in the subcutaneous tissues and serous cavities.

The cardiac output in failure tends to be fixed. It does not increase during exercise; indeed it may fall. The reduction in perfusion tends to be evenly distributed among body organs, with the exception that renal blood flow is disproportionately reduced. The marked reduction in glomerular filtration rate leads to altered handling of sodium, and therefore water; renal excretion of sodium may total less than 1 mEq in 24 hr. There is increased aldosterone secretion in congestive heart failure, but it is probably of less import than the altered renal handling of sodium. Inadequate perfusion of the kidneys also results in urea retention, since decreased flow through the proximal tubules permits resorption of an increased proportion of filtered urea. This is an example of prerenal azotemia.

Retention of sodium and water increases the blood volume and extracellular fluid volume. Edema fluid collects in the dependent portions of the body and where tissue pressure is lowest, and large volumes may accumulate in the pleural, pericardial, and peritoneal cavities. Since vascular permeability is normal, the specific gravity and protein content of edema fluid are low. During daytime hours, edema tends to be most marked in the pretibial and ankle areas. At night, the edema tends to shift to the sacral region, although the improved cardiac function at rest may allow diuresis of excess fluid. Fluid also shifts to the lungs, and is responsible for symptoms of orthopnea and paroxysmal nocturnal dyspnea. With progression of congestive heart failure, pulmonary edema becomes diurnal as well as nocturnal.

Table 15.1 shows typical data for a patient in congestive heart failure due to rheumatic mitral stenosis. As cardiac output falls, oxygen extraction increases in the tissues, and the arteriovenous oxygen difference rises. The pressure values obtained by cardiac catheterization reflect severe pulmonary hypertension and right ventricular hypertrophy, as well as biventricular failure. The rise in blood urea nitrogen is not accompanied by a proportional rise in creatinine. This is because creatinine is not resorbed in the proximal tubules. A disproportionate rise in urea nitrogen often suggests a perfusion defect, rather than intrinsic renal disease. The findings of respiratory alkalosis reflect hyperventilation, a common occurrence in patients with pulmonary edema.

Table 15.1
Findings in Congestive Heart Failure (CHF) due to Mitral Stenosis

	CHF	Normal
Blood volume (liters)	7.0	4.6
Cardiac output (liters/min)	3.0	5–8
Cardiac index (liters/min/m^2)	1.8	3–4
Arteriovenous oxygen difference (vol %)	8.3	<5.0
Left ventricular ejection fraction (%)	43	>50
Mitral valve area (cm^2)	0.45	>3.5
Pressures (mm Hg)		
Right atrium (mean)	12	1–5
Right ventricle	100/15	25/4
Pulmonary artery	100/50	25/9
Pulmonary capillary wedge (mean)	45	9
Left ventricle	100/20	130/9
Renal blood flow (ml/min)	300	1200
Glomerular filtration rate (ml/min)	56	120
Sodium excretion (mEq/24 hr)	<1	>100
Potassium excretion (mEq/24 hr)	30	70
Blood urea nitrogen (mg/dl)	80	7–18
Creatinine (mg/dl)	2.8	0.9–1.5
Blood pH	7.48	7.33–7.43
Arterial pCO$_2$ (mm Hg)	30	35–45

The Lungs

Early in congestive heart failure, the lungs may show little more than congestion of pulmonary vessels and interstitial or alveolar edema. With time, however, there is evidence of progressive injury. The alveolar septa become thickened and fibrotic, particularly in the dependent portions of the lung. The accumulation of large numbers of hemosiderin-laden macrophages in the alveolar spaces is indicative of repeated episodes of alveolar hemorrhage (Fig. 15.1). Prolonged pulmonary hypertension is reflected in arteriolar thickening and in atherosclerotic lesions of the pulmonary arteries.

The Splanchnic Circulation

Increased oxygen extraction, particularly in the intestine, results in low oxygen content of portal vein blood. The cells in the central regions of the hepatic lobules show ischemic changes, triglyceride accumulation, atrophy, and occasional necrosis (see Fig. 6.2). Central lobular congestion and loss of liver cells give the liver a *nutmeg* appearance (Fig. 15.2). If hemorrhage and necrosis have occurred repeatedly, there may be considerable fibrosis, starting in the central areas and distorting the hepatic architecture. Despite often dramatic morphologic findings, the functional changes in chronic passive congestion are usually rather mild, and do not lead to hepatic failure.

The spleen in congestive heart failure is often enlarged, weighing 2 or 3 times the normal weight. The sinusoidal architecture is often accentuated by the deposition of fibrous tissue (Fig. 15.3). As is true in all instances of splenic enlargement, there may be evidence of hypersplenism, with increased destruction of red cells, white cells, and platelets.

A serious and often fatal complication of congestive heart failure is the

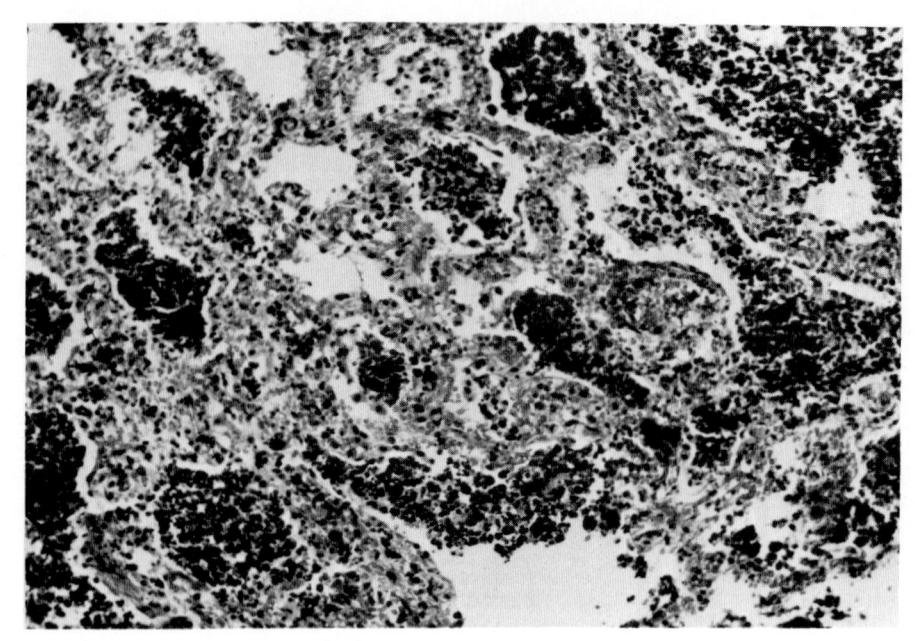

Figure 15.1. Chronic passive congestion of lung. The alveolar septa are markedly thickened and contain an increase in fibrous tissue. The alveolar spaces contain many pigment-laden macrophages ("heart failure cells").

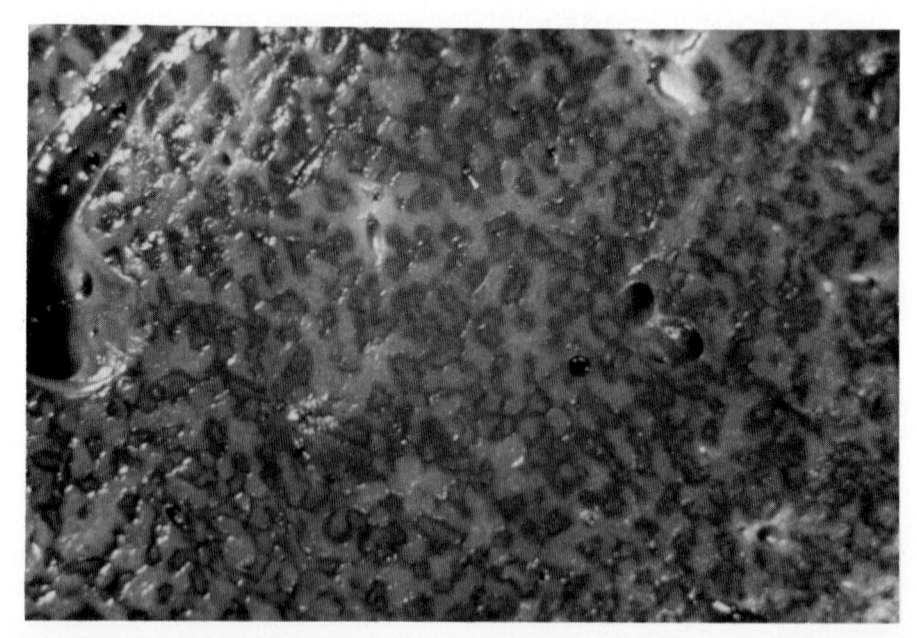

Figure 15.2. Gross appearance of chronic passive congestion of liver. The central lobular areas are markedly congested, giving the cut surface a nutmeg appearance.

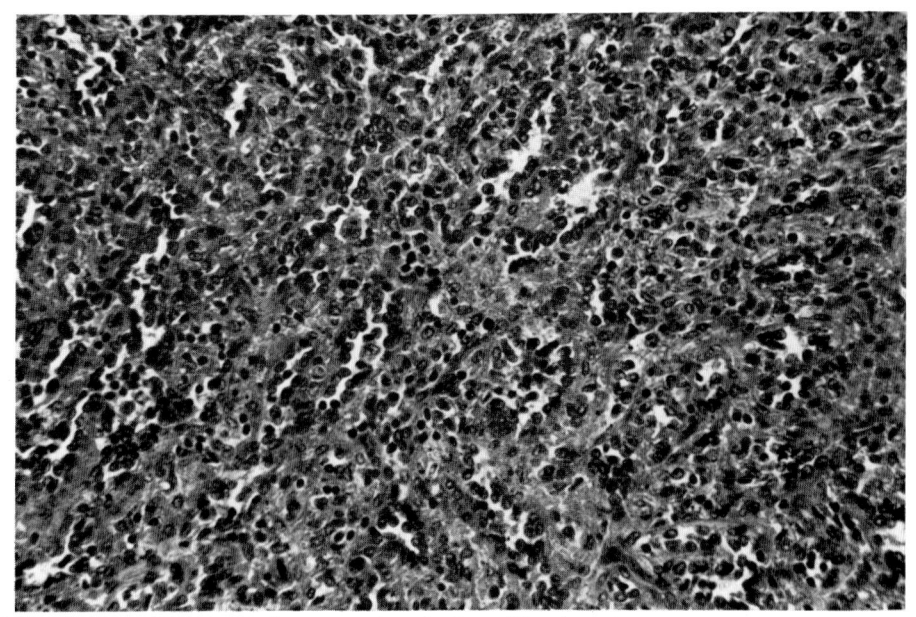

Figure 15.3. Chronic passive congestion of spleen. The sinusoidal architecture of the red pulp is accentuated by the addition of considerable fibrous tissue.

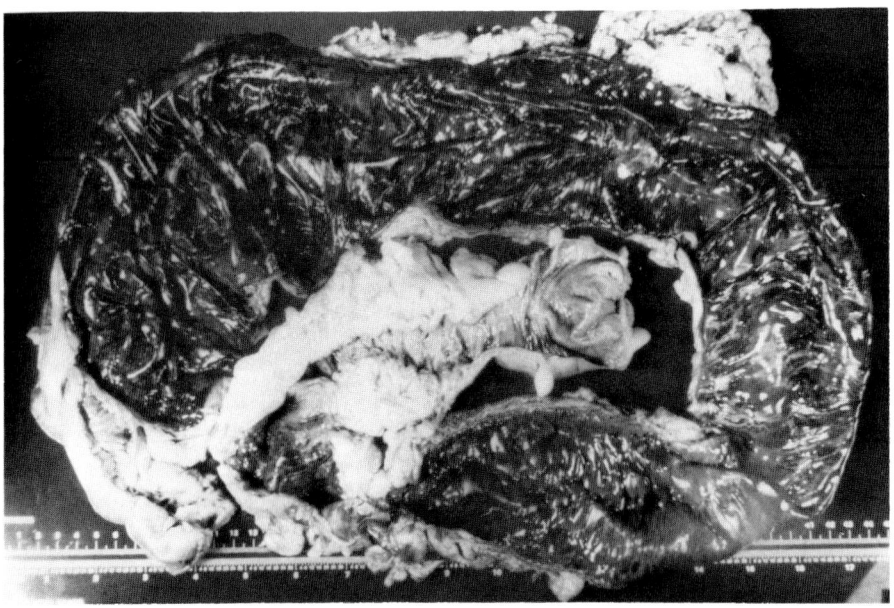

Figure 15.4. Ischemic colitis. The mucosa of the entire colon is devitalized and deeply congested or hemorrhagic.

development of a *hemorrhagic enteropathy*, in which ischemia is responsible for devitalization and hemorrhage of the intestinal mucosa (Fig. 15.4). Patients may suffer a paralytic ileus or severe hemorrhagic diarrhea, and enteric microorganisms may gain access to the portal system.

Central Nervous System

Patients in congestive heart failure have an increased incidence of infarction of the brain (*encephalomalacia*) and cerebral hemorrhage. Aside from neurologic deficits associated with these lesions, patients often manifest irritability, restlessness, and loss of concentrating ability.

Thromboembolic Disease

A distended venous system and a prolonged circulation time predispose patients with congestive heart failure to vascular thrombosis and embolism. Prolonged periods of bedrest, with pooling of blood in the lower extremities and pelvic veins, further increase the hazard. Pulmonary embolism and infarction are not infrequent causes of death.

Right and Left Ventricle Failure

Although both ventricles are insufficient in most instances of congestive heart failure, there are times when failure of one or the other is predominant. The right ventricle becomes hypertropied and may fail as a result of such destructive pulmonary lesions as emphysema and fibrosing lung disease, in obstructive deformities of the chest, in the aftermath of repeated pulmonary emboli, and in primary pulmonary hypertension. Right heart enlargement in these situations is a consequence of increased resistance to pulmonary blood flow, and is referred to as *cor pulmonale*. Left ventricular failure, by elevating pulmonary vascular pressure, is the most frequent cause of right ventricular failure.

Acute left ventricular failure, as may occur in patients with myocardial infarction, is often associated with *cardiogenic shock* rather than congestive failure. There is rapid outpouring of edema fluid into the lungs, with resulting hemoconcentration and reduction of blood volume.

ISCHEMIC HEART DISEASE

Ischemic heart disease refers to altered myocardial function due to inadequate coronary blood flow. For practical purposes, the term is virtually synonymous with the effects of atherosclerosis of the coronary arteries, although markedly insufficient coronary blood flow is occasionally encountered on the basis of emboli, hypotension and shock, extension of an acute aortic dissection to involve the proximal coronary vessels, narrowing of the coronary ostia due to syphilitic aortitis, some inflammatory vascular lesions involving the coronary arteries, and spasm. Atherosclerosis is discussed in Chapter 16. Suffice it here to say its most important expression in terms of human morbidity and mortality is coronary artery disease.

The most important consequence of coronary artery disease is myocardial infarction. *Angina pectoris*, precordial or substernal pain due to focal myocardial ischemia, is generally thought of as a reflection of reversible myocardial injury unassociated with morphologic change, although there is much evidence to suggest that small areas of myocardial necrosis occur. If coronary artery disease results in diffuse and generalized myocardial ischemia and fibrosis, congestive heart failure may be the clinical presentation. This pattern of injury, more frequent in elderly patients, is referred to as *ischemic cardiomyopathy*. Coronary artery disease may also be a cause of sudden death, presumably the result of a fatal cardiac arrhythmia triggered by ischemia.

Myocardial Infarction

Ischemic heart disease is the leading cause of death in the United States. The age-adjusted death rate was over 330 per 100,000 men in 1968, but there has been a slow but steady decline to about 264 in 1977. Myocardial infarction accounts for the vast majority of ischemic heart disease deaths, killing some 600,000 per year. The death rate in Japan is less than one-fourth that in this country, and even lower death rates are encountered in some so-called underdeveloped countries. Myocardial infarction is much more frequent in men than women, although sex differences decrease with advancing age. Infarction is infrequent in women under 50, but oral contraceptive agents and cigarette smoking have significantly increased the incidence.

Although myocardial infarction is almost always associated with coronary atherosclerosis, infarction may be triggered by increased myocardial activity and by diminished oxygen transport capacity of the blood, as in severe anemia. In the clinical entity of *variant angina pectoris*, ischemia and frequent infarction are thought to result from changing vascular supply rather than changing need. The basis is marked spasm of the coronary arteries, with or without underlying atherosclerosis. The anginal pain is usually prolonged, associated with diaphoresis, hypotension, arrhythmias, mitral insufficiency, and electrocardiographic changes of severe transmural ischemia.

The gross and histologic features of myocardial infarction were described in Chapter 3, and need not be repeated here. Atherosclerosis usually involves the coronary arteries before their entrance into the myocardium, and is usually most marked in the first 1 to 2 cm of the right coronary artery or the principal branches of the left. Infarction is most frequent in the anterior wall of the left ventricle and anterior septum, related to severe occlusive disease of the left anterior descending artery. The posterior wall of the left ventricle and posterior septum are infarcted when there is severe disease of the proximal right coronary artery, and the lateral left ventricular wall is infarcted when there is severe restriction of blood flow through the left circumflex artery. Infarction involving the right ventricle is not unusual, and is particularly likely to occur in the presence of right ventricular hypertrophy. The relationship of severe occlusive disease to the site of infarction may not be so simple as stated, since, as has been known for many years, the progression of coronary atherosclerosis is associated with the development of an extensive collateral circulation. Because of this, it is not uncommon to find several complete old occlusions of coronary vessels with no evidence that infarction has occurred.

Although acute coronary artery occlusion by a thrombus complicating an atherosclerotic plaque or by hemorrhage within a plaque is frequently observed, it is important to recognize that many infarctions occur without acute occlusion, and acute occlusion does not necessarily lead to infarction. It is unlikely that a thrombus will be found when infarction is triggered by excessive exertion, anxiety, shock, or anemia.

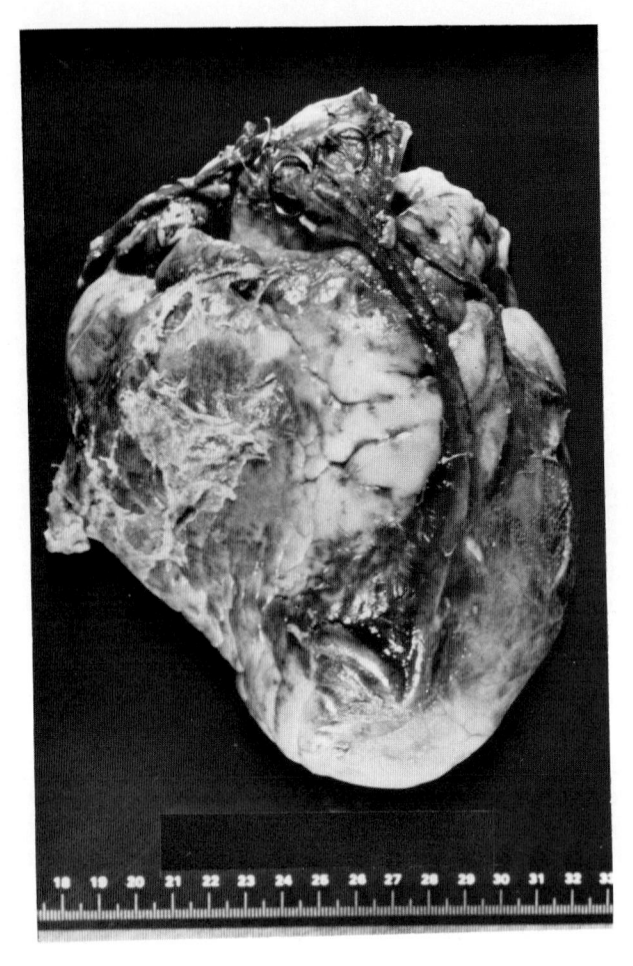

Figure 15.5. Saphenous vein bypass graft. A venous graft is shown running from the aortic root above to the cardiac apex. This vessel is thrombosed, a not infrequent complication of bypass surgery. Two other vein grafts are seen, their points of origin marked by the small metallic rings at the root of the aorta.

Complications of Myocardial Infarction

The mortality for acute myocardial infarction is about 40%, and nearly half of the deaths occur within the first 2 hr after onset of symptoms. Arrhythmias, particularly those resulting in inadequate ventricular filling and cardiogenic shock (ventricular tachycardia and ventricular fibrillation), occur in nearly half of patients with left ventricular infarction. They are most likely to occur in the first few hours after onset.

Congestive heart failure is a most serious complication, and can occur acutely or occasionally during convalescence. Papillary muscle dysfunction is often the precipitating cause of failure. It is due to infarction of a papillary muscle or the adjacent free wall of the left ventricle. Occasionally, there is complete rupture of the papillary muscle. Papillary muscle dysfunction is manifested by severe insufficiency of the mitral valve.

Rupture of a transmural infarction and sudden cardiac tamponade may occur as early as the first day of illness, but is more likely to happen between the fourth and seventh days. Rupture of the interventricular septum may also occur, with development of an acute left to right shunt and rapid cardiac failure.

Mural thrombi overlying areas of infarction are not uncommon, and can embolize to the lungs and to organs of the systemic circulation.

Late complications include the formation of ventricular aneurysms, and at any time, of course, the area of infarction may extend or new infarction can occur.

The postmyocardial infarction syndrome (*Dressler's syndrome*) is observed in some patients a few weeks after infarction. It consists of fever and inflammation of the pericardium and pleura, with pain and accumulation of serous fluid. It is thought to represent an autoimmune reaction to altered myocardial muscle fibers.

Bypass Surgery

Saphenous vein bypass grafts connect the aorta to the distal epicardial segments of the coronary arteries, bypassing the most severe occlusive disease in the proximal segments (Fig. 15.5). This procedure is being done more and more, particularly in the acute stage of myocardial infarction; however, its total impact on the morbidity and mortality of coronary artery disease remains to be seen. It appears most successful in prolonging life in those with severe disease of all three coronary vessels.

CARDIOMYOPATHIES

The cardiomyopathies are a group of disorders of the myocardium that are not relatable to coronary artery disease, hypertension, or valvular disease. Some are primary, *i.e.*, of unknown etiology, while others are secondary to disease elsewhere in the body. All are associated with cardiac hypertrophy and slowly progressive congestive heart failure that is relatively unresponsive to therapy.

Cardiomyopathies are also categorized on the basis of their hemodynamic consequences as *restrictive*, *congestive*, or *obstructive*. Restrictive lesions are those that stiffen the myocardium and interfere with diastolic filling. The hemodynamic effect is comparable to that in constrictive pericarditis, and the end result is low output failure. Congestive cardiomyopathy is the most common and is characterized by a flabby, dilated myocardium, weak pumping action, and biventricular failure. Obstructive cardiomyopathy is rare, the best known example being *idiopathic hypertrophic subaortic stenosis*.

Idiopathic Congestive Cardiomyopathy

This disorder is uncommon, sometimes familial. It is characterized by a large flabby heart with some hypertrophy, but mostly dilatation and patchy fibrosis of all four chambers. There is slowly progressive congestive heart failure. Mitral and aortic valvular insufficiency may result from dilatation of the valve rings. Mural thrombi may be present in any of the chambers, and pulmonary or systemic emboli can occur.

Idiopathic Hypertrophic Subaortic Stenosis

In this anomaly, there is marked hypertrophy of the interventricular septum which is often twice as thick as the left ventricular free wall, and there is disarray of the myofibers. The left ventricle is small, and the anterior leaflet of the mitral valve is pushed against the septum and becomes fibrotic. Obstruction to left ventricular outflow tends to be intermittent. Left ventricular pressure is very high and may force incompetence of the mitral valve. Patients with this disorder may have angina pectoris, and are prone to arrhythmias and sudden death. More than half of cases are familial, and in these there is genetic linkage to HLA antigens.

Toxic Cardiomyopathy

Daunorubicin and doxorubicin, anthracyclines used in the treatment of neoplastic disease, interfere with DNA systhesis and inhibit DNA and RNA polymerases in cardiac muscle fibers. Abnormal fibrils are noted by electron microscopy in the nucleus, and cell contractility is markedly impaired. This is a congestive cardiomyopathy.

Alcoholic cardiomyopathy is observed in some chronic alcoholics, particularly "binge" drinkers. It is due to direct toxic effects of alcohol on the myocardium, although it may be complicated by nutritional deficiency of proteins and B vitamins. Again, the cardiomyopathy is congestive, with dilated, fibrotic, and flabby chambers. The high incidence of cardiac failure in beer drinkers in Quebec and Nebraska has been attributed to excessive cobalt intake.

Cardiac Amyloidosis

Amyloid is a fibrillary protein deposited in the connective tissue between parenchymal cells. In the heart, interstitial deposition may be extensive and cause atrophy of myocardial fibers. Amyloid fibers may contain immunoglobulin light chains, and their deposition can be a reflection of altered immunoglobulin synthesis (Chapter 24). The myocardium is firm and rubbery, and the hemodynamic result is restrictive.

Miscellaneous Cardiomyopathies

There are many other causes of cardiomyopathy, including metabolic, nutritional, and endocrine disturbances, and the myocardium may be involved in various virus and parasitic infections. Cardiac involvement in sarcoidosis is not unusual, and, because of extensive fibrosis, is a restrictive lesion.

VALVULAR DISEASE

Rheumatic fever and rheumatic heart disease are discussed in this section, since the major long term effects involve the cardiac valves. Other entities included are isolated aortic stenosis, the floppy valve syndrome, and infective endocarditis.

Rheumatic Fever and Rheumatic Heart Disease

Rheumatic fever is an acute illness that can injure all parts of the heart. Rheumatic heart disease is a late sequel to rheumatic fever, and results from healing with scarring of the injuries.

Acute Rheumatic Fever

Acute rheumatic fever is a multisystem disease, clinically manifested by fever, polyarthritis, skin rashes, subcutaneous nodules, occasionally chorea, and, most importantly, a pancarditis. It is a recurring disease, usually starting between the ages of 5 and 15, although an initial episode can occur at any age. It is, in all likelihood, an immunologically mediated disorder, although the mechanism is incompletely understood. There is virtually always a preceding Group A β-hemolytic streptococcal infection, usually a pharyngitis. Although organisms may still be present in the pharynx at the time of onset of rheumatic fever, they are never found in the lesions of the heart or joints. Antibodies to components of the streptococcal cell wall have been shown to cross-react with myocardial fibers, and perhaps also with smooth muscle and skeletal muscle. The lesions of rheumatic fever, however, arise in connective tissue, and they do not show consistent evidence of an immunologic pathogenesis.

The heart involvement is a pancarditis: pericarditis, myocarditis, and endocarditis. The pericarditis is a fibrinous or "bread and butter" inflammation, that usually heals with little scarring. The highly characteristic lesion of the myocardium is the *Aschoff nodule*, consisting of an area of fibrinoid necrosis of connective tissue, surrounded at first by polymorphonuclear leukocytes, plasma cells, and lymphocytes, but later by large mononuclear phagocytes (Aschoff cells) and Anitschkow myocytes, peculiar cells thought to be derived from fibroblasts (Fig. 15.6). The endocarditis consists of small bead-like vegetations along the lines of valvular closure (Fig. 15.7). The vegetations consist of platelets and fibrin deposited over an area of connective tissue degeneration and covered by endothelium. They are firmly attached and do not embolize. Similar vegetations form over the chordae tendineae. Involvement of mitral and aortic valves is most

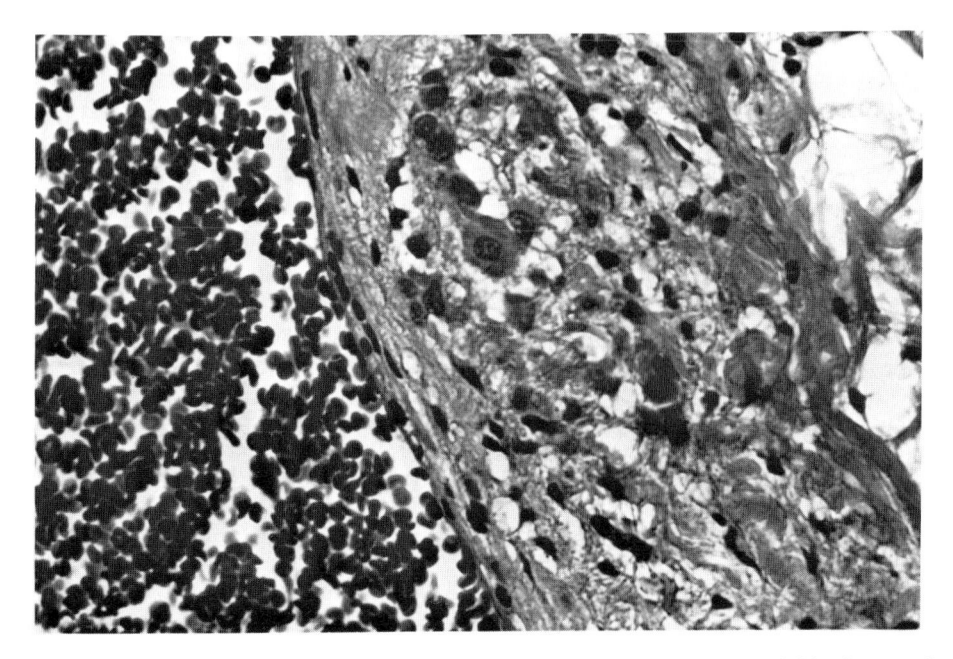

Figure 15.6. Aschoff nodule. The lesion occupies the *right central portion* of this photograph. There is degeneration of connective tissue, and an infiltration by large mononuclear cells with deep staining cytoplasm. This nodule is in a subendocardial location of the left atrium.

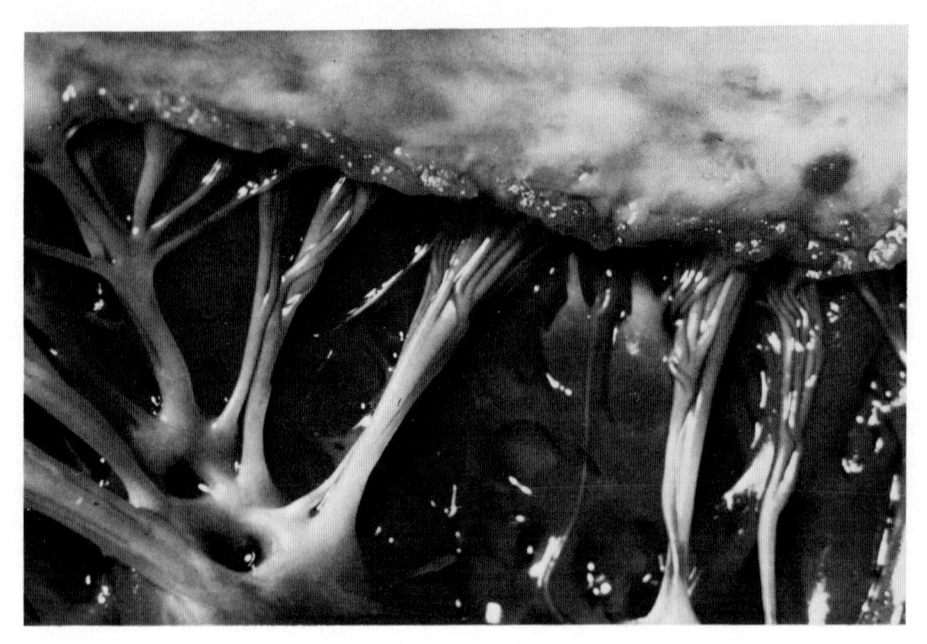

Figure 15.7. Acute rheumatic endocarditis. The line of closure of this mitral valve leaflet is covered by small thrombotic vegetations that are being organized and are firmly attached.

frequent, although the tricuspid valve may also show lesions. Aschoff nodules are occasionally encountered within the substance of the valves, and may also involve the pericardial tissues.

In terms of functional disturbance, the myocarditis is by far the most serious involvement, and death during an episode of acute rheumatic fever is usually due to congestive heart failure.

The Aschoff nodule has usually been considered evidence of rheumatic activity. Its presence, however, in perhaps half of patients years after any clinical evidence of active disease, seriously questions its significance. An alternative interpretation is that rheumatic fever is usually a progressive and smoldering disease whose activity is not made apparent by clinical manifestations.

The incidence of rheumatic fever has dropped drastically in this country during the past generation. This is in part attributable to a decrease in severe streptococcal infections, but predominately results from prompt and effective treatment of these infections, and long term antibiotic prophylaxis to prevent recurrences in those who have had rheumatic fever.

Rheumatic Heart Disease

The most important late consequence of rheumatic fever is valvular scarring, causing functional stenosis or regurgitation. The mitral valve is involved alone in 40% of patients, mitral and aortic valve in 50%, and mitral, aortic, and tricuspid in 10%. If several episodes of rheumatic fever occur during childhood, the first evidence of mitral valve involvement, *i.e.*, systolic and/or diastolic murmurs, might be noted in the early 20's, and symptoms of congestive heart failure would probably start between the ages of 35 and 45. The classical appearance of the mitral valve includes fibrous thickening and often calcification of the leaflets, thickening, shortening, and fusion of the chordae tendineae, and marked compromise of the valve opening (Figs. 15.8 and 15.9). The valve is both stenotic and incompetent. The normal mitral valve has an opening of at least 3.5 cm^2, and there is no gradient across the valve, even with maximum flow of blood. If the opening is reduced to 1.5 to 2.5 cm^2, there may be dyspnea on marked exertion, and early left atrial enlargement. At 1.0 to 1.5 cm^2, symptoms occur with mild exertion, and orthopnea and paroxysmal nocturnal dyspnea are common. When the opening is less than 1.0 cm^2, there are symptoms of failure at rest, a fixed cardiac output, and a strong tendency to atrial fibrillation and complicating embolic phenomena. There is marked enlargement of the left atrium, pulmonary hypertension, and right ventricular hypertrophy or failure. Tricuspid regurgitation is often noted. The pulmonary changes of chronic passive congestion, described earlier, are often most severe in patients with mitral stenosis.

The aortic valve is never involved alone in rheumatic heart disease, but always together with the mitral valve. The valve leaflets become thickened and fused, and there is often marked calcification in the sinuses of Valsalva. Aortic valve involvement tends to be more severe in men, mitral involvement in women.

Isolated Calcific Aortic Stenosis

Isolated aortic stenosis can be due to a congenitally deformed valve, or to hemodynamic wear and tear (Figs. 15.10 and 15.11). Unicuspid valves result in

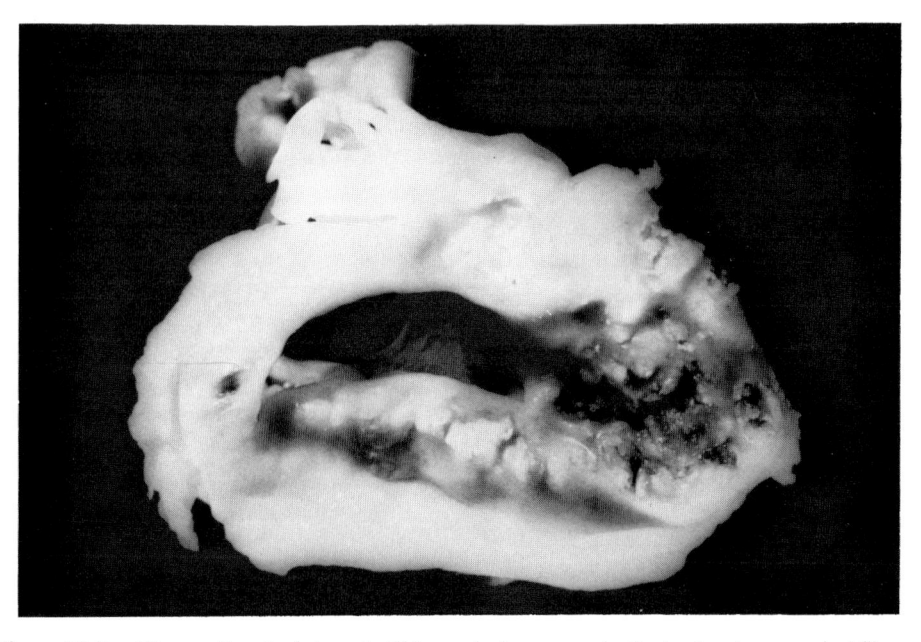

Figure 15.8. Rheumatic mitral stenosis. This surgically removed mitral valve shows marked fibrous thickening and calcification of its leaflets. The opening of the valve is small and flattened, often referred to as a "fish mouth" opening. The valve is both stenotic and incompetent.

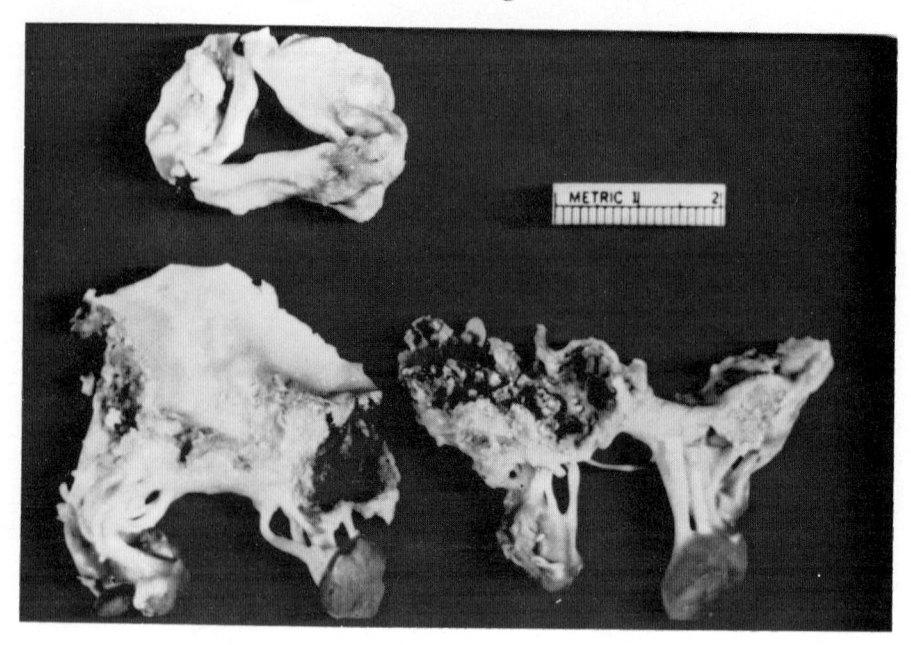

Figure 15.9. Rheumatic involvement of mitral and aortic valves. These valves, removed at surgery, show striking fibrosis and calcification of their leaflets. The marked thickening and fusion of the chordae tendineae of the mitral valve (*below*) is apparent.

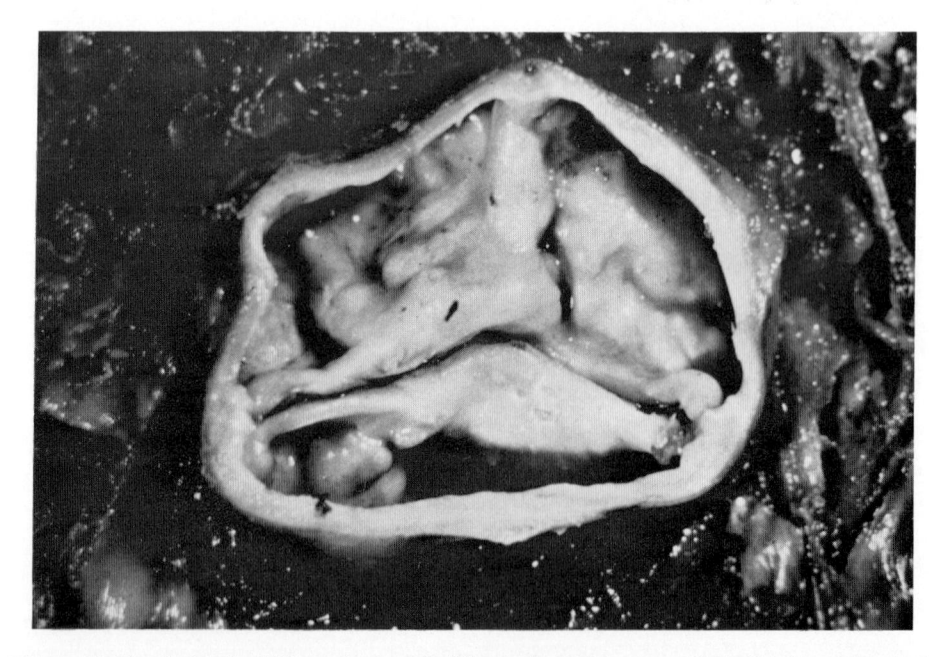

Figure 15.10. Isolated calcific aortic stenosis. The marked thickening and calcification of the aortic valve leaflets are viewed from the aortic side. This valve is tricuspid, and the changes are attributed to hemodynamic wear and tear.

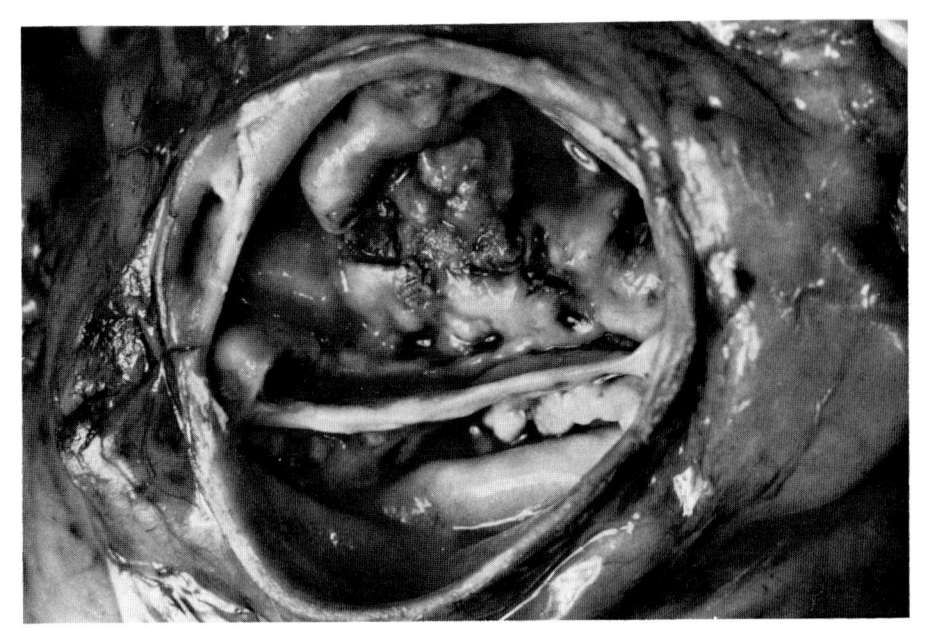

Figure 15.11. Isolated calcific aortic stenosis. This congenitally bicuspid aortic valve shows marked calcification and scarring of its leaflets. The valve is viewed from the aortic side.

early stenosis, with manifestations often appearing before the age of 15. Bicuspid valves become stenotic later, but are usually symptomatic before 65, whereas wear and tear stenosis, a common occurrence, becomes apparent after age 65.

Aortic stenosis causes a systolic pressure gradient across the valve, and a loud ejection murmur. There is concentric hypertrophy, often marked, of the left ventricle. Congestive heart failure may be the first clinical manifestation, although syncope and angina pectoris are also common.

Mitral Valve Prolapse

Commonly referred to as the floppy mitral valve syndrome, or *Barlow's syndrome*, mitral valve prolapse is characterized by a ballooning of the valve leaflets, particularly the posterior leaflet, with functional incompetence (Fig. 15.12). The disorder is much more frequent in women than men, and affects some 1 in 20. The physical findings usually become apparent during the second or third decades, and include a midsystolic click and a late systolic mitral murmur. If severe, congestive heart failure is likely, but arrhythmias and infection of the valve leaflets also occur.

Some patients with prolapsed mitral valves have the generalized connective tissue disorder Marfan's syndrome (p. 96), but, in most, findings are confined to the mitral valve.

Infective Endocarditis

Infection can occur on normal valves, on valves scarred by disease, around prostheses, and on such congenital defects as ventricular septal defects. The

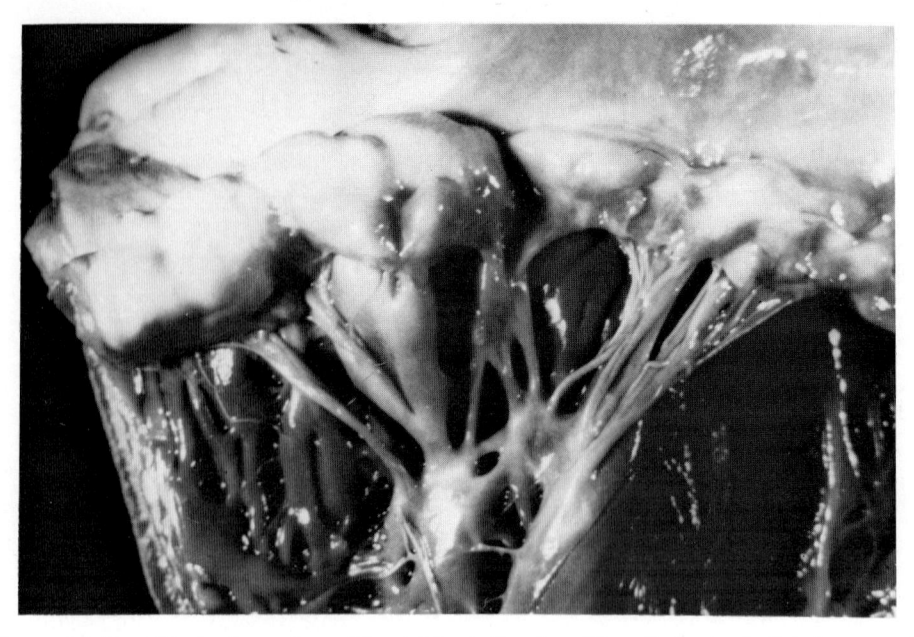

Figure 15.12. Mitral valve prolapse. The striking ballooning of the mitral valve leaflets is apparent. This valve is functionally incompetent.

microorganisms, circulating in the bloodstream, probably settle out and colonize minute foci of endocardial injury covered by platelet and fibrin thrombi. Vegetations form, composed of thrombotic material and masses of organisms, and there are attempts at organization by ingrowth of granulation tissue from the valvular or endocardial connective tissue. The vegetations are often bulky and friable, and embolization is almost the rule (Fig. 15.13). Valve leaflets may be perforated or destroyed, or infection may remain superficial and result only in some fibrous thickening (Fig. 15.14).

Endocarditis used to be encountered principally as a complication of rheumatic heart disease, and was most often due to *Streptococcus viridans*, an organism of low pathogenicity. Destructive endocarditis due to virulent organisms occurred most often on normal valves or aortic valves injured by syphilis. It is now seen increasingly in immunosuppressed patients and patients who have received prosthetic valves, and a wide spectrum of organisms may be recovered, including *Candida* and cryptococcal fungi. Organisms are particularly likely to be introduced into the bloodstream in association with dental procedures and placement of indwelling catheters.

The mitral valve is most often involved; the aortic valve is second. Tricuspid endocarditis is particularly likely to occur in heroin addicts and as a complication of gonococcal infections.

Endocarditis due to organisms of low pathogenicity does not usually destroy the valves, and embolic manifestations are usually bland, *i.e.*, sterile infarcts. Once the organisms leave their protected environment on the endocardium, they appear to be destroyed readily by body defenses. A notable exception is the formation of infected or "mycotic" aneurysms.

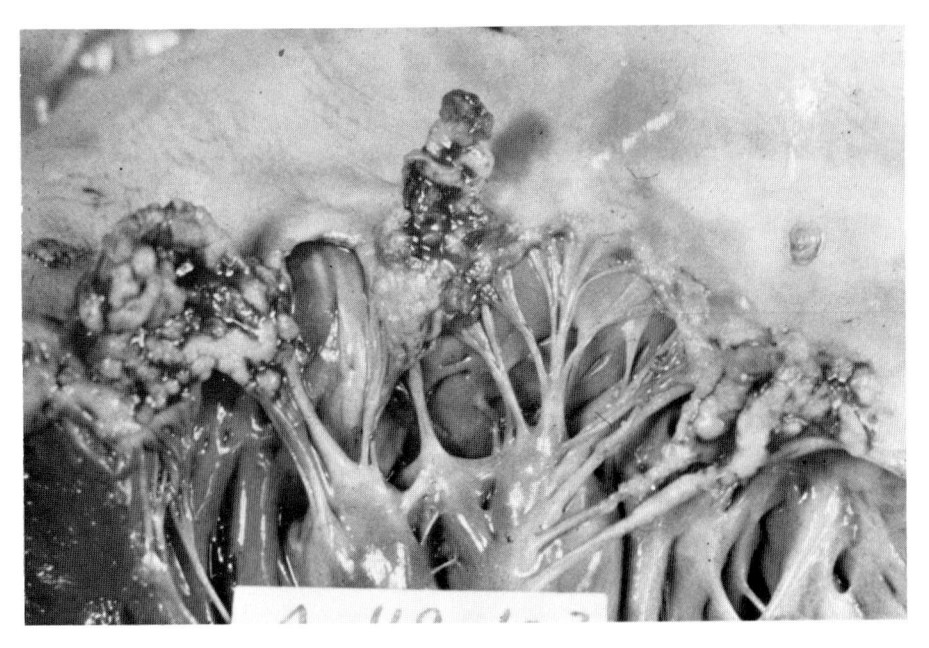

Figure 15.13. Bacterial endocarditis due to *Streptococcus viridans*. Many soft friable vegetations are seen over the mitral valve leaflet and its chordae tendineae.

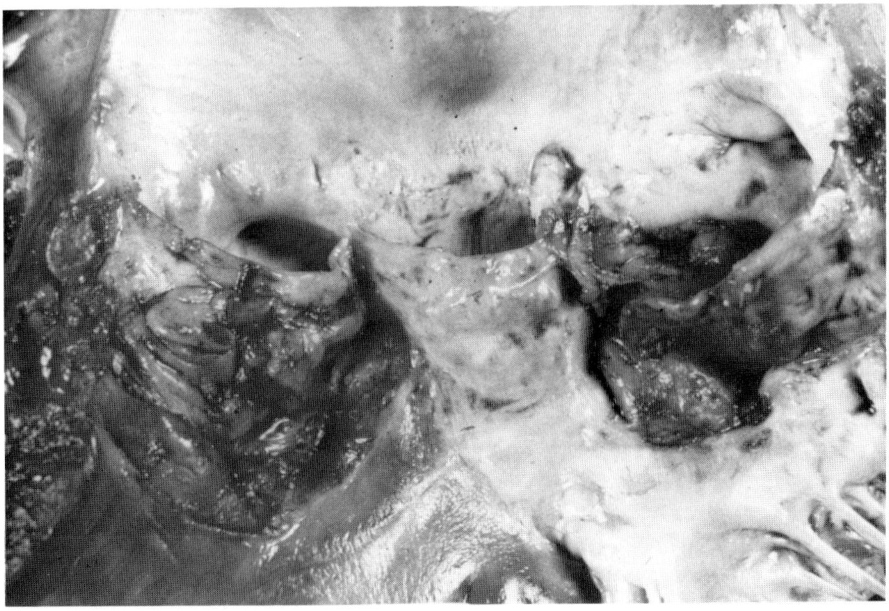

Figure 15.14. Pneumococcal endocarditis. This aortic valve has been extensively destroyed by infection of its leaflets. Large perforations are seen in two leaflets, communicating with the sinuses of Valsalva. This patient died of uncontrollable congestive heart failure.

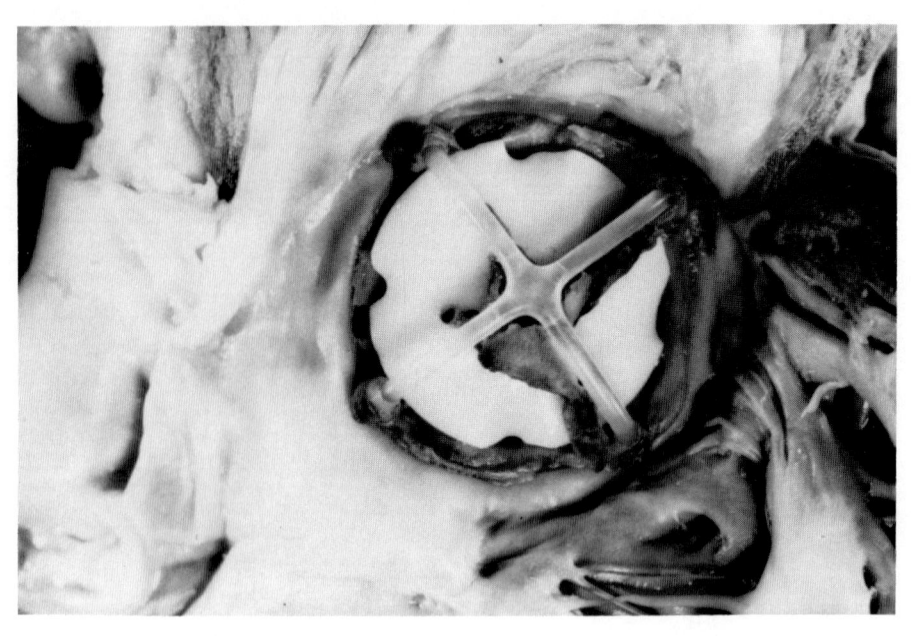

Figure 15.15. Deterioration of a prosthetic disc valve. This valve, in place for several years, shows deterioration and tearing of the disc, and thrombosis over the roughened areas and the suture line.

Virulent organisms are likely to be highly destructive within the heart, and emboli are usually septic. Cerebral, splenic, and other infarcts become abscesses. Valve ring abscesses are found in the heart, and are a mechanism of spreading infection from one valve to another. In addition to the clinical manifestations of severe systemic infection, endocarditis due to virulent organisms can cause severe valvular incompetence and rapidly progressive heart failure. Surgical intervention, with removal of diseased valves and placement of prostheses, may be the only successful therapeutic approach.

CONGENITAL HEART DISEASE

Congenital heart defects are encountered in some 7 of every 1000 live births. As recently as 1940, only patent ductus arteriosus could be corrected surgically. Now, most defects are amenable to surgery, and deaths from congenital heart disease have been dramatically reduced.

Consideration is given here to the more important defects that are surgically correctable. It should be noted that the effects of congenital heart disease on the pulmonary circulation are key to both prognosis and operability. If there is obstruction to pulmonary blood flow, and shunting of blood from the right side of the heart to the left, arterial blood is inadequately oxygenated and there is cyanosis, compensatory polycythemia, and growth retardation. If shunting of blood is from left to right, the pulmonary circuit is overloaded, and, sooner or later, pulmonary hypertension becomes severe and obstructive, and reversal of the shunt is likely to occur. Left ventricular failure can complicate left-to-right shunts, although pulmonary hypertension may prevent this by reducing the degree of shunt, and right ventricular failure occurs with intracardiac or pulmonary obstruction to right ventricular output. In addition to changes in blood flow and blood pressure, the lungs show increased susceptibility to infection. Infective endocarditis occurs in association with many forms of congenital heart disease.

Atrial Septal Defects

Several types of atrial septal defects are seen. Some consist of persistence of a large fossa ovalis (septum secundum defect). Lower defects (septum primum) are likely to be associated with endocardial cushion defects (see below).

Shunting of blood is from left atrium to right atrium. There is volume overload of the pulmonary circulation and increased pulmonary blood flow, right ventricular hypertrophy, and, at times, right ventricular failure. Pulmonary hypertension and the development of pulmonary vascular constriction are usually late developments.

Ventricular Septal Defects

Most ventricular septal defects create communication between the subaortic region of the left ventricle and the infundibulum of the right ventricle, and are located in the membranous septum. They are usually below the parietal limb of the crista supraventricularis. Defects may also occur in the lower or muscular septum. Shunting of blood is from left to right, depending on the size of the defect. Small defects may close spontaneously, usually during the first year of life. Large defects may permit so great a shunt as to cause left ventricle failure. The pulmonary blood flow is increased and there is both volume and pressure overload, so that right ventricular hypertrophy and pulmonary hypertension can be early manifestations. The small pulmonary arteries and arterioles at first show medial hypertrophy and intimal thickening; later, plexiform lesions are seen at major branches. The vascular changes are irreversible and obstructive, and pulmonary hypertension often exceeds systemic pressures, with reversal of the shunt from right to left (Fig. 15.16). This is called the *Eisenmenger syndrome.*

Endocardial Cushion Defect

Endocardial cushion defect, or common atrioventricular canal, is the most frequent cardiac defect in children with Down's syndrome (p. 101). There is a single opening between the atria and ventricles, together with a low (ostium primum) atrial septal defect and a high membranous ventricular septal defect (Fig. 15.17). Leaflets representing both tricuspid and mitral valves are present, but are often abnormally attached, so that insufficiency is marked. The septal defects and valvular regurgitation combine to produce a striking left-to-right shunt, frequent left ventricular failure, and a greatly increased pulmonary blood flow. Pulmonary hypertension and pulmonary obstructive vascular disease occur early.

Patent Ductus Arteriosus

In most examples of patent ductus arteriosus, the ductal opening is small, and, although there is a left-to-right shunt, aortic pressures are not transmitted to the pulmonary circulation, and obstructive pulmonary vascular disease does not

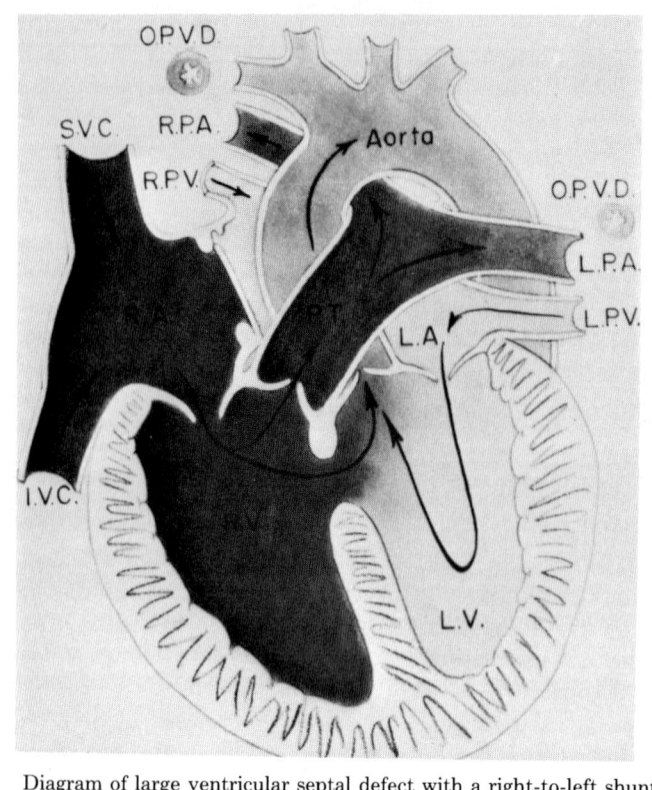

Figure 15.16. Diagram of large ventricular septal defect with a right-to-left shunt resulting from occlusive pulmonary vascular disease.

develop. If a patent ductus is large, and permits unobstructed shunting from left to right, the effects are the same as those of a large ventricular septal defect.

Tetralogy of Fallot

Tetralogy of Fallot consists of a membranous ventricular septal defect, dextroposition of the aorta so that it receives blood from both ventricles, obstruction of the pulmonary outflow tract, and right ventricular hypertrophy. In most instances, obstruction to pulmonary flow is sufficiently marked to cause a right-to-left shunt. The obstruction may be in part the result of pulmonic valve deformity or stenosis, but is usually due primarily to stenosis of the infundibulum. Right ventricular pressure is greater than left ventricular pressure, and venous blood shunts to the left heart and through the overriding aorta (Fig. 15.18). There is cyanosis, clubbing of fingers, and growth retardation. Sudden episodes of severe cyanosis with unconsciousness and convulsions are attributable to infundibular spasm that effectively prevents pulmonary blood flow. Brain injury may occur during these episodes.

Chronic hypoxia results in hyperplasia of erythroid elements in the bone marrow and compensatory polycythemia. Blood viscosity is increased, and there is predisposition to vascular thrombosis, particularly in the cerebral circulation. Severe infections, including brain abscesses, may be related to infective endocar-

The Heart 163

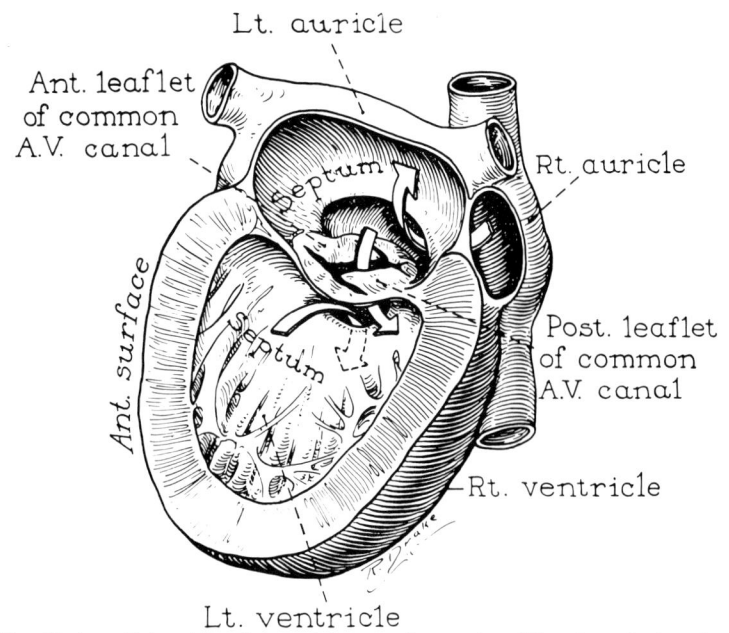

Figure 15.17. Endocardial cushion defect of the complete variety. View from the interior of the left side of the heart. Characteristically, there is a crescent-shaped defect in the lowermost part of the atrial septum. An atrioventricular valve common to both sides of the heart and a subvalvular ventricular septal defect are other features of the complex.

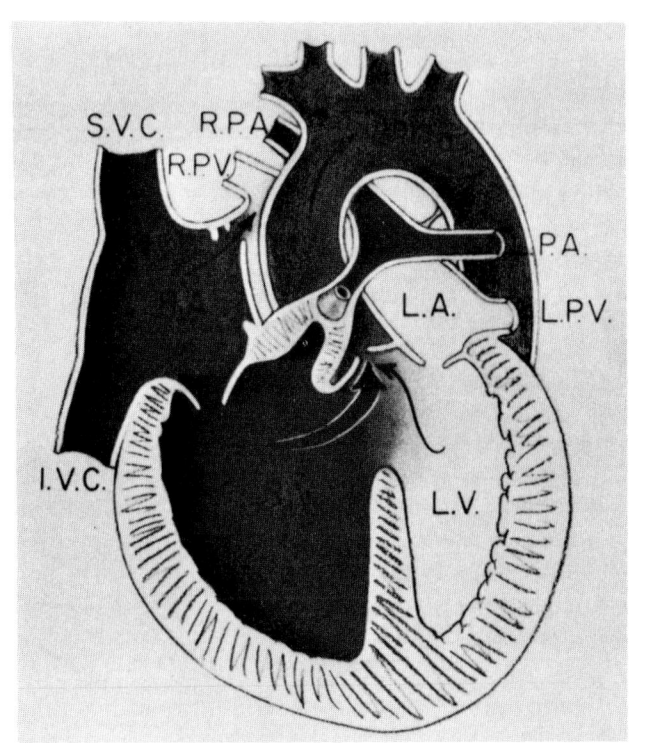

Figure 15.18. Diagram of the central circulation in classical tetralogy of Fallot, where pulmonary stenosis of severe degree is associated with a right-to-left shunt into the aorta.

164   Pathology: Understanding Human Disease

ditis or to bacteremia in which the protective effects of the pulmonary circulation are short-circuited.

Coarctation of the Aorta

Most coarctations of the aorta consist of a defect of the media that produces a localized membrane-like stenosis or obstruction of the aorta at or near the junction of the arch and the descending aorta. The consequences are generally milder if the coarctation is located distal to the ductus arteriosus. The lower parts of the body are dependent upon a collateral circulation developing from branches of the subclavian arteries. Other forms of aortic obstruction include a tubular narrowing, usually distal to the left subclavian artery, and a total lack of continuity between the arch and descending aorta.

Coarctation is often associated with a bicuspid aortic valve which is prone to bacterial infection, and, in time, to calcific aortic stenosis.

MISCELLANEOUS DISORDERS

Endocardial fibroelastosis is an uncommon disorder of unknown etiology, characterized by diffuse or patchy opaque thickening of the mural endocardium (Fig. 15.19). The left side of the heart is more often involved than the right. The thickened endocardium is composed of collagen and elastic fibers, often arranged in orderly parallel rows. Mitral and aortic valves may show similar thickening, with evidence of stenosis. Some instances of endocardial fibroelastosis appear to

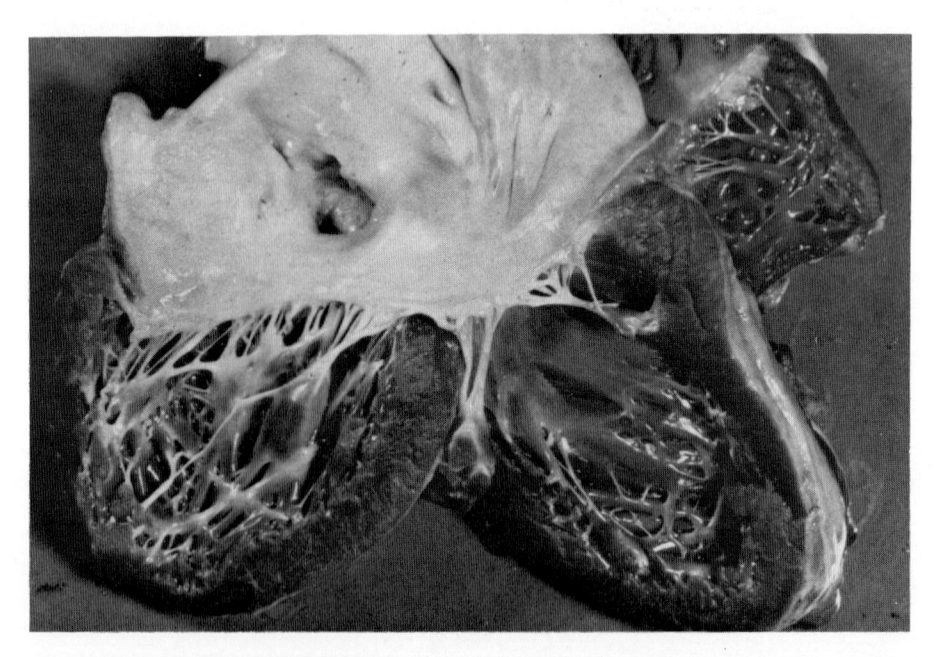

Figure 15.19. Endocardial fibroelastosis. There is striking opaque thickening of the mural endocardium of the left atrium, and some thickening over the papillary muscles of the left ventricle. This heart is from a young adult who died in congestive heart failure.

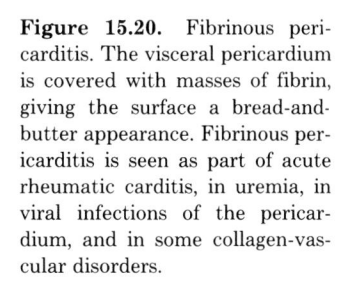

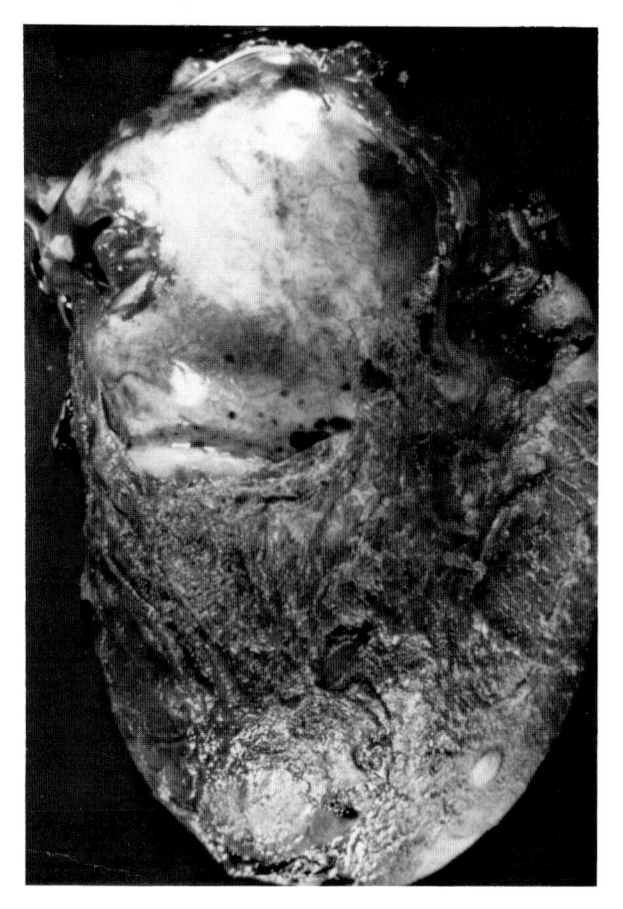

Figure 15.20. Fibrinous pericarditis. The visceral pericardium is covered with masses of fibrin, giving the surface a bread-and-butter appearance. Fibrinous pericarditis is seen as part of acute rheumatic carditis, in uremia, in viral infections of the pericardium, and in some collagen-vascular disorders.

be familial, and some are associated with other cardiac defects. This disorder is a cause of rapidly fatal congestive heart failure in infants and young children, and of more slowly progressing failure in older children and young adults.

Syphilitic involvement of the heart has become rare. It is a manifestation of late or tertiary syphilis, and its effect is on the aortic valve. Aortitis involving the proximal aorta consists of an obliterative arteritis of the vasa vasorum, with resulting loss of muscle and elastic fibers of the media. Dilatation of the aorta involves the aortic valve ring, separating the commissures, and producing an incompetent valve. The valve leaflets show rolling of the free edges, and occasional rupture.

Thrombotic, nonbacterial, or marantic endocarditis occurs most often in elderly debilitated patients, although it may occasionally be observed in young, well nourished individuals. Vegetations are found at the lines of closure, particularly of the mitral and aortic valves. These vegetations are sterile, composed of platelets and fibrin, and evoke little reaction from the underlying valve tissue. They are friable, and can cause embolic phenomena, although this disorder is usually a manifestation of very terminal disease.

Suggested Reading

Edwards JE. Survey of operative congenital heart disease. Am. J. Pathol. *82:* 407, 1976.
Kirklin JW. The replacement of cardiac valves. N. Engl. J. Med. *304:* 291, 1981.
Roberts WC. The coronary arteries and coronary heart disease, morphologic observations. Pathobiol. Ann. *5:* 249, 1975.
Roberts WC, Ferrans VJ. Pathologic anatomy of the cardiomyopathies. Human Pathol. *6:* 287, 1975.
Wagner S, Cohn K. Heart failure. Arch. Intern. Med. *137:* 675, 1977.
Weinstein L. "Modern" infective endocarditis. JAMA *233:* 260, 1975.

Chapter 16

Vascular Disorders

The disorders discussed in this chapter include atherosclerosis, acute aortic dissection, Mönckeberg's medial sclerosis, fibromuscular dysplasia, various examples of vasculitis, and thrombophlebitis. Arteriolar sclerosis is considered in Chapter 18.

Arterial diseases assume functional significance when they impair blood flow to body tissues. The lesions of a disease may gradually impinge upon and occlude the arterial lumens, or more rapid occlusion can result from hemorrhage into the lesions or from luminal thrombosis subsequent to endothelial injury. Arterial disease may also result in *aneurysm* formation, *i.e.*, localized areas of saccular, fusiform, or cylindrical dilatation. Aneurysms are of frequent occurrence in patients with atherosclerosis and syphilitic arteritis, may result from septic embolization from infective endocarditis (*mycotic* aneurysm), and may follow focal injury to arterial walls in such arteritides as polyarteritis nodosa. Vascular trauma may result in aneurysm formation as well as in abnormal arteriovenous communication. Some aneurysms are congenital, including most intracranial aneurysms. The latter are discussed in Chapter 20. Regardless of cause, aneurysms may rupture and cause massive hemorrhage, or they may compress and interfere with the functions of vital structures.

The principal complications of diseases affecting veins are thrombosis and embolism. Pulmonary embolism alone accounts for some 50,000 deaths each year in this country.

ATHEROSCLEROSIS

The prevalence of atherosclerosis, its intimate relationship to ischemic heart disease, and some data concerning epidemiology were discussed in Chapter 15. In this chapter, particular attention is given to the pathogenesis of atherosclerosis, its morphology, and its complications.

A variety of risk factors have been shown to affect the incidence and severity of atherosclerosis. The most important are disturbances of lipid metabolism (hyperlipoproteinemias), obesity, and hypertension. Diabetes mellitus, cigarette smoking, and the use of oral contraceptive agents involve additional risk. Genetic determinants clearly play a role in several of these predisposing factors.

The hallmark of atherosclerosis is the *intimal plaque*. As observed in the aorta, it is a rather well circumscribed yellowish or grayish thickening of the intima, measuring from a few millimeters to 2 or 3 cm in diameter (Fig. 16.1). Microscop-

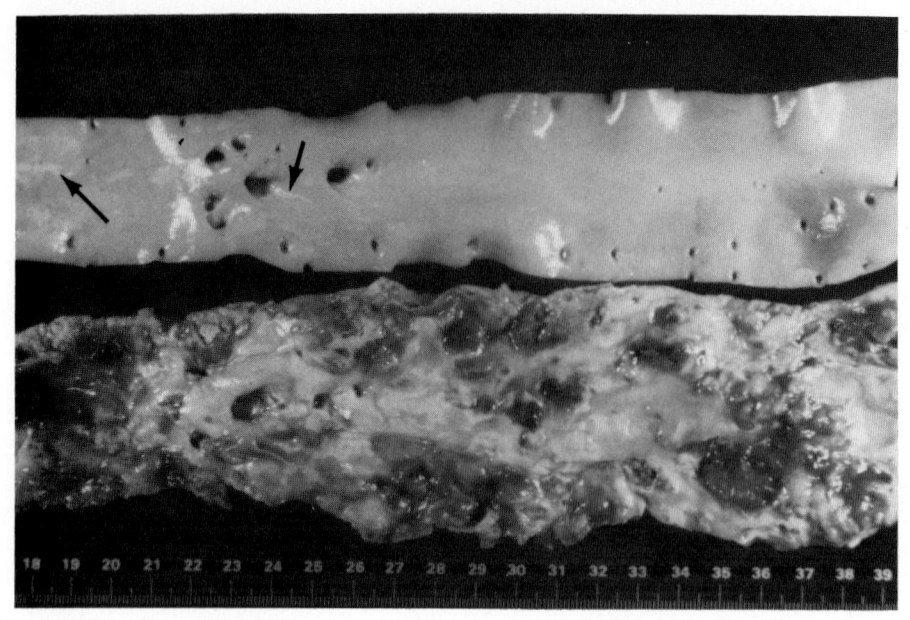

Figure 16.1. Aortic atherosclerosis. The *lower* aorta is from a 65-year-old man. There are a great many intimal plaques, most appearing yellowish gray in color, but many have been the site of endothelial ulceration and overlying thrombus formation. The *upper* aorta is from an 18-year-old man. The *arrows* point to delicate fatty streaks, an almost universal finding in aortas of the young.

ically, there is deposition of lipid material, often in mononuclear phagocytes ("foam cells"), cholesterol crystals, cellular debris, and a proliferation of fibroblasts and smooth muscle cells (Fig. 16.2). There may be an increase in vascularity, and calcification is common.

The pathogenesis of the atherosclerotic plaque has not been clearly defined. A possible precursor lesion is the *fatty streak* seen in the aorta of virtually all children. These consist of very slightly elevated, longitudinally oriented linear streaks, 1 or 2 mm wide, composed of lipid accumulations in foam cells and smooth muscle cells (Fig. 16.1). In contrast to the atherosclerotic plaque, the fatty streak is observed in all global population groups, and it is most marked in the proximal aorta. The vast majority of fatty streaks are probably resorbed, and it is debatable if they ever progress to atheroma formation.

It is thought by many observers that the initial pathogenetic event is an injury to the vascular endothelium that alters its permeability to plasma components and leads to platelet adherence and thrombus formation. A growth factor released by platelets stimulates smooth muscle migration and proliferation as well as fibroblastic growth. Smooth muscle cells ingest lipid released by platelets and leukocytes or derived from plasma reaching the intima through the injured endothelium. Plasma lipids may themselves promote further smooth muscle proliferation and migration. Smooth muscle growth ceases with repair of the endothelial injury, and the entire process may revert to normal; repeated injury, however, would lead to atheroma formation. This hypothesis is attractive, since several of the risk factors for atherosclerosis are known to increase the frequency of endothelial injuries. There is also evidence that platelet function is abnormal

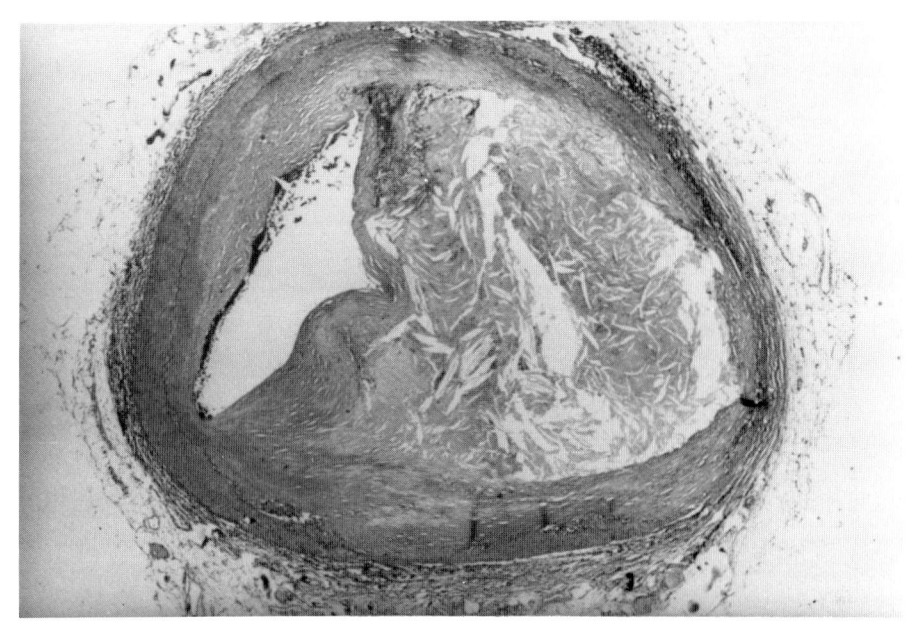

Figure 16.2. Atherosclerosis of coronary artery. This vessel shows a large plaque, occupying most of the former lumen, composed of fibrous tissue and containing many cleft-like spaces representing cholesterol deposits. The atherosclerotic plaque is predominantly an intimal lesion, but at the *right* it has extended to involve the media. The lumen, at the *left*, is markedly reduced in caliber.

in patients with severe atherosclerosis. Platelet life span is decreased, and there is an increase in the plasma of such platelet products as a growth factor, Platelet Factor 4, and β-thromboglobulin.

It has also been proposed that smooth muscle proliferation can be the initial change in the genesis of the atherosclerotic plaque. This could represent a mutation and a monoclonal growth of smooth muscle.

Atherosclerosis tends to be most marked in large and medium-sized arteries: the descending aorta and vessels of the lower extremities, the coronary arteries, and the internal carotid and cerebral arteries. Its principal expressions are ischemic heart disease, cerebral ischemia and infarction, and peripheral vascular insufficiency. Wherever they are found, atherosclerotic plaques are likely to become calcified. They often show areas of hemorrhage. Large plaques frequently undergo surface endothelial necrosis and ulceration, followed by mural thrombus formation, and possible embolization. Thrombotic occlusion of the distal aorta and iliac vessels causes severe exertional ischemia of the legs (Leriche syndrome).

In the aorta and the proximal portions of its largest branches, extension of atherosclerosis to involve the media results in loss of elastic tissue and possible aneurysm formation. Atherosclerotic aneurysms are much more common in men than women, and usually appear after age 50. The abdominal aorta distal to the origins of the renal arteries is the most frequent site (Fig. 16.3). The aneurysms, which may be multiple, are usually fusiform in shape. They are frequently filled with partially organized thrombotic material, with marked reduction in the caliber of the aortic lumen. Rupture, with massive retroperitoneal hemorrhage, is a not infrequent cause of death.

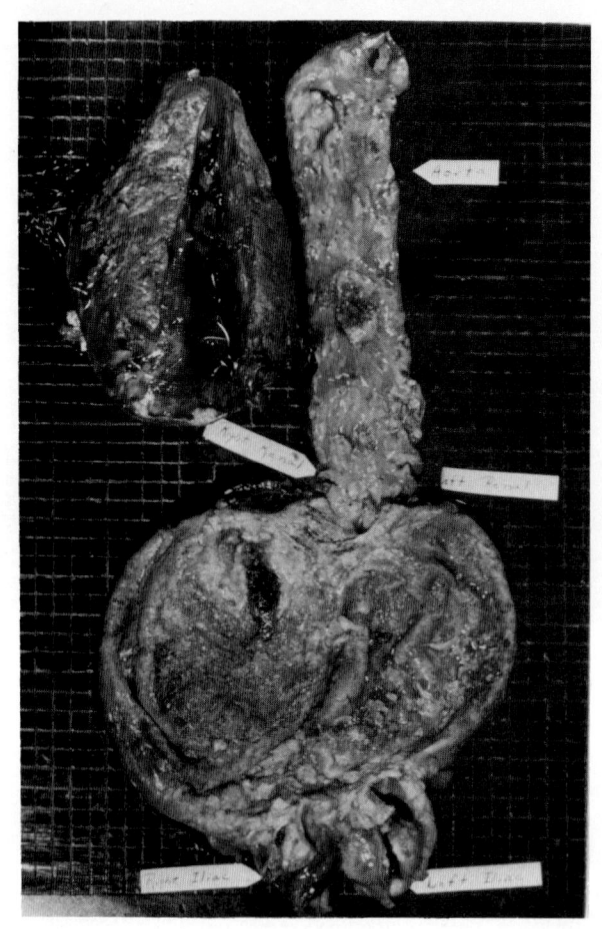

Figure 16.3. Atherosclerotic aneurysm of aorta. There is a large saccular aneurysm located between the renal arteries and the aortic bifurcation. The aneurysm had been largely filled with thrombotic material, seen at the *upper left*.

ACUTE AORTIC DISSECTION

Acute aortic dissection (or *dissecting aneurysm*) consists of a mural hemorrhage that spreads rapidly through the wall of the aorta, usually creating a new channel between the outer and middle thirds of the media. There is often little dilatation of the aorta, and the lesion is not, properly speaking, an aneurysm.

Aortic dissection is twice as frequent in men as in women, although it may occur as a complication of pregnancy. It usually occurs in individuals over 40, and is almost always associated with hypertension. It is noteworthy, however, that aortic dissection is probably the most frequent cause of death in patients with Marfan's syndrome.

Although absent in some 10% of dissections, there is most often a transverse tear of the intima, typically in the ascending aorta or arch. From here, the dissection may extend proximally to involve the root of the aorta and the coronary ostia. It most commonly proceeds distally, and may extend through the entire length of the aorta and into the iliac arteries. It can involve the entire circumference or only a part (Fig. 16.4). Branches, such as the neck vessels, often show dissection; others, such as intercostal and renal arteries, may be sheared from

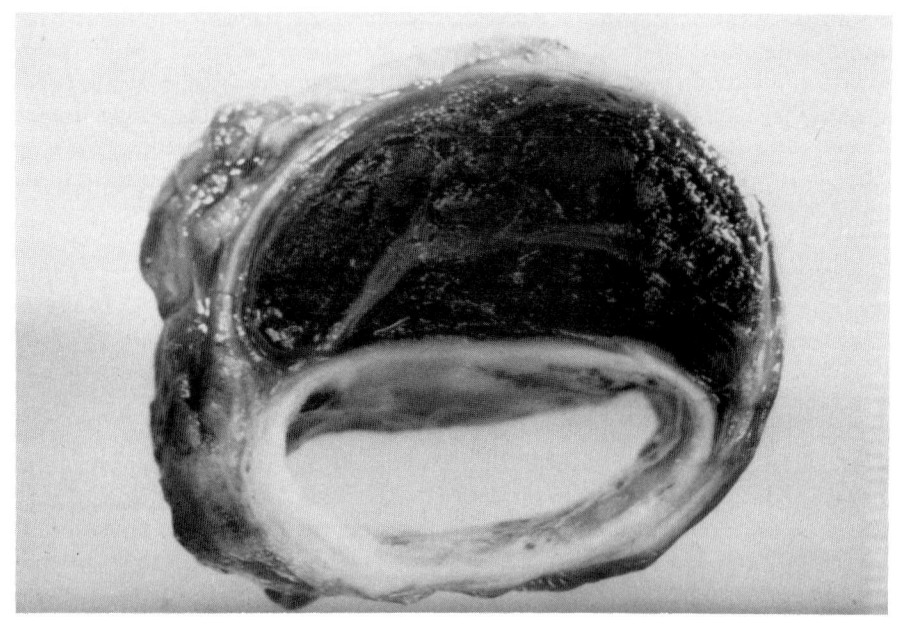

Figure 16.4. Acute aortic dissection. This cross-section of thoracic aorta shows a large area of hemorrhage in the media, involving one-half of the aortic circumference. This aortic dissection involved the entire length of the aorta from the aortic valve ring past the bifurcation.

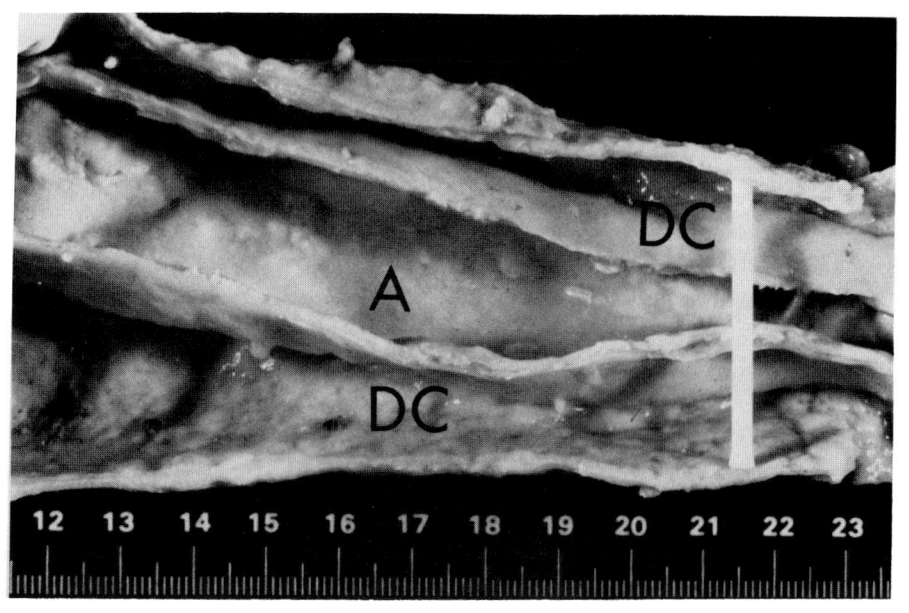

Figure 16.5. Aortic dissection. This dissection occurred 1 year before the patient's death. The original aortic channel (*A*) is seen in the center. It is surrounded by the dissected channel (*DC*). The dissected channel has become endothelialized; indeed, it shows lesions of atherosclerosis.

their ostia. A re-entry of the dissecting channel into the aortic lumen is often found in one of the iliac arteries, occasionally in a neck vessel; this creates a functioning double barreled aorta. The most frequent cause of death is rupture and massive hemorrhage, usually into the pericardium, pleura, or peritoneum. Those dissections that ascend to the aortic root (Type A) generally carry a poor prognosis for recovery with or without surgical intervention. Those that start beyond the left subclavian artery and extend distally only (Type B) have a better outlook (Figs. 16.5 and 16.6).

The principal manifestation of aortic dissection is severe pain, often starting in the precordium, and gradually shifting to the back and then the legs. Involvement of the aortic root may result in acute insufficiency of the aortic valve, and encroachment on the coronary ostia can cause myocardial infarction. Involvement of the renal arteries may be reflected in hematuria and oliguria.

A disorder of the aortic media, *medial cystic necrosis,* can be identified in most, but not all, instances of aortic dissection, and may be of etiologic and pathogenetic significance (Fig. 16.7). This lesion consists of lake-like accumulations of mucopolysaccharide together with disruption and fragmentation of elastic fibers. It may result from the effects of hypertension on the aortic vasa vasorum. Its presence, often striking, in patients with Marfan's syndrome (p. 96), however, suggests that medial cystic necrosis may be part of a generalized disturbance of collagen and elastic tissue. Medial accumulation of mucopolysaccharides may also be prominent in the presence of severe hypothyroidism.

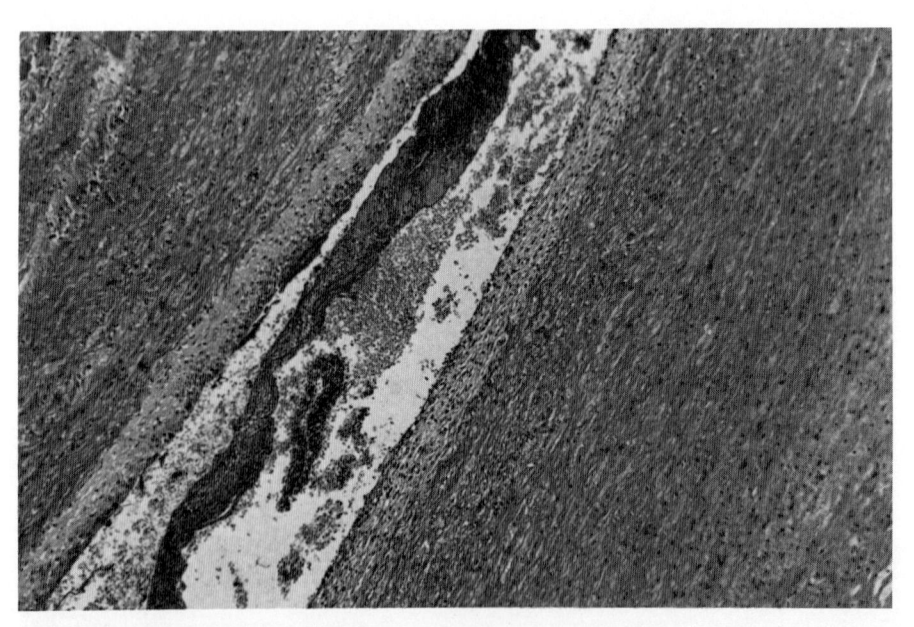

Figure 16.6. Aortic dissection. This dissection took place 1 month before the patient's death. The dissected channel, running through the *center* of the photograph, has formed new intimal structures over the exposed media.

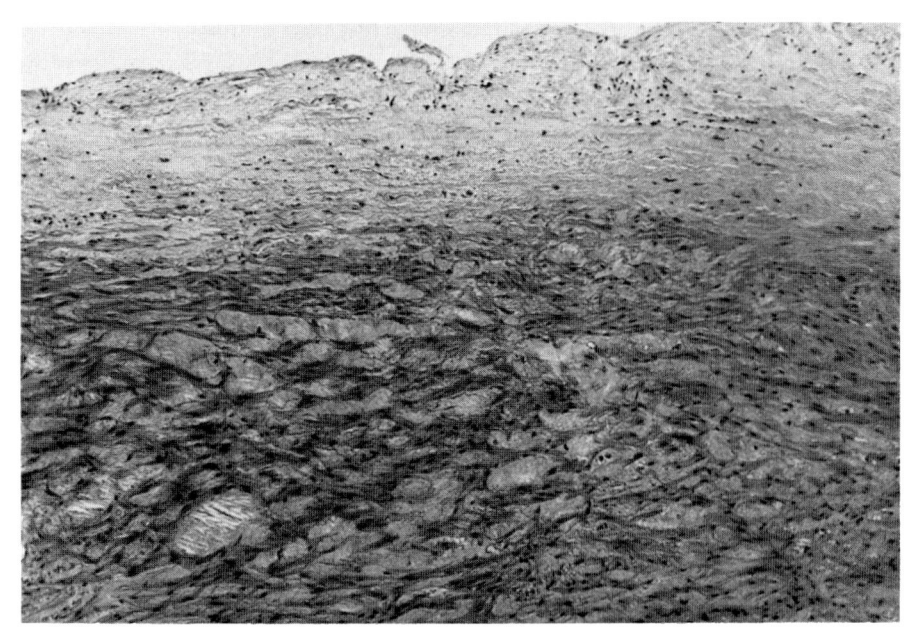

Figure 16.7. Medial cystic necrosis of aorta. The media shows multiple cyst-like spaces filled with mucopolysaccharide. There is resulting disruption of elastic fibers.

MÖNCKEBERG'S SCLEROSIS

Mönckeberg's medial sclerosis consists of calcification of medium-sized muscular arteries, and is particularly prominent in vessels of the extremities. Individual arteries show circumferential calcification, restricted to the media, often with metaplastic bone and bone marrow formation. The intima is not involved, and the lumen is not reduced.

Although this disorder may not be a specific entity, it can be distinguished from atherosclerosis, even when the two coexist in the same artery. It is observed principally above the age of 50, and is thought to be related to prolonged arterial spasm.

FIBROMUSCULAR DYSPLASIA

This is an uncommon arterial disorder, but it has assumed importance as a cause of renal ischemia and hypertension. Involvement of the renal arteries is often unilateral, and removal of an ischemic kidney may alleviate or cure hypertension. The lesion is characterized by areas of medial hypertrophy or fibrosis, resulting in focal stenosis. Arteriographic study may show a beaded appearance, due to alternating foci of stenosis and dilatation.

VASCULITIS

There are many causes of vasculitis, including infections, immunologically mediated injury, and injury by ionizing radiation, toxic substances, and trauma.

Only a few examples of vasculitis, principally arteritides, are mentioned here, and these but briefly.

Vasculitis in Infections

Vasculitis is prominent in many infections. Reference has already been made to the widespread acute endothelial injury in rickettsial disease. Vasculitis may also be prominent in many bacterial diseases, particularly Gram-negative infections, but also in such disorders as tuberculosis. Emboli arising in infective endocarditis may injure peripheral arterial walls, with the formation of mycotic aneurysms. In all of these lesions, thrombosis is a frequent consequence of vessel injury.

Syphilitic Arteritis

The characteristic vascular lesion of syphilis is an obliterative endarteritis. It consists of intimal proliferative narrowing of the lumens of small arteries, and is observed in all stages of syphilis: the chancre, mucocutaneous lesions of secondary syphilis, and in the gumma and such other tertiary manifestations as aortitis and meningovascular syphilis. Vasculitis does not appear to play a role in general paresis or tabes dorsalis.

Aortitis results from endarteritis of the vasa vasorum. It is most marked in the ascending and upper thoracic aorta, and consists of a loss of elastic tissue and weakening of the wall. Longitudinal wrinkling gives a tree bark appearance, and grayish fibrous plaques of the intima may be prominent. Dilatation of the aortic root and aortic valve ring are responsible for incompetence of the valve. The valvular commissures appear separated, and the free edges of the leaflets are rolled. The coronary ostia may be sufficiently narrowed by the aortitis to interfere with coronary artery flow.

Aneurysms of the ascending aorta and arch are often the result of syphilitic aortitis, as are many occurring in the descending thoracic aorta. Syphilitic aneurysms are usually saccular and are likely to compromise mediastinal structures (Fig. 16.8). The esophagus may be compressed, and respiratory function may be impaired. Left recurrent laryngeal nerve paralysis is frequent. Pulsating aneurysms may erode the vertebral bodies and ribs.

Polyarteritis Nodosa

Polyarteritis nodosa is an immune complex-mediated disorder of small and medium-sized arteries. It is primarily a disease of young adults, and shows a male predominance of at least 2:1.

The lesions of polyarteritis nodosa are characterized by focal areas of fibrinoid necrosis, often involving only part of the circumference of an artery. There is an inflammatory cell infiltration through the entire vessel wall and surrounding connecting tissue, consisting of polymorphonuclear leukocytes and mononuclear phagocytes (see Fig. 8.5). Eosinophils are often prominent. Thrombosis of the lumen is frequent, causing distal areas of infarction. The eccentric distribution of injury can be responsible for aneurysm formation. Lesions are usually widespread among small arteries, but may also be observed in the renal, mesenteric, coronary, or cerebral arteries.

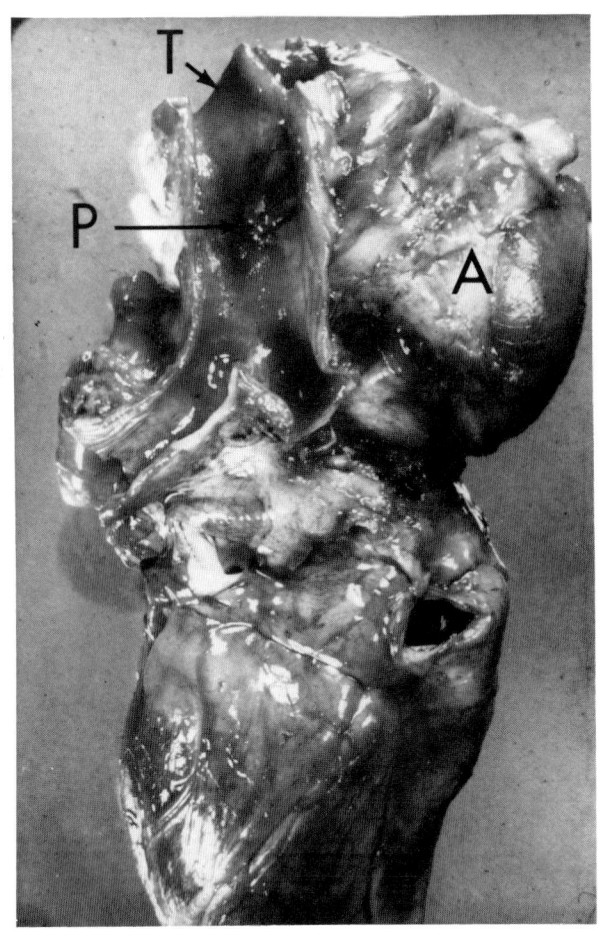

Figure 16.8. Syphilitic aneurysm of aorta. The unopened heart is seen *below*. A large aneurysm (*A*) has arisen from the ascending aorta. The trachea (*T*) has been opened posteriorly, revealing perforation of the aneurysm into the trachea (*P*). This was the cause of death.

Clinical evidence of illness varies, but often includes fever, hypertension, abdominal pain, peripheral neuritis, hematuria, and renal failure. Increased numbers of circulating eosinophils are often noted.

Polyarteritis nodosa is often a manifestation of hypersensitivity to drugs or foreign sera. Hepatitis B antigen may be the sensitizing substance in as many as one-third of patients; there is a high incidence of hepatitis B surface antigenemia, and immune complexes containing the antigen can be identified in the circulation.

The term *hypersensitivity angiitis* is often used to describe lesions similar to polyarteritis involving arterioles, capillaries, and venules. Hypersensitivity to sulfonamides is particularly associated with this finding. Renal involvement may be severe, and lead to rapid renal failure.

Arterial lesions with many of the feature of polyarteritis nodosa may be encountered in patients with rheumatoid arthritis and rheumatic fever.

Wegener's Granulomatosis

This disorder is characterized by arterial lesions similar to those of polyarteritis nodosa, most prominent in the lungs and upper respiratory tract, and associated with granuloma formation. Chronic sinusitis, nasopharyngeal ulcers, and pulmonary cavities are frequent findings. Focal necrotizing lesions may be found in many renal glomeruli and death may be due to renal failure.

Although Wegener's granulomatosis is thought to be immunologically mediated, immune complexes, as a rule, are not demonstrable in its lesions.

Giant Cell Arteritis

Giant cell arteritis, also termed *temporal arteritis*, consists of scattered granulomatous lesions of medium-sized and small arteries, with a striking predilection to involve the temporal and other cranial arteries. Clinical findings include fever, headache, visual disturbances (blindness, diplopia), and redness and tenderness over the involved arteries.

The granulomas are seen close to the internal elastic membrane, and generally involve the entire circumference (Fig. 16.9). Giant cells are numerous. The intima is greatly thickened and the lumen compromised.

Although immune complexes are occasionally demonstrable in the lesions, the etiology of giant cell arteritis is obscure. It occurs most often in the elderly, and there is a moderate female predominance.

Pulseless Disease

This disorder, first described by Takayasu, is probably not a specific entity, but a syndrome characterized by occlusive narrowing of the proximal branches of

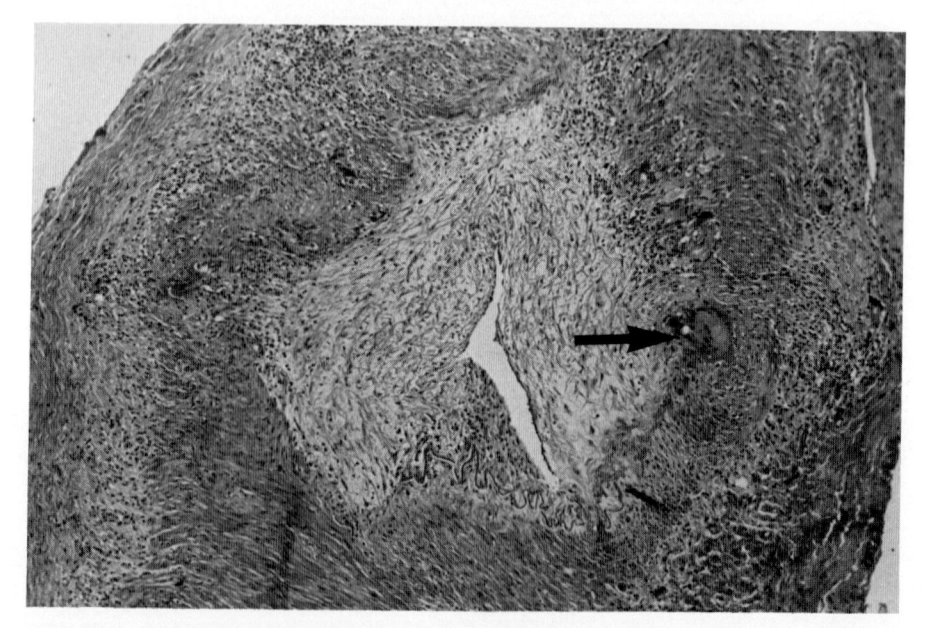

Figure 16.9. Giant cell arteritis. This section of temporal artery shows granulomatous inflammation concentrated in the region of the internal elastic membrane. A giant cell is seen at the *right* (*arrow*). There is marked intimal fibrosis, with compromise of the lumen.

the aorta, and manifested by ischemia of the head and upper extremities. The lesions may resemble atherosclerosis, syphilis, or giant cell arteritis, but there is a marked female predominance, and the onset of disease is usually before the age of 30.

Thromboangiitis Obliterans

Thromboangiitis obliterans or *Buerger's disease* is an occlusive peripheral vascular disease, often apparent by age 35, and showing a dramatic male predominance. It is observed almost exclusively in tobacco smokers.

The lesions start as an acute arteritis, often with luminal thrombosis, and progress to involve adjacent veins and nerve trunks. Extensive fibrosis accompanies healing, with obliteration of arterial and venous channels. The popliteal vessels are the most often involved, but any small or medium-sized arteries, including the mesenterics, may be affected.

The etiology is obscure; immune complexes are not seen. A genetic predisposition is supported by a high incidence of certain HLA haplotypes.

Thrombophlebitis

Thrombophlebitis is the only primarily venous disorder included in this chapter. It is characterized by thrombosis and inflammation of the venous wall. Veins may be injured by spread from adjacent infections; indeed, venous involvement is an important mechanism of dissemination of infection to contiguous and distant tissues. In most circumstances, however, thrombosis appears to occur first (*phlebothrombosis*), and inflammation is part of the local reaction preceding organization.

Causes of thrombosis were reviewed in Chapter 7. Thrombosis, often followed by embolism, is particularly likely to occur in association with congestive heart failure, prolonged immobilization, the postoperative state, neoplastic disease, and use of oral contraceptive agents. The vessels most often involved include the deep leg veins and the pelvic veins. Involved veins, when palpable, are warm and tender, and the overlying skin may be reddened.

A *migratory thrombophlebitis*, often affecting small subcutaneous vessels, may be an early clinical manifestation of occult neoplastic disease.

Suggested Reading

Benditt EP. The origin of atherosclerosis. Sci. Am. *236:* 74, 1977.
Buja LM, Kovanen PT, Bilheimer DW. Cellular pathology of homozygous familial hypercholesterolemia. Am. J. Pathol. *97:* 327, 1979.
Cooper RA, Shattil SJ. Membrane cholesterol—is enought too much? N. Engl. J. Med. *302:* 49, 1980.
Dawber TR. Risk factors for atherosclerotic disease. Kalamazoo, MI, The Upjohn Company, 1975.
Weiss HJ. Platelets and ischemic heart disease. N. Engl. J. Med. *302:* 225, 1980.

Chapter 17

The Kidneys

This chapter includes discussions of the pathology and pathophysiology of chronic renal failure, and the nephrotic and nephritic syndromes. The many disorders initially affecting the glomeruli are summarized, largely in tabular form. Presentation of interstitial and tubular disorders emphasizes pyelonephritis, interstitial nephritis, and acute tubular necrosis, and brief consideration is given to several congenital and neoplastic conditions. The effects of hypertension on the kidneys and the role of the kidneys in initiating or sustaining hypertension is discussed in Chapter 18. Diabetic nephropathy is described in Chapter 26.

RENAL FAILURE

Renal failure is a disturbance of function in which the kidneys fail to maintain the volume and composition of body fluids under conditions of normal fluid and electrolyte intake. Renal failure may be acute or chronic. Focus here is placed on chronic failure; acute renal failure is discussed later in this chapter.

Some of the more important causes of chronic renal failure are listed in Table 17.1. Chronic renal failure implies bilateral disease, most often manifested morphologically by shrunken, granular kidneys, with a symmetrical loss of parenchyma.

The nephron is the functional and structural unit of the kidney; both the number of nephrons and their integrity are prerequisite to normal function. Although there are varying pathways to renal failure, all progressive renal diseases result in loss of nephrons. Hypertension affects the kidney by first altering the small arteries and afferent arterioles, glomerulonephritis by injuring the glomerular filter, and pyelonephritis by attacking the interstitium. All eventually affect entire nephrons, and can lead to the functional disorder of renal failure. Since all can cause a symmetrical loss of nephrons, the morphologic result, or "end stage kidney," may be remarkably similar.

If a normal adult loses a kidney, the contralateral organ undergoes a structural and functional hypertrophy, limited to an increase of some 25 to 30%. Renal function, as measured by creatinine clearance, would fall from 120 ml per min to 60 immediately following loss of a kidney. Over a period of several months, clearance would increase to approximately 75 ml per min. No new nephrons are formed; the response is entirely a hypertrophy.

Nephrons are lost gradually in the course of progressive renal disease. This loss is compensated for a considerable period of time by hypertrophy of remaining

Table 17.1
Some Causes of Renal Failure

Vascular disorders	Metabolic disorders
Nephrosclerosis, benign and malignant	Diabetic nephropathy
Bilateral cortical necrosis	Amyloidosis
Infection	Gout
Pyelonephritis	Nephrocalcinosis
Immunologic injuries	Congenital disorders
Acute glomerulonephritis	Hereditary nephropathy
Membranoproliferative glomerulonephritis	Polycystic kidneys
Rapidly progressive glomerulonephritis	Renal hypoplasia
Membranous glomerulonephritis	Obstructive uropathy
Chronic nonspecific glomerulonephritis	Ionizing radiation
Systemic lupus erythematosus	Analgesic abuse
Polyarteritis nodosa	Acute tubular necrosis
Systemic sclerosis	Disseminated intravascular coagulation
Acute interstitial nephritis	

nephrons, with increased glomerular filtration and tubular maxima *per nephron*. Normal function is at first maintained, but, when no more hypertrophy is possible, functional loss becomes evident. When function is reduced to less than 50% of normal, retention of urea, creatinine, and other products can be noted, and, with each further 50% reduction, levels of retained metabolites tend to double. This may convey the impression that disease is progressing rapidly, when, in fact, the course has been gradual and prolonged.

Since progressive renal disease results in the loss of entire nephrons, there is a balanced loss of glomerular and tubular functions. Renal function in renal failure is characterized by an osmotic diuresis (per functioning nephron) due to retained urea. This diuresis is responsible for excretion of a large fraction of the glomerular filtrate so that the urine approaches the composition of plasma. There is poor conservation of sodium, and a decreased concentrating capacity. The alterations of nephron function are summarized in Figure 17.1.

An important consequence of these adaptations is that it is difficult to distinguish among the major chronic kidney diseases on the basis of altered function.

The End Stage Kidney

The morphologic changes that characterize the end stage kidney result from a progressive loss of nephrons, often associated with previously existing or superimposed vascular disease. The kidney is usually small, with a granular cortical surface composed of small pitted scars and grayish elevated nodules (Figs. 17.2 and 17.3). The cortical mass is reduced. The glomeruli show loss of their delicate filter structure, and progressive solidification. Many of the tubules are atrophic and scarred, while others are strikingly hypertrophied and dilated (Figs. 17.4 to 17.6). Afferent arteriolar hyalinization and intimal thickening of interlobular arteries may be prominent if hypertension was an important clinical manifestation.

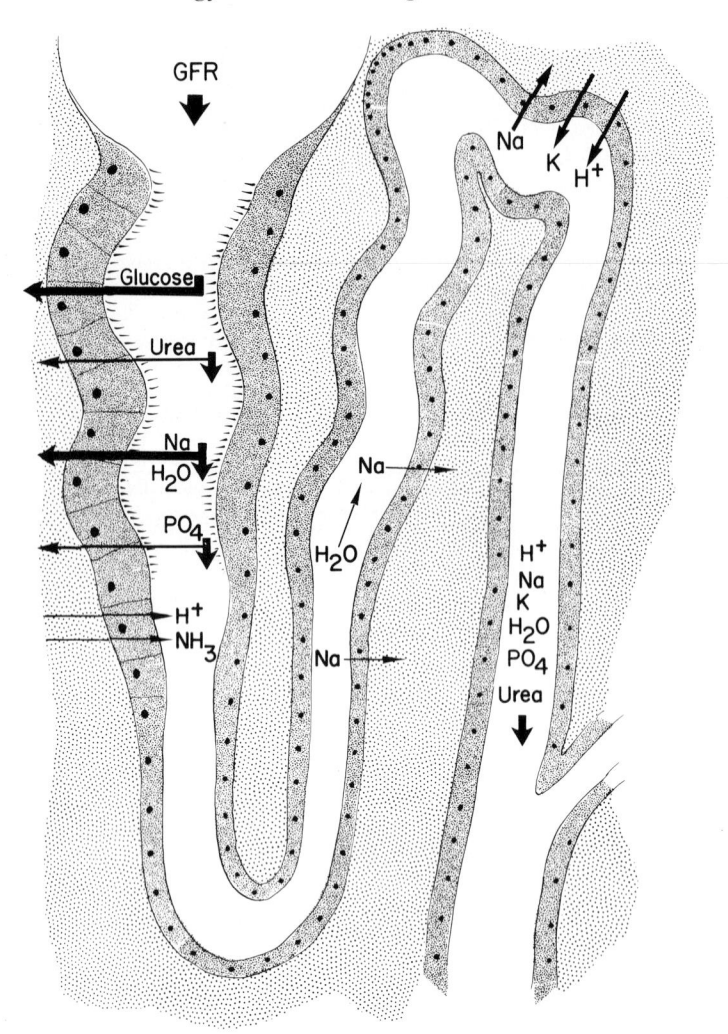

Figure 17.1. Schematic diagram of the nephron in renal failure. There is a reduced number of nephrons, and glomerular filtration rate is increased in each functioning nephron. There is proximal tubular hypertrophy and the resorptive capacity is increased, so that despite the increased filtered load per nephron, all glucose is resorbed. An increased quantity of urea is filtered and escapes resorption. An increased amount of salt and water also escapes proximal resorption. There is increased parathyroid hormone activity, and the tubular resorption of phosphate is decreased. Hydrogen ions entering the tubular lumen are buffered by the increased amount of phosphate. Ammonia production is not proportionally increased, and hydrogen ions are excreted more as titratable acid than buffered by ammonia. Sodium resorption occurs in the ascending limb of the loop of Henle, allowing for dilution of the urine, but the quantitative reduction in the number of nephrons and the osmotic diuresis decrease maximal urinary concentration. Sodium is resorbed by exchange for potassium in the distal tubule. The increased quantity of sodium delivered per nephron to this site allows for a relatively large quantity of potassium to be excreted. The final urine often reflects more urea, water, potassium, sodium, hydrogen ion, and phosphate per nephron than occurs when there is a normal number of healthy nephrons.

The Kidneys

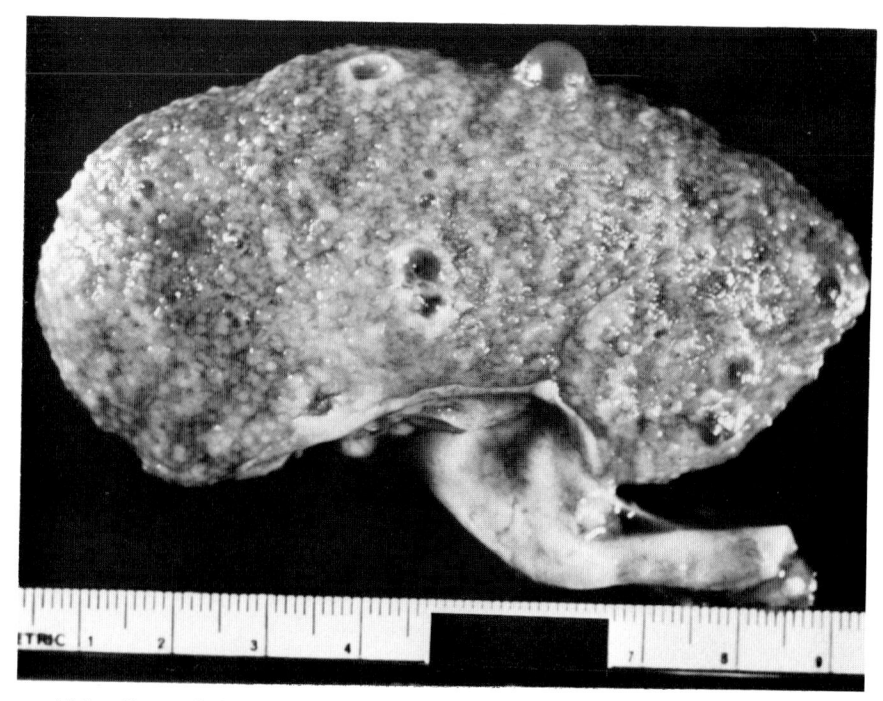

Figure 17.2. External view of kidney weighing 60 g from a patient dying of chronic renal disease. There is symmetrical loss of parenchyma. The cortical surface is diffusely granular, with grayish elevated nodules separated by pitted scars.

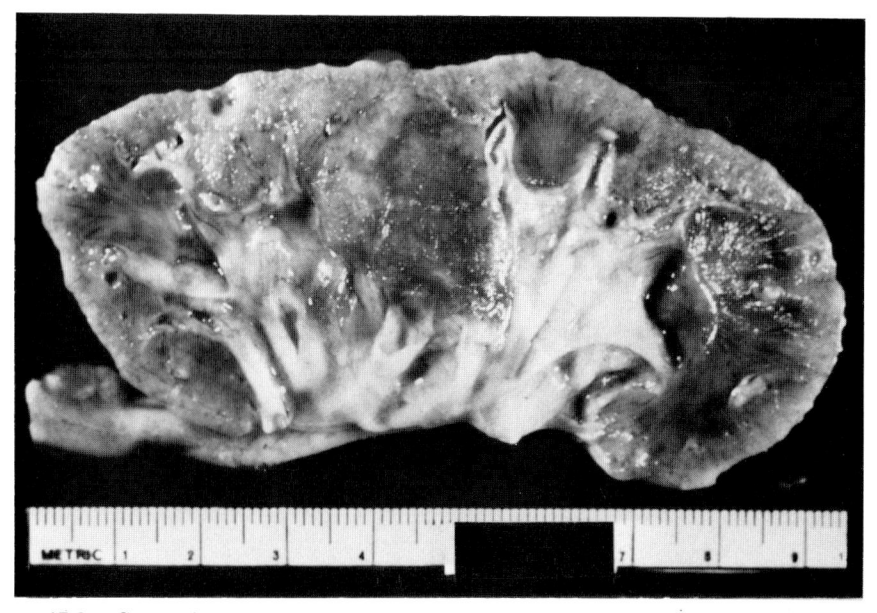

Figure 17.3. Cut section of kidney shown in Figure 17.2. The thin cortex is poorly demarcated from the medulla.

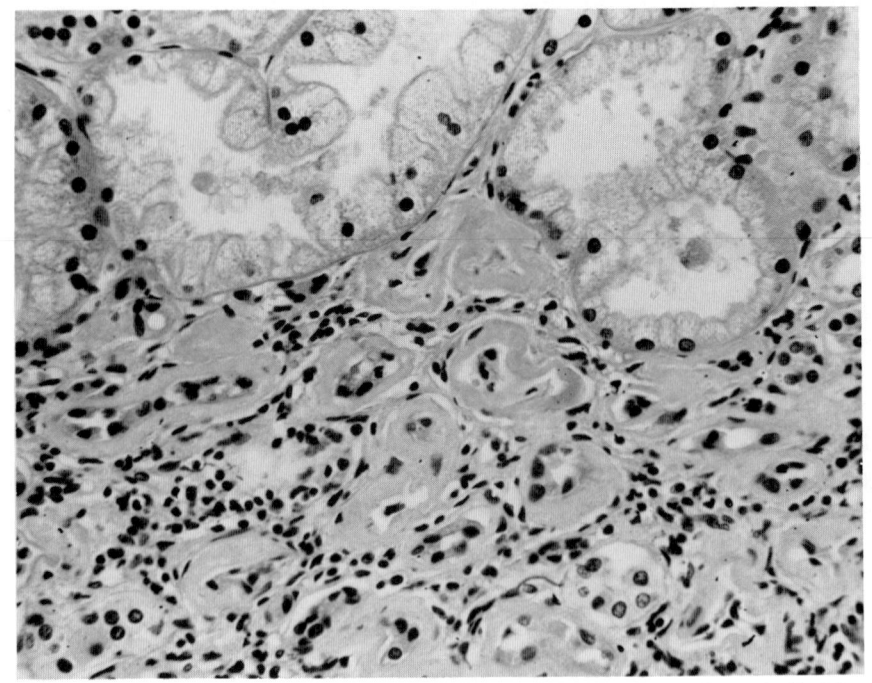

Figure 17.4. Tubular atrophy in chronic renal disease. The tubules in the *lower half* of the field are shrunken and display atrophic lining cells together with markedly thickened basement membranes. The tubules in the *upper half* are normal or slightly enlarged in caliber, and are lined by prominent cells with granular cytoplasm.

Azotemia and Uremia

Azotemia is an elevation of blood urea concentration. Uremia is the symptom complex that results from the retention of nitrogenous products in patients with renal failure.

Azotemia (and occasionally uremia) can occur in the absence of intrinsic renal disease. This is usually the result of decreased renal perfusion, as in congestive heart failure, the hepatorenal syndrome, or shock, but it can also follow gastrointestinal hemorrhage or excessive protein intake, presenting the kidneys with an inordinate urea load.

In addition to azotemia, patients with advanced renal failure show retention of creatinine, uric acid, phosphate, sulfate, and organic anions. Metabolic acidosis is due to retention of hydrogen ions. The serum potassium may be dangerously elevated, due in part to retention and in part to release of cellular potassium because of acidosis. Sodium and water retention is variable, depending in large part on intake, since both the capacity to excrete and to conserve are impaired.

The Uremic Syndrome

The manifestations of the uremic syndrome include disturbed function of most body systems. There is generalized weakness, weight loss, and poor appetite. There may be symptoms of water intoxication or sodium depletion. The brain is

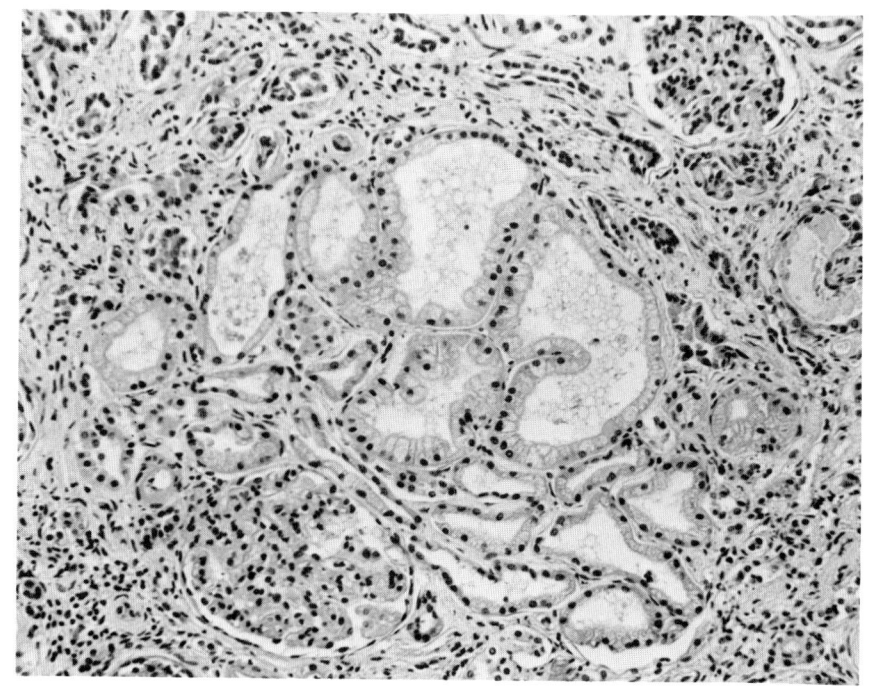

Figure 17.5. Hypertrophied tubules. The tubules in the *center* are dilated, and are lined by prominent epithelial cells. Glomeruli are noted at the *upper right* and *lower left*.

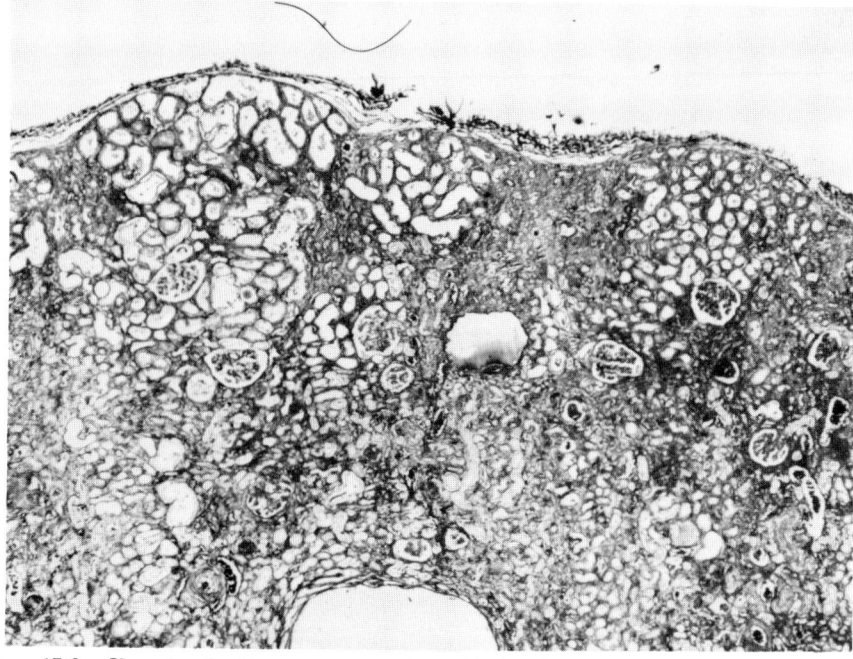

Figure 17.6. Hypertrophied tubules beneath the cortical surface correspond to the elevated nodules seen in Figure 17.2. The intervening pitted areas are atrophic and scarred.

often edematous, with petechial hemorrhages, and patients show poor mental concentration, lethargy, and occasionally convulsions. Central nervous system depression is often associated with neuromuscular irritability.

Fibrinous pericarditis is seen in severe renal failure. Congestive heart failure often complicates the uremic syndrome; this may be due to a uremic cardiomyopathy or to coexisting hypertension. Uremic pneumonitis is a centrally distributed edema, typically of high protein concentration, with hyaline membrane formation.

Gastrointestinal lesions include stomatitis, esophagitis, gastritis, and a hemorrhagic ulcerative colitis. Focal pancreatitis is common, but may not be clinically apparent.

Skin changes include pruritis, easy bruising, and a maculopapular eruption. The skeleton is likely to show renal osteodystrophy, a severe and often painful metabolic disturbance, described in Chapter 31.

Anemia always accompanies chronic renal failure, and is proportional to the severity of azotemia. It can result from decreased marrow activity secondary to the loss of erythropoietin, from a shortened red cell life span, or both, and is often aggravated by bleeding. Platelet function is often depressed, and thromboembolic phenomena are less common than anticipated in patients so ill. There may be significant blood loss, particularly through the gastrointestinal tract.

Death is most often due to infection, complications of severe hypertension, congestive heart failure, or hemorrhage.

THE NEPHROTIC SYNDROME

The clinical manifestations of the nephrotic syndrome include proteinuria in excess of 3 g per 24 hr, hypoproteinemia, edema, lipiduria, and hypercholesterolemia. Systemic blood pressure more often than not is normal, and azotemia is not usually observed, at least early in the course.

There are many diseases that are associated with the nephrotic syndrome, but all have in common a primary alteration of the glomerular filter apparatus that permits passage of excessive protein. The glomerular changes are usually readily recognized, but may be subtle and visible only by electron microscopy. Table 17.2 lists the principal causes of the nephrotic syndrome. Nephrotic patients with renal vein thrombosis are usually found to have glomerular changes indistinguishable from membranous glomerulonephritis.

Proteinuria, which may reach 25 or 50 g per 24 hr, is usually nonselective; *i.e.*, several or all plasma proteins are present. It may be selective, however, limited to albuminuria. The edema of the nephrotic syndrome, particularly in children, may be prominent in the facial and periorbital tissues. *Anasarca*, or generalized

Table 17.2
Principal Causes of the Nephrotic Syndrome

Membranoproliferative glomerulonephritis	Hereditary nephropathy
Membranous glomerulonephritis	Diabetic glomerulosclerosis
Lipoid nephrosis	Systemic lupus erythematosus
Poststreptococcal glomerulonephritis	Amyloidosis
Focal glomerulonephritis	Renal vein thrombosis

edema, may be massive, including fluid accumulations in the serous cavities. Pulmonary edema, however, is uncommon; if present, it usually indicates superimposed congestive heart failure.

As plasma albumin decreases, plasma cholesterol levels increase. Hyperlipidemia results from impaired lipid binding and transport, and increased hepatic production of lipoproteins. Lipids in the urine take the form of doubly refractile cholesterol esters, and desquamated lipid-containing tubular epithelial cells ("oval fat bodies").

Hypoproteinemia leads to a decreased plasma volume and a decrease in glomerular filtration rate. Retained sodium and water further dilute the plasma, and tend to pass to the interstitial fluid compartment. The low plasma volume stimulates aldosterone secretion, producing further sodium retention and edema. In addition to the effects of altered glomerular filtration and the secretion of aldosterone, edema formation in the nephrotic syndrome can be promoted by increased proximal tubular resorption of sodium.

It is important to recognize the nephrotic syndrome because of its diagnostic and prognostic implications. It is unlikely to remain unchanged for prolonged periods. It may subside, with a return of renal function to normal; more often, it represents a stage in progressive renal disease, and presages eventual renal failure.

THE NEPHRITIC SYNDROME

The nephritic syndrome is an acute illness characterized by hematuria, red cell casts, proteinuria (usually less than 2 g per 24 hr), hypertension, oliguria, and, frequently, azotemia. It always indicates glomerular injury. Acute poststreptococcal glomerulonephritis is the classical example of this syndrome, but it is also observed in many patients with membranoproliferative glomerulonephritis, rapidly progressive glomerulonephritis, and systemic lupus erythematosus.

Glomerulonephritis may become manifest with an abrupt onset of gross hematuria, sometimes tea-colored or dark brown as a result of hemolysis in an acid urine. Microscopic examination of the urine shows red blood cell casts, pointing to bleeding high in many nephrons. Granular casts and casts containing polymorphonuclear leukocytes may also be present. In other patients, edema may be the sign that signals disease. In children, it is likely to be facial or periorbital. Hypertension is usually mild or moderate, but hypertensive encephalopathy with convulsions or coma can occur. Congestive heart failure is a not infrequent complication. Some retention of nitrogenous products is usual, and severe acute nephritis may lead to uremia.

DISORDERS PRIMARILY AFFECTING THE GLOMERULUS

A considerable number of disorders injure the renal glomerulus. Some present clinically as an acute nephritis, others with the nephrotic syndrome, and several may present either way.

The study of glomerular disease has been made unduly difficult by a nomenclature that is, at best, irrational. The name poststreptococcal glomerulonephritis implies etiology, while rapidly progressive glomerulonephritis indicates a clinical course; membranoproliferative glomerulonephritis defines morphologic changes, and Berger's disease is an eponym.

Table 17.3
Summary of Diseases Primarily Affecting the Glomerulus

Disease	Age Predominance	Clinical Presentation	Serum Complement	Light Microscopy	Electron Microscopy	Immunofluorescent Findings	Course
Acute poststreptococcal glomerulonephritis	Children, young adults	Nephritic syndrome	↓C3	Proliferation Monocyte or granulocyte infiltration	Subepithelial "humps"	Granular deposits; IgG, IgM, C3	Complete recovery in 85–95% of children, over 50% of adults
Membranoproliferative glomerulonephritis Type I	Children, young adults	Acute nephritis; occasional nephrotic syndrome	↓C3, persistent in many. ↓C4	Mesangial proliferation; thickened capillary walls Lobular simplification	Split basement membranes Subendothelial and subepithelial deposits	Granular deposits; IgG, IgM, C3	Nephrotic syndrome in most Renal failure in 50% within 10 yr
Membranoproliferative glomerulonephritis Type II (dense deposit disease)	Children, young adults	Acute nephritis; occasional nephrotic syndrome	↓C3, persistent	Same as Type I	Dense, linear intramembranous deposits	Deposits containing C3; no immunoglobulins	Same as Type I
Rapidly progressive glomerulonephritis	10–40 yr	Insidious onset, nephritic, often nephrotic	N	Crescentic glomerulonephritis	Fibrin deposits in Bowman's space Glomerular destruction	Some have anti-glomerular basement membrane antibodies Others have scattered granular deposits	Relentless progression to renal failure in weeks or months, if untreated
Lipoid nephrosis	Children	Nephrotic syndrome, often abrupt Selective albuminuria	N	Usually normal	Foot process fusion	Negative	Relapsing, but with complete recovery in 95%

The Kidneys

Focal segmental sclerosis (?variant of lipoid nephrosis)	Children	Nephrotic syndrome Nonselective proteinuria	N	Focal, segmental injury and solidification, especially in juxtamedullary glomeruli	Focal IgM and C3 fluorescence	Slowly deteriorating renal function, hypertension and death in 3–15 yr
Membranous glomerulonephritis	15–50 yr	Nephrotic syndrome Hypertension and hematuria may appear early	N or ↓C3	Diffuse capillary wall thickening	Extensive subepithelial granular deposits	Progression to renal failure, often over 10 to 15 yr period
IgA nephropathy (Berger's disease)	6–40 yr	Mild or gross hematuria and selective proteinuria	N or ↓C3	Focal prominence of mesangium	Mesangial deposits	Prolonged benign course; 15% progress to renal failure
Systemic lupus erythematosus	Young women	Nephritic syndrome, without hypertension Nephrotic syndrome	↓C1q ↓C3 ↓C4	Various focal and diffuse proliferative or necrotizing lesions	Mesangial complexes containing C3, IgA, and some IgG Deposits containing IgG, IgA, IgM, C3, C4 Extensive subendothelial deposits Myxovirus-like particles	Slow or rapid progression to renal failure, if untreated
Chronic glomerulonephritis	Adults	Hematuria and proteinuria Hypertension	N	Progressive glomerular obsolescence Obliteration of glomeruli by basement membrane-like material or collagen	Scattered small complexes	Slow progression to renal failure in 3–30 yr

In nearly all of these disorders, glomerular injury is immunologically mediated. Immune complex deposition is the most frequent mechanism, but antiglomerular basement membrane antibodies are the basis of injury in some examples of rapidly progressive glomerulonephritis, including Goodpasture's syndrome. There is no laboratory or morphologic evidence of immune mechanisms in lipoid nephrosis.

Table 17.3 is an attempt to simplify the presentation of the glomerular diseases. Most of the salient features are found in this table or in the illustrations, permitting brief discussion in the text.

Acute Poststreptococcal Glomerulonephritis

Acute poststreptococcal glomerulonephritis is an important disease of children and young adults. It is preceded by a recognizable infection with one of the nephritogenic types of Group A β-hemolytic streptococci, particularly Types 12, 1, 4, 25, and 49. Prior streptococcal infection may be documented by the presence of circulating antibodies to streptococcal antigens. Acute glomerulonephritis may occasionally follow other bacterial or viral infections.

Acute glomerulonephritis presents as the nephritic syndrome. Many patients will have moderate hypertension, and impaired renal function will be manifested by azotemia, decreased renal clearances, and metabolic acidosis. In severe cases, necrosis and thrombosis of glomerular capillaries will be reflected by marked oliguria or anuria (Figs. 17.7 and 17.8).

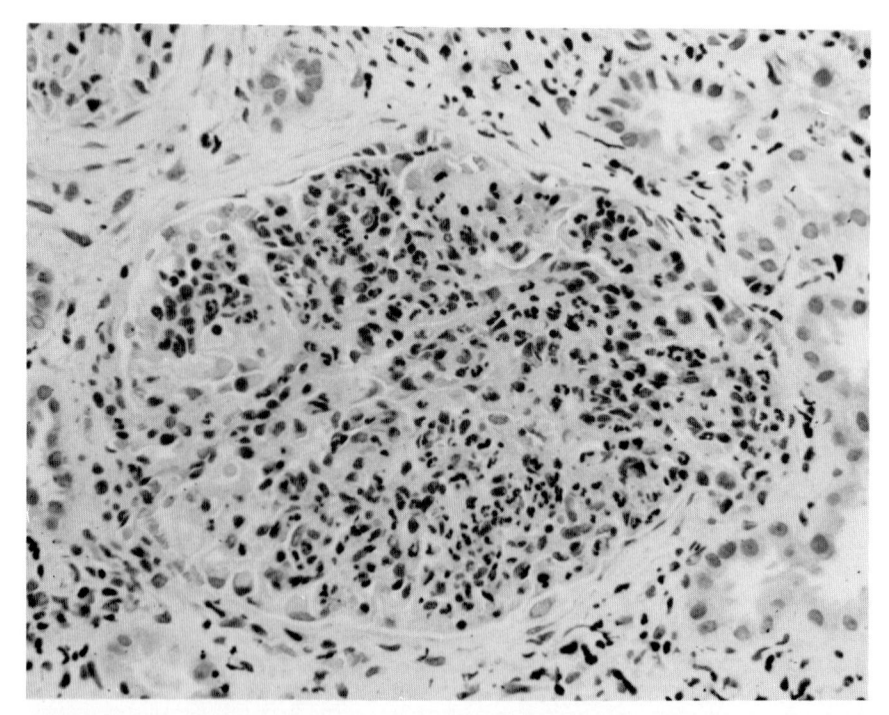

Figure 17.7. Acute glomerulonephritis. There is a striking increase in cellularity, predominately endothelial and mesangial, although many monocytes and polymorphonuclear leukocytes are also present.

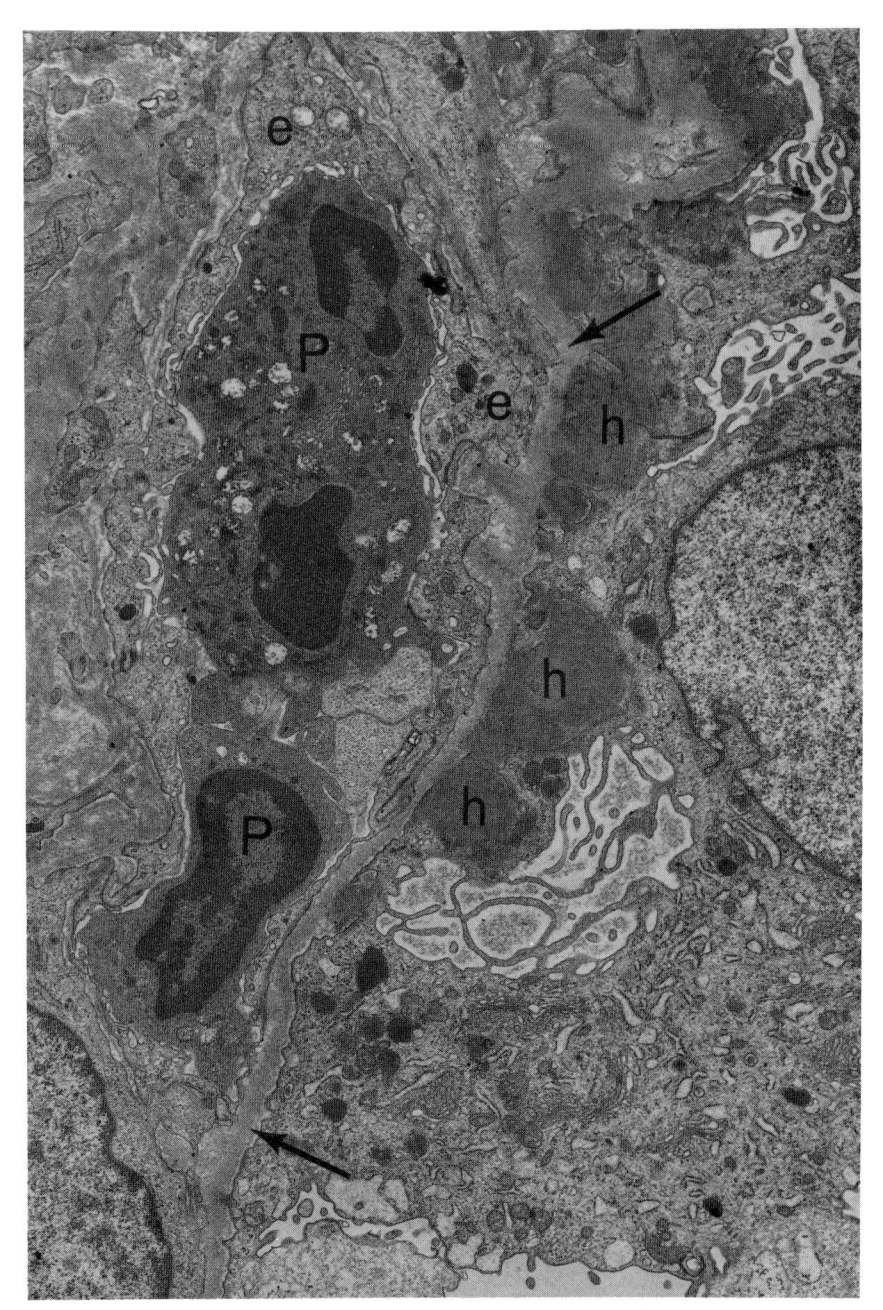

Figure 17.8. Acute glomerulonephritis. Several large hump-like subepithelial deposits (*h*) are seen. There is overlying epithelial foot process fusion. The capillary basement membrane (*arrows*) is normal, but the endothelial cytoplasm (*e*) is thickened. Two leukocytes (*P*) appear to fill the capillary lumen.

The vast majority of children with acute glomerulonephritis will recover completely, although disappearance of all clinical and laboratory evidence of disease may take as long as 2 years. The recovery rate is lower in adults, and poor in the elderly. If death occurs during acute glomerulonephritis, it is most often due to the effects of hypertension and sodium retention on the heart, but severe hypertensive encephalopathy and uremia may also occur.

Membranoproliferative Glomerulonephritis

It is important to differentiate membranoproliferative glomerulonephritis from acute poststreptococcal glomerulonephritis. Membranoproliferative glomerulonephritis tends to involve the same age group, and may present in a very similar manner with a nephritic picture, but it is a progressive disease and eventuates in renal failure. Hypertension is less frequent at the onset. Very occasionally, it appears to follow a streptococcal infection. The nephrotic syndrome may appear early, or be the presenting manifestation, and three-fourths of patients become nephrotic at some point in their illness.

There are two forms of membranoproliferative glomerulonephritis, indistinguishable clinically or on light microscopy (Fig. 17.9). Type I shows granular deposits containing IgG, IgM, and complement at the periphery of the lobules. In Type II, there are dense linear intramembranous deposits containing C3, but no immunoglobulins. In patients with Type II, or dense deposit disease, a nephritic factor, C3neF, is thought to trigger the alternative pathway of complement

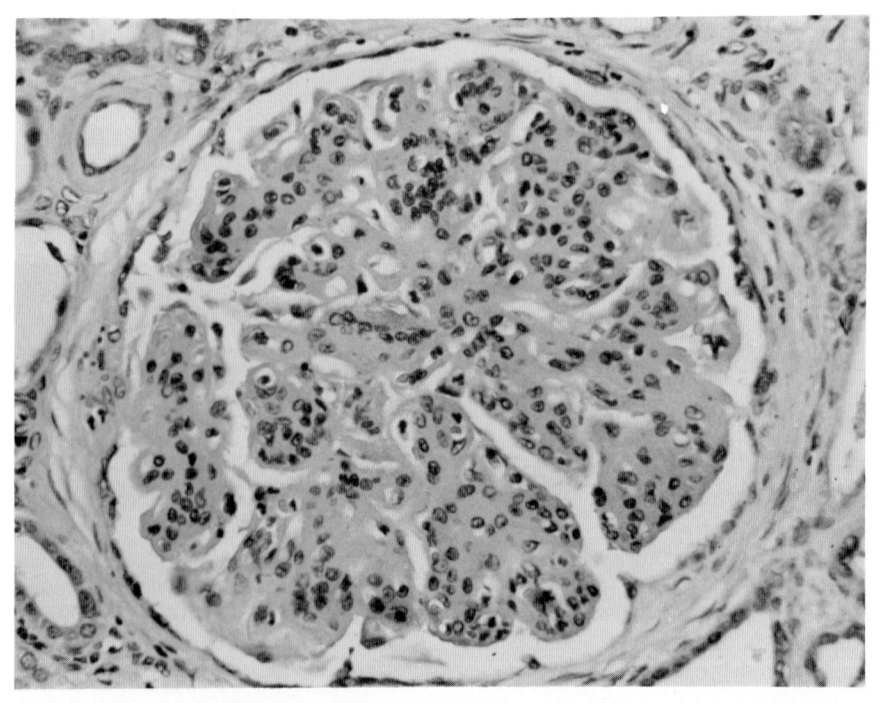

Figure 17.9. Membranoproliferative glomerulonephritis. The glomerulus is large. The proliferation of mesangial cells has produced a lobular simplification of the glomerular architecture. Striking thickening of the capillary walls is noted.

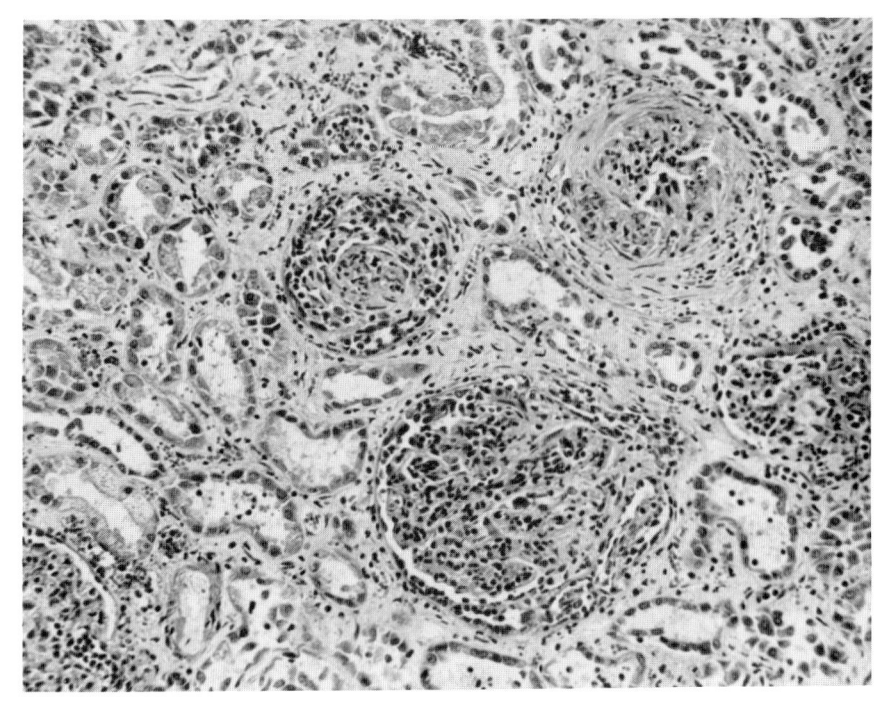

Figure 17.10. Rapidly progressive glomerulonephritis. All of the glomeruli show shrinkage of their tufts, with variable necrosis and polymorphonuclear leukocytic infiltration, and prominent epithelial proliferation with crescent formation.

activation. Hypocomplementemia (C3) may be striking and persistent, particularly in Type II disease.

Rapidly Progressive Glomerulonephritis

Rapidly progressive glomerulonephritis generally has an insidious onset, but shows a steady and rapid progression to death in renal failure in a few weeks or months. The key morphologic feature is the proliferative epithelial crescent, a response to fibrin deposition in Bowman's space, with destruction of the glomerulus (Fig. 17.10).

Immunofluorescence studies show antiglomerular basement membrane antibodies in some patients with this disorder. Goodpasture's syndrome consists of a rapidly progressive glomerulonephritis and pulmonary hemorrhages and hemosiderosis, often following a flu-like illness. Antiglomerular basement membrane antibodies are present, and they appear to react also with pulmonary alveolar basement membranes. Other patients with rapidly progressive glomerulonephritis show immune complex deposition. This is true when rapidly progressive glomerulonephritis occurs in the course of Henoch-Schönlein purpura or polyarteritis nodosa.

Lipoid Nephrosis

Lipoid nephrosis is by far the most frequent cause of the nephrotic syndrome in children, and it is responsible for some 10 to 20% of adult cases. Although there are no morphologic or serologic findings to suggest an immunologically mediated injury, the onset of disease is often relatable to such antigenic stimuli as bee stings and poison ivy, and onset may follow respiratory infections.

The paucity of structural changes in the glomeruli is reflected in the alternative terms *nil disease* and *miminal change disease.* The only consistent finding is foot process fusion on electron microscopy, and this may be a consequence rather than a cause of proteinuria.

Although lipoid nephrosis often follows a relapsing, polycyclic course, the outlook for eventual full recovery of children is highly favorable, particularly with adrenal steroid therapy.

Focal segmental sclerosis is, in all likelihood, a variant of lipoid nephrosis. The glomeruli, starting in the juxtamedullary region, show focal areas of scarring with

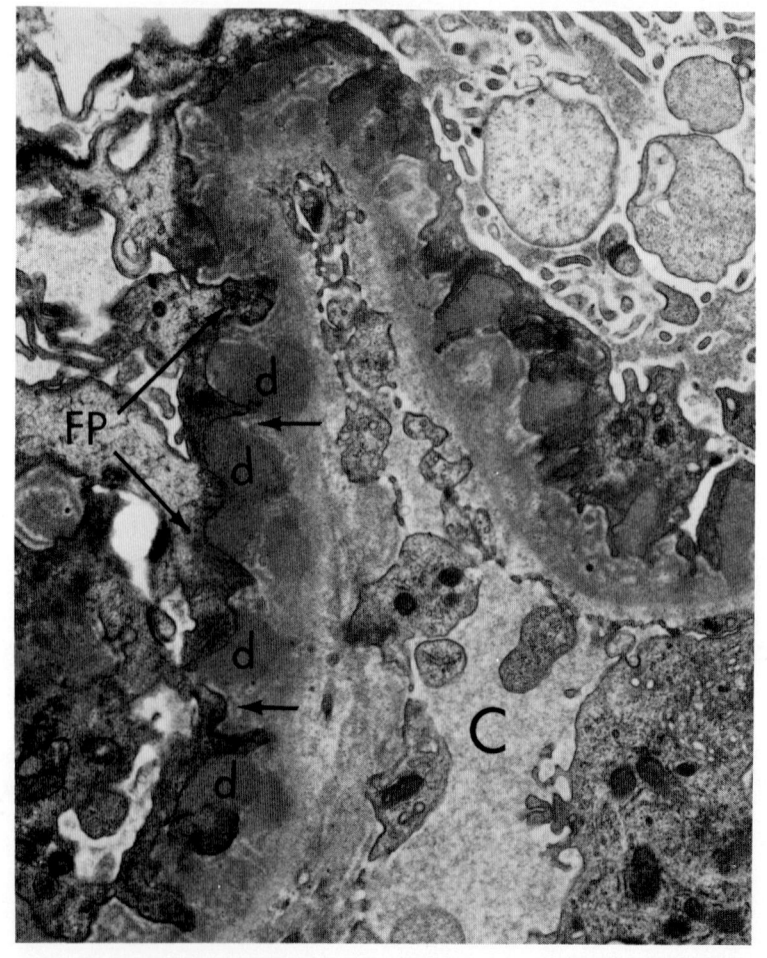

Figure 17.11. Idiopathic membranous glomerulonephritis. This electron micrograph shows a single capillary loop (*C*). There are numerous electron-dense deposits (*d*), mostly subepithelial in location. The basement membrane is thickened and shows spike-like extensions between deposits (*arrows*). There is diffuse fusion of epithelial foot processes (*FP*).

IgM and C3 deposits. In these patients, proteinuria is nonselective (in contrast to the pure albuminuria of lipoid nephrosis), and hematuria occasionally occurs. Hypertension is often present, and patients show a gradual deterioration of renal function, with renal failure after 3 to 15 years.

Another likely variant of lipoid nephrosis has been called *mesangioproliferative glomerulonephritis*, since the glomeruli show a diffuse increase in mesangial matrix and cellularity. Children with this finding tend to respond poorly to adrenal steroid therapy, and suffer progressive renal injury.

Membranous Glomerulonephritis

Membranous glomerulonephritis accounts for some 30% of adult onset nephrotic syndrome, and a very small percentage of childhood disease. It is characterized by extensive subepithelial deposition of large numbers of immune complexes which become incorporated in a thickened basement membrane (Figs. 17.11 and 17.12). It is usually of unknown etiology, although some cases have been related to hepatitis B antigen, tumor-associated antigens, or cryoglobulins. It is the glomerular lesion usually found in nephrotic patients with renal vein thrombosis.

The nephrotic syndrome often begins gradually. The proteinuria is nonselective. Hematuria is frequent, and hypertension develops during the course of disease in many patients. The outlook for recovery is poor, and, although renal

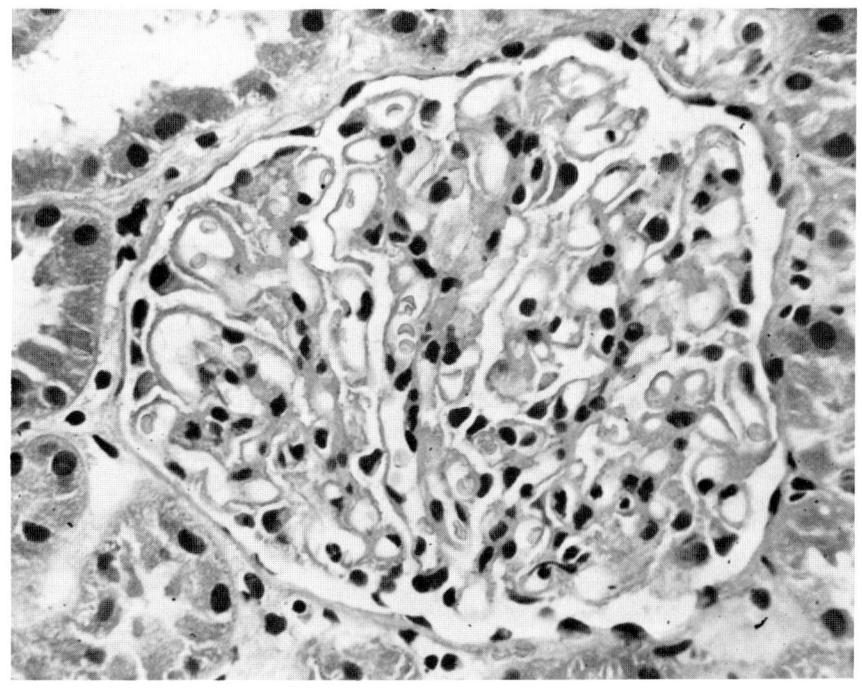

Figure 17.12. Idiopathic membranous glomerulonephritis. There is striking diffuse thickening of the glomerular basement membrane. The capillaries are widely patent, and there is no change in cellularity.

function may remain static for prolonged periods, renal failure is likely to develop after 10 or 15 years.

Berger's Disease

Berger's disease, or *IgA nephropathy*, is thought to be caused by IgG antibodies against IgA. There are large complexes containing IgA, some IgG, and C3 in the mesangium, and there is proliferation of mesangial cells and matrix.

The principal manifestations are hematuria, characteristically appearing within 3 days of an upper respiratory infection, and mild selective proteinuria. The course of disease is usually prolonged and mild, but a few patients progress to renal failure.

Glomerular Disease in Systemic Lupus Erythematosus

There is evidence of kidney involvement in more than 50% of patients during the course of systemic lupus erythematosus. The prognosis is distinctly worsened in those with such severe glomerular changes as diffuse proliferative or membranous glomerulonephritis or widespread mesangial alterations. Patients with only focal lesions usually follow a prolonged and mild course. Immune deposits, often numerous, contain IgA, IgM, IgG, and several complement components. The deposits are usually subendothelial in location (Fig. 8.4). Myxovirus-like particles are often seen in glomeruli.

Therapy with adrenal steroids or immunosuppressive agents is successful in many patients, and proliferative and necrotizing lesions may heal. Some patients, despite therapy, die in renal failure.

Chronic Glomerulonephritis

Chronic glomerulonephritis may be the end result of several of the disorders considered in this section, but it more often represents *de novo* disease. It is but rarely a sequel to poststreptococcal disease. Chronic glomerulonephritis is likely the result of exposure to small doses of antigen over a prolonged period of years.

There is progressive destruction of glomeruli and tubules. Scattered small immune complexes are seen on immunofluorescence microscopy, and electron microscopy shows collapsed capillary walls, and replacement of the normal architecture by masses of basement membrane-like material.

The course is slowly progressive, characterized by hematuria, proteinuria, edema, and hypertension, and renal failure is likely in between 3 and 30 years. In patients receiving transplants, the disease can soon become apparent in the graft.

Other Glomerular Injuries

Extensive thrombosis of glomerular capillaries occurs in disseminated intravascular coagulation (DIC). *Thrombotic thrombocytopenic purpura*, probably a variant of DIC, is often manifested by azotemia and uremia. The *hemolytic uremia syndrome* is characterized by a microangiopathic hemolytic anemia, thrombocytopenia, and acute renal failure, and may also represent a form of DIC. It is observed most often in children, and may follow an upper respiratory infection or diarrhea. There is an extensive acute glomerular injury, and, at times, thrombosis of afferent arterioles and glomerular capillaries.

Systemic amyloidosis frequently involves the glomeruli as well as the renal interstitium and vasculature. Glomerular amyloid infiltration is often associated with the nephrotic syndrome and renal failure, usually without hypertension.

Polyarteritis nodosa (p. 174) frequently involves the kidneys and may lead to renal failure. Glomerular lesions may be focal, or take the pattern of rapidly progressive glomerulonephritis. Involvement of renal artery branches may result in multiple infarcts of cortex and medulla. A focal form of glomerulonephritis is also encountered in Henoch-Schönlein purpura (anaphylactoid purpura). It may heal, or progress gradually. This disorder was also mentioned above as a cause of a rapidly progressive glomerulonephritis. Patients with Wegener's granulomatosis (p. 176) frequently show a focal necrotizing glomerulonephritis.

Patients with chronic bacteremia from bacterial endocarditis or infected arteriovenous shunts may develop a diffuse proliferative glomerulonephritis, indistinguishable from poststreptococcal disease, or a focal form of glomerulonephritis. Although this is often called *embolic glomerulonephritis*, it is more likely the result of circulating immune complexes.

TUBULAR AND INTERSTITIAL DISORDERS

Acute and Chronic Pyelonephritis

The pathogenesis of acute pyelonephritis due to *Escherichia coli* was discussed in Chapter 5, and emphasis was placed on the role of obstructive lesions of the urinary tract and the mechanisms that enable coliform organisms to injure the kidney. Table 17.4 lists some of the more frequently encountered causes of urinary

Table 17.4
Some Causes of Urinary Tract Obstruction

Urethral obstruction
  Congenital valves
  Stricture
  Prostatic hyperplasia and tumors
Bladder obstruction
  Bladder neck hypertrophy
  Chronic cystitis
  Stones
  Bladder tumors
  Neurogenic bladder
Ureteral obstruction
  Ureterovesical scarring or compression by tumors
  Pregnancy
  Stones
  Clots
  Intrinsic and extrinsic tumors
  Adhesive bands
  Anomalous vessels
  Anomalous collecting system
Intrarenal obstruction
  Nephrolithiasis
  Tumors of renal pelvis and parenchyma
  Polycystic kidneys
  Intratubular crystallization
  Nephrocalcinosis
  Chronic renal disease

tract obstruction. Such obstructive lesions are present in the majority of patients with acute pyelonephritis. Although *E. coli* is most often the causative organism, infection may also be due to *Aerobacter aerogenes*, proteus organisms, *Pseudomonas aeruginosa*, and *Streptococcus faecalis*. Pyelonephritis due to *Staphylococcus aureus* is usually part of a generalized sepsis. Viruses may also cause pyelonephritis, and fungi are occasionally identified.

Acute pyelonephritis may be a fulminant infection, with high fever, flank pain, frequency, and dysuria, or it may be associated with few manifestations of illness. The urine contains many polymorphonuclear leukocytes, often included in casts, occasional red blood cells, protein, and large numbers of microorganisms. Urine culture usually reveals more than 100,000 organisms per ml, particularly if enteric species are found. Azotemia and hypertension are uncommon during an acute episode, and antibiotic therapy usually results in a prompt subsidence of the disease. There is, however, a marked predilection for recurrence.

Acute pyelonephritis may involve the kidneys in a patchy manner, or infection may be diffuse. It may be unilateral or bilateral. Infection is first evident in the interstitium, with polymorphonuclear leukocytic infiltration and frequent abcess formation (see Figs. 5.1 and 5.2). The tubules are secondarily involved, but the glomeruli are generally spared. The renal pelvic tissues are virtually always affected.

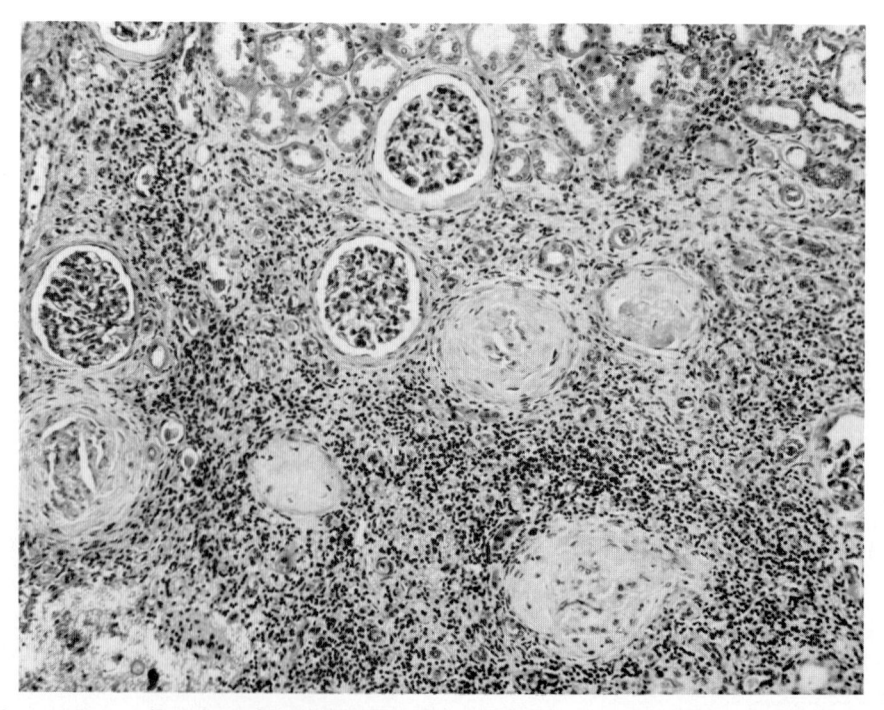

Figure 17.13. Chronic pyelonephritis. Five fibrotic obsolescent glomeruli are recognized. Three other glomeruli appear more normal, but are surrounded by fibrous tissue. In the entire *lower portion* of the field, there is marked loss of tubules and striking infiltration by lymphocytes and some plasma cells.

Chronic pyelonephritis is a progressive disease that may destroy the renal parenchyma and terminate in renal failure. It may be the eventual result of repeated episodes of acute pyelonephritis, but, unless the urinary tract is structurally abnormal, this is a rare occurrence. The same factors important in the pathogenesis of acute pyelonephritis apply to chronic pyelonephritis. Although some microorganisms may persist for prolonged periods in the renal interstitium, it is suggested that it is bacterial antigens that persist and may be responsible for evoking an autoimmune process.

The kidneys in chronic pyelonephritis are generally small and scarred, often showing asymmetry of involvement. There is chronic inflammation, fibrosis, and progressive destruction of nephrons (Fig. 17.13). There is always inflammation and scarring of the calyces and pelves. These structures may be markedly dilated (*hydronephrosis*) in the presence of chronic urinary tract obstruction (Fig. 17.14).

The manifestations of chronic pyelonephritis are variable, but include such findings of renal failure as anemia and impaired handling of sodium and water. Pyuria and proteinuria are often present. Although severely impaired, renal function may remain stable for prolonged periods.

Hypertension is a prominent finding in between one-half and three-fourths of patients with pyelonephritis. Generalized renal vascular changes indistinguishable from those seen in arterial and arteriolar nephrosclerosis (Chapter 18) are found in chronic pyelonephritis and are particularly severe in areas of dense scarring. Patients with chronic pyelonephritis who are not hypertensive may demonstrate vascular changes only in areas of greater involvement, but do not have generalized

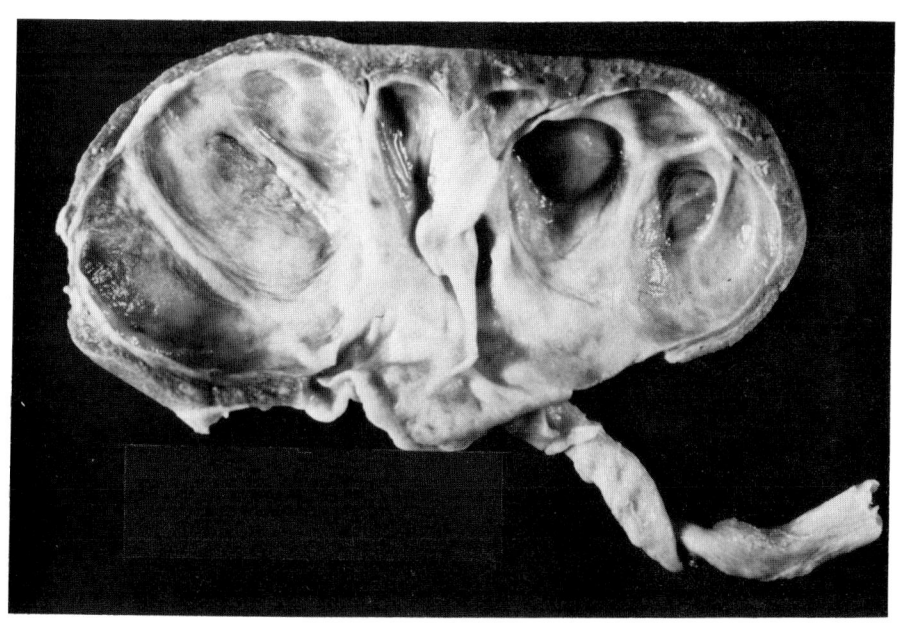

Figure 17.14. Chronic pyelonephritis and hydronephrosis. There has been extensive destruction of the parenchyma. There is marked dilatation of pelvis and calyces, the result of long standing obstruction in the lower urinary tract.

vascular disease. Although the mechanism of hypertension in chronic pyelonephritis is not clear, it is thought that healing of pyelonephritis entraps blood vessels, and that renal blood flow is impaired.

Interstitial Nephritis

Although the interstitium is involved in any progressive renal disease, and is the initial site of infection in pyelonephritis, the term interstitial nephritis refers to a group of disorders characterized by diffuse inflammatory cell infiltration, usually with a predominance of mononuclear phagocytes, lymphocytes, plasma cells, and sometimes eosinophils (Fig. 17.15). A clinically acute interstitial nephritis occurs in patients hypersensitive to penicillin, sulfonamides, rifampin, phenytoin, and other drugs. The kidneys are enlarged and swollen, and renal function impaired. Recovery may be complete, but some patients experience acute renal failure and death in uremia.

Chronic interstitial nephritis is a progressive disorder with destruction of the renal parenchyma, eventuating in renal failure and kidneys that are basically indistinguishable from those of chronic pyelonephritis. One of the most important causes is abuse of analgesic drugs, especially phenacetin and salicylate combinations. There is a very high incidence of necrotizing papillitis, which may represent the initial injury to the kidney.

ACUTE RENAL FAILURE

Acute renal failure results from an abrupt loss of renal function. It is most often a reflection of acute injury to the renal tubules, but may also follow bilateral

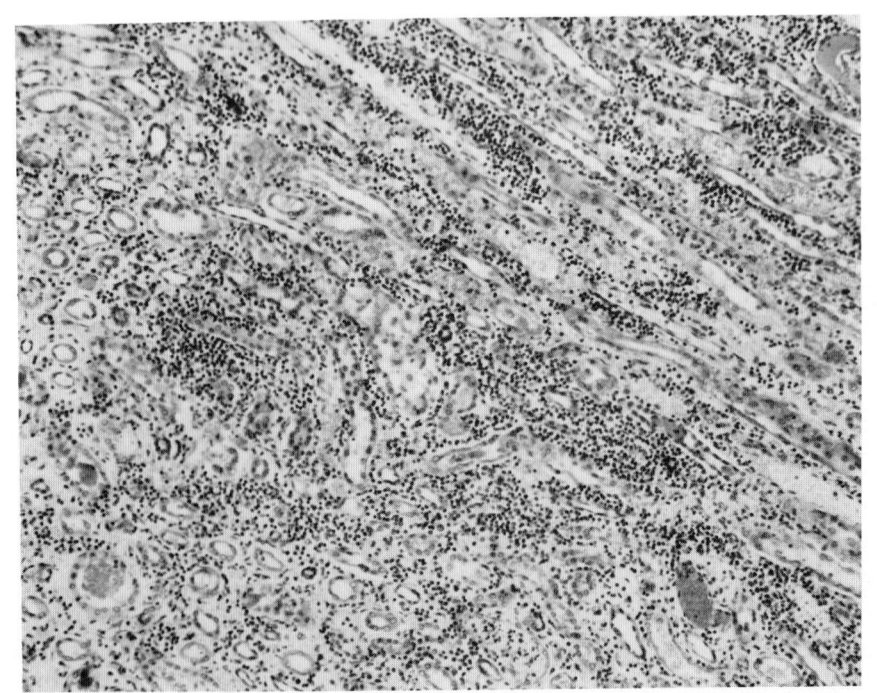

Figure 17.15. Acute interstitial nephritis. There is diffuse infiltration of the interstitium by lymphocytes, plasma cells, and mononuclear phagocytes. The tubules appear uninjured.

cortical necrosis, an uncommon disorder associated with severe hemorrhage and shock. Acute renal failure occasionally signals severe necrotizing glomerular injury in several forms of glomerulonephritis or in malignant hypertension.

Acute Tubular Necrosis

Acute tubular necrosis is most often observed in young healthy individuals following exposure to toxic substances or as a complication of shock. Toxic substances that can injure renal tubules include bichloride of mercury, carbon tetrachloride, sulfonamides, glycols, organic iodides, and aminoglycoside antibiotics. Shock associated with hemolysis, infection, and hemoconcentration is particularly likely to result in ischemic tubular injury. Acute tubular necrosis can also follow shock during surgical procedures, postpartum shock, severe burns, crush injuries, and transfusion reactions.

Oliguria is the usual presenting symptom, urine volume being between 100 and 400 ml per day. There may be evidence of fluid overload. The urine is poorly concentrated, but may contain considerable sodium and protein. Manifestations of uremia may appear within a few days. Potassium retention is characteristic and represents the principal threat to life; it is aggravated by a severe metabolic acidosis, with loss of cellular potassium to the extracellular fluid.

The kidneys are large, edematous, and swollen, and the cortex appears pale. Severe injury with necrosis of tubules resulting from toxic substances is usually easily recognized. The findings following ischemic injury are more subtle. The tubules are markedly dilated and may show prominent nuclei and basophilic

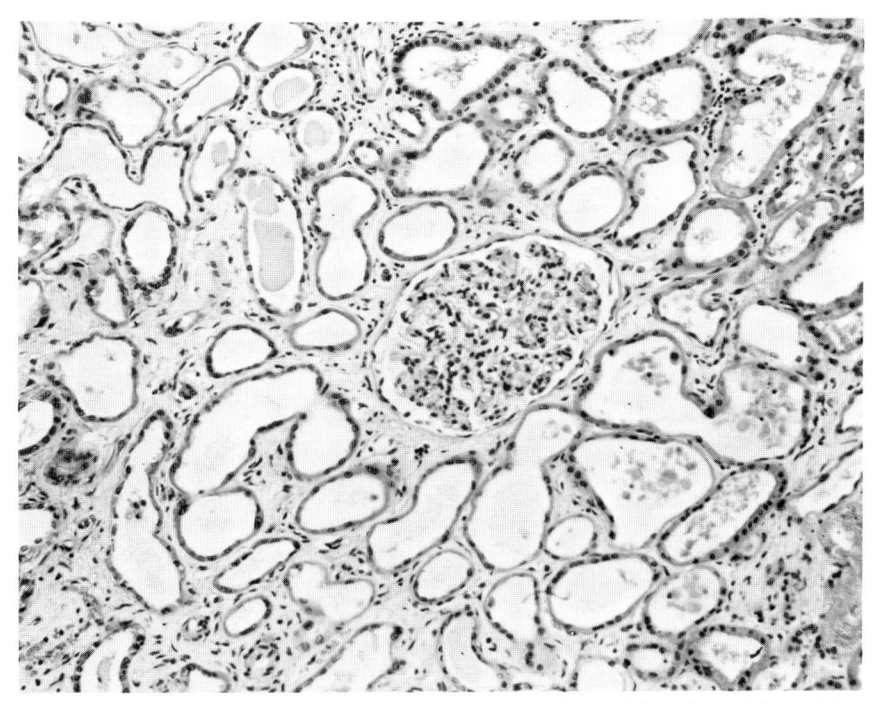

Figure 17.16. Ischemic tubular injury. There is moderate interstitial edema. The tubules are markedly dilated and several show basophilic staining and increased numbers of nuclei. The glomerulus appears normal.

cytoplasm, changes that may represent regenerative activity (Fig. 17.16). Interstitial edema is prominent.

The pathogenesis of acute renal failure in acute tubular necrosis is poorly understood. Explanations based on tubular obstruction by casts, back leakage of tubular contents, increased interstitial pressure, a lower glomerular capillary filtration coefficient, and decreased renal blood flow are not proven.

Oliguria may persist for only 1 or 2 days, or for as long as 8 or 10 weeks. Recovery is heralded by a diuresis, often massive, reflecting fluid overload and the osmotic effects of urea retention. The diuresis is indiscriminate, and there may be severe depletion of sodium and potassium. Tubular functions return to normal or near normal over a prolonged period of time, often 1 or 2 years. Complete morphologic recovery, as evaluated by electron microscopy, is also a slow and gradual process.

MISCELLANEOUS RENAL DISORDERS

Hereditary Nephropathy

There are several forms of hereditary nephropathy. One of these, *Alport's syndrome*, is characterized by glomerular changes with hematuria and proteinuria, and associated nerve deafness and occular abnormalities (cataract, nystagmus, severe myopia). It is transmitted as an autosomal dominant. Males are more severely involved than females, and often progress to renal failure in childhood. Females are affected later and the disorder is less severe. The principal early glomerular change noted on electron microscopy is a poorly formed and fragmented basement membrane. Later changes may be indistinguishable from those of chronic glomerulonephritis.

Polycystic Disease

Adult polycystic disease is transmitted as an autosomal dominant. Multiple cysts, involving all parts of the tubules, are responsible for gross enlargement of both kidneys, which may weigh several kilograms (Fig. 17.17). There is gradual destruction of remaining nephrons, and renal failure may occur during middle years, or, occasionally, late in life. Hypertension is frequent, and polycythemia may result from excessive erythropoietin. There are often associated cysts of the liver, lined by biliary epithelium, and congenital aneurysms of the cerebral arteries.

An infantile form of polycystic disease is inherited as an autosomal recessive, and is usually rapidly fatal.

Medullary Sponge Kidney

In this disorder, there is cystic dilatation of collecting ducts within the medulla and papillae. It is usually noted during adult life, associated with renal calculi. Unless intrarenal obstruction results in a chronic pyelonephritis, the course is benign.

Medullary Cystic Disease

This recessively inherited disease is characterized by numerous cysts in the medulla. Teenaged patients usually present with advanced renal failure and small

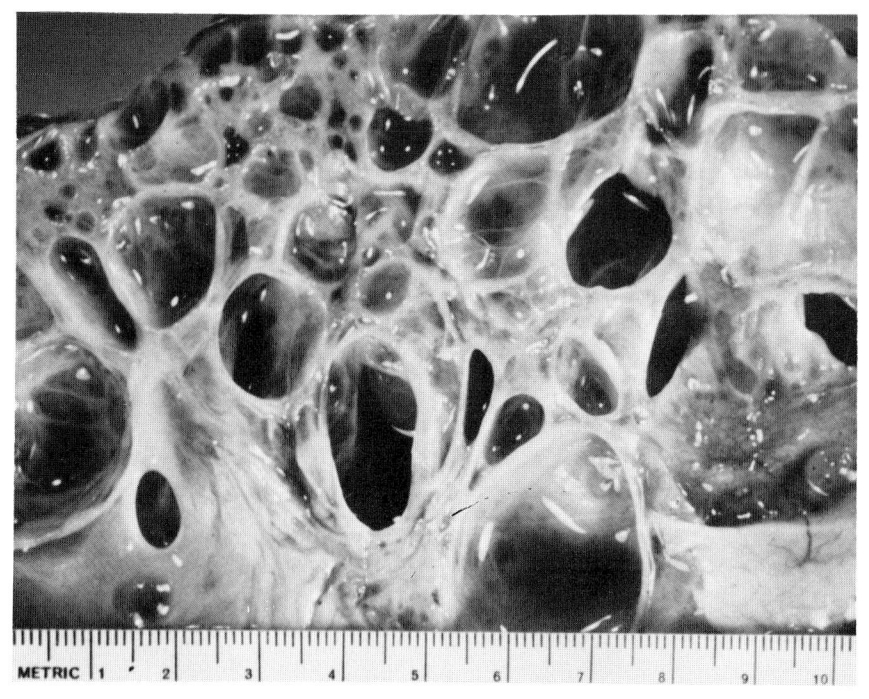

Figure 17.17. Polycystic kidney. Part of the cut surface of a 2000-g kidney. The obstructive nature of the enlarging cysts often leads to superimposition of pyelonephritis.

atrophic kidneys. The blood pressure is normal or low because of severe salt wasting.

Congenital Hypoplasia

Hypoplasia, particularly unilateral hypoplasia, is of significance chiefly as a possible renal cause of hypertension. Hypoplastic kidneys often weigh less than 10 g, have a reduced number of calyces, and show a marked reduction in the number of mature nephrons.

Tumors

The most important tumors of the kidney are the renal cell carcinoma (hypernephroma), Wilms' tumor (nephroblastoma), and carcinoma of the renal pelvis. Wilms' tumor occurs almost exclusively in infants and young children, and is discussed in Chapter 35. Carcinoma of the renal pelvis is identical in appearance and biologic behavior with the more common urothelial carcinoma of the urinary bladder. In the renal pelvis, there may be obstruction to urine flow, or the tumor may invade the renal vein early in its course. Urothelial tumors may be multicentric in origin, with involvement of kidneys, ureters, and bladder.

Renal cell carcinoma (Fig. 17.18) is by far the most frequent malignant kidney tumor of adults. There is a marked male preponderance, and an increased frequency among tobacco smokers. The tumor is solitary, often quite large, usually arising in one of the poles. It may be associated with hematuria, hypertension, or polycythemia due to erythropoietin production. At times, low grade

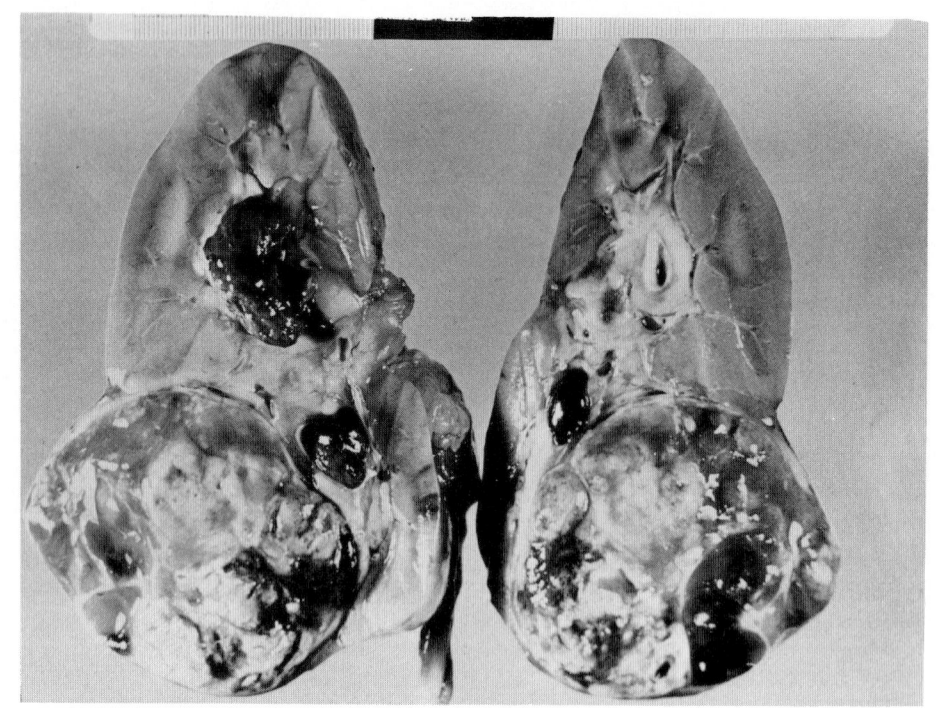

Figure 17.18. Renal cell carcinoma. This bisected kidney shows a large tumor mass occupying the lower pole. The tumor had areas of yellow coloration, but other areas of hemorrhage and necrosis. It appears to be well circumscribed, but the renal vein has been invaded. There is hemorrhage in the upper portion of the pelvis.

fever may be the only clinical manifestation. The tumor usually has areas of yellow coloration, and this, together with the frequent histologic appearance of large clear cells, suggested an adrenal rest origin, and is responsible for the persistent term hypernephroma. There is often early invasion of the renal vein tributaries and metastasis to lungs, bone, or brain. Occasional cure has been achieved by surgical excision of a solitary lung metastasis together with the primary renal mass. Of great interest is the recent report of a balanced translocation of chromosomes 3 and 8 in members of a family with a very high incidence of renal cell carcinoma.

Suggested Reading

Carpenter CB. HLA and renal transplantation. N. Engl. J. Med. *302:* 860, 1980.
Golden A, Maher JF. The Kidney. Baltimore, Williams & Wilkins, 1977.
Heptinstall RH. Interstitial nephritis. Am. J. Pathol. *83:* 214, 1976.
Kashgarian M, Hayslett JP, Spargo BH. Renal disease (a teaching monograph). Am. J. Pathol. *89:* 183, 1977.
Salant DJ, Belok S, Stilmant MM, Darby C, Couser WG. Determinants of glomerular localization of subepithelial immune deposits. Lab. Invest. *41:* 89, 1979.

Chapter 18

Hypertension

Arterial hypertension is one of the most important disorders of man. It is an abnormal physical measurement rather than a disease, but it is the single most useful risk factor in predicting severe vascular disease. Although the overall incidence of hypertension in this country is about 5%, it increases to some 25% of individuals by age 50.

Hypertension is usually defined as a sustained elevation of blood pressure above the accepted normal values of 140 mm mercury systolic and 90 mm diastolic. A more meaningful definition might be that level of blood pressure at which therapeutic intervention alters morbidity and mortality. Lowering a diastolic pressure of 105 mm or greater can be shown to decrease the likelihood of cerebrovascular accidents and congestive heart failure. Evidence that lowering a diastolic pressure of between 90 and 105 mm alters the course of vascular disease is not as yet convincing, and the level of systolic pressure that warrants therapy has not been established.

Hypertension is classified as primary, or *essential*, when its cause is unknown, and as secondary when of known etiology. Some known causes of hypertension are shown in Table 18.1. Although at least 90 to 95% of hypertensive patients fall into the category of essential hypertension, it is important to recognize those in whom hypertension can be prevented or cured by surgery.

Hypertension is also characterized as *benign* or *malignant*, depending on the severity of its manifestations and their rapidity of progression. Benign hypertension is a misnomer, since, in most instances, it has clearly deleterious effects on both health and longevity. Although some patients live out a normal life span,

Table 18.1
Some Known Causes of Hypertension

Endocrine causes	Congenital disorders of renal parenchyma
Pheochromocytoma	Polycystic kidneys
Primary aldosteronism	Unilateral hypoplasia
Cushing's syndrome	Acquired parenchymal disease
Oral contraceptive agents	Chronic pyelonephritis
Tumors of juxtaglomerular apparatus	Acute glomerulonephritis
Coarctation of the aorta	Chronic glomerulonephritis
Renal artery obstruction	Diabetic nephropathy
Atherosclerosis	Intrarenal arterial disease
Fibromuscular dysplasia	Atherosclerosis
Vascular anomalies	Polyarteritis nodosa
	Scleroderma

half will die of myocardial infarction, and others will succumb to congestive heart failure, or cerebral infarcts or hemorrhage. Five per cent will die in renal failure. Malignant or accelerated hypertension can occur as a complication of benign hypertension or as *de novo* disease. It is characterized by high levels of diastolic pressure, often above 140 mm mercury, and by evidence of organ damage. Kidney involvement tends to be severe and rapidly progressive, and, if untreated, most patients die in uremia, often with severe central nervous system manifestations.

Both genetic and environmental factors play a role in the incidence of hypertension. The extent of genetic influence is variously estimated to be between 30 and 80%, and it is thought to be polygenic. Environmental factors include body weight and salt intake, and the questionable effects of societal tensions.

Mechanisms of Hypertension

Blood pressure is determined by two variables: the cardiac output and peripheral vascular resistance. Hypertension can result either from an increased arteriolar tone or an increased plasma volume due to sodium and water retention. The latter causes an increased cardiac output, but the autoregulation of the vascular system increases peripheral resistance, and returns cardiac output to normal at the expense of hypertension. The cardiac output is generally normal in patients with sustained, but uncomplicated hypertension. Hypertensive patients may also demonstrate an exaggerated natriuresis when presented with a saline load.

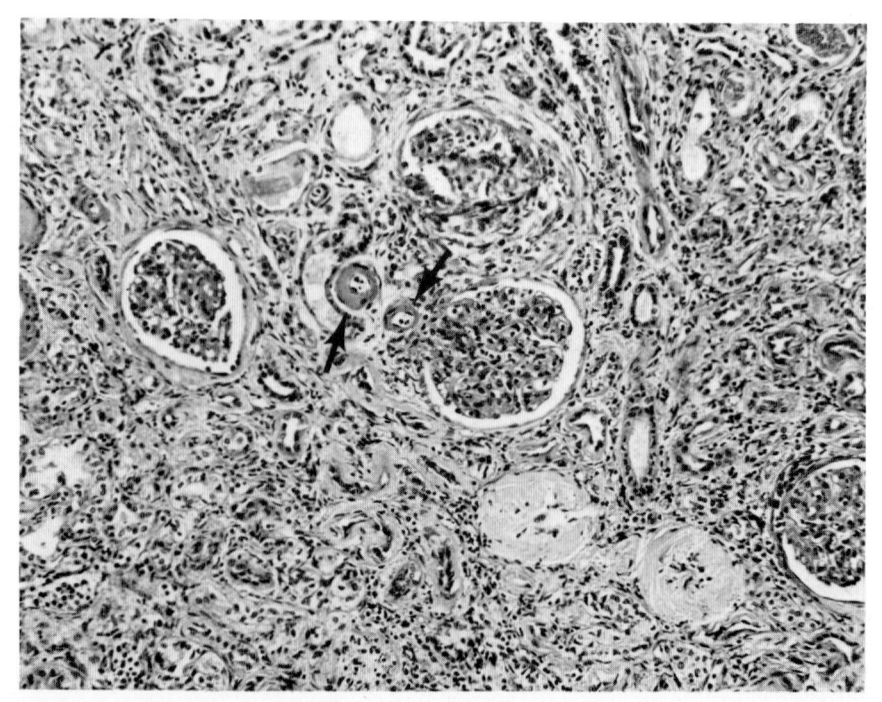

Figure 18.1. Arteriolar sclerosis. The two arterioles in the *center* of the field (*arrows*) show thickened, homogeneous, or hyalinized walls. The effect of these vascular lesions is renal ischemia. There is striking tubular atrophy, and several scarred glomeruli are seen.

Many mechanisms are involved in the control of blood pressure. They include arterial baroreceptors, regulators of body fluid volume, catecholamines, prostaglandins, and the renin-angiotensin system. Aldosterone and cortisol promote renal sodium and water retention, and may increase peripheral arteriolar tone through increasing the sodium content of arteriolar walls. Angiotensin II directly affects arteriolar tone, and it also acts through increased aldosterone secretion. The renin-angiotensin system is controlled by renal baroreceptors, by the tubular concentration of sodium, by β-adrenergic receptors in the kidney, and by a feedback effect of angiotensin II. This system is an important means of maintaining blood pressure in hypovolemia resulting from sodium depletion, and it is the mechanism of hypertension in patients with coarctation of the aorta and in renal vascular hypertension. It probably contributes to the maintenance of hypertension in malignant hypertension and in some patients with chronic glomerulonephritis and chronic pyelonephritis. Blood pressure tends to be elevated after bilateral nephrectomy. This "renoprival" hypertension may result from loss of the normal threshold mechanism for renal excretion of sodium and water and from loss of renal prostaglandins.

BODILY EFFECTS OF HYPERTENSION

Vascular Disease

Hypertension is associated with changes in arterioles throughout the body, called *arteriolar sclerosis*. The arteriolar walls are thickened, they have a

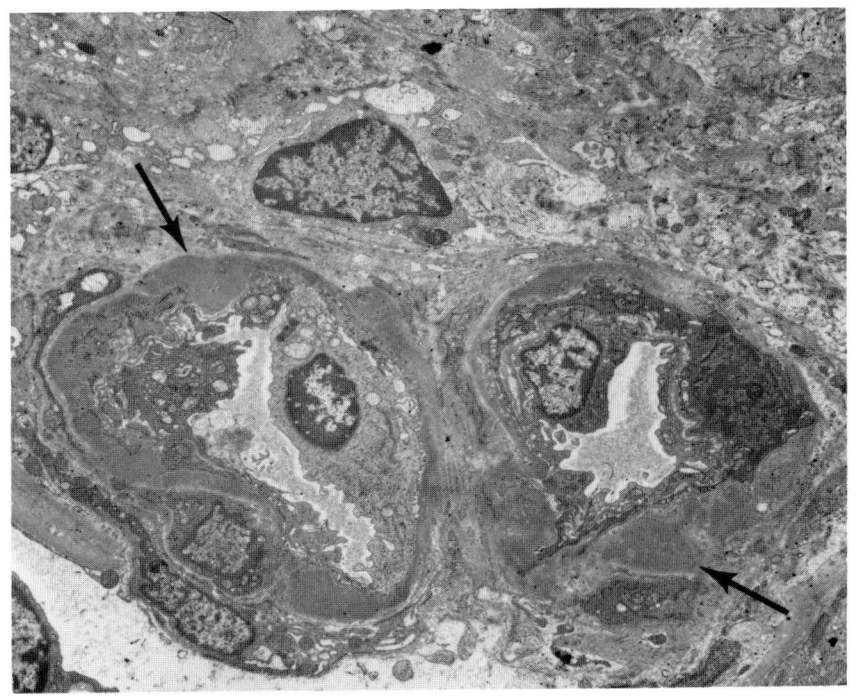

Figure 18.2. Arteriolar sclerosis. Electron micrograph showing arterioles containing intramural deposits of protein (*arrows*), responsible for their hyaline appearance on light microscopy.

homogeneous or "hyalinized" appearance, and their lumens are compromised (Fig. 18.1). Electron microscopy indicates that the principal alteration is incorporation of plasma proteins in the wall (Fig. 18.2). The basement membrane is thickened. Although arteriolar sclerosis may occasionally be observed in nonhypertensive patients, it is almost always a direct result of hypertension. It is not a cause of hypertension, although, in the kidney, it may result in ischemia and contribute to sustaining hypertension. Severe hypertension may cause hyperplastic changes in arterioles and small arteries. These vessels have thickened walls showing increased numbers of smooth muscle cells and thickened basement membranes. They may have an "onion skin" appearance (Fig. 18.3). Fibrin deposition in the wall can give the appearance of fibrinoid necrosis, and thrombosis is not uncommon (Fig. 18.4).

Hypertension is a major risk factor for atherosclerosis; it accelerates the development of its lesions, and augments its effects. Patients with hypertension are likely to die of complications of atherosclerosis, particularly myocardial infarction and cerebral infarction.

Acute aortic dissection (p. 170) occurs predominately in hypertensive patients. Medial cystic necrosis, the underlying lesion in most aortic dissections, may result from arteriolar sclerosis of adventitial vessels or may reflect a congenital connective tissue defect.

The heart in hypertension characteristically shows prominent concentric hypertrophy of the left ventricle (see Fig. 13.2). Many patients develop congestive heart failure during the course of hypertension, and show the changes described in Chapter 15.

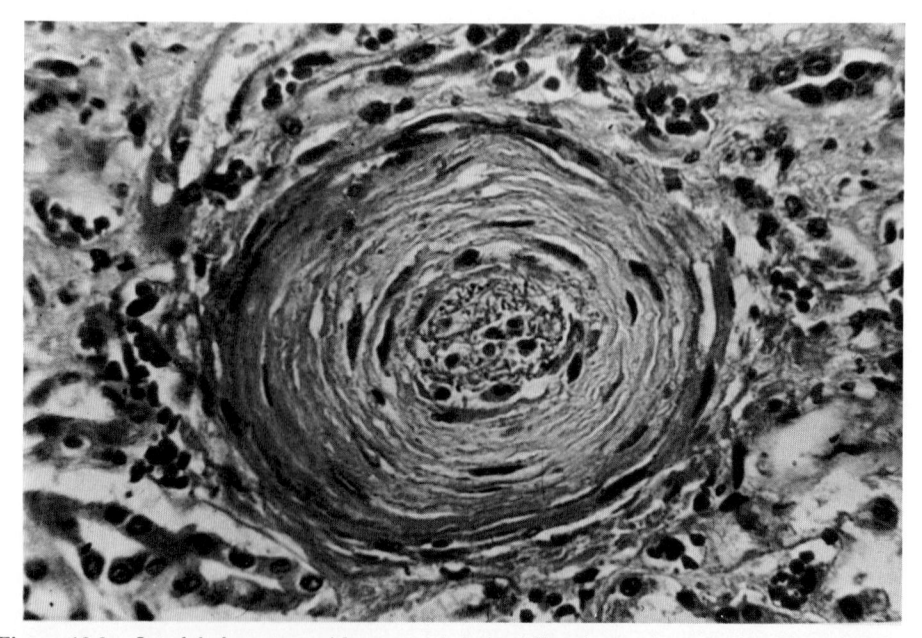

Figure 18.3. Interlobular artery with concentric intimal fibrosis creating an onion skin appearance. This is a characteristic finding in patients with severe hypertension.

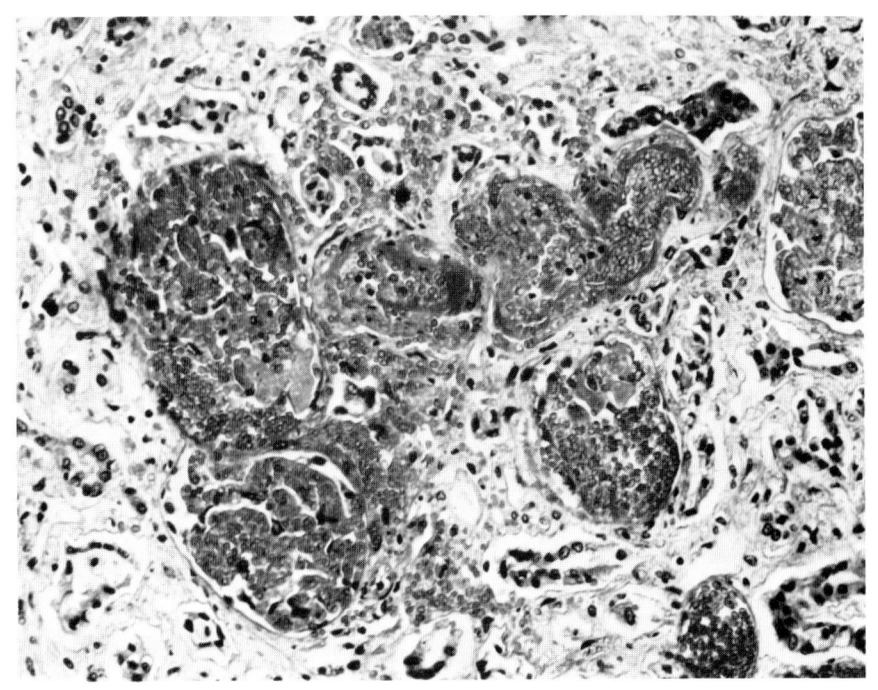

Figure 18.4. Fibrinoid necrosis of arterioles. Necrosis of the arteriole seen at the *upper right* has resulted in hemorrhagic infarction of the two glomeruli at the *left*.

The Central Nervous System

Cerebral infarction, or *encephalomalacia*, a result of atherosclerosis of internal carotid and cerebral arteries, is an important cause of morbidity and death in hypertensive patients. Cerebral hemorrhage is another serious complication, and a frequent cause of death. It results from rupture of small saccular or fusiform aneurysms, called *Charcot-Bouchard* aneurysms, especially of branches of the lenticulostriate arteries. The putamen is the most frequent site of hemorrhage, and death often follows rupture into the ventricular system. Hypertension also greatly increases the likelihood that congenital, or "berry," aneurysms of the major cerebral arteries will rupture, causing subarachnoid hemorrhage.

Hypertensive encephalopathy occurs in patients with malignant hypertension. It consists of transient focal neurologic signs, including seizures and stupor or coma. There is generalized cerebral edema and patchy arteriolar injury with leakage of plasma proteins into their walls. Encephalopathy may result from a reflex constriction of these arterioles and consequent ischemia.

The Retina

Retinal changes are observed in both benign and malignant hypertension. In benign hypertension, the arterioles appear narrowed, and there is nicking of veins where crossed by arterioles. Retinal changes in malignant hypertension include papilledema, cotton wool exudates, and linear hemorrhages.

HYPERTENSION AND THE KIDNEYS

By producing the same arteriolar sclerosis in the kidneys as in the rest of the body, hypertension can have profound effects on renal structure and function. On the other hand, the kidneys can cause hypertension, either by retaining sodium and water or through the renin-angiotensin system. Furthermore, in any established hypertension, kidneys injured by arteriolar sclerosis can act to sustain or perhaps augment the level of hypertension.

Arteriolar sclerosis results in atrophy of nephrons. Tubular atrophy is initially most striking, but progressive deposition of collagen internal to Bowman's capsule accompanies shrinkage of the glomerular tufts (Fig. 18.1). The interlobular arteries may also show changes relatable to hypertension: intimal proliferation with or without smooth muscle hyperplasia (Fig. 18.5). Involvement of the kidney is not homogeneous, and less involved nephrons become hypertrophied; the end result is the contracted, granular kidney described in Chapter 17 (Figs. 17.2 and 17.3). These changes are referred to as *arteriolar nephrosclerosis*. It is the almost inevitable result of sustained hypertension.

Malignant hypertension is usually associated with more severe renal injury. The interlobular arteries show striking concentric intimal proliferation and fibrosis, conveying an onion skin appearance. There may also be a loose mucinous

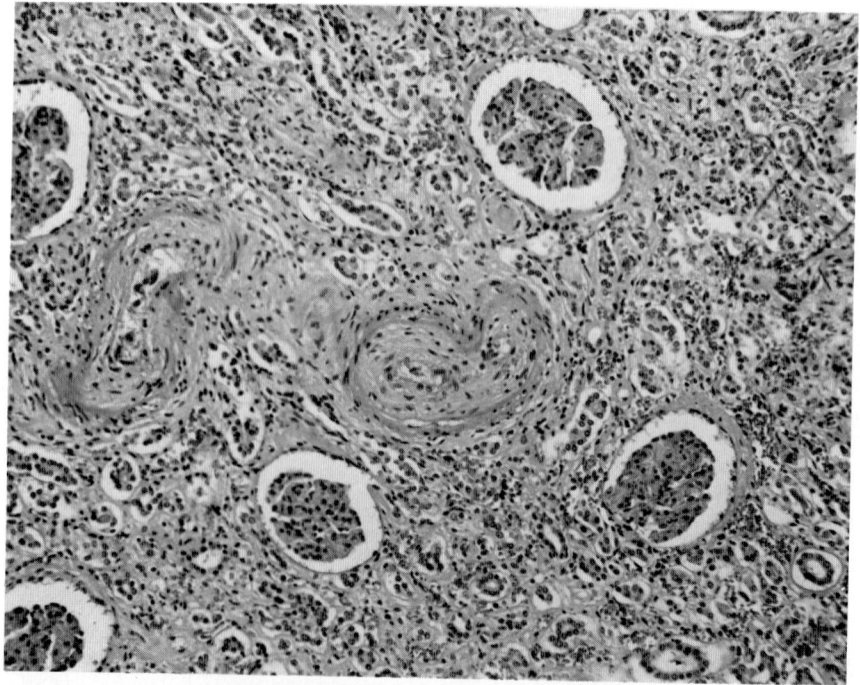

Figure 18.5. Arteriolar nephrosclerosis. There is striking thickening of the wall of the interlobular artery in the center of the field. The thickening is primarily intimal. This lesion adds to the ischemia of the kidney, and there is striking tubular atrophy in this area.

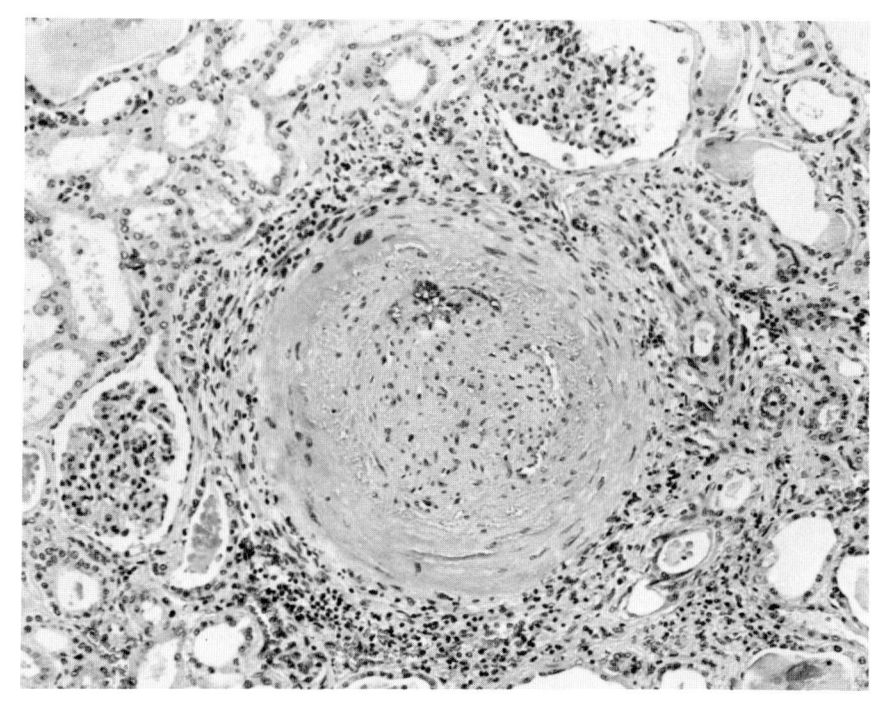

Figure 18.6. Severe interlobular artery disease in a patient with malignant hypertension. There is marked thickening of the intima, which has a mucinous appearance, suggesting an organized thrombus. Similar vascular changes have been described in patients with acute renal failure following pregnancy and in some patients receiving oral contraceptive agents.

thickening of the intima, believed to represent organization of thrombi (Fig. 18.6). The afferent arterioles characteristically reveal fibrinoid necrosis and thrombosis, with hemorrhage and infarction of glomeruli and ischemic necrosis of tubules (Fig. 18.4). Functionally, there is acute renal failure with hematuria, red cell casts, oliguria, azotemia, and a striking fall in clearances. The renal lesions described here, called *malignant nephrosclerosis*, may be superimposed upon benign nephrosclerosis or can occur in previously normal kidneys. It is important to caution that malignant hypertension and malignant nephrosclerosis are not synonymous or interchangeable terms. Clinically malignant hypertension can occur without concurrence of arteriolar necrosis and its consequences. Conversely, marked changes of the interlobular arteries are often observed in patients with severe but not malignant hypertension.

Renal Vascular Hypertension

Renal vascular hypertension results from disease of the renal artery or its major branches and ischemic atrophy of the kidney. The vascular disease is usually atherosclerosis, but fibromuscular dysplasia and congenital anomalies are other important causes. Involvement is almost always unilateral, and there is striking reduction in kidney size compared to the contralateral organ. The atrophic kidney has a smooth surface; the contralateral kidney usually demonstrates the granular kidney of arteriolar nephrosclerosis, since it is exposed to the effects of hypertension. Hypertension caused by unilateral renal vascular disease results from continuous activation of the renin-angiotensin system. The diagnosis must be established by showing a difference in renal vein renin concentration from the two kidneys.

Although renal vascular hypertension accounts for very few instances of mild hypertension, it appears more significant as a cause of severe hypertension. It is of importance because it is often curable by surgery, and because it has helped clarify a mechanism of hypertension of renal origin.

Suggested Reading

Haber E. The renin-angiotensin system and hypertension. Kidney Int. *15:* 427, 1979.
Kaplan NM. The control of hypertension: a therapeutic breakthrough. Am. Sci. *68:* 537, 1980.

Chapter 19

The Lungs

Following a discussion of the pathophysiology of respiratory failure and a description of pulmonary defense mechanisms, the many important disorders of the lung are presented in groups that reflect major functional abnormalities: chronic obstructive pulmonary disease, fibrosing (restrictive) disease, the adult respiratory distress syndrome, lung infections, and malignant tumors. Brief mention is made of several lesions of the larynx.

RESPIRATORY FAILURE

Respiratory function serves to maintain a normal oxygen saturation in pulmonary venous and systemic arterial blood and to remove carbon dioxide from blood returning to the lungs. Failure of normal respiration leads to impaired function of body organs and, eventually, to an inability to sustain life. A partial pressure of oxygen (PaO_2) in arterial blood below 60 mm mercury (normal, 80 to 100) or a $PaCO_2$ above 50 mm mercury (normal, 35 to 45) generally signals the presence of respiratory failure.

There are three major components of respiratory function, and failure can result from a deficiency of each or from an altered balance among them. *Ventilation* of the lungs brings atmospheric air to the alveoli. *Perfusion* delivers pulmonary arterial blood to the alveolar wall capillaries. *Diffusion* is the exchange of oxygen and carbon dioxide between capillary blood and alveolar air.

Respiratory failure can be classified as ventilatory or hypoxic. *Ventilatory failure*, or *alveolar hypoventilation*, results in retention of carbon dioxide in the blood, and a corresponding decrease in PaO_2. The clinical manifestation is carbon dioxide narcosis, and oxygen administration serves only to suppress ventilation further. In *hypoxic failure*, the PaO_2 of arterial blood is reduced. The $PaCO_2$ may be normal, but is often lowered as a result of hyperventilation. Patients with hypoxic failure generally benefit from oxygen administration.

Alveolar Hypoventilation

Marked retention of carbon dioxide, together with a moderate drop in arterial PaO_2, is indicative of a pure ventilatory defect. Although alveolar hypoventilation can be due to obstruction of the pulmonary airways, it is most often the result of extrapulmonary disorders. Ventilation is impaired by drugs that depress central nervous system activity, by infections of the brain (encephalitis), and by metabolic alkalosis. Respiratory muscles may be affected in poliomyelitis and myasthenia gravis, and the thoracic cage has restricted expansion in ankylosing spondylitis.

Severe obesity can reduce tidal volume to the point of inducing somnolence and carbon dioxide narcosis (*Pickwickian syndrome*).

Hypoxic Respiratory Failure

Hypoxic respiratory failure can be the result of an alveolar wall abnormality that interferes with normal diffusion of oxygen. A much more frequent cause, however, is an imbalance between alveolar ventilation and perfusion.

Diffusion Defect

The term *alveolar capillary block* has been used to designate a generalized impairment of oxygen diffusion across abnormal alveolar walls. This is probably a rather uncommon circumstance, however, as most of the disorders thought to act through this mechanism fail to show significant alveolar wall abnormalities. Sarcoidosis is the principal exception. It can cause diffuse alveolar fibrosis and respiratory failure based on impaired diffusion.

Ventilation-Perfusion Imbalance

By far the majority of pulmonary disorders that lead to respiratory failure do so through an imbalance between ventilation and perfusion. Normal respiratory function implies that all respiratory units are both normally ventilated and normally perfused. Normal air exchange averages 4 liters per min, pulmonary blood flow 5 liters, and this relationship tends to remain rather constant. Imbalance can result from alveolar dead space, from shunting of blood through unventilated lung, and from disturbances of both ventilation and perfusion.

Alveolar dead space is pulmonary tissue that is normally ventilated but not perfused. Embolic obstruction of branches of the pulmonary artery is an obvious example. There may be a striking fall in PaO_2, but hyperventilation largely compensates for carbon dioxide retention in the dead space areas. This is true whenever the PaO_2 falls below 50 mm mercury.

Occlusion of bronchi by abnormal secretions, foreign bodies, or tumors can result in shunting of blood through unventilated lung tissue. Cystic fibrosis is a dramatic example of shunting due to extensive bronchial obstruction by viscid, mucoid secretions.

In many of the most important chronic pulmonary diseases, one observes a mixture of normal, hypoventilated, and hyperventilated alveoli. This is true in emphysema, chronic bronchitis, and chronic fibrosing disorders. Hypoventilated alveoli produce a shunt, whereas hyperventilated alveoli are at least relatively poorly perfused and represent dead space. These focal inequalities between ventilation and perfusion, when widespread in the lungs, result in severe respiratory failure.

PULMONARY PROTECTION FROM INJURY

The respiratory apparatus is remarkably able to protect itself from injury, considering the quantities of toxic particulate matter and microorganisms that enter with inspired air. The components of its defense mechanism include the mucociliary apparatus of the trachea, bronchi and bronchioles, the distal respiratory unit, the alveolar macrophage, and the respiratory membrane.

The trachea, bronchi, and bronchioles are lined by ciliated respiratory epithelium; mucus-secreting goblet cells constitute nearly half of the lining cells, but are absent in terminal bronchioles. Particulate matter less than 5 μ in diameter is trapped in a layer of mucus and swept upward by the synchronized beating of cilia. Larger particles do not reach the lung, but are generally cleared in the upper respiratory passages. The mucociliary apparatus is impaired in cystic fibrosis, where an abnormally viscid mucus and the loss of coordinated ciliary function relatable to a circulating polypeptide causes trapping of mucus and bacteria in small bronchi and bronchioles. Mucociliary function is severely altered by chronic inflammation of the bronchial tree in response to cigarette smoke and other air pollutants. Chronic inflammation is often associated with squamous metaplasia of respiratory epithelium and a striking hyperplasia of mucus-secreting cells.

The distal respiratory unit, consisting of a single respiratory bronchiole with its alveolar ducts and alveolar sacs, tends to react as a unit, becoming overdistended or collapsed, contributing to ventilation-perfusion imbalance. Viruses, including cytomegalovirus and influenza virus, tend to affect primarily the respiratory bronchioles, producing an obstructive bronchiolitis. Disordered function of the respiratory bronchiole and the distal respiratory unit is key to the pathophysiology of emphysema.

Alveolar macrophages are derived from the bone marrow, but are modified to function at an air-tissue interface. They are directly exposed to inhaled microorganisms and air pollutants, and constitute the first line of defense against these particles. They are essential to phagocytosis of foreign material and its conveyance to the mucociliary apparatus for disposal. Alveolar macrophage have receptors for the Fc fragment of IgG and for C3, important to particle attachment and ingestion. Viruses, dusts, and pollutants, as well as alcohol ingestion, appear to depress macrophage function, and predispose the lung to bacterial infection. It is likely that alveolar macrophages must be activated as part of a cell-mediated immune response, and that macrophages may stimulate lymphocytes to produce specific antibodies. Pulmonary alveolar macrophages may also be important in the pathogenesis of emphysema. Cigarette smoke causes excessive macrophage secretion of elastases that injure the alveolar architecture. This is especially detrimental in patients with α-1-antitrypsin deficiency who manifest defective neutralization of elastolytic enzymes.

The respiratory membrane, or alveolar septum, is composed of the endothelial cells lining the alveolar capillaries, the epithelial Type I or Type II pneumocytes, and the joined epithelial and endothelial basement membranes. The epithelial cells can be injured by toxic gases, cytotoxic agents, and certain viruses. The endothelium is sensitive to high oxygen tension, ionizing radiation, and shock. The basement membrane may be injured by immunologic mechanisms, as in Goodpasture's syndrome (p. 191). The effect of injury, wherever in the alveolar septum it occurs, is an increased permeability, with passage of plasma and blood cells into the alveolar space, often with protein condensation and hyaline membrane formation. The respiratory membrane has considerable capacity for repair, although Type I pneumocytes may be replaced by Type II, and repair may involve connective tissue organization of the alveolar interstitium and alveolar spaces.

Pathology: Understanding Human Disease

CHRONIC OBSTRUCTIVE PULMONARY DISEASE

The term "chronic obstructive pulmonary disease (COPD)" denotes a group of intrinsic disorders of the lung that are characterized by obstruction to airflow, ventilation-perfusion abnormality, and hypoxic respiratory failure. These important disorders include emphysema, chronic bronchitis, bronchiectasis, "small airways disease," and bronchial asthma.

Emphysema

The diagnosis of emphysema is based on morphologic changes in the lung: enlargement of air spaces distal to the terminal bronchiole, with destruction of alveolar walls. Enlargement of air spaces compensatory to loss of a lung or a lobe, but without destruction of alveolar tissue, is not emphysema.

Emphysema is a common disorder, present to some degree in nearly half of all adults. Although relatively few have manifestations of diminished pulmonary function, severe emphysema, particularly when coexistent with chronic bronchitis, is the principal cause of chronic respiratory failure in the American population.

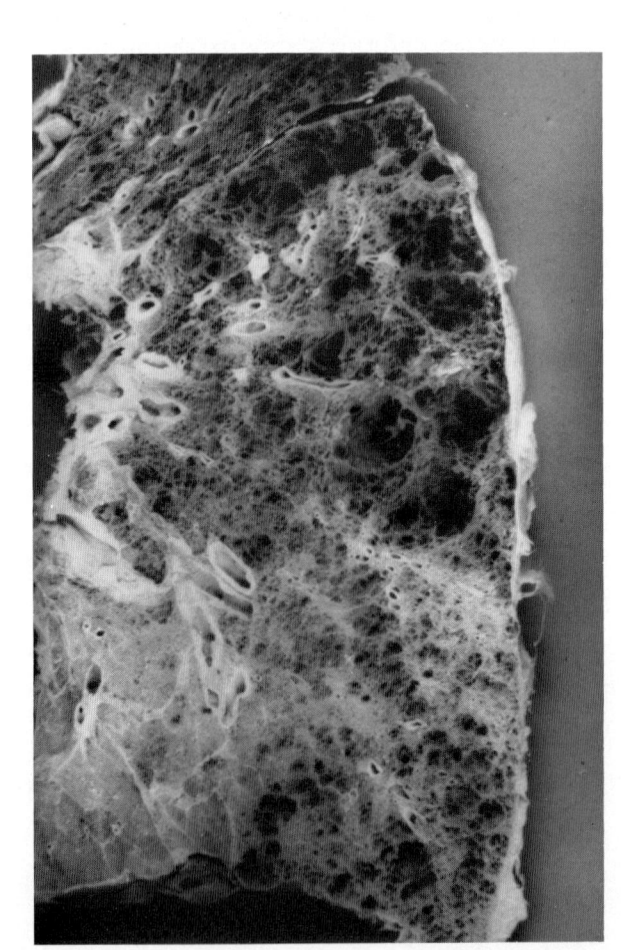

Figure 19.1. Centrilobular emphysema. There is striking cystic dilatation at the center of the lobules. The findings are most marked in the upper lobe and in the upper portion of the lower lobe.

The Lungs

In normal lungs, the alveolar septa have a tethering effect in keeping small airways (respiratory bronchioles) open during expiration. In emphysema, these airways tend to collapse, and there is obstruction to the outflow of air. There is no obstruction during inspiration. The loss of elastic tissue in emphysema results in large, flabby lungs, with increased compliance, increased static total lung capacity and functional reserve capacity, but a markedly diminished 1-sec forced expiratory volume, expressed as a fraction of forced vital capacity (FEV_1/FVC).

The two major forms of emphysema are designated centrilobular and panacinar. Centrilobular emphysema is the more common.

Centrilobular Emphysema

In centrilobular emphysema, the lesions are seen primarily at the center of the pulmonary lobules (Fig. 19.1). (A lobule consists of several terminal bronchioles and their branches demarcated by fibrous connective tissue.) There is a striking tendency to greater involvement of the upper lobes or upper portions of lower lobes. The enlarged spaces consist primarily of injured respiratory bronchioles, rather than alveoli. Centrilobular emphysema occurs virtually exclusively in

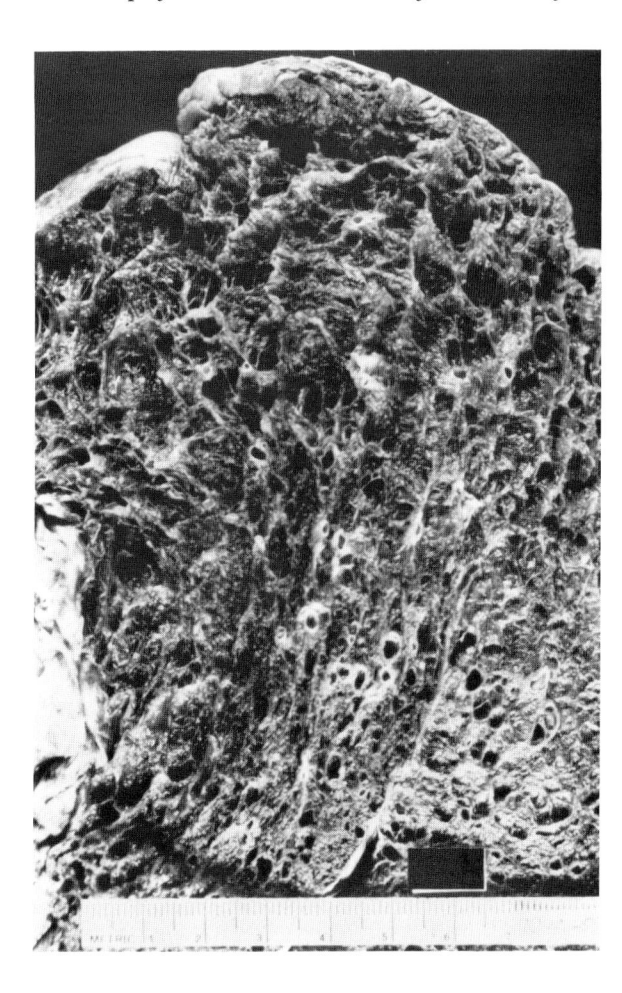

Figure 19.2. Panacinar emphysema. There is diffuse involvement of the entire pulmonary architecture. Compare with Figure 19.1.

cigarette smokers. Many patients with this form of emphysema also suffer from chronic bronchitis.

Panacinar Emphysema

Panacinar emphysema tends to involve all portions of the lobules and all lobes of the lungs, although the lower portions may show somewhat greater involvement (Fig. 19.2). There is less of an association with cigarette smoking, but a generally greater association with aging. Half of patients below the age of 50 who have clinically manifest panacinar emphysema have an impaired ability to counteract proteolytic enzymes, particularly trypsin and elastases, released by alveolar macrophages and other leukocytes. This usually takes the form of α-1-antitrypsin deficiency, and a deficiency of this protease inhibitor should be strongly suspected in any young patient with panacinar emphysema. Some 3% of the American population is heterozygous for this trait; homozygosity occurs in fewer than 1 in 3000.

Chronic Bronchitis

Chronic bronchitis is defined in functional rather than anatomic terms. It is present in any individual who has a persistent productive cough for 3 months of the year during at least 2 consecutive years, in the absence of other specific cause. Chronic bronchitis is clearly associated with cigarette smoking, and exacerbations often follow bacterial or viral infections of the respiratory tract.

The bronchial walls are thickened by connective tissue and infiltrated by inflammatory cells. The mucous glands are markedly increased, and there is striking goblet cell hyperplasia of lining cells. Obstruction of airflow is due in part to mucus plugging, but the replacement of surfactant in the peripheral airways by mucus leads to collapse of these passages and further obstruction.

Chronic bronchitis and emphysema, particulary centrilobular emphysema, coexist in many patients, and together constitute the principal form of obstructive pulmonary disease. If emphysema is the dominant component, there is dyspnea and hyperventilation, with little disturbance of blood gases and little sputum production. Those in whom chronic bronchitis predominates tend to be severely hypoxic, cyanotic, and polycythemic, and usually produce copious amounts of sputum. Cor pulmonale and right ventricular failure are frequent in patients with severe chronic bronchitis.

Bronchiectasis

Bronchiectasis is an abnormal dilatation of bronchi and bronchioles. It may be generalized or localized to one or more segments of the lung (Fig. 19.3). In most instances, it results from bronchial obstruction together with a necrotizing infection. Obstruction is followed by atelectasis (collapse) distal to the obstruction, so that negative inspiratory pressure is applied directly to bronchial walls. The resulting dilatation becomes permanent if infection is superimposed.

Bronchiectasis may occur with obstruction by foreign bodies or bronchogenic tumors, chronic bronchitis, and cystic fibrosis. It may be a sequel to atelectasis occurring in such childhood diseases as measles and pertussis. If infection can be controlled, bronchiectasis may remain static and nonprogressive.

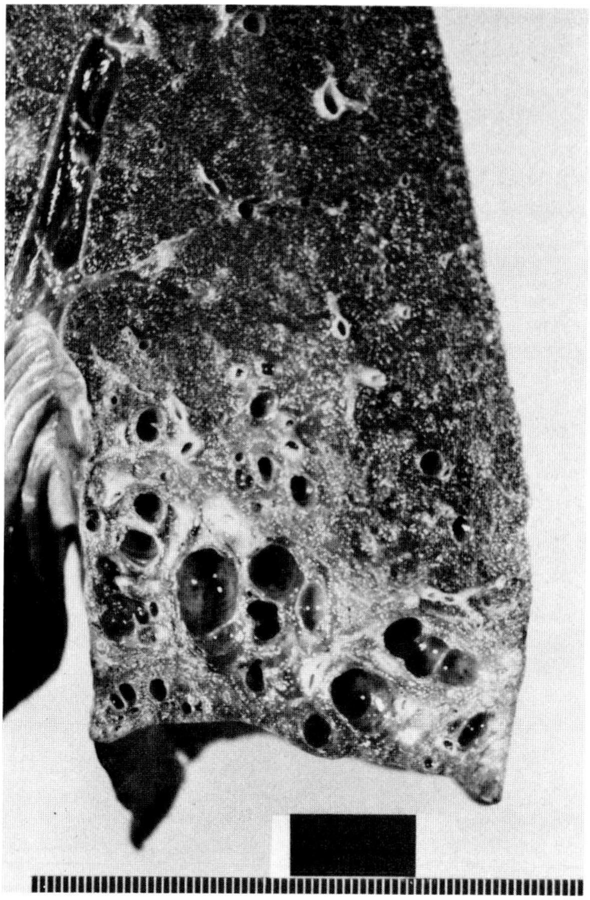

Figure 19.3. Bronchiectasis. There is striking dilatation of the bronchi of the lowermost portion of the lower lobe. The surrounding lung tissue is collapsed and fibrotic.

Small Airways Disease

This term applies to mucus plugging or narrowing of bronchioles less than 2 mm in diameter. It is associated with chronic bronchitis and emphysema, and may be an early manifestation of injury from cigarette smoking. Under normal circumstances, the small airways are responsible for only 10% of pulmonary resistance to airflow, so that considerable disorder of these airways would have little noticeable effect on total resistance. Ventilation-perfusion abnormalities would be more significant consequences of small airways disease.

Asthma

Asthma is characterized by paroxysmal narrowing of airways. Attacks are characterized by wheezing and marked respiratory difficulty, particularly during expiration. The PaO_2 is reduced, due to ventilation-perfusion inequalities, but the $PaCO_2$ may remain normal as a result of hyperventilation.

The bronchi and bronchioles are often plugged with mucus and show basement membrane thickening, hyperplasia of the smooth musculature, enlargement of mucous glands with hypersecretion of mucus, edema, and infiltration of inflammatory cells, notably polymorphonuclear eosinophils.

Asthma is often relatable to immunologic mechanisms. It may be mediated by IgE (atopic asthma) or by immune complexes. Aspirin may precipitate asthma in some patients, perhaps through interference with prostaglandin synthesis. Regardless of cause, there is hyperirritability of the airways of all asthmatic individuals.

FIBROSING LUNG DISEASE

Fibrosing lung disease is the end result of a large group of pulmonary injuries, and is characterized by diffuse interstitial and, at times, alveolar fibrosis. Other terms used in describing this group include chronic interstitial pneumonia, fibrosing alveolitis, diffuse infiltrative lung disease, diffuse interstitial fibrosis, Hamman-Rich syndrome, and restrictive lung disease.

Regardless of etiology, fibrosing lung disease is manifested by markedly reduced lung volumes (total lung capacity, functional reserve capacity, vital capacity), decreased compliance, and ventilation-perfusion inequality. There is no obstruction to airflow. In addition to fibrosis, the lungs may have a honeycomb appearance, due to cystic dilatation proximal to the terminal respiratory bronchioles (Fig. 19.4).

Some of the causes of fibrosing lung disease are shown in Table 19.1. Only a few are discussed.

Pneumoconioses

Asbestosis results from inhalation of fibrous hydrated silicates, particularly disilicates and metasilicates. Exposure to these compounds is widespread among workers in the insulation, building materials, construction, and automobile in-

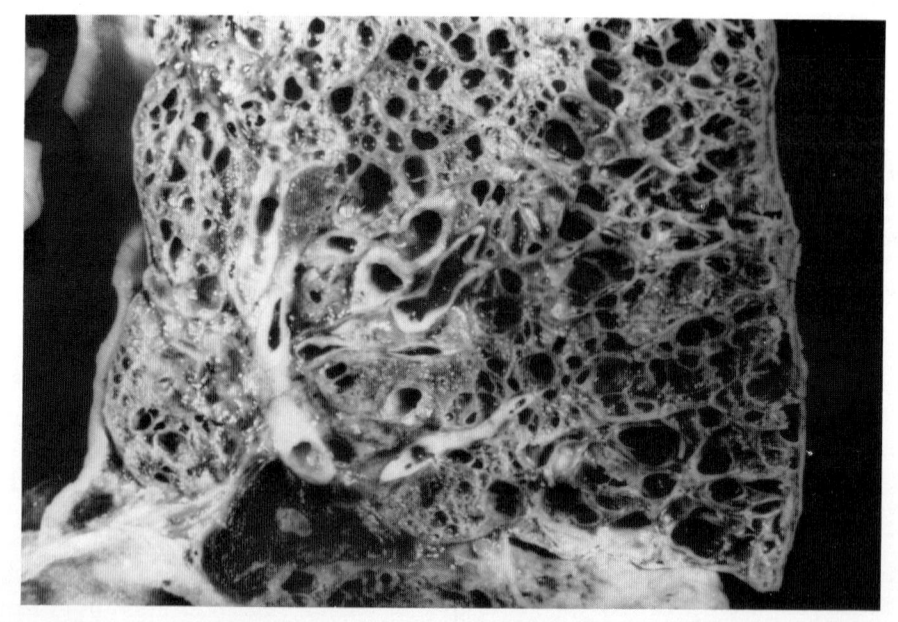

Figure 19.4. Fibrosing lung disease. There is marked fibrosis, and the lungs have a honeycomb appearance due to cystic dilatation proximal to the terminal respiratory bronchioles.

Table 19.1
Some Causes of Fibrosing (Restrictive) Lung Disease

Pneumoconioses	Left ventricular heart failure
Silicosis	Immunologic lung diseases
Beryllosis	Hypersensitivity pneumonitis
Asbestosis	Farmer's lung
Cytotoxic agents	Autoimmune disorders
Myleran	Systemic lupus erythematosus
Cytoxan	Rheumatoid arthritis
Bleomycin	Wegener's granulomatosis
Ionizing radiation	Goodpasture's syndrome
Noxious gases	Sarcoidosis
Nitrogen dioxide	Pulmonary hemosiderosis
Ozone	Idiopathic interstitial fibrosis
Oxygen toxicity	Diffuse neoplasms
Infections	
Tuberculosis	
Histoplasmosis	

dustries. The fibers are inhaled into the respiratory bronchioles and alveoli and provoke a mononuclear, often granulomatous response. There is progressive fibrosis of these lesions and interstitial fibrosis of surrounding alveolar septa. The asbestos fibers themselves become coated with protein and iron, forming the *ferruginous bodies* that aid in diagnosis (see Fig. 12.1). Asbestosis is a slowly progressive disorder, usually asymptomatic for many years. The most serious consequences, appearing 20 to 40 years after the diagnosis is first established, are bronchogenic carcinomas and mesotheliomas of the serous cavities.

Silicosis is caused by exposure to silica (silicon dioxide) dust of small enough size to reach the periphery of the lung. It occurs most often among miners, stone cutters, sandblasters, foundry, and pottery workers. The particles are ingested into phagosomes by alveolar macrophages which soon die and release their constituents, including the silica particles. There is repeated phagocytosis and cell death, formation of granulomatous nodules, and extensive fibrosis. Foundry workers are likely to have a diffuse, non-nodular form of disease. Silicosis increases susceptibility to tuberculous infection.

Coal worker's pneumoconiosis is observed among workers in various occupations related to coal. "Primary dust macules," consisting of coal dust and silica surrounded by fibrous tissue, are scattered through the lungs. These nodules may remain discrete or they may coalesce. Fibrosis is generally not marked, but progressive massive fibrosis, with restrictive lung disease, occasionally complicates severe involvement. Chronic bronchitis and proximal acinar emphysema are frequently observed, as well as a high incidence of tuberculosis and other lung infections. It is difficult to define a specific coal worker's pneumoconiosis apart from silicosis and the effects of cigarette smoking. The existence of "black lung" as a disabling pulmonary disease directly related to coal mining is very much in doubt.

Immunologic Lung Diseases

All four types of immunologically mediated injury are observed in the lung. Type I reactions are involved in many patients with asthma. Most of these reactions are mediated by IgE, but certain IgG antibodies may also function as reagins in some asthmatic patients. Goodpasture's syndrome (p. 191) is an example of cytotoxic antibody-mediated disease (Type II). Immune complex deposition is the mechanism of lung injury in patients with rheumatoid arthritis and in many with idiopathic interstitial fibrosis. Complex deposition is observed in other pulmonary lesions, but may not represent the mechanism of injury. Cell-mediated immunity is, of course, present in tuberculous infection. It also appears to be the basis of pulmonary injury in patients receiving nitrofurantoin.

Allergic bronchopulmonary aspergillosis and hypersensitivity pneumonitis from inhalation of organic dusts are clearly immunologically mediated. The former involves both Type I and Type III reactions, the latter Types III and IV. Pulmonary lesions are encountered in such systemic immunologically mediated diseases as polyarteritis nodosa (p. 174). *Wegener's granulomatosis* (p. 176) consists of the triad of granulomatous vasculitis of both upper and lower respiratory tracts, focal glomerulonephritis, and a generalized necrotizing vasculitis. Although the pathogenesis is not clear, many findings implicate an immune disorder.

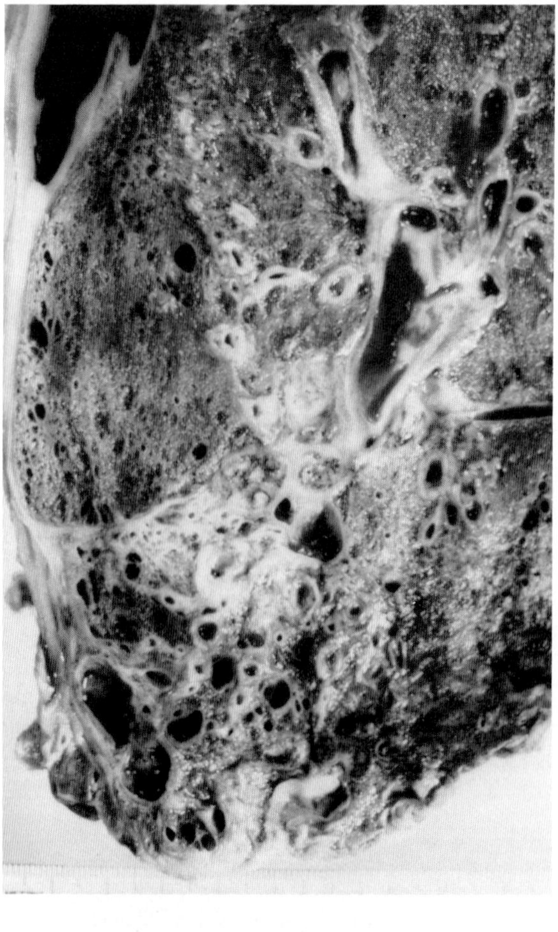

Figure 19.5. Pulmonary sarcoidosis. There is patchy severe fibrosis as well as areas of cystic dilatation. Hilar lymph nodes tend to be enlarged and replaced by granulomatous inflammation.

Sarcoidosis, a systemic granulomatous disease of unknown etiology, often has its most devastating effects in the lung, leading to extensive fibrosis and hypoxic respiratory failure (Fig. 19.5). Patients with sarcoidosis have evidence of decreased T cell function and increased B cell activity. Hypergammaglobulinemia, the frequent presence of rheumatoid factor, and high antibody titers to various viral antigens suggest that abnormal B cell function may play a pathogenetic role in this disease.

THE ADULT RESPIRATORY DISTRESS SYNDROME

The adult respiratory distress syndrome, often called "shock lung," is an acute respiratory failure due to noncardiogenic pulmonary edema. There is severe hypoxia, unresponsive to oxygen administration, dyspnea, and cyanosis. Left atrial and pulmonary venous pressures are normal; there is no airflow obstruction. The lungs are heavy, firm, and congested. Histologically there is striking intra-alveolar edema, with extensive hyaline membrane formation (Fig. 19.6). The hyaline membranes consist of fibrinogen and fibrin together with debris derived from necrotic alveolar lining cells. With time, there is proliferation of Type II pneumocytes, and organization of alveolar contents may result in alveolar and interstitial fibrosis.

There are many disparate causes of the adult respiratory distress syndrome, some of which are outlined in Table 19.2. Whatever the etiology, the basic mechanism is injury to the respiratory membrane. Some agents affect the epithelium, some the endothelium, and some the basement membrane, but all lead to injury to the entire membrane and abnormal permeability to constituents of the blood.

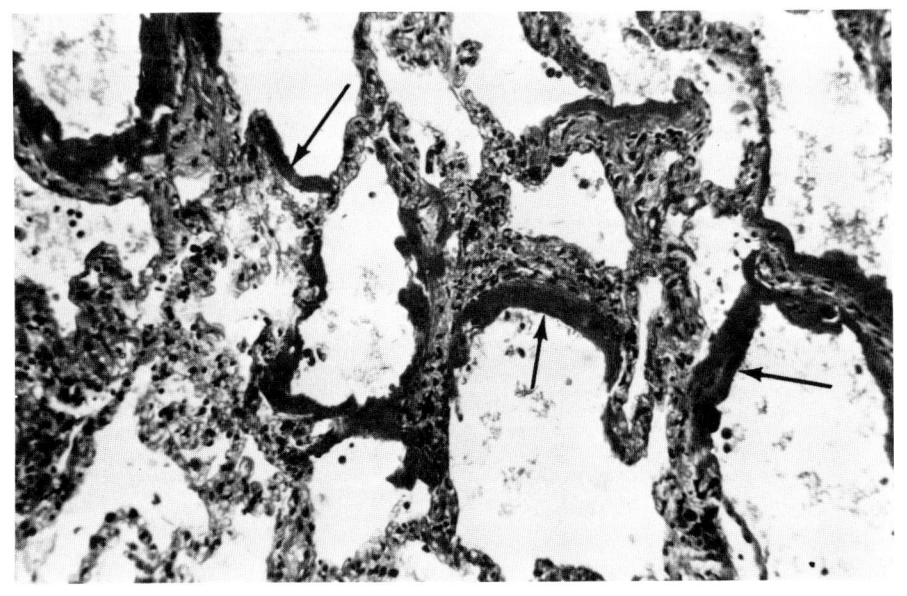

Figure 19.6. Adult respiratory distress syndrome. The alveolar walls are thickened by edema fluid and some mononuclear cell infiltration. Some protein precipitate is seen in the alveolar spaces, and there is striking hyaline membrane formation (*arrows*).

Table 19.2
Some Causes of Adult Respiratory Distress Syndrome

Shock	Toxic gases
Uremic pneumonitis	Phosgene
Radiation pneumonitis	Nitrogen dioxide
Viral pneumonia	Chlorine
Gram-negative sepsis	Disseminated intravascular coagulation
Drowning	Head trauma
Drug overdose	Postcardiopulmonary bypass
Heroin	Pancreatitis, acute
Barbiturates	Burns
Oxygen toxicity	

PULMONARY INFECTIONS

Many of the important infections of the lung have already been discussed. Pneumococcal pneumonia and staphylococcal lung abscess were presented in Chapter 4, tuberculosis and pneumocystis pneumonia in Chapter 5. Only a few other types of infection are considered here. Lobar pneumonia, although the classical form of pneumonia, is seen today much less frequently than *bronchopneumonia*, a patchy consolidation of the lungs, usually involving several lobes, and bilateral. Many microorganisms are associated with bronchopneumonia, particularly in debilitated patients and patients receiving immunosuppressive and adrenal cortical drugs. These include *Pseudomonas aeruginosa*, staphylococci, streptococci, pneumococci, *Haemophilus influenzae*, and enteric organisms. Many fungus infections of the lung have a bronchopneumonic distribution. The nodules of consolidation show intense polymorphonuclear infiltration and fibrin deposition in bronchi, bronchioles, and alveoli. Ulceration of bronchial mucosa is frequent, as are necrosis of alveolar septa and microabscess formation. Although healing by resolution can occur, at least some organization and fibrosis are likely.

Other pulmonary infections show an interstitial pattern, with inflammation of the alveolar septa. The alveoli reflect altered septal permeability, but may be free of inflammation. Interstitial pneumonia is characteristic of certain viral and mycoplasma pneumonias.

Legionnaires' Disease

Legionnaires' disease has been recognized only since the 1976 outbreak in Philadelphia. The etiologic agent, *Legionella pneumophilia*, fails to grow on routine bacteriologic media, and requires silver impregnation for light microscopic demonstration in tissue sections.

The morphologic findings in fatal cases consist of a confluent bronchopneumonia, occasionally a lobar consolidation, marked intra-alveolar exudation of macrophages and polymorphonuclear leukocytes, red blood cells, and fibrin. Areas of coagulation necrosis of lobular tissues may also be seen. Evidence of healing by organization is seen if the acute phase of illness is survived.

Legionnaires' disease can be sporadic or affect groups of people. It can also constitute a very serious nosocomial infection.

A pneumonia in many ways similar to Legionnaires' disease has been described recently in immunosuppressed patients. The causative organism has been called

Pittsburgh pneumonia agent, and shares several characteristics with *L. pneumophilia*.

Viral Pneumonia

Many viruses have the capacity to cause pulmonary infection. Among them are the influenza viruses, rhinoviruses, respiratory syncytial viruses, Coxsackie, and ECHO viruses. The pneumonia they produce is usually patchy, but may involve several lobes. The inflammatory process is predominantly interstitial, within the alveolar septa, which appear thickened, edematous, and infiltrated by mononuclear cells, principally macrophages. The alveolar spaces may contain a few inflammatory cells, but generally show edema fluid and prominent hyaline membranes, similar to findings in the adult respiratory distress syndrome (Fig. 19.7).

Although death may occur in uncomplicated viral pneumonia, it is more usually relatable to secondary bacterial pneumonia. This was particularly true in the great influenza epidemic at the end of World War I, when staphylococcal and streptococcal pneumonias took a heavy toll.

A pneumonic process indistinguishable from viral pneumonia can be caused by *Mycoplasma pneumoniae*. Other *Mycoplasma* organisms have assumed importance as etiologic agents in vaginitis and nonspecific urethritis.

PULMONARY HYPERTENSION

Pulmonary hypertension can result from congestive heart failure, many intrinsic pulmonary diseases, multiple pulmonary emboli, and congenital cardiovascular

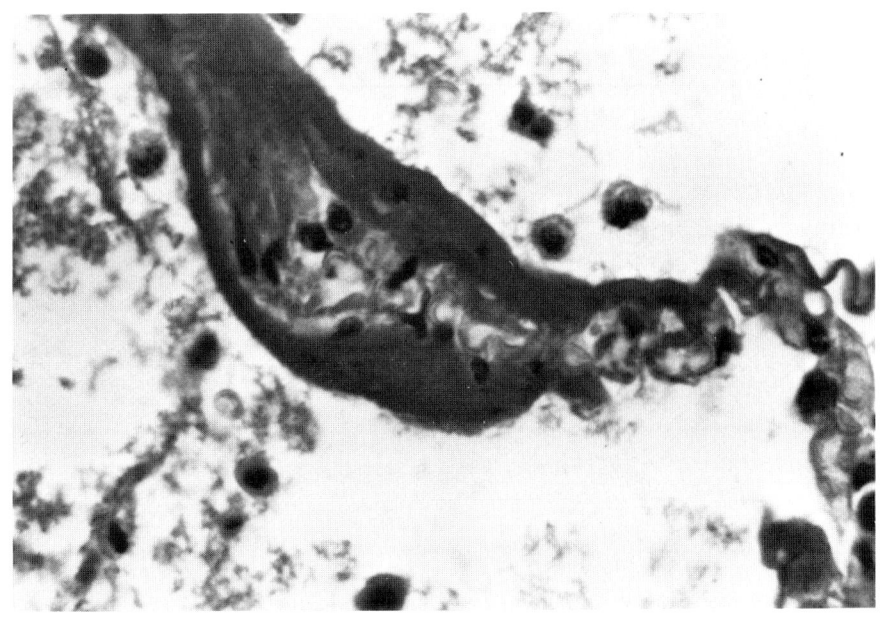

Figure 19.7. Influenza pneumonia. This field shows an alveolar septum covered by hyaline membrane and containing a few mononuclear cells. Some mononuclear phagocytes are also seen in the alveolar spaces.

224   Pathology: Understanding Human Disease

defects that shunt left ventricular blood into the pulmonary artery or overload the pulmonary circuit. Pulmonary hypertension can occasionally be a primary disorder of unknown etiology.

As in the systemic circulation, the most striking vascular changes due to hypertension are in the arterioles. There is medial thickening and compromise of the lumen and a tendency with time to form plexiform lesions (Fig. 19.8). Small and medium-sized arteries show medial hypertrophy and thickening and splitting of the internal elastica. The main pulmonary artery and its proximal branches are likely to contain elevated atherosclerotic plaques, although these are never comparable in magnitude to aortic lesions.

LUNG TUMORS

Primary malignant tumors of the lung comprise 20% of all malignancies in men and account for one-fourth of all cancer deaths. Their incidence has increased $2\frac{1}{2}$ times in men since 1950. The incidence in women, some one-fourth that in men, is also increasing steadily.

Particular attention was paid in Chapter 12 to the relationship between lung cancer and cigarette smoking. Other environmental pollutants contribute to the risk. Asbestosis increases the incidence by a factor of at least 5, asbestos and tobacco together by a factor of 92. Nickel, beryllium, and other metals have a significant, if less dramatic, role. Tumors may also arise in relation to pulmonary scars of old tuberculosis or other infections.

Malignancies arising in bronchi constitute the overwhelming majority of primary lung tumors. In order of frequency, they are squamous cell carcinoma,

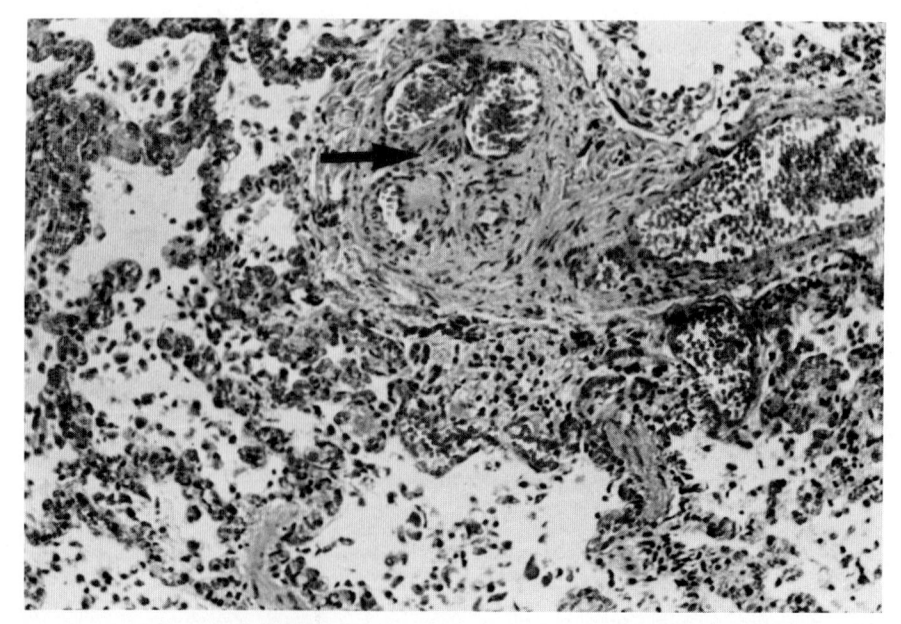

Figure 19.8. Pulmonary hypertension. The *arrow* points to a plexiform vascular lesion that is thought to be a sequel to thrombosis of small arteries or arterioles.

adenocarcinoma, small cell ("oat cell") anaplastic carcinoma, large cell anaplastic carcinoma, and bronchial adenoma. Bronchiolar-alveolar carcinomas account for less than 5%.

Bronchogenic Carcinoma

Squamous cell carcinomas and anaplastic carcinomas most often arise in the hilar region, from the bifurcation of the trachea to the third order bronchi (Fig. 19.9). Adenocarcinomas are more likely to arise in the periphery of the lung, particularly if associated with scars (Fig. 19.10). The point of origin of either may be the bronchial mucosa or the peribronchial glands. Tumor growth may project into and occlude the bronchial lumen, or it may invade through the bronchial wall to the peribronchial tissues. From here, it may extend centrally to involve mediastinal structures (Fig. 19.11) or, peripherally, following the course of the bronchial tree. At other times, a large mass is formed that surrounds bronchi and pulmonary vessels. Hemorrhage and necrosis of tumor tissue are prominent.

Metastasis from bronchogenic carcinomas occurs by both lymphatic and vascular paths. Hilar and mediastinal nodes are involved early, particularly in the anaplastic tumors, and the scalene nodes are positive for metastasis in half of patients. Hematogenous spread to distant organs may occur before the primary site has produced symptoms. The adrenal glands show metastasis in at least half of patients, and brain, bone, liver, and kidneys are frequent metastatic sites.

Squamous cell carcinoma shows a male predominance and is most closely associated with cigarette smoking. It appears to arise following squamous meta-

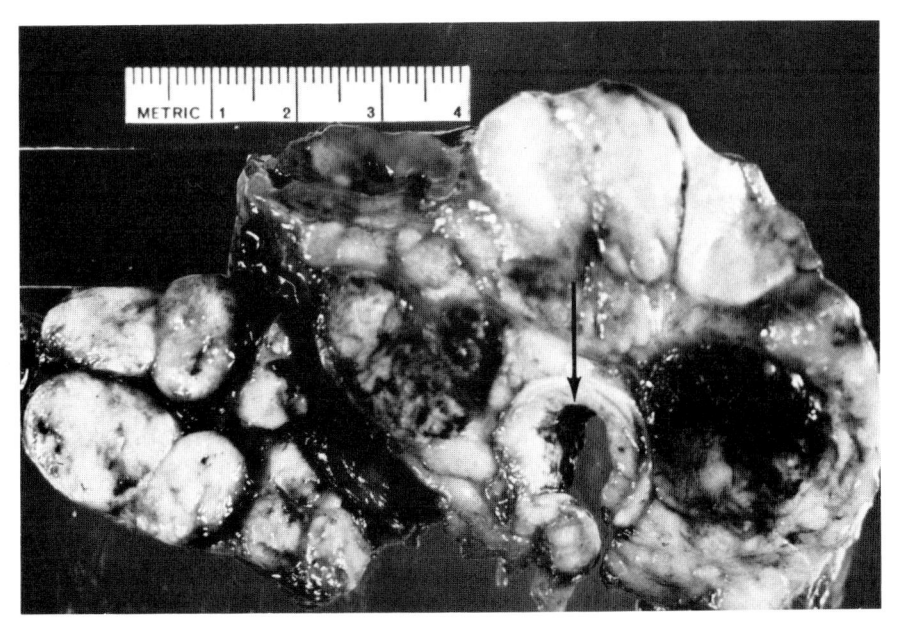

Figure 19.9. Anaplastic bronchogenic carcinoma. The mucosa of a large bronchus (*arrow*) has been replaced by an anaplastic carcinoma. There has been extensive metastasis to hilar and mediastinal lymph nodes.

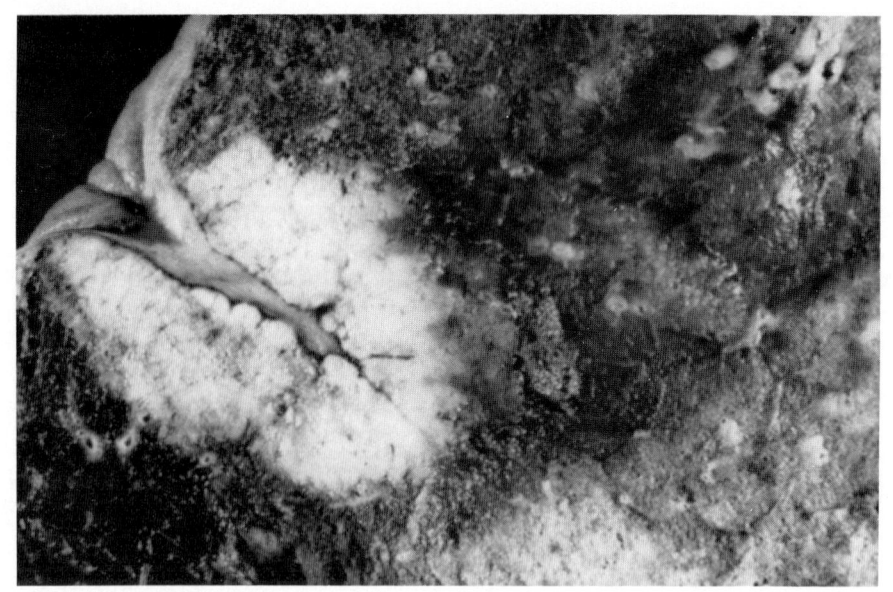

Figure 19.10. Adenocarcinoma arising in a scar. The retracted scar tissue is surrounded by firm grayish tumor tissue. It is poorly circumscribed from the surrounding pulmonary tissue.

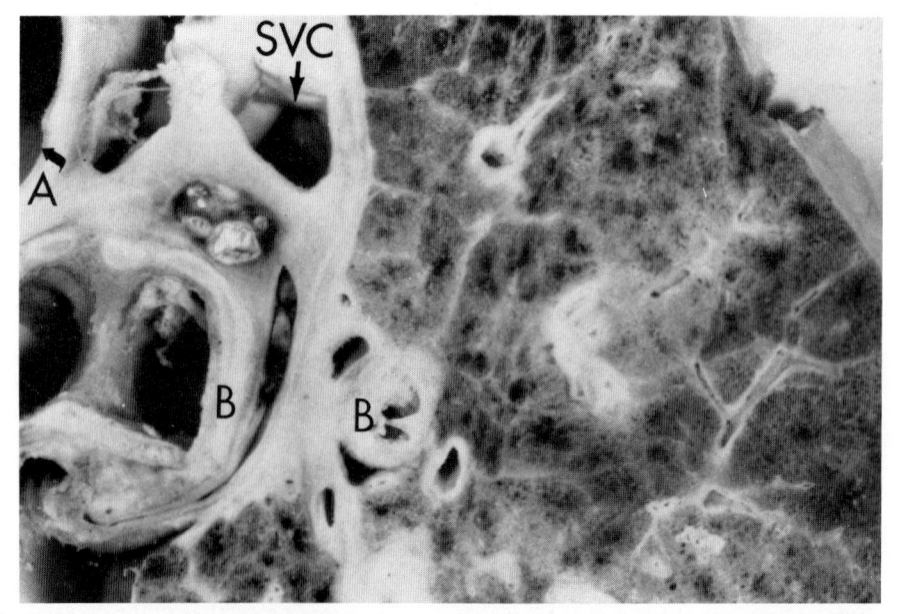

Figure 19.11. Anaplastic small cell carcinoma. There is extensive involvement of the bronchial mucosa (*B*) and extension into the mediastinum to surround the superior vena cava (*SVC*) and the aorta (*A*).

plasia of bronchial epithelium. This change, as well as *in situ* malignancy, are often discernible adjacent to a squamous tumor.

Adenocarcinoma shows no sex dominance. It tends to arise in peripheral lung tissue, and progresses more slowly than squamous carcinoma. It may be well differentiated or poorly differentiated, tends to secrete mucin, and may assume a papillary configuration. Its association with tobacco smoking is not so well established as in squamous carcinoma.

Small cell, or oat cell, anaplastic carcinoma is the most malignant of all primary lung tumors (Fig. 19.12). Its cells contain neurosecretory granules, and are part of the APUD system (p. 350). They have been known to secrete most of the polypeptide hormones. Origin from APUD cells suggests that small cell carcinoma is a highly malignant variant of the less aggressive bronchial carcinoid, but some observations tend to link it more with squamous cell precursors.

Large cell anaplastic carcinoma may show suggestive differentiation toward squamous cell carcinoma or adenocarcinoma. The tumor cells are very large and pleomorphic, and tumor giant cells are frequent.

Bronchogenic carcinomas may call attention to themselves in several ways. A small lesion may produce bronchial obstruction, causing distal atelectasis and bronchitis, complicated by bronchiectasis or lung abscess. Other tumors invade and compress such mediastinal structures as the superior vena cava. Tumors arising near a lung apex may invade the brachial plexus and interfere with cervical sympathetic nerves, producing a Horner's syndrome. The symptoms of many bronchogenic carcinomas relate to polypeptide hormone secretion. Small cell anaplastic carcinomas often secrete adrenocorticotrophic or antidiuretic hormone, and may secrete calcitonin, gonadotrophins, or serotonin. Parathyroid hormone may be secreted by squamous tumors. Bronchogenic tumors may be first manifest by their metastases or by such systemic symptomatology as myopathy, neuropathy, or clubbing of fingers and toes.

Although progress has been made in surgical, radiologic, and chemotherapeutic

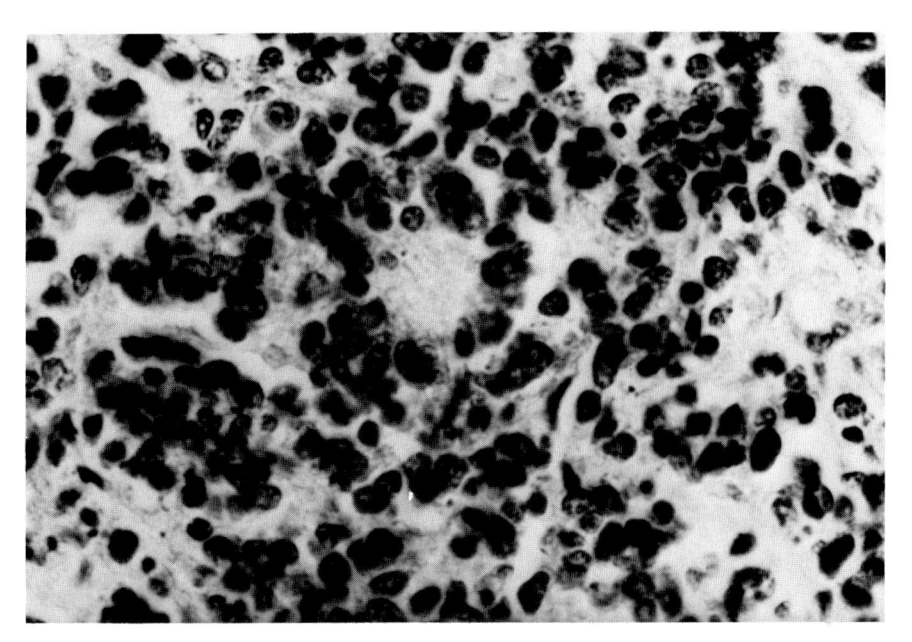

Figure 19.12. Anaplastic small cell carcinoma. The cells are uniform, have little cytoplasm, and show no evidence of differentiation.

Bronchiolar-Alveolar Carcinoma

This tumor arises in terminal bronchioles or alveolar septa. Its distribution and appearance in the lung are often more suggestive of a pneumonic consolidation, and it may be bilateral (Fig. 19.13). The tumor is usually well differentiated, composed of tall, columnar, mucin-secreting cells. Growth usually takes advantage of the existing connective tissue structure of the lung, tumor cells appearing to replace normal alveolar epithelium (Fig. 19.14). Mucus secretion may be the most prominent manifestation of the tumor.

Bronchiolar-alveolar carcinoma tends to spread primarily in the lung tissue, and metastases are likely to occur only late in the course.

Bronchial Adenoma

Bronchial adenomas are misnamed, since they are all low grade malignancies. The majority have a carcinoid structure, while others resemble salivary gland tumors. They tend to project into bronchi, are highly vascular, and bleed easily. Carcinoid tumors may secrete serotonin or other polypeptide hormones.

Secondary (Metastatic) Tumors

Tumors metastatic to the lung are more common than primary tumors. They tend to be more peripheral in location and are often multiple. Differentiating primary and metastatic tumors in the lung, however, can be difficult both clinically and morphologically.

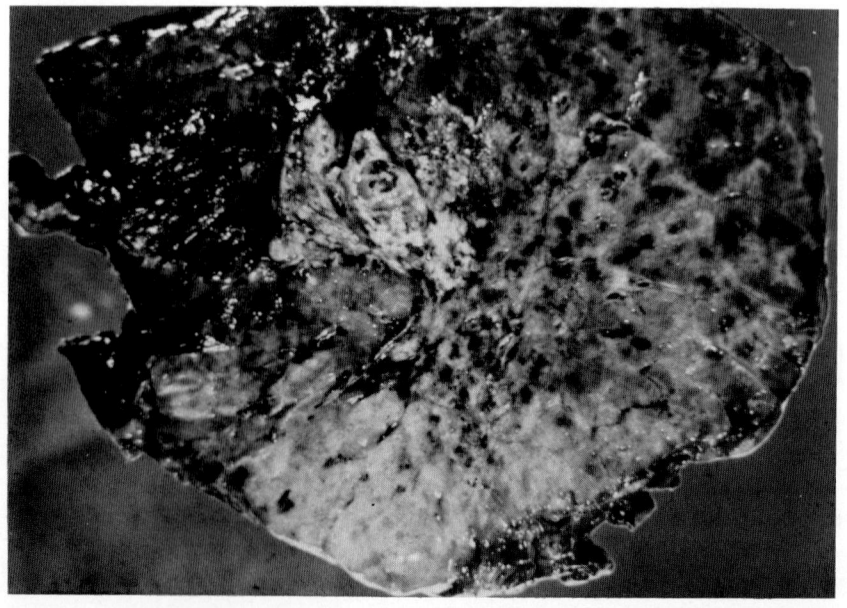

Figure 19.13. Bronchiolar-alveolar carcinoma. The cut surface of the lung is largely consolidated, and it has a distinctly mucoid appearance.

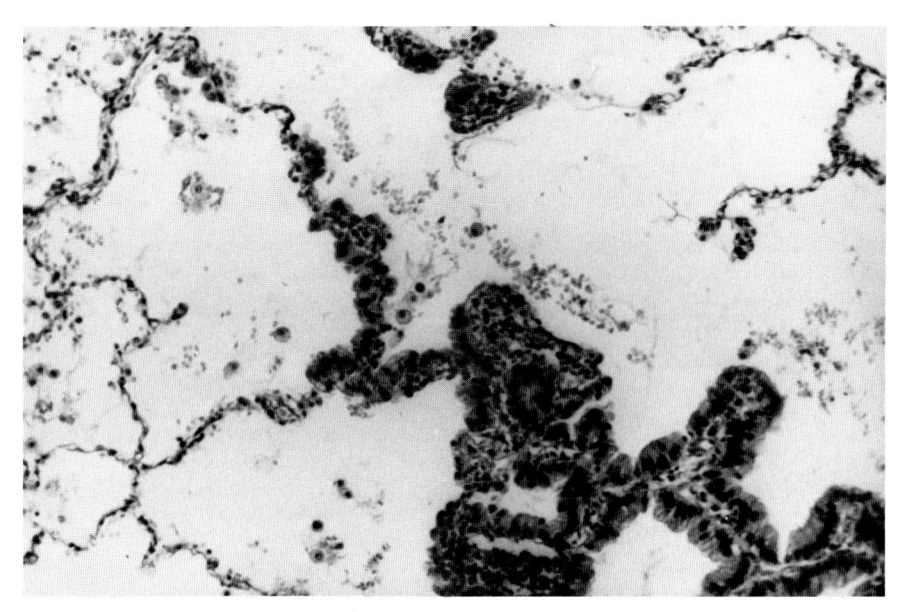

Figure 19.14. Bronchiolar-alveolar carcinoma. The tumor is well differentiated, showing a single layer of mucus-producing cells. The tumor appears to be growing along the normal alveolar architecture, replacing normal lining cells with neoplastic cells.

Mesothelioma

Mesotheliomas are generally malignant tumors that arise from the mesothelial lining of the serous cavities. They tend to spread through a serous cavity, may invade adjacent organs by continuity, but usually do not metastasize to distant sites. Their histologic appearance may suggest a sarcoma or a papillary adenocarcinoma that secretes acid mucopolysaccharides.

Workers exposed to asbestos have a much higher than expected incidence of mesotheliomas, appearing some 20 to 40 years after first exposure. Conversely, evidence of asbestosis can be found in most patients with mesotheliomas.

THE LARYNX

Several important lesions of the larynx are inserted at this point.

Laryngeal *polyps* are small, round, pedunculated, or sessile nodules of the true cords. They occur equally often in men and women, and are associated with cigarette smoking. The nodules are composed of fibrous or myxomatous connective tissue. Sometimes referred to as singer's nodes, their principal manifestation is hoarseness. They are probably not true neoplasms.

Laryngeal *papillomas* are usually small polypoid lesions, often ulcerated. Multiple papillomas may occur in children, but tend to regress at puberty.

Squamous cell carcinoma has a marked male predominance and a close association with cigarette smoking. Asbestosis and other environmental carcinogens may also bear on the incidence. Laryngeal carcinomas may arise on or near the cords, on the epiglottis, in the pyriform sinuses, or in the aryepiglottic folds. The frequency of dysplastic changes in the laryngeal mucosa makes early recognition of carcinoma extremely difficult.

Suggested Reading

Carrington CB, Gaensler EA. Clinical-pathologic approach to diffuse infiltrative lung disease. In: Thurlbeck WM, Abell MR, eds. The lung. Baltimore, Williams & Wilkins, 1978.

Ebert RV. Small airway disease of the lung. Ann. Intern. Med. *88:* 98, 1978.

Hocking WG, Golde DW. The pulmonary alveolar macrophage. N. Engl. J. Med. *301:* 580, 639, 1979.

Ioachim HL. Present trends in lung cancer. In: Thurlbeck WM, Abell MR, eds. The lung. Baltimore, Williams & Wilkins, 1978.

Murray JF. Mechanisms of acute respiratory failure. Am. Rev. Respir. Dis. *115:* 1071, 1977.

Niewoehner DE, Cosio MG. Chronic obstructive lung disease: the role of airway disease, with special emphasis on the pathology of the small airways. In: Thurlbeck WM, Abell MR, eds. The lung. Baltimore, Williams & Wilkins, 1978.

Schatz M, Patterson R, Fink J. Immunologic lung disease. N. Engl. J. Med. *300:* 1310, 1979.

Chapter 20

The Central Nervous System

WILLIAM R. MARKESBERY, M.D.

This chapter includes discussion of the more important areas of neuropathology; basic reactions and herniation, cerebrovascular disease, brain tumors, central nervous system infections, degenerative and demyelinating diseases and traumatic disorders. Some subjects, such as CNS malformations, have been omitted.

BASIC CELLULAR AND TISSUE REACTIONS AND BRAIN HERNIATION

Like other organ systems the nervous system has a limited number of ways it reacts to injury. The basic pathologic processes of neoplasia, inflammation, and ischemia are not significantly different from those of other tissues. Only because of the complexity of the cellularity of the nervous system is the process rendered less easily understood.

Neuronal Reactions

Neurons can undergo a variety of reactions to injury. They are the most vulnerable of all CNS cellular elements to pathologic processes. Loss of neurons occurs in numerous different disorders and is almost always accompanied by an astrocytic reaction. Assessment of neuronal loss is difficult and a loss of up to 30% of cortical neurons can remain undetected.

Acute ischemic neuronal change is characterized by retraction of the cell body, eosinophilic cytoplasm, loss of Nissl substance, and pyknotic, hyperchromatic nuclei. This is an irreversible alteration occurring as a result of oxygen depletion.

Simple neuronal atrophy is seen in progressive degenerative diseases. It is characterized by shrinkage and diffuse cytoplasmic basophilia and shrunken hyperchromatic nuclei. These cells subsequently die.

Central chromatolysis of neurons is a reaction of the cell body to axonal injury. In this the cell body is enlarged, Nissl substance disappears from all but the periphery of the cytoplasm, and the nucleus is displaced to the periphery. Recovery or progression of the neuronal change depends on the reversibility of the axonal lesion.

Neurons accumulate abnormal lipids and carbohydrates in a variety of lysosomal storage diseases. This results in swelling of the perikarya and displacement of Nissl granules and nucleus.

Alzheimer's neurofibrillary tangles are variably shaped, silver-positive, neuronal intracytoplasmic fibrillary structures composed of paired helical filaments. Although found in the aging brain, when seen in large numbers throughout the cerebral cortex they are diagnostic of Alzheimer's disease.

The presence of large eosinophilic intranuclear inclusions displacing the nucleus, surrounded by a halo (Cowdry A inclusions), is characteristic of but not pathognomonic of viral infection. They are found in herpes simplex, cytomegalovirus and varicella zoster encephalitis, and subacute sclerosing panencephalitis. Cytoplasmic inclusions are found in neurons in a variety of specific disease states. Negri bodies are small eosinophilic cytoplasmic inclusions found in 70% of patients with rabies. Lewy bodies are eosinophilic inclusions found in the cytoplasm of pigmented neurons in idiopathic parkinsonism.

Glial Reactions

Astrocytes are divided into fibrous type, occurring largely in the white matter, and protoplasmic type, occurring primarily in gray matter. The former have long, thin, infrequent branching processes containing abundant glial filaments while the latter have more frequent, shorter processes with fewer filaments. Astrocytic processes extend to the pial and ependymal surfaces and around blood vessels and neurons. They function to give structural support, insulate receptor surfaces of neurons, regulate extracellular ions, form part of the anatomic blood-brain barrier and aid in repair of injured neural tissue. In the latter role, they react by hyperplasia, hypertrophy, and formation of more extensive fibrillary processes. The primary stimulus to astrocytic reaction is destruction of CNS tissue, irrespective of cause. In many situations astrocytes react by hypertrophy of the cell body. Formation of abundant 8- to 9-nm glial filaments usually accompanies hyperplasia and hypertrophy. When they form large, round eosinophilic, hyaline cytoplasmic bodies they are called gemistocytes. In response to most stimuli, protoplasmic astrocytes become transformed into reactive fibrillary astrocytes. An exception to this is the Alzheimer's Type II astrocyte reaction which occurs primarily in hepatic and renal failure. In these conditions, protoplasmic astrocytes develop enlarged vesicular nuclei, glycogen granules, and prominent nuclear membranes.

Microglial cells are mesenchymal elements, not true glial cells. They are the primary phagocytic cells of the CNS and can be a prominent component of the reaction to disease. In acute conditions (vascular disorders, trauma, etc) they become enlarged and rounded and play a phagocytic role. However, autoradiographic studies have shown that the majority of phagocytes in acute brain injury originate from circulating mononuclear cells. In chronic conditions such as tertiary syphilis and some subacute conditions, abundant rod-shaped microglial cells develop. In viral encephalitis or CNS rickettsial infection, clusters of elongated or round microglial cells termed microglial nodules are found.

Oligodendroglia function to form and maintain CNS myelin. In gray matter, oligodendroglia often form satellite cells around neurons. Oligodendroglia occasionally undergo degeneration in which the nucleus becomes pyknotic, and the cytoplasm swells and develops a mucinous change, termed acute swelling. Although oligodendroglia contain inclusions in subacute sclerosing panencephalitis and progressive multifocal leukoencephalopathy, for practical purposes they do not exhibit reactive changes which provide useful criteria for diagnostic evaluation.

To understand better how the CNS cells participate in overall tissue reactions, consider the events that occur in an area of infarction. The order of susceptibility of cellular elements to ischemia is: neurons, myelin and axon, oligodendroglia, astrocytes, microglia, and blood vessels. Following total occlusion of a cerebral artery, ischemia develops in its region of supply. After 12 to 24 hr the tissue is soft and edematous and neurons show eosinophilic cytoplasmic change and eccentric nuclei. By 24 to 72 hr, blood vessels are congested and neutrophilic leukocytes migrate into the infarction. After 72 hr there is an increase in microglial cells which slowly evolve into rounded macrophages. Other macrophages develop from circulating mononuclear cells which have migrated into the infarct. At the margin of the infarct, astrocytes survive and by 5 to 10 days they increase in number and show mild cytoplasmic enlargement. By 2 to 3 weeks the center of the infarct is liquefied and macrophages contain abundant ingested necrotic debris. By this time reactive hypertrophied astrocytes are prominent at the margin of the infarct. By 6 weeks the lipid-laden macrophages are being resorbed and diminish in number. After several months a multilayered scar of astrocyte processes circumscribe the infarct cavity. Subsequently the area is an empty cavity surrounded by a glial scar.

BRAIN HERNIATIONS

Most intracranial masses or severe focal or generalized cerebral edema can result in shifting of brain parenchyma from one intracranial compartment to another, spoken of as brain herniation. The direction and degree of shift are related to the location of the expanding mass. The most important form of herniation is transtentorial herniation (Fig. 20.1). Expanding supratentorial masses, especially of the temporal or posterior frontal lobes and middle cranial fossa, cause displacement of the uncus and parahippocampal gyrus medially over the free edge of the tentorium. This results in compression of the third nerve and nucleus, compression of the posterior cerebral arteries against the tentorium which can cause hemorrhagic infarction in the medial occipital lobes, compression of the homolateral or contralateral cerebral peduncle resulting in corticospinal tract dysfunction, and caudal shift of the brainstem resulting in altered venous and arterial blood flow leading to hemorrhages in the midbrain and pons. These events proceed acutely and are associated with a series of predictable clinical findings: homolateral pupillary dilatation and failure to move the eye laterally, loss of "doll's eye" movements and caloric reflexes, alteration in respiratory pattern, contralateral or homolateral hemiparesis with decorticate posturing progressing to decerebrate posturing, and altered consciousness progressing to deep coma. These signs appear in an advancing pattern of rostral-caudal deterioration.

Cerebellar tonsillar herniation (Fig. 20.2) through the foramen magnum can occur with posterior fossa mass lesions or diffuse increased intracranial pressure. It causes compression of the medulla resulting in vasomotor collapse and respiratory arrest.

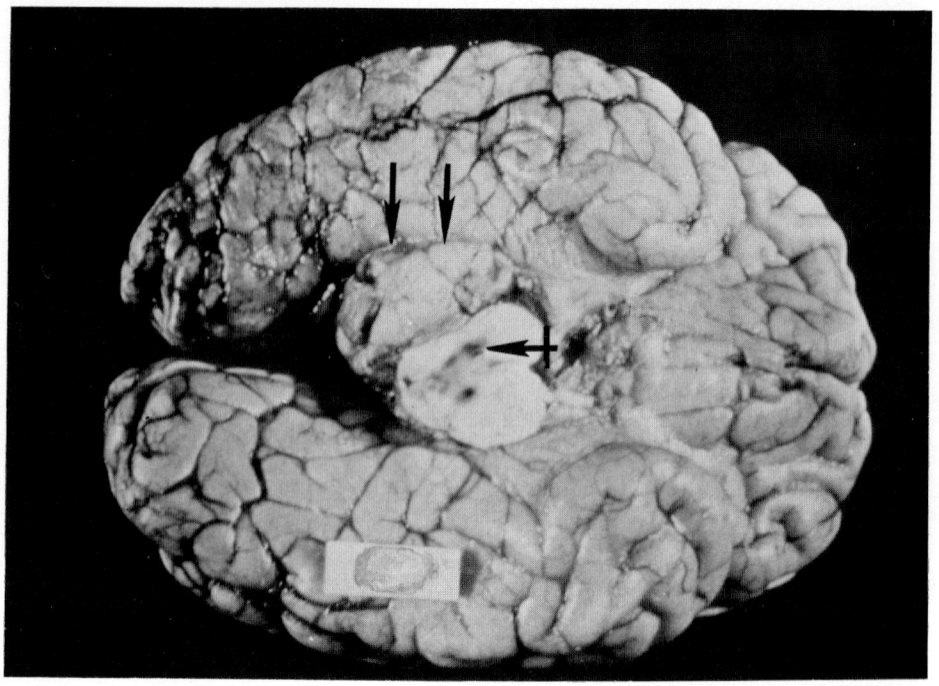

Figure 20.1. Transtentorial herniation. A large mass in the right temporal lobe has caused herniation of the uncus and parahippocampal gyrus (*arrows*) through the tentorial opening compressing the midbrain. Note the Duret hemorrages (*crossed arrow*) in the midbrain.

Cingulate gyrus herniation beneath the free edge of the falx cerebri is seen in unilateral lesions of the frontal or parietal lobe. It has no clinical signature but may be valuable in diagnostic radiologic studies.

VASCULAR DISEASE OF THE CNS

Cerebrovascular disease is the most common cause of neurologic disability and is the third most common cause of death in this country. "Stroke" or "cerebrovascular accident" are terms applied to the clinical manifestations of vascular disease of the brain. The pathologic changes can be classified into pale or hemorrhagic cerebral infarction, intracerebral hemorrhage, and subarachnoid hemmorrhage. In a community of 100,000, it has been estimated that there are 190 cerebral infarctions, 35 intracerebral hemorrhages, and 25 subarachnoid hemorrhages per year.

Cerebral Infarction

Cerebral infarction denotes the irreversible necrosis of brain parenchyma caused by inadequate blood supply or intereference with oxygen availability. This is the most common of all cerebrovascular diseases. Cerebral infarctions are classified as pale (Fig. 20.3) or hemorrhagic (Fig. 20.4).

The most common cause of intracranial vascular occlusion is atherosclerosis (Chapter 16). It commonly involves the vessels of the circle of Willis and their

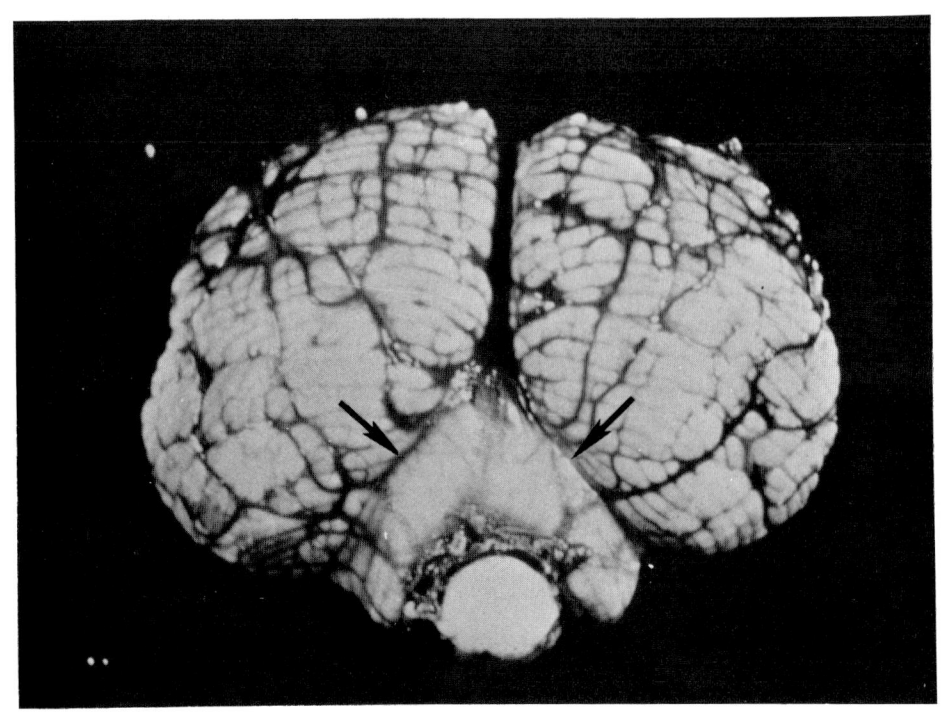

Figure 20.2. Cerebellar tonsillar herniation. Note the large grooves (*arrows*) in the caudally displaced cerebellar tissue.

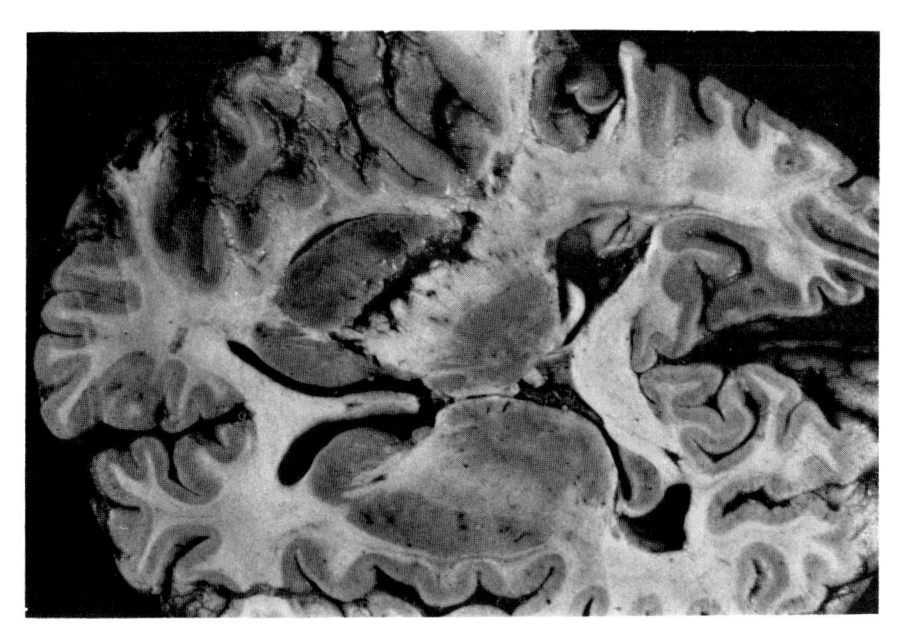

Figure 20.3. Recent infarction in the distribution of the right middle cerebral artery. The infarcted tissue is softened, slightly discolored, and edematous.

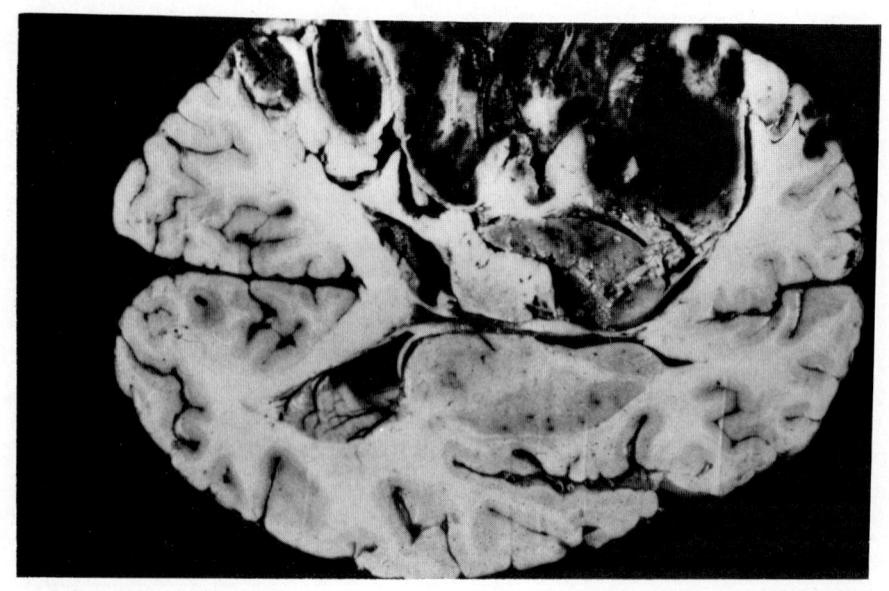

Figure 20.4. Hemorrhagic infarction in left middle cerebral artery territory, presumed to be due to embolus. Hemorrhage predominately located in cortex with some confluent hemorrhages. Note edema of left hemisphere with compression of lateral ventricle. Anterior and posterior cerebral artery territories are spared.

proximal branches, although in association with hypertension it may extend into small cerebral vessels. Extracranial stenosis or occlusions of the carotid or vertebral arteries cause approximately one-third of cerebral infarctions. Ulceration of atheromatous plaques of cervical vessels may be a source of cerebral emboli. Rare causes of cerebral infarction include syphilis, granulomatous arteritis, collagen-vascular disease, sickle cell anemia, polycythemia vera, thrombotic thrombocytopenic purpura, and many others.

The extent of an infarction is determined by a number of factors including the site of occlusion, size of the occluded vessel, duration of the occlusion, and the collateral circulation. Once infarction occurs, autoregulation is abolished and there is vasoparalysis. The vessels are maximally dilated, blood flow varies with the perfusion pressure, and there is no response in the infarcted area to CO_2 or vasoactive drugs. The specific neurologic findings depend on the artery involved. General clinical manifestations of cerebral infarction include prodromal transient ischemia attacks, stuttering onset, occurrence during sleep or upon arising in the morning, and predominance in older individuals with systemic atherosclerosis, diabetes, or hypertension.

Occlusion of small deep penetrating arteries causes small irregular shaped infarctions called lacunae. They are most commonly found in the anterior pons, centrum semiovale, putamen, thalamus, and cerebellar white matter. They are associated with combined hypertension and atherosclerosis.

Cerebral Embolism

The majority of cerebral emboli arise from the heart but ulcerated atheromatous plaques of the cervical arteries are also a common source. Emboli usually involve smaller arteries than thrombi and are frequently found at bifurcation points or where vessel lumens become narrow.

Cardiac causes of cerebral emboli are arrhythmias (primarily atrial fibrillation), myocardial infarction associated with mural thrombi, acute and subacute bacterial endocarditis, nonbacterial thrombotic endocarditis, complications of cardiac surgery, and myocarditis.

Infarctions from cerebral embolization may be massive when major vessels are occluded, but are more often smaller and sometimes multiple. Emboli more commonly reach the brain through the internal carotid artery and proceed into the middle cerebral artery branches. They may cause pale, hemorrhagic (Fig. 20.4), or a mixed pattern of infarction. It is generally held that hemorrhagic infarction is primarily caused by embolization. Hemorrhagic infarction may result from fragmentation and distal movement of emboli, allowing for reflow of blood into damaged vessels and leakage into infarcted parenchyma. The microscopic picture of cerebral embolization is similar to that described previously for infarction except for the presence of abundant blood or hemosiderin pigment.

The neurologic findings in cerebral embolization depend on the artery involved and the site of obstruction. Cerebral embolization causes a more rapid onset of symptoms than other forms of stroke and usually has no prodromal episodes. Occasionally embolization to several different cerebral vessels or to other organs, such as the kidney or the extremities, is seen.

Intracranial Hemorrhage

Many of the causes of intracranial hemorrhage are listed in Table 20.1.

Hypertensive Intracerebral Hemorrhage

Except for CNS trauma, the most common cause of intracranial hemorrhage is hypertension. The true nature of the vascular lesion leading to arterial rupture in hypertension is not fully known but it has been hypothesized that microaneurysms (Charcot-Bouchard aneurysms) which develop on small intraparenchymal arteries, are the source of many hemorrhages. Large hemorrhages occur in the following sites: basal ganglia (Fig. 20.5), 50%; thalamus, 10%; cerebellum, 10%; pons, 10%; and miscellaneous sites, 20%. Most of these hemorrhages produce massive destruction and distortion of neural parenchyma. In the white matter the blood tends to dissect along fiber tracts. The hematomas accumulate rapidly and may act as a mass resulting in displacement of neural parenchyma and to

Table 20.1
Causes of Intracranial Hemorrhage (Intracerebral and Subarachnoid)

Trauma
Hypertension
Ruptured saccular aneurysms
Ruptured vascular malformations
Blood dyscrasias (leukemias, aplastic anemia, thrombocytopenic purpura, hemophilia, etc.)
Inflammatory disorders of arteries and veins
Hemorrhage into metastatic or primary brain tumors
Mycotic aneurysms
Anticoagulant therapy
Cerebral vein and venous sinus thrombosis

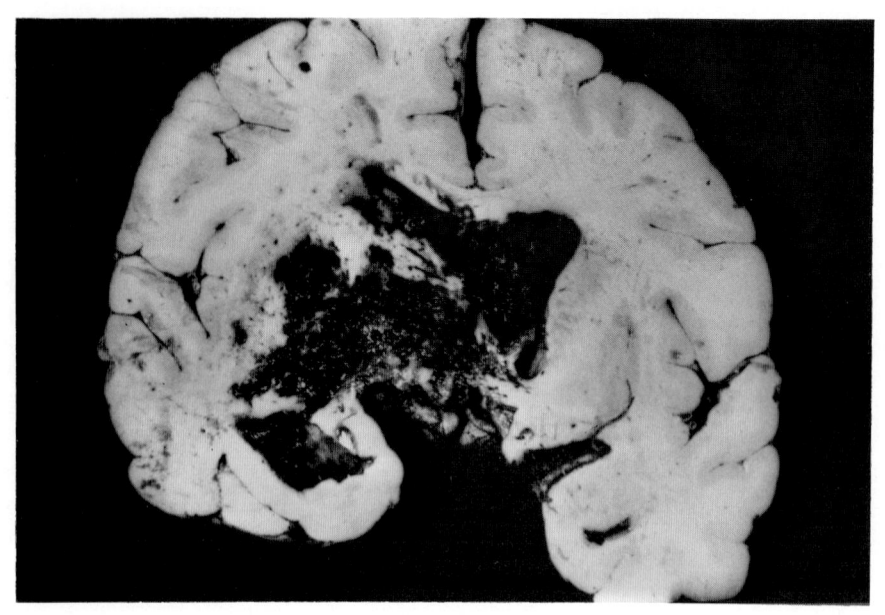

Figure 20.5. Large hypertensive hemorrhage in the left basal ganglia and internal capsule with rupture into the ventricular system.

herniation. They may rupture into the ventricular system or subarachnoid space. Occasionally small slit hemorrhages occur in the lateral basal ganglia or subcortical white matter.

After several days, the hemorrhage begins to liquify and change from red to brown. Subsequently yellowish orange pigment is found around the hematoma. Resorption of the major portion of the hematoma takes months. Eventually a cavity will form and the walls will contain hemosiderin pigment and an astrocytic scar similar to that described above.

Hypertensive intracranial hemorrhages occur more commonly during the daytime, without prodromal symptoms, and have a relatively rapid onset of headache, stupor or coma, and focal neurologic signs. Large basal ganglia hemorrhages present with a dense hemiplegia and stupor progressing to coma and carry a grave prognosis. Those that rupture into the lateral ventricles usually have a rapidly fatal course. Pontine hemorrhages usually cause cranial nerve and pyramidal tract signs, coma, and a rapid demise. Cerebellar hemorrhages can cause tonsillar herniation and medullary compression leading to death.

Subarachnoid Hemorrhage

Ruptured saccular aneurysms are the most common cause of primary subarachnoid hemorrhage. Vascular malformations and mycotic aneurysms are much less common.

Saccular aneurysms are found in approximately 2 to 3% of adults. These small, thin walled outpouchings arise at the bifurcations of the major cerebral arteries (Fig. 20.6), and approximately 90% occur in the anterior part of the circle of Willis or its major branches. The common sites of saccular aneurysms are: anterior communicating-anterior cerebral artery, internal carotid-middle cerebral artery bifurcation, internal carotid-posterior communicating bifurcation, and middle cerebral artery trifurcation (Fig. 20.6). They are multiple in approximately 20% of affected individuals. Aneurysms vary in size from 2 mm to 3 or 4 cm in diameter.

The pathogenesis of aneurysms is disputed, but they are thought to arise from congenital defects in the internal elastic membrane and media at branching points of cerebral arteries. Detractors from this hypothesis point out that these defects are commonly found at autopsy without associated aneurysms and are also present in the posterior circulation where aneurysms are less frequent. A combination of hemodynamic factors and atherosclerosis may also play a role in their formation and development.

Aneurysms most commonly cause symptoms by rupturing into the subarachnoid space. If the point of rupture is directed toward the parenchyma an intracerebral hematoma may develop. Rupture through the arachnoid membrane can occur, producing a subdural hematoma. Blood in the subarachnoid space may block the Pacchionian granulations causing acute hydrocephalus. It may also cause fibrosis of the leptomeninges and chronic hydrocephalus. Subarachnoid blood can also cause intense vasospasm which in turn reduces cerebral blood flow, leading to ischemia and infarction.

Ruptured aneurysms occur more often during periods of exertion with the acute onset of severe headache, occasional loss of consciousness, and subsequent nuchal rigidity. There is often a paucity of localizing signs. Death occurs in approximately 50% of cases in the first 6 weeks.

Atherosclerotic aneurysms are large segmental dilatations of the basilar artery or the subclinoid portion of the internal carotid arteries. They cause symptoms by compression of adjacent structures.

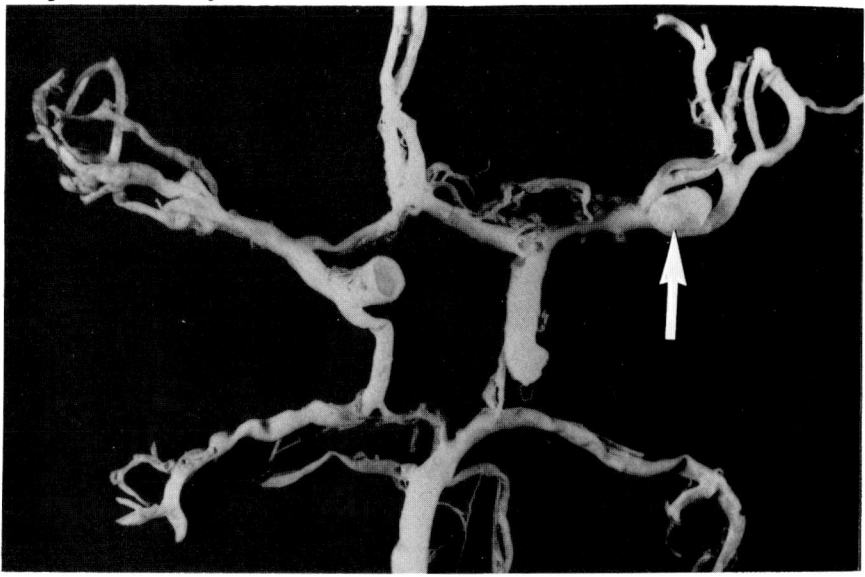

Figure 20.6. Dissected circle of Willis showing round saccular aneurysm (*arrow*) at the trifurcation of the middle cerebral artery.

Cerebrovenous Occlusive Disease

Thrombosis of the cerebral venous system or dural venous sinuses is relatively rare compared to arterial occlusive disease. It is most often seen in association with malnutrition, dehydration, cachexia, head injury, and meningitis. Thrombosis is most commonly found in the superior sagittal sinus and superior cerebral veins. Venous thrombosis causes hemorrhage into the subarachnoid space, hemorrhagic infarction, and large confluent hemorrhages in the underlying cortex and white matter.

TUMORS OF THE CNS

Primary brain tumors form about 9% of all neoplasms and account for about 1% of all autopsies. The site and type of intracranial tumor are dependent on the patient's age. In children approximately 70% of intracranial neoplasms are infratentorial and in adults about 70% are supratentorial. The frequent infratentorial tumors in children are cerebellar and brainstem astrocytomas, medulloblastomas, and ependymomas. In adults, glioblastoma multiforme, astrocytomas, meningiomas, and pituitary adenomas are the most frequent types of supratentorial tumors.

Brain tumors are similar to tumors arising elsewhere except that they grow in a cavity with rigid walls, where there is little room for expansion, and they rarely metastasize. Their intracranial location is of prime importance since histologically benign tumors near vital centers or interfering with cerebrospinal fluid (CSF) flow can threaten life early in their course. Most cause cerebral edema which adds to the mass effect of the neoplasm.

Clinical manifestations of tumors are focal and generalized. Focal signs depend on the location of the neoplasm. Generalized effects include headache, nausea, vomiting, papilledema, abducens nerve palsies, and somnolence and are, in general, due to increased intracranial pressure.

Gliomas

Neoplasms derived from astrocytes, oligodendrocytes, and ependymal cells are referred to as gliomas. They represent the largest group of primary intracranial neoplasms.

A variety of different types of astrocytomas occurs in various sites in the CNS and in different age groups. All infiltrate widely and destroy brain tissue. They vary from well differentiated, less malignant tumors (Grades 1 or 2) to markedly anaplastic, highly malignant tumors (Grades 3 or 4). Some astrocytomas occur in specific anatomic sites and represent well defined clinicopathologic entities. Cerebellar astrocytomas are either cystic or solid, more often occur in childhood and most have a benign course. Juvenile piloid astrocytomas occur most commonly in the pons, hypothalamus, and optic nerves or chiasm in childhood. Diffuse cerebral astrocytomas are more frequently seen in adults.

Glioblastoma multiforme is the most common primary glioma (Fig. 20.7). They occur in adults, with a peak incidence in the sixth decade. They are highly malignant and the average postoperative survival is approximately 9 months. They occur most frequently in the frontal, temporal, and parietal lobes. Origin in

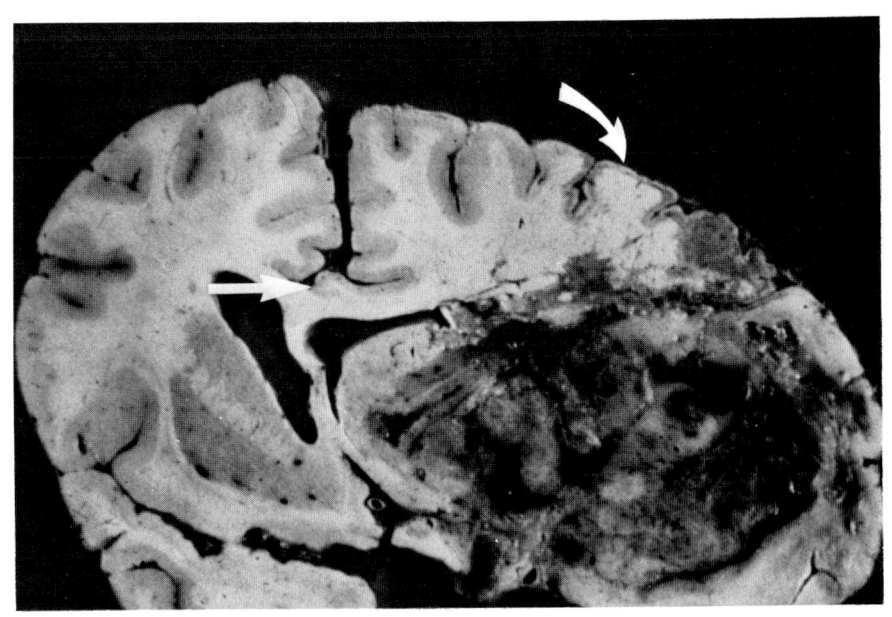

Figure 20.7. Glioblastoma multiforme. This large necrotic, hemorrhagic neoplasm has infiltrated the temporal and frontal lobes, basal ganglia, and internal capsule. Note the marked enlargement of the right hemisphere and the right cingulate gyrus herniation (*arrow*). Just superior to the neoplasm is an area of infarction (*curved arrow*) caused by compression of the middle cerebral artery by the neoplasm.

or spread across the corpus callosum is not unusual. Histologically, they exhibit hypercellularity, pleomorphism, frequent mitotic figures, necrosis, and endothelial proliferation. They are thought to arise from previously existing astrocytomas.

Oligodendrogliomas make up about 5% of gliomas and primarily occur in adults. They are usually located in the cerebral hemispheres and may contain considerable calcification. They have a variable biologic behavior, but many grow slowly. Histologically they are composed of sheets of uniform cells with clear perinuclear halos. Mixed oliodendrogliomas and astrocytomas are common.

Ependymomas, derived from the ependymal cells lining the ventricles, make up 5% of all intracranial gliomas. They occur most commonly in the posterior fossa of children, but are found in all age groups. They are well circumscribed and grow slowly. They are composed of sheets of well differentiated ependymal cells that occasionally form ependymal or true rosettes or perivascular pseudorosettes.

Medulloblastomas are primitive neuroectodermal neoplasms arising in the cerebellum in childhood or young adults. In children, they usually are found in the midline vermis while in young adults they are in the lateral cerebellar hemispheres. They are thought to be derived from undifferentiated cells of the persistent fetal external granular layer. In children, they often block the fourth ventricle, causing hydrocephalus, ataxia, and increased intracranial pressure. Histologically they are composed of highly cellular sheets of small dark cells with dense nuclei and scanty cytoplasm. They often form pseudorosettes characterized by cells surrounding eosinophilic centers containing fibrillary material. The neoplasm has a tendency to spread throughout the subarachnoid space. It responds well to radiation therapy, but has a tendency to recur, with eventual fatal termination.

Tumors of Meninges

Meningiomas are discrete, slowly growing, extraparenchymal, benign neoplasms thought to arise from arachnoidal cells. They account for approximately 15% of all intracranial neoplasms and primarily occur in adults. Meningiomas compress rather than invade the adjacent brain and occasionally penetrate contiguous bone or cause hyperostosis. The most common subtypes are meningotheliomatous, transitional, fibroblastic, and angioblastic. They occur most commonly in the parasagittal region (Fig. 20.8), over the cerebral convexities, along the sphenoid ridge or olfactory groove, and in the cerebellopontine angle and foramen magnum. They are surgically removable, do not respond to radiation therapy, and have a tendency to recur. Primary sarcomas can also occur in the meninges but are quite rare.

Tumors of Nerve Roots and Peripheral Nerve

Schwannomas (neurilemmomas) are benign tumors arising from Schwann cells that occur along the course of cranial, spinal, or peripheral nerves. The most common intracranial site is the eighth nerve in the cerebellopontine angle. They arise from the nerve sheath and act to compress rather than to infiltrate the nerve. They are encapsulated and grow slowly. They commonly occur in the spinal canal, arising most frequently from dorsal nerve roots.

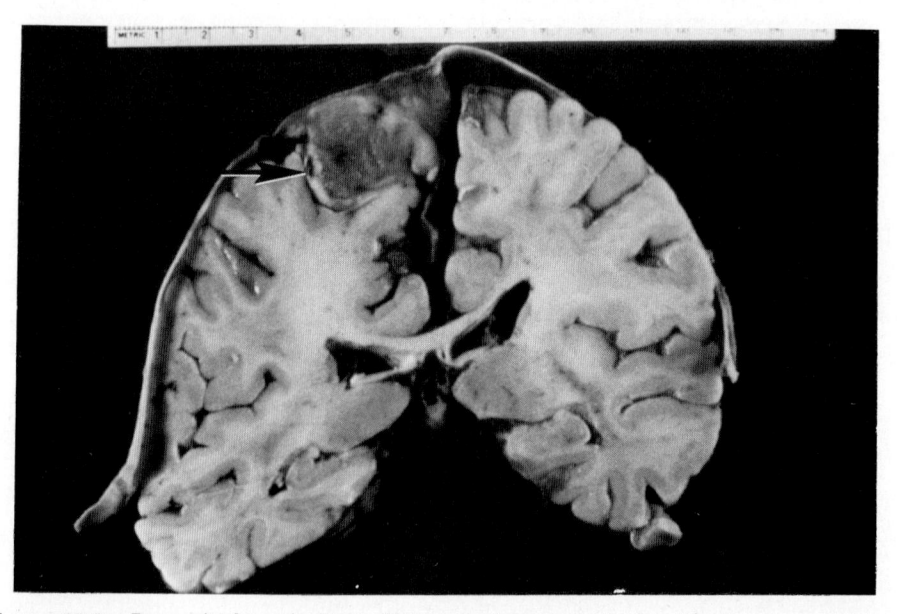

Figure 20.8. Parasagittal meningioma. This well circumscribed, globoid, discrete meningioma (*arrow*) is attached to the dura and falx. It compresses rather than invades the underlying superior frontal gyrus.

Neurofibromas also develop on cranial, spinal, and peripheral nerves. They may be derived from Schwann cells, fibroblasts, or perineural cells. They are primarily seen in association with von Recklinghausen's disease and are commonly multiple. They infiltrate and expand the involved nerve. In a small percentage of cases, malignant neurofibrosarcomas develop.

Metastases to the Central Nervous System

Metastatic neoplasms make up about 50% of all intracranial tumors. The most common sources of intracranial metastases are lung, breast, kidney, and gastrointestinal carcinomas. Malignant melanomas, although less common, frequently metastasize to the brain. It is not uncommon for a CNS metastatic tumor to cause the initial symptom of the disease. CNS metastases are usually blood-borne. The most common sites are the cerebral hemispheres, where they are located at the junction of the cortex and white matter, or in the cerebellum. They are frequently necrotic, occasionally are the site of hemorrhage, and commonly are associated with severe focal edema. Meningeal carcinomatosis is a diffuse spread of metastatic tumor through the subarachnoid space and usually involves multiple cranial and spinal nerves. This can be associated with low CSF glucose. Metastases to skull, vertebra, dura, and the spinal epidural space are not uncommon.

INFECTIOUS DISEASES OF THE CNS

The CNS is normally sterile and is well protected from microorganisms by its coverings, the brain-barrier systems, and the body defense mechanisms. Most CNS infections result from focal or generalized systemic infections. The most common route of infection to the CNS is via the bloodstream. Infection may spread by direct extension along veins (thrombophlebitis) from diseases of the middle ear, mastoid air cells, paranasal sinuses, nasopharynx, scalp, and face. Direct implantation of infection from skull fractures and dural tears or extension from osteomyelitis also occurs. Spread along axons, Schwann cells, or epineural space of peripheral nerves occurs in some viral diseases.

Acute Bacterial Meningitis (Leptomeningitis)

Leptomeningitis is an inflammation of the arachnoid and pia mater. Although most bacteria can produce meningitis, the common organisms vary with the age of the patient. Group B *Streptococcus* and Gram-negative enteric organisms most commonly cause neonatal meningitis. In children, *Haemophilus influenzae*, *Streptococcus pneumoniae*, and *Neisseria meningitidis* are the common causitive organism. In adults *S. pneumoniae* and *N. meningitidis* are the most common causes of meningitis. The majority of these organisms reach the CNS via a hematogenous route. Young children, the elderly, alcoholics, and those with immunosuppressive diseases are most commonly susceptible to meningitis.

Grossly, the subarachnoid space over the brain and spinal cord contains a white or yellow-white purulent exudate (Fig. 20.9). It is most pronounced along leptomeningeal vessels and in sulci, basilar cisterns, and the lumbar sac. Microscopically there is initial predominance of polymorphonuclear leukocytes. After 2 to 3 days arachnoidal phagocytes appear and subsequently many lymphocytes, larger mononuclear cells, and fibrin. In the majority of cases the infection is confined to

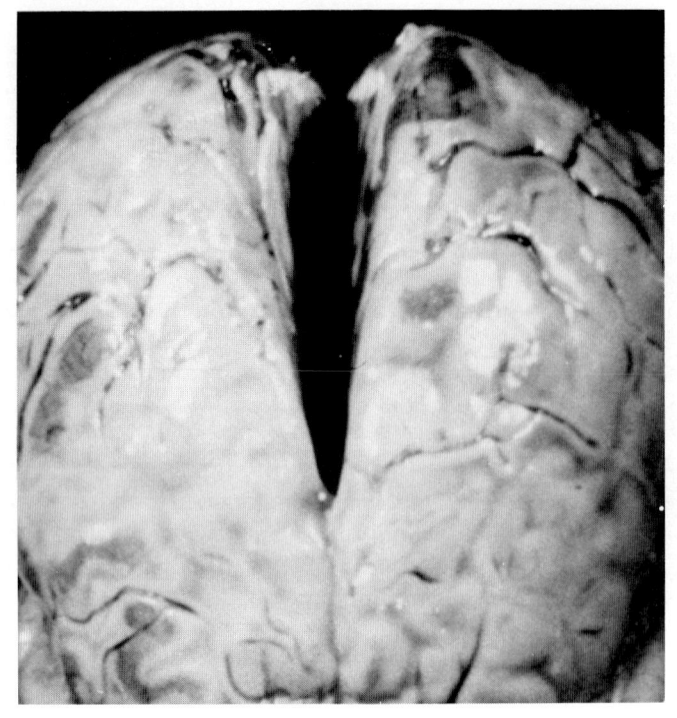

Figure 20.9. Acute bacterial meningitis. Superior view of the cerebral hemisphere showing purulent material in subarachnoid space.

the subarachnoid space except for extension along the Virchow-Robin spaces.

The clinical manifestations of uncomplicated meningitis include fever, headache, photophobia, nuchal rigidity, lethargy, irritability, confusion, vomiting, and positive Kernig's and Brudzinski's signs. The CSF is under increased pressure and contains 500 to 50,000 leukocytes per mm^3 (predominately polymorphonuclear cells), a reduced glucose content (0 to 30 mg per dl), and an elevated protein content (45 to 1,000 mg per dl).

Brain Abscess

A significant number of brain abscesses develop from local pericranial infections of the middle ear, mastoid, or paranasal sinuses or from osteomyelitis of the skull. These produce abscesses by direct extension through contiguous structures or via septic thrombophlebitis. Ear infections lead to cerebellar or temporal lobe abscesses and paranasal sinusitis can cause frontal lobe abscesses (Fig. 20.10). Penetrating wounds of the cranial vault give rise to a small percentage of abscesses. Up to 50% of abscesses result from blood-borne systemic infections associated with bronchiectasis, pulmonary abscesses, bacterial endocarditis, congenital heart disease, and others. Multiple cerebral abscesses usually result from metastases from systemic infections. The most common organisms found in brain abscesses are the Streptococcus and Staphylococcus species, anaerobic streptococci, coliform bacilli, diphtheroids, and bacteroides, although in many instances

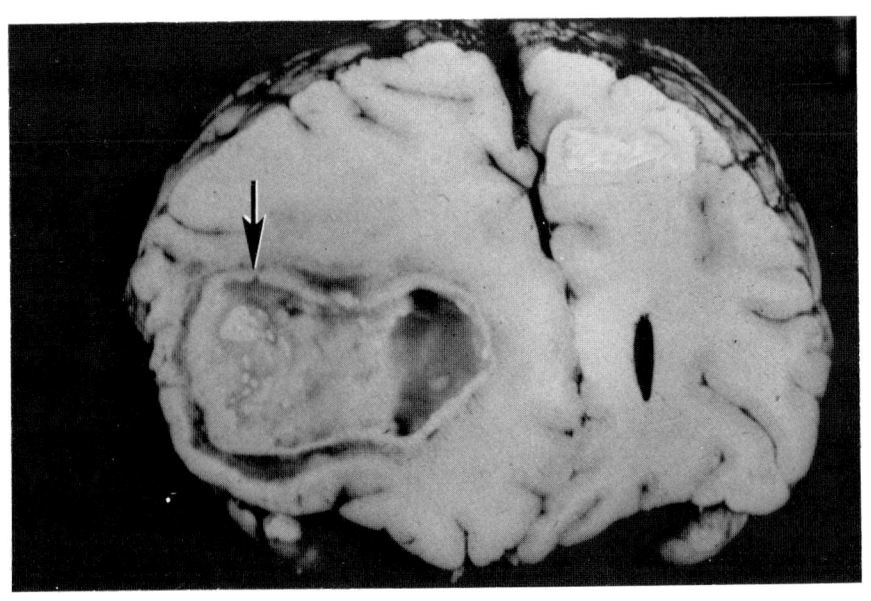

Figure 20.10. Brain abscess. This frontal lobe abscess has a well formed capsule (*arrow*) surrounding an area of liquefaction necrosis. Note the edema surrounding the abscess.

no organisms are cultured.

In the earliest stage of an abscess the infected brain tissue is soft, congested, and swollen. Subsequently, the tissue liquifies, the purulent exudate increases in amount, and the lesion becomes encapsulated. Microscopically three zones can be identified. The inner zone is composed of necrotic tissue, neutrophils, and fibrin. Next is a zone of macrophages, lymphocytes, small proliferating vessels, and hyperplastic fibroblasts, which has the appearance of granulation tissue. A fibrous capsule is formed from this layer. A third layer is composed of reactive astrocytes, perivascular lymphocytes, and edematous compressed parenchyma. The fibrous capsule begins to develop in 3 to 5 days and is moderately well developed by 2 weeks when it reaches 2 mm in thickness.

The clinical manifestations of a brain abscess are like those of any mass lesion. Rupture of the abscess into a ventricle or increased intracranial pressure with temporal lobe or cerebellar tonsillar herniation are common modes of death from cerebral abscesses.

Tuberculous Infection

Although less common than in the past, tuberculosis of the CNS is still prominent in some regions of the world. Tuberculosis produces meningitis, tuberculomas of brain parenchyma, or spinal epidural granulomas. Tuberculous meningitis occurs most frequently in childhood and in debilitated or immunosuppressed individuals. It is thought to reach the brain by hematogenous dissemination where small tubercles develop which communicate with the leptomeninges and cause a generalized meningitis. The granulomatous exudate is most pronounced at the base of the brain where it can involve cranial nerves and arteries.

The clinical course of tuberculous meningitis is more indolent and chronic. Patients develop headache, low grade fever, apathy, and mental changes. The CSF is under increased pressure and contains up to 1000 cells per mm^3 (primarily lymphocytes), a protein content of 100 to 200 mg per dl or more, and glucose levels of 20 to 40 mg per dl.

Fungus Infections

Mycotic infections of the CNS have increased in frequency in recent years although they are much less common than CNS bacterial infections. A large number of fungi are capable of causing a CNS infection, although the most common are the cryptococcus, coccidioides, blastomyces, actinomyces, nocardia, mucorales, histoplasma, and candida. CNS invasion by fungi can result in meningitis, meningoencephalitis, abscess, granuloma, or arterial thrombosis. Mycotic infections of the CNS occur more frequently in patients with debilitating diseases such as diabetes or malignancies or in those on immunosuppressive therapy.

Virus Infections

Viruses are capable of causing a variety of different diseases in the CNS. Acute viral infections may produce a mild meningitis (aseptic meningitis) or a meningoencephalitis. Chronic or "slow" virus infections can cause slowly progressive disorders simulating degenerative neurologic diseases or demyelinating disorders. Malformation of the fetal brain can be produced by viruses in humans and experimental animals.

Acute viral infections of the human CNS are most commonly caused by herpes simplex, arboviruses, ECHO, Coxsackie, the mumps agent, and lymphocytic choriomeningitis virus. The route of entry for viruses is via animal, mosquito, or tick bites, through the respiratory, enteric, or genital mucosa, or across the placenta. After setting up a focal or systemic infection, viruses spread to the CNS via peripheral nerves, olfactory nerves, the choroid plexus, or the brain vascular endothelium. Certain areas of the brain are more susceptible to specific viruses than others. For example, herpes simplex affects the orbitofrontal and medial temporal lobes, polio affects motor neurons, and herpes zoster involves sensory ganglia. Some viruses have a propensity for involving white matter (leukoencephalitis) while others primarily involve gray matter (polioencephalitis).

The characteristic general microscopic findings in acute viral encephalitis are mononuclear inflammatory cells in the subarachnoid space and perivascular sites, neuronophagia, microglial nodules, intranuclear (Fig. 20.11) or intracytoplasmic inclusion bodies, and fibrous astrocytic response.

The clinical manifestations of viral meningoencephalitis are headache, fever, stiff neck, photophobia, drowsiness, confusion, stupor or coma, seizures, involuntary movement, and hemiparesis. The CSF usually contains less than 500 cells per mm^3, a mild increase in protein content (100 mg per dl or less), and normal glucose content.

Chronic, "slow," or unconventional virus infections are characterized by a long latency period of months to several years, a protracted clinical course, and lesions in only a single organ system. Kuru and Creutzfeldt-Jakob disease were the initial

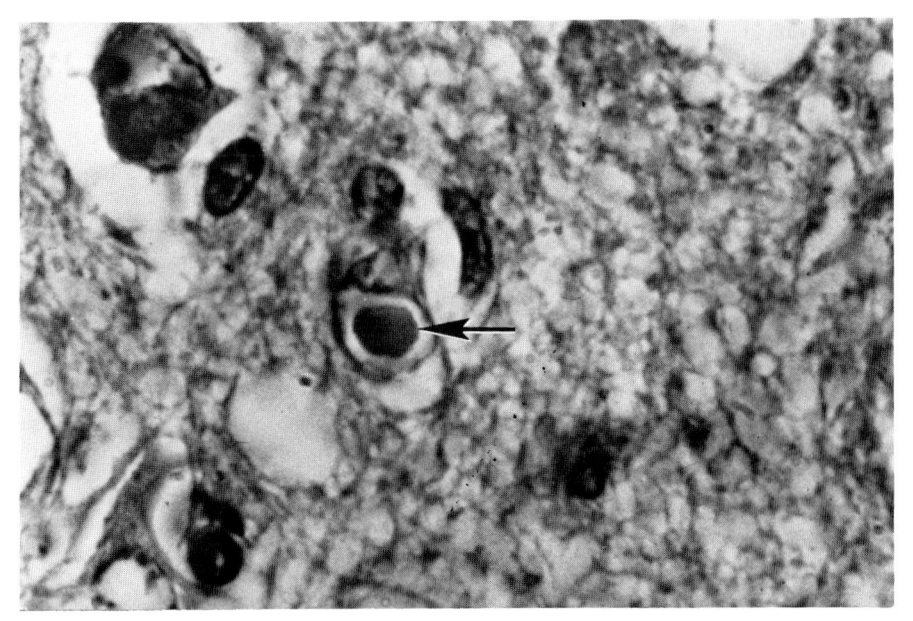

Figure 20.11. Inclusion (*arrow*) filling much of a neuronal nucleus (Cowdry Type A) in viral encephalitis.

examples of what are now called transmissible spongiform encephalopathies. Kuru, a progressive disease with cerebellar ataxia, dysarthria, dysphagia, and tremor occurring in the Fore tribes of New Guinea, was found to be related to cannibalism. The disease has been transmitted to chimpanzees but the specific agent has not been isolated. The brain of these patients shows a vacuolar or spongiform change, neuronal degeneration, and a marked astrocytosis.

Creutzfeldt-Jakob disease or subacute spongiform encephalopathy is characterized by dementia, pyramidal and extrapyramidal signs, myoclonic jerks, ataxia, lower motor neuron signs, and a rapidly progressive fatal course, usually within 1 year. Microscopically there is neuronal degeneration, an astrocytosis, and diffuse spongiform change. The disease has been transmitted to chimpanzees, guinea pigs, and mice by brain inoculations. Accidental transmission from human to human via corneal transplant has been documented.

Subacute sclerosing panencephalitis is a diffuse encephalitis occurring in children under 18 years of age, caused by a paramyxovirus similar to the measles virus. It has a slowly progressive course with intellectual deterioration, myoclonic jerks, seizures, extrapyramidal signs, and visual changes. Microscopically, there are alterations in the cortex and white matter.

Progressive multifocal leukoencephalopathy is a progressive demyelinating disease occurring in individuals with lymphomas, leukemias, sarcoidosis, and collagen-vascular diseases and in immunosuppressed patients. Pathologically there are focal areas of demyelination in the white matter in which there is a loss of oligodendroglia, bizarre large hyperplastic astrocytes, and intranuclear inclusions in oligodendroglia. Papovavirus particles are present in inclusions and several antigenically similar viruses have been isolated from these patients. It has been postulated that this disease results from an opportunistic virus infections of oligodendroglia which cause demyelination in an immunoincompetent host.

DEGENERATIVE DISEASES

This group of diseases is of unknown etiology, has a gradually progressive course, primarily involves neurons and their axons, has a hereditary basis in some and an acquired basis in others, and develops clinical manifestations after many years of normal life. There is a predilection for these disorders selectively to involve specific anatomic and physiologic systems of the nervous system. Some primarily involve the cerebral cortex, others the basal ganglia, while others have a predilection for the brainstem, cerebellum, or spinal cord. We consider here a degenerative cortical disease which gives rise to progressive dementia, degeneration of the basal ganglia which causes involuntary movements, spinocerebellar degeneration which causes ataxia, and motor neuron degeneration causing weakness and atrophy.

Cortical Degenerative Disease

Alzheimer's disease in the presenium (onset prior to age 65) and senile dementia of the Alzheimer type (onset after age 65) differ only in their age of onset and are collectively referred to as Alzheimer's disease (AD). It has been estimated that there are over 1,000,000 persons with AD in the United States and, although it usually does not appear on death certificates, it may be the fourth or fifth most common cause of death in this country. Clinically AD is

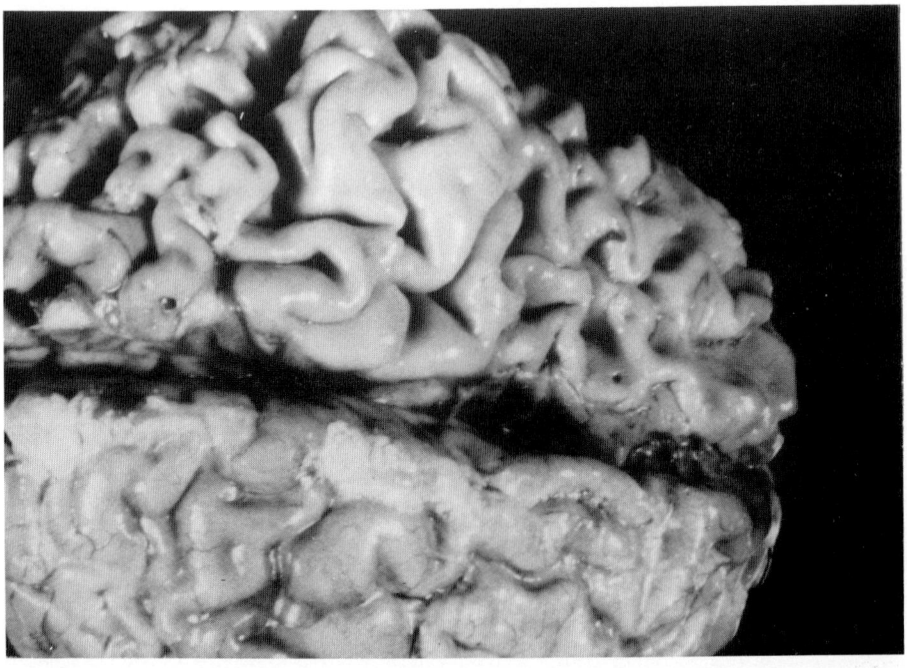

Figure 20.12. Alzheimer's disease. View of exposed left cortex showing severe atrophy.

characterized by gradually progressive loss of memory and other cognitive functions. Pathologically there is generalized atrophy of the cerebral cortex (Fig. 20.12) and enlargement of the ventricular system (hydrocephalus *ex vacuo*). Microscopically there is formation of neurofibrillary tangles in cortical neurons and senile (neuritic) plaques (Fig. 20.13). It has been shown that there is a high degree of correlation between the concentration of these microscopic lesions and dementia. Granulovacuolar degeneration, cytoplasmic membrane-bound vacuoles, occurs primarily in the hippocampus. All of these changes also develop in the brains of aged individuals without significant dementia, but are more limited to the temporal lobe and are less numerous. Recent biochemical studies have shown that choline acetyltransferase and acetylcholinesterase synthesis are diminished in the brain in AD, but that muscarinic cholinergic receptor binding sites are normal. The etiology of the disease is not known although recent studies have suggested toxic factors such as aluminum, errors in neuronal protein synthesis, or a chronic viral infection.

Basal Ganglia Degenerative Diseases

Parkinson's disease is a sporadic disease occurring most commonly in the sixth and seventh decade, manifest clinically by tremor, cogwheel rigidity, and bradykinesia. It has a prevalence rate of approximately 160 per 100,000. There are three major types of parkinsonism: symptomatic, postencephalitic, and idiopathic. The former occurs after carbon monoxide intoxication, manganese poisoning, trauma,

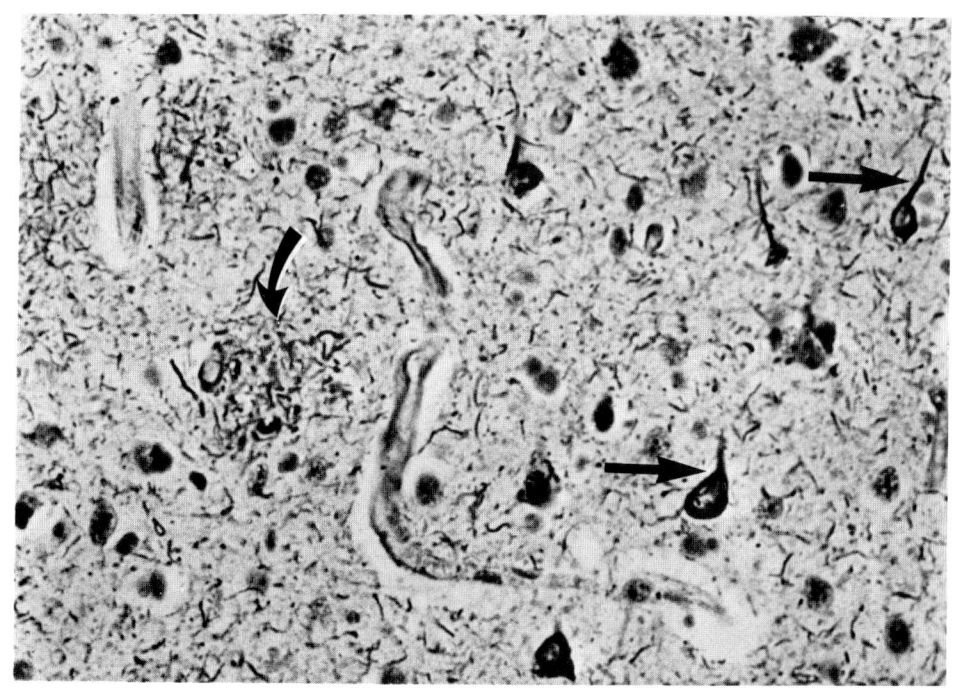

Figure 20.13. Light micrograph of the cerebral cortex showing neurofibrillary tangles (*arrows*) and senile plaque (*curved arrow*) in Alzheimer's disease.

250 Pathology: Understanding Human Disease

and use of various psychotrophic drugs. Postencephalitic parkinsonism followed von Economo's encephalitis in the 1918 to 1923 pandemic. Most cases of parkinsonism do not have a known cause and are referred to as idiopathic. The major gross morphologic finding in this disorder is depigmentation of the substantia nigra (Fig. 20.14) and locus ceruleus. Microscopically, there is a loss of pigmented neurons in these nuclei and the presence of neuronal, intracytoplasmic, eosinophilic inclusions called Lewy bodies. In postencephalitic parkinsonism neurofibrillary tangles are found in the substantra nigra and Lewy bodies are rarely found. The neuromelanin-containing cells of the substantia nigra produce the inhibitory neurotransmitter, dopamine. A decrease of dopamine in the caudate nucleus and putamen has been found in Parkinson's disease. This may cause an imbalance of output to the globus pallidus and from there to the thalamus where an influence on the corticospinal tract causes some of the symptoms of the disease.

Huntington's chorea is characterized by choreoathetoid movements, mental changes, and an autosomal dominant inheritance pattern. The mean age of onset is 37 years and the mean survival is approximately 15 years. There is marked atrophy of the caudate nucleus and putamen. Histologically there is a severe loss of the small Golgi Type 2 neurons in these nuclei with relative sparing of the larger neurons and a reactive fibrillary astrocytosis. Biochemically a decrease in γ-aminobutyric acid and glutamic acid decarboxylase has been found in the

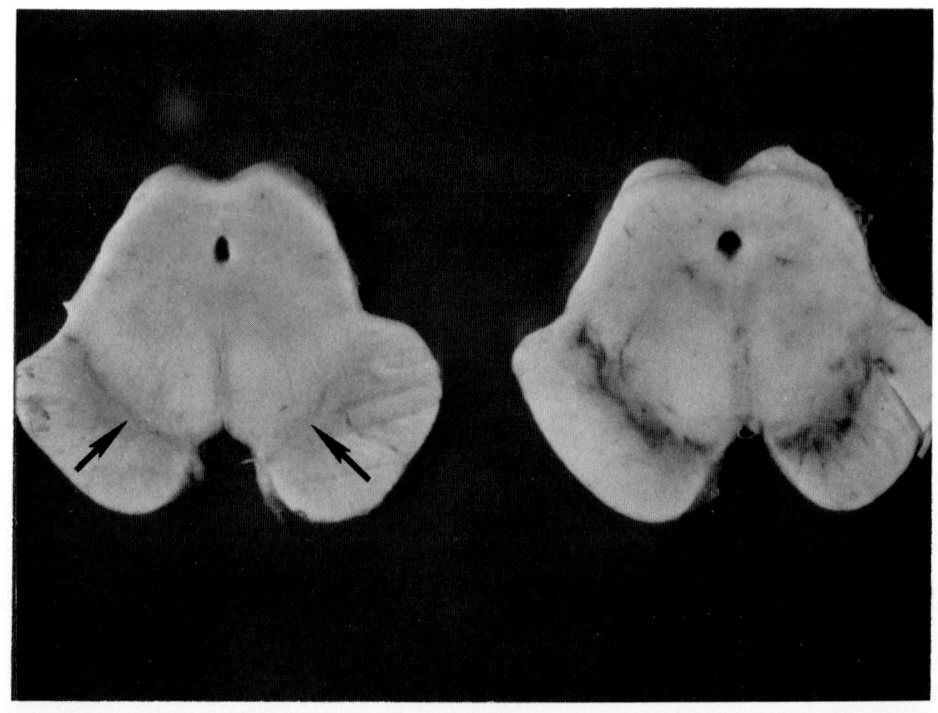

Figure 20.14. Parkinson's disease. Section of midbrain showing depigmentation of substantia nigra in Parkinson's disease on *left* (*arrows*) and normal substantia nigra on *right*.

Spinocerebellar Degeneration

This is a complicated group of inherited disorders predominately involving the cerebellum, its afferent connections, and the spinal cord. Several distinct forms are described, but many intermediate forms exist. The most common form is Friedreich's ataxia.

Friedreich's ataxia is inherited as an autosomal dominant trait. It is characterized clinically by gait, limb, and trunkal ataxia, loss of vibration and position sense, and deep tendon reflexes, extensor plantar responses, dysarthria, nystagamus, kyphoscoliosis, cardiomyopathy, and occasionally optic atrophy. Onset is in the first and second decade. There is loss of myelin and axons in the posterior columns, corticospinal tracts, and spinocerebellar tracts (Fig. 20.15) and a neuronal loss from Clarke's column and the dorsal root ganglia. Purkinje cell loss is present in some cases. Death is often from cardiac arrhythmias or congestive heart failure.

Spinal Cord and Brainstem Degenerative Disorders

Amyotrophic lateral sclerosis (ALS), the most common form of *motor neuron disease*, is a pure motor system degeneration involving both the upper and lower motor neuron. ALS usually occurs sporadically and the onset is most common in the fifth and sixth decades. It is more common in males and has a relatively rapid progression with death ensuing in 3 to 5 years of onset. It is characterized by a combination of symptoms of lower motor neuron degeneration (atrophy, loss of reflexes, fasciculations) and upper motor neuron degeneration (spasticity, hyper-

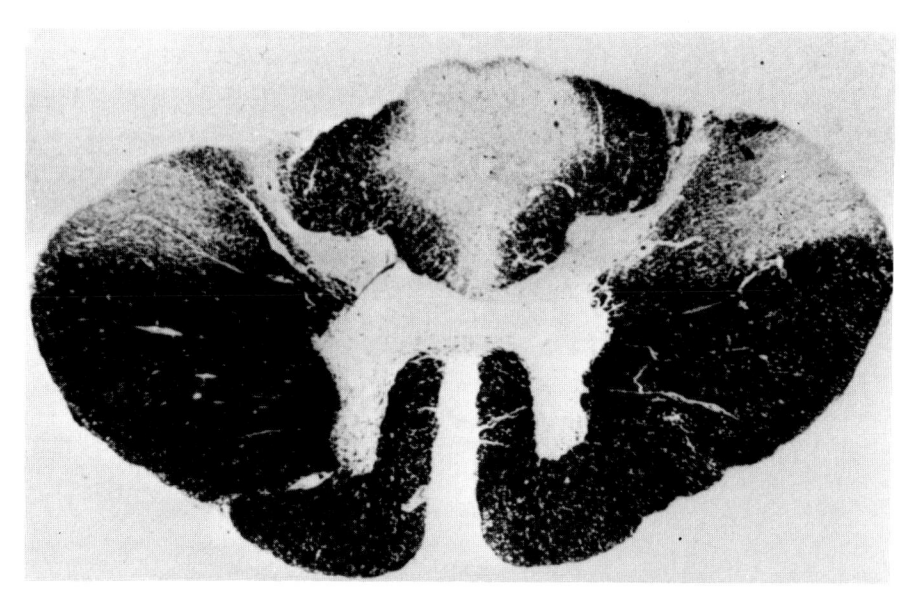

Figure 20.15. Friedreich's ataxia. Section of thoracic spinal cord showing loss of myelin in posterior columns, corticospinal tracts, and dorsal spinocerebellar tracts. (Myelin stain.)

reflexia, and pathologic reflexes). There is also difficulty swallowing and chewing. Grossly, the major change is atrophy of the anterior nerve roots of the spinal cord. Microscopically, there is a loss of anterior horn cells and cranial nerve motor nuclei, loss of myelin sheaths and axons in the pyramidal tracts of the spinal cord (Fig. 20.16) and brainstem and the anterior nerve roots, and a mild reactive gliosis. The etiology of this disease is not known. Several other variants of motor neuron disease exist in which brainstem nuclei are primarily affected (progressive bulbar palsy) or anterior horn cells and roots are selectively involved (progressive spinal muscular atrophy) or the corticospinal tracts are affected (primary lateral sclerosis). All of these entities are much less frequent than ALS.

A childhood form of motor neuron disease inherited as an autosomal recessive trait is called infantile progressive spinal muscular atrophy or *Werdnig-Hoffmann disease*. It becomes manifest soon after birth by severe generalized weakness and hypotonia. The course is generally rapidly progressive and leads to death within 1 to 2 years. Pathologically, changes similar to those described in ALS without involvement of the corticospinal tract are found. There are other forms of chronic spinal muscular atrophy with much slower rates of progression.

DEMYELINATING DISEASES

Although myelin is destroyed in a variety of CNS lesions, there is a group of disorders in which myelin damage is the most prominent histologic finding. In

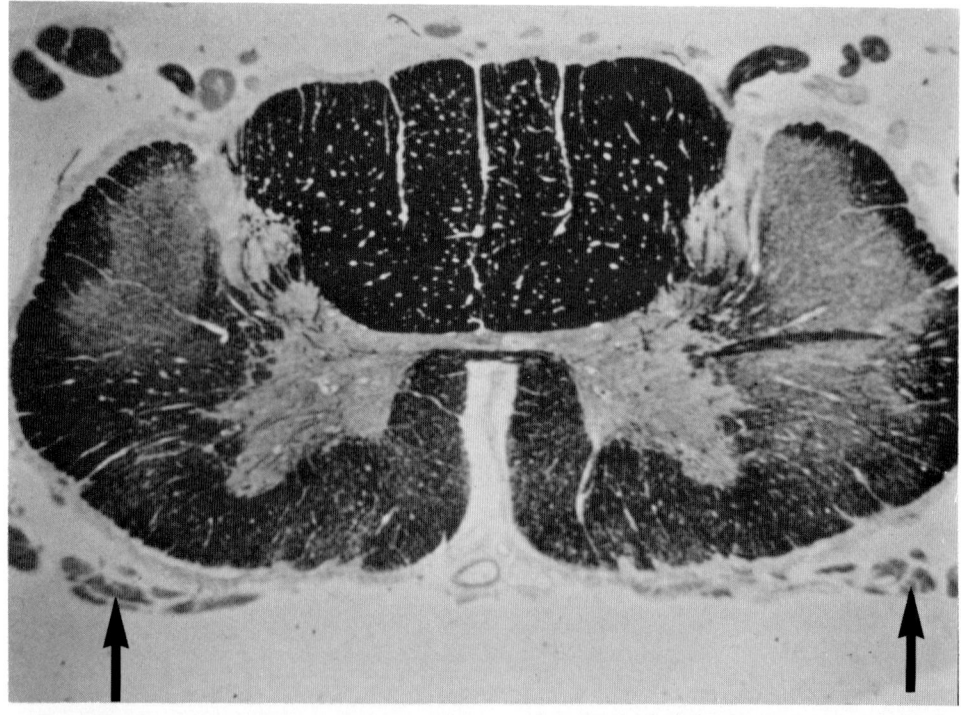

Figure 20.16. Amyotrophic lateral sclerosis. Section of cervical spinal cord showing demyelination of corticospinal tracts and degeneration of anterior roots (*arrows*). (Myelin stain.)

primary demyelinating disorders, there is destruction of normally developed myelin and oligodendroglia cells with relative preservation of axons. Multiple sclerosis and acute disseminated encephalomyelitis are examples of this type of disease. In dysmyelinating diseases, myelin is not formed properly or myelin turnover is abnormal. The leukodystrophies, usually occurring in childhood, are examples of this type of disorder. Other diseases in which myelin is lost are not so readily classified.

Multiple sclerosis (MS), the most common demyelinating disorder, is one of the major debilitating neurologic diseases of young adults. It has an incidence of 40 to 60 per 100,000 in northern climates and 10 to 15 per 100,000 in southern climates. It is more prevalent in females than males. Onset is most commonly between ages 20 and 40 years. It is characterized by remissions and relapses and involvement of different areas of the nervous systems, *i.e.*, spinal cord, optic nerves, brainstem, and cerebellum. The most common initial manifestations are motor weakness, paresthesias, visual impairment, diplopia, ataxia, and bladder dysfunction. Average life expectancy after onset is 20 years or longer. In some instances there is a long latency period between the initial attack and the next exacerbation, while in approximately 10% of patients there is a chronic progressive course.

The CSF in multiple sclerosis contains a few mononuclear inflammatory cells (<50 per mm^3) and approximately one-fourth of patients have a slight elevation of protein content (<100 mg per dl). An elevation of γ-globulin (IgG) above 13% is present in two-thirds of patients. Antibodies against oligodendroglial cells and myelin are also found. CSF measles antibody titers are elevated in a large percentage of patients.

The pathologic hallmark of MS is the plaque, an irregular shaped area of demyelination with sharp borders (Fig. 20.17). Recent plaques are yellowish, while chronic plaques are gray and retracted. They have a predilection for the angles of the lateral ventricles (Fig. 20.17), optic nerves, spinal cord, tegmentum of the brainstem, and cerebellar peduncles. In acute plaques there is loss of oligodendroglial cells, breakdown of myelin, perivascular mononuclear inflammatory cells, and macrophages containing lipid of myelin origin. Many axons remain intact. As the plaque ages, few macrophages are found and fibrous astrocytes abound. Older plaques show severe demyelination and gliosis (sclerosis). The etiology and pathogenesis of MS are not known, although a slow or latent virus or an autoimmune disorder have been hypothesized.

Acute disseminated encephalomyelitis is a rare disorder usually occurring in children or young adults after exanthematous diseases (measles, chickenpox, smallpox), following vaccination against smallpox or rabies, or after nonspecific infections. Neurologic symptoms develop within 4 to 14 days after initial infection or inoculation. The clinical manifestations depend on the area of the brain or spinal cord involved. The acute onset with convulsions, confusion, headache, stiff neck, and subsequent focal neurologic signs is typical. The mortality is variable but averages 10 to 20%. Histologically there are diffuse perivenous foci of demyelination containing infiltrates of lymphocytes, plasma cells, and macrophages.

It is thought that this disease is produced by an autoimmune reaction against

254   *Pathology: Understanding Human Disease*

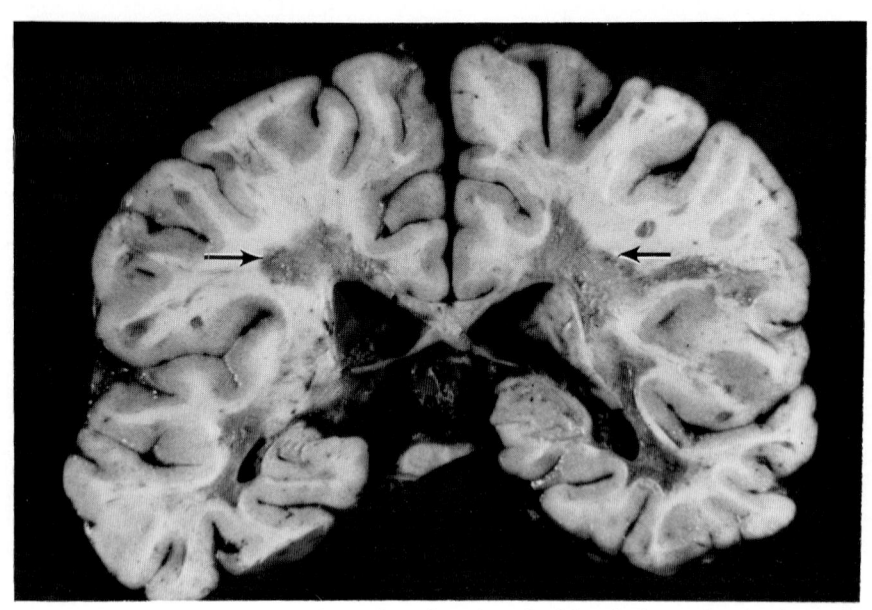

Figure 20.17. Multiple sclerosis. Coronal section of cerebral hemispheres showing large, sharply demarcated plaques adjacent to the bodies of the lateral ventricles (*arrows*). Other plaques are found adjacent to the temporal horns and smaller plaques are present in the subcortical white matter and centra semiovales.

myelin. Experimental allergic encephalomyelitis, an animal model of this disease, is produced by subcutaneous injection of myelin basic protein with Freund's adjuvant.

Diffuse Scleroses

The *leukodystrophies* are a group of diseases usually inherited as Mendelian recessive traits, with onset in early childhood, characterized by mental deterioration, visual loss, and spasticity. Pathologically, they show a severe lack of, or destruction of, white matter of the cerebral and cerebellar hemispheres in a relatively symmetrical pattern. Some have alterations in peripheral nerves. They have been called dysmyelinating diseases because the myelin is not formed or maintained properly. In all, the lack of myelin is most pronounced in the centra semiovales of the cerebral hemispheres. Subcortical arcuate fibers are relatively spared in most. Oligodendroglial cells are diminished in number. Accumulation of abnormal products of myelin metabolism are found in macrophages. Axons may be initially spared but are ultimately lost and there is a diffuse fibrillary gliosis. The two most well studied leukodystrophies are metachromatic leukodystrophy and globoid cell leukodystrophy.

Metachromatic leukodystrophy is the most common of the leukodystrophies. Its onset is usually between 1 and 2 years of age. Biochemically the brain shows a marked increase in sulfatides, a deficiency of cerebrosides, and deficiency of arylsulfatase A. Intracellular and extracelluar metachromatic granules are present throughout the white matter. They are also seen in peripheral nerves and various visceral organs.

Globoid cell leukodystrophy (Krabbe's disease) has its onset in early infancy and is characterized biochemically by deficiency of galactocerebroside-β-galactosidase. Microscopically, numerous large, occasionally multinucleated histiocytes (globoid cells) are present throughout the white matter. The disease progresses rapidly with death by 2 years.

TRAUMATIC LESIONS OF THE CNS

Head injuries are classified as *closed*, in which there is no perforation of the skull or dura, and *penetrating*, in which the skull and/or brain are directly violated. To understand closed head injuries better, it must be appreciated that the brain does not completely fill the bony cavity. After an injury to the head, when the moving head stops abruptly, the brain continues until it strikes the adjacent bone. When the head accelerates quickly, as a result of an injury, the brain lags behind and is struck by the skull. Coup lesions are those that develop at the site of the traumatic impact. Contracoup lesions are lesions that develop contralateral to the site of the traumatic impact. In general contracoup lesions are more extensive than coup lesions.

Epidural hemorrhage is a collection of blood between the inner table of the skull and the dura usually as a consequence of laceration of meningeal arteries or rarely from tears in the venous sinuses. The blood increases in volume quickly and causes focal compression of the brain with increased intracranial pressure leading to early transtentorial herniation. A typical clinical sequence is loss of consciousness with the head injury, followed by a lucid interval and, as the compression increases, loss of consciousness again, with hemiplegia, subsequent herniation, and death.

Subdural hemorrhage is a collection of blood between the dura and the arachnoid membrane (Fig. 20.18), usually resulting from tearing of superficial cortical veins that cross the subdural space to the superior sagittal sinus. It can be caused by penetrating or closed head injury. It occurs most frequently in the elderly, infants, and alcoholics. Because they are venous in origin, the hematoma may enlarge slowly. After 2 to 3 weeks the hematoma is encapsulated. Recurrent bleeding from newly formed vessels can be a source of enlargement of the hematoma. In chronic subdural hematomas symptoms may appear days, weeks, or even months after head injury and are primarily due to compression of the cerebral hemisphere. Acute subdural hematomas are often associated with lacerations of the underlying brain and have a more rapid evolution of symptoms and a higher mortality.

Concussion is a transient loss of consciousness of instantaneous onset with temporary loss of brainstem reflexes following closed head trauma. Patients usually have complete recovery with amnesia for the event. No demonstrable pathologic lesions are seen grossly or microscopically. The pathogenesis has not been fully established.

Contusion refers to bruising of the brain surface consequent to head injury. They are associated with tearing of capillaries and necrosis, usually on the crest of gyri. They are wedge-shaped with the base toward the pia. They occur more commonly in the frontal and temporal poles and inferior surfaces of the frontal

256 Pathology: Understanding Human Disease

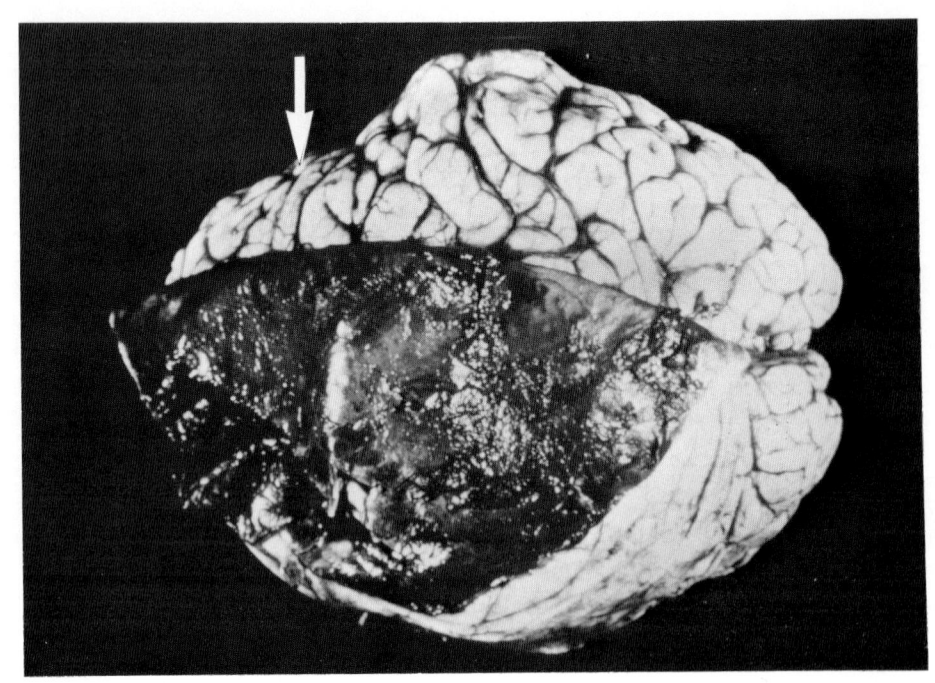

Figure 20.18. View of superior surface of brain showing subdural hematoma (dura folded back) and compression of right frontal region (*arrow*).

lobes, especially near bony ridges or prominences. Old contusions are shrunken, wrinkled, and rust-colored (plaques jaune) and can serve as epileptogenic foci.

Lacerations or tears in the brain parenchyma are caused by penetrating objects, fractured bone, or impact. They are associated with hemorrhage and marked edema, and a high mortality. Sizable traumatic intracerebral hemorrhages can occur without laceration. They are usually located in the cerebral hemispheres and are well limited, circumscribed hemorrhages.

Cerebral edema is a common accompaniment of severe head injury. Loss of the blood-brain barrier and increased permeability of blood vessels accompany contusions, lacerations, and hemorrhages.

METABOLIC AND NUTRITIONAL DISORDERS OF THE CNS

Many acquired systemic metabolic disorders, such as hepatic encephalopathy (Chapter 21), uremic encephalopathy, myxedema, hypoxia, hypoglycemia, and others, are capable of causing considerable neurologic derangement. Hypoxia and hypoglycemia produce neuronal loss in the third and fifth cortical layers, Sommer's sector of the hippocampus, neostriatum, and Purkinje cells. Many inherited metabolic diseases of the CNS have been described. The aminoacidurias such as phenylketonuria and homocystinuria and the neuronal lysosomal storage diseases such as the sphingolipidoses, mucopolysaccharidoses, and the ceroid lipofuscinoses are the prototypes of this form of disorder.

A variety of nutritional disorders affects the nervous system. The most common of these are the alcohol-associated conditions: alcoholic peripheral neuropathy, cerebellar degeneration, Marchiafava-Bignami disease, central pontine myelinolysis, Korsakoff's psychosis, and Wernicke's encephalopathy. The latter disorder is characterized clinically by extraocular muscle palsies, gait ataxia, and disturbance of mentation, and pathologically by lesions of the mammillary bodies, periaqueductal gray matter, and periventricular region of the thalamus and hypothalamus. The disease is caused by a deficiency of thiamine.

Suggested Reading

Burger PC, Vogel SF. Cerebrovascular disease. Am. J. Pathol. *92:* 257, 1978.
Fishman RA. Cerebrospinal fluid in diseases of the nervous system. Philadelphia, W.B. Saunders Co, 1980.
Lewis AJ. Mechanisms of neurological disease. Boston, Little, Brown and Co, 1976.
Lindenberg R. Trauma of meninges and brain. In: Minckler J, ed. Pathology of the nervous system. Vol. 2. New York, McGraw-Hill, 1971.
Rubinstein LJ. Tumors of the central nervous system. In: Atlas of tumor pathology. Washington DC, Armed Forces Institute of Pathology, 1972.
Terry RD. Senile dementia. Fed. Proc. *37:* 2837, 1978.

Chapter 21

The Liver and Gall Bladder

This chapter first considers hepatic failure and the end stage, or cirrhotic, liver. The various forms of injury to the basic functional unit of the liver are presented, emphasizing viral hepatitis and its complications, alcoholic hepatitis, and drug-induced hepatitis, but including α-1-antitrypsin deficiency, hemochromatosis, biliary cirrhosis, Wilson's disease, certain circulatory injuries, and the hereditary defects of bilirubin metabolism. There are brief discussions of primary carcinoma of the liver and of cholecystitis and cholelithiasis.

HEPATIC FAILURE

Hepatic failure denotes loss of the metabolic and excretory functions of the liver to the extent that homeostasis cannot be maintained. Hepatic failure implies diffuse disease, since basal functional needs can be met by as little as 10% of the liver, providing that that portion is entirely normal. Failure can be acute or chronic; emphasis here is placed on chronic, progressive failure.

The simplest functional unit of the liver can be conceived as a hepatocyte, a sinusoidal capillary, and a bile canaliculus. This unit can be attacked at any point. Table 21.1 outlines the more important forms of liver injury. They include infections, immunologically mediated injuries, and toxic, mechanical, and hemodynamic injuries. The majority affect the hepatocyte directly; others act through the hepatic vasculature or the biliary system. As was true of the nephron, and of the alveolar respiratory membrane, persistent injury at any point in the functional unit results, in time, in injury to the entire unit. Thus, many disparate injuries tend to be expressed in a common structural end result—the end stage liver, or *cirrhosis*—and the common functional result—hepatic failure. This is not to say that the end results of all chronic, progressive, liver diseases are identical, but rather that their similarities heavily outweigh their differences.

Cirrhosis—The End Stage Liver

The cirrhotic liver is the end result of chronic, progressive, liver disease. It represents an abnormal regeneration of the lobular architecture. In addition to atypical parenchymal nodules, there is an increase in fibrous tissue, frequent bile stasis, an altered vasculature, and varying degrees of inflammation.

The nodules of liver cells may have formed by regeneration within the confines of a single lobule or they may represent several or many lobules (Figs. 21.1 and 21.2). In the latter case, multiple portal and central areas are recognized within

Table 21.1
Some Causes of Liver Injury

Injury to Hepatocyte

Toxins
  Alcohol
  Phosphorus
  Carbon tetrachloride
  Benzene derivatives
  Mushroom poisoning

Drug toxicity
  Primarily cholestatic
    Methyl testosterone
    Oral contraceptives
  Cholestasis and hepatocyte necrosis
    Sulfonamides
    Thiouracil
    Phenothiazines
    Chlorpromazine
    Erythromycin
  Primarily hepatocyte necrosis
    Halothane
    Penthrane
    Isoniazid
    p-Aminosalicylate
    Indomethacin
    Methotrexate
    Acetaminophen
    Furosemide
    Allopurinol
    Methyldopa
    Tetracycline

Infection
  Viral hepatitis A, B, non-A non-B

Metabolic
  Hemochromatosis, hemosiderosis
  Wilson's disease
  Cystic fibrosis
  α-1-antitrypsin deficiency
  Intestinal bypass surgery

Immunologic
  Chronic active hepatitis
  Aldomet
  ? Halothane

Injury to Biliary System

Mechanical obstruction
  Extrahepatic; stones, pancreatic carcinoma
  Intrahepatic; metastatic carcinoma
Primary biliary cirrhosis

Injury via Vasculature

Congestive heart failure
Disseminated intravascular coagulation
Budd-Chiari syndrome
Hereditary telangiectasia

---

each nodule. The hepatic plates are irregular in distribution and often of two-cell thickness. The individual liver cells may show evidence of regeneration; they appear as large cells with prominent, often multiple, nuclei.

Fibrous tissue septa may surround individual parenchymal nodules, or they may bisect them by connecting portal areas with central veins (Fig. 21.3). Septa may form by collapse of preexisting stroma, which stimulates new fibrous tissue deposition, or by simple reparative fibrosis. When portal and central vessels are connected through fibrous septa, blood flow may largely bypass the sinusoidal network.

One of the major consequences of the cirrhotic process is the development of hypertension in the portal system. Portal hypertension exists when there is a pressure gradient across the liver in excess of 10 to 12 mm mercury. Several factors are thought responsible: compression of hepatic vein tributaries by parenchymal nodules or by fibrous septa, abnormal communications of hepatic arteries

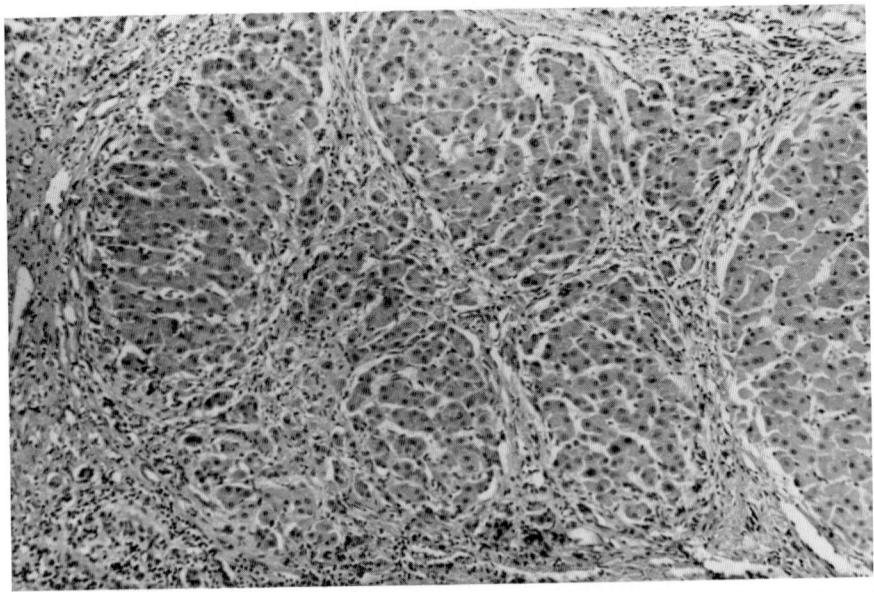

Figure 21.1. Regenerating liver nodules. Multiple nodules are seen. The liver cell plates are irregular, and central veins are not recognizable. The nodules are separated by loose fibrous tissue containing some bile ducts and scattered inflammatory cells.

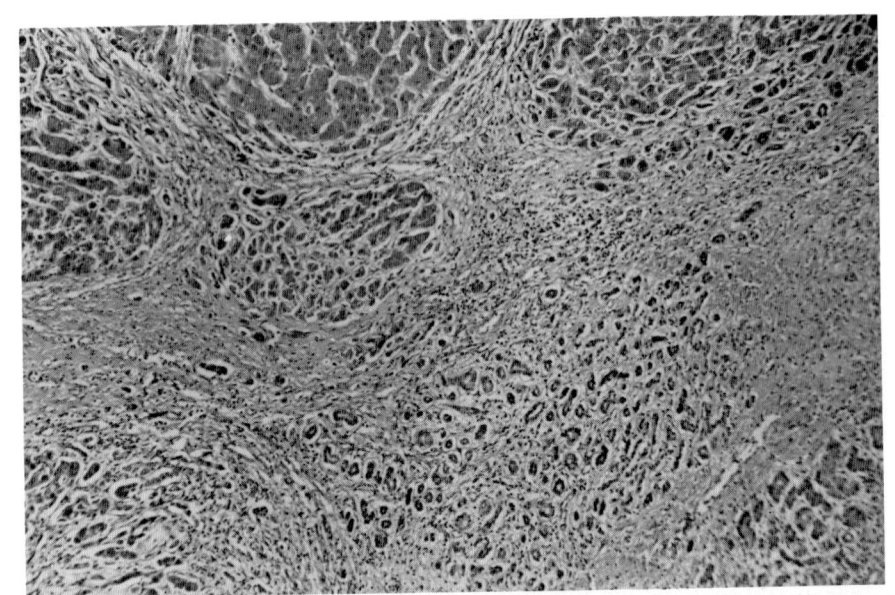

Figure 21.2. Cirrhosis. Several nodules of regenerating liver cells are seen, particularly at the periphery of this field. The central area shows stromal collapse, proliferation of fibrous tissue, and many small bile ducts.

and arterioles with portal vein branches, scarring of portal tracts and an increased portal blood flow related to an enlarged, congested, spleen.

The cirrhotic process shunts portal venous blood away from the hepatocytes. This is in large part due to marked enlargement of extrahepatic anastomoses

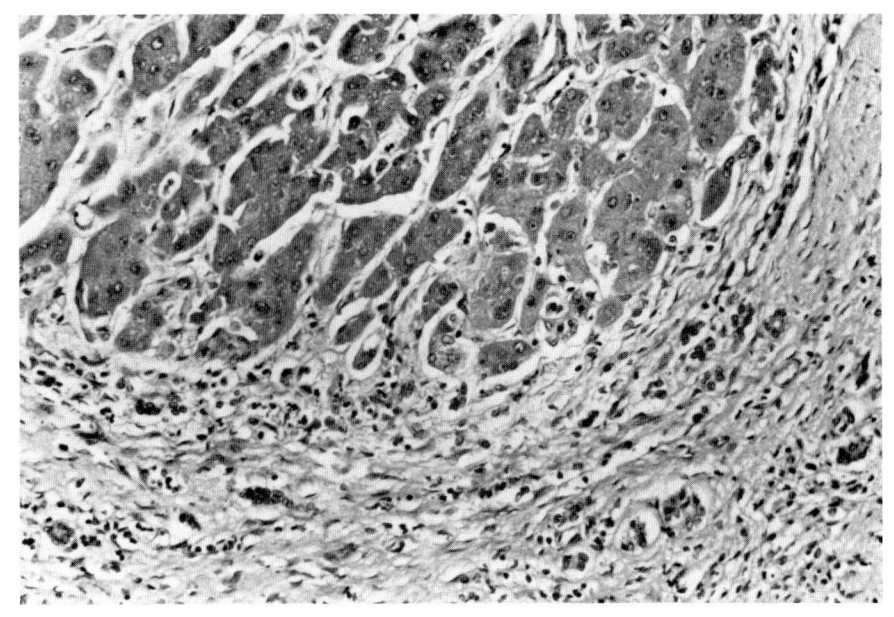

Figure 21.3. Cirrhosis. This field shows the margin of a regenerating nodule. The irregularity of the liver plates is apparent. There is surrounding active fibrous tissue production and moderate numbers of inflammatory cells.

between the portal system and the systemic venous circulation in response to the high pressure gradient. It relates also to intrahepatic anastomoses or abnormal connections between portal and hepatic venules within fibrous septa that permit bypass of the sinusoidal network, and alterations within the sinusoids themselves. These hemodynamic changes reduce hepatocyte function, but also permit enteric organisms and endotoxins to bypass the liver and its Kupffer cells and enter the general circulation. Endotoxins may explain such manifestations of hepatic failure as hypotension and impaired renal perfusion.

Bile stasis may be due to mechanical obstruction by periductal scarring or by the altered lobular architecture, and may also reflect excessive secretion related to high sinusoidal pressure (Fig. 21.4).

Cirrhosis is usually classified as predominantly *micronodular*, when the parenchymal nodules are each derived from a single hepatic lobule (Figs. 21.5 and 21.6), or *macronodular*, when nodules represent several or many lobules (Figs. 21.7 and 21.8). Micronodular cirrhosis is also called Laënnec's or portal cirrhosis; macronodular cirrhosis is referred to as postnecrotic. These divisions are not sharp, and intermediate or mixed patterns are common. There is a moderately good correlation of type of cirrhosis with etiology, although many exceptions occur. Micronodular cirrhosis is associated with alcohol abuse, intestinal bypass surgery, and dose-related methotrexate toxicity. It is also the pattern observed in hemochromatosis and Wilson's disease. Macronodular cirrhosis occurs in relation to viral hepatitis and many drug reactions.

Cirrhosis is being described here as an end stage condition, but it should be noted that some evidence suggests at least partial reversibility of the process when the causative agent can be totally eliminated.

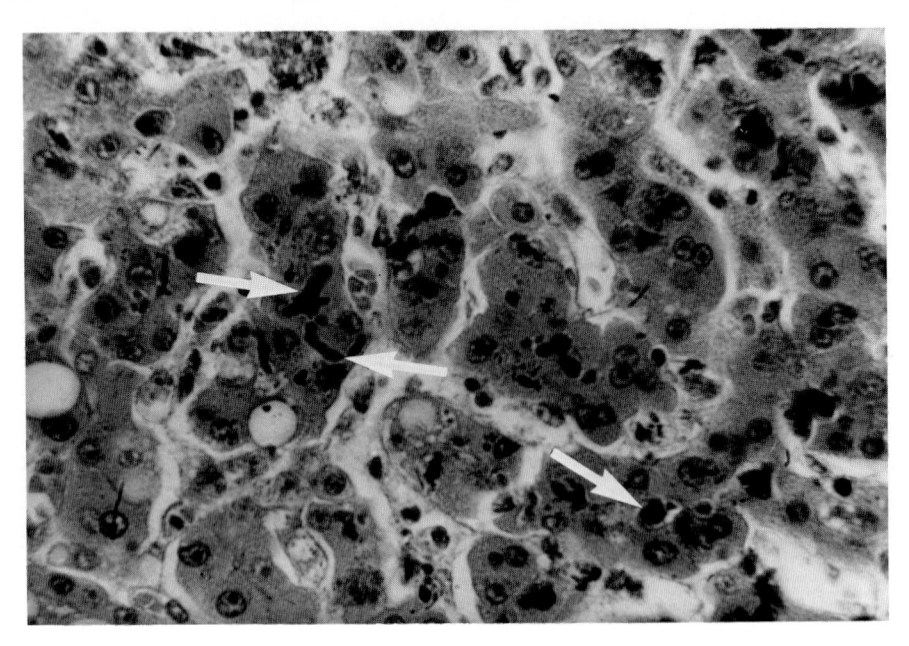

Figure 21.4. Bile stasis. This field shows part of a regenerating liver nodule. Many of the bile canaliculi are distended with bile (*arrows*).

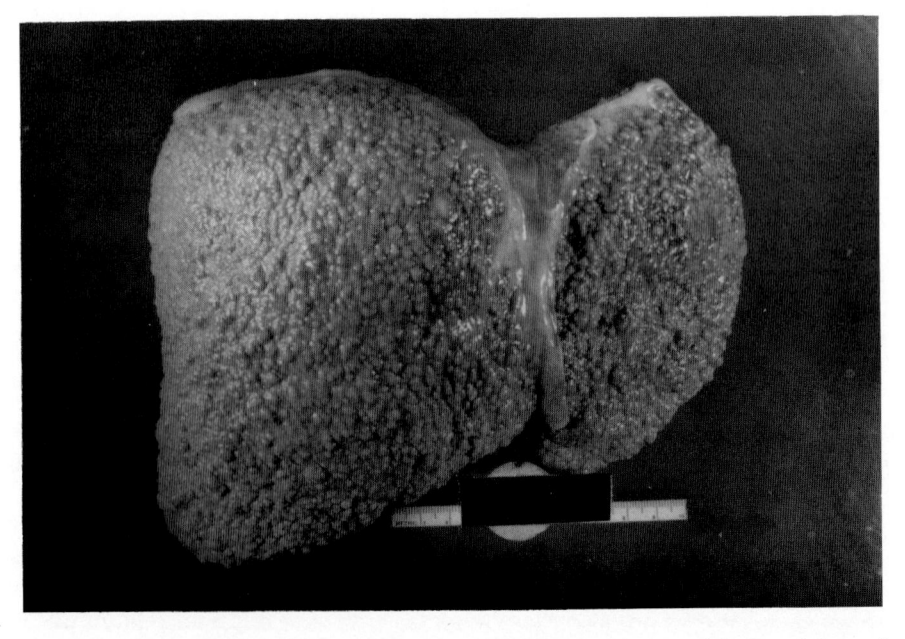

Figure 21.5. Micronodular cirrhosis. This liver, weighing 1500 g, shows a strikingly nodular surface. It was very firm in consistency.

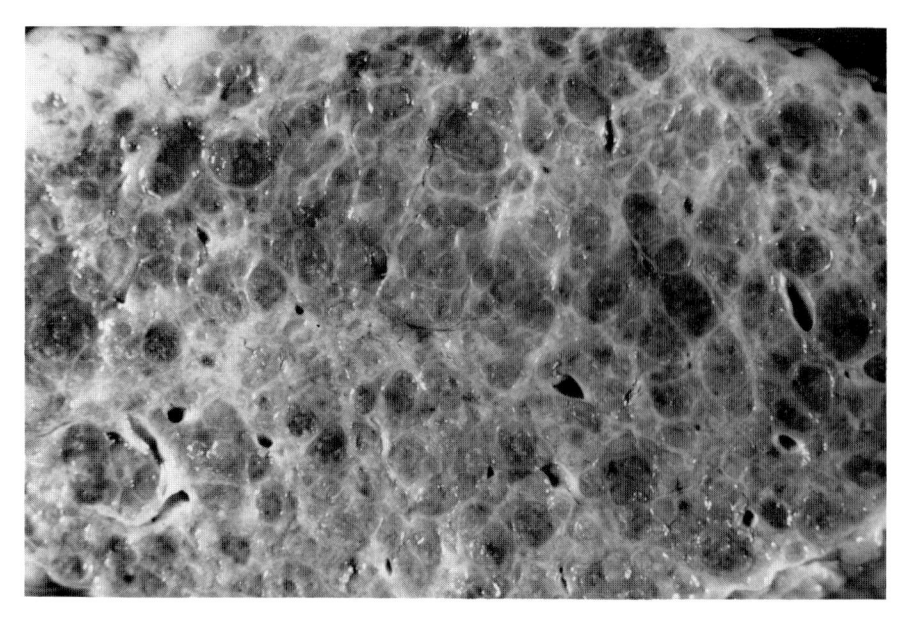

Figure 21.6. Micronodular cirrhosis. This close-up view of a cut surface shows the highly nodular configuration of the cirrhotic liver. The nodules vary in size between 2 and 5 mm. Delicate bands of fibrosis are apparent between nodules.

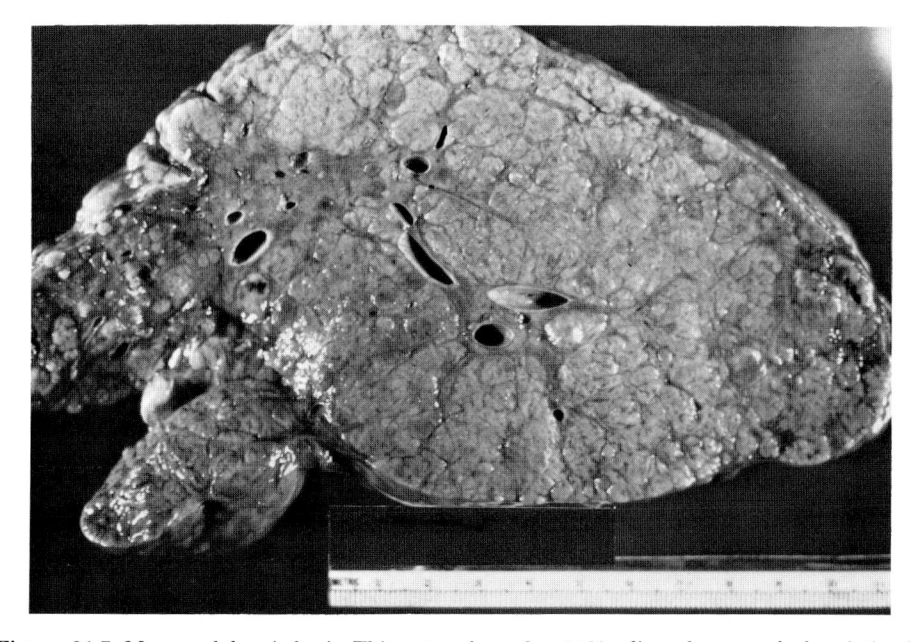

Figure 21.7. Macronodular cirrhosis. This cut surface of an 1100-g liver shows marked variation in the size of regenerated nodules. The left lobe, seen at the *lower left*, is severely involved and shrunken.

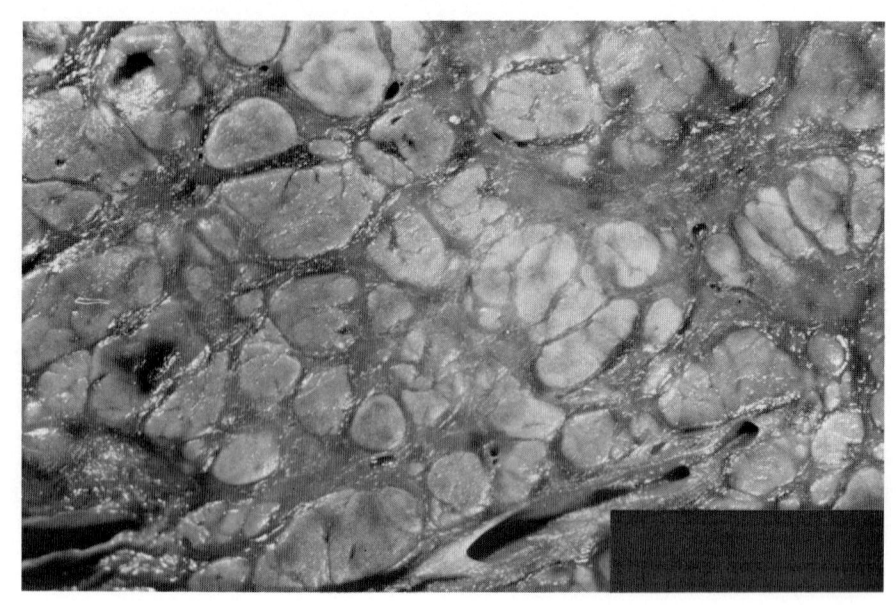

Figure 21.8. Macronodular cirrhosis. A close-up view of a cut surface shows marked variation in the size of nodules, from 1 or 2 mm to as large as 2 cm. The intervening tissue appears soft and sunken. It consists largely of collapsed stroma, although there is a moderate increase in fibrous tissue.

The Syndrome of Hepatic Failure

Although loss of function may at first reflect the site of initial injury to the liver, in virtually all chronic, progressive, liver disease there is an admixture of the manifestations of hepatocyte failure, disturbed excretory function, and altered hemodynamics in the portal venous system. These manifestations are discussed as segregated aspects of hepatic failure, but it should be remembered that they are usually coexistent.

Impaired Hepatocyte Function

The varied manifestations of loss of hepatocyte function reflect the diversity of that cell's normal functions. There is generalized malnutrition with wasting of musculature and, usually, loss of weight. Decreased caloric intake, intestinal malabsorption, and increased catabolism contribute to malnutrition. A diet high in alcohol is associated with deficient protein, folic acid, ascorbic acid, B vitamin, and mineral intake.

Protein synthesis is deficient, since the liver synthesizes all proteins except immunoglobulins and Factor VIII. Serum albumin concentration is decreased. The prothrombin time is prolonged, and there is a bleeding tendency. Immunoglobulin concentrations may be quite elevated, because of frequent bacteremia and, perhaps, viremia, consequent to shunting of blood away from the liver.

The synthesis of urea from ammonia is impaired, and levels of blood urea concentration are often reduced. Striking elevation of serum ammonia may follow gastrointestinal bleeding or a high protein intake.

Interference with glycogenolysis and gluconeogenesis, particularly in the presence of alcohol, can lead to episodes of hypoglycemia. On the other hand, poor uptake of glucose and glycogen synthesis are reflected in a diabetic glucose tolerance curve.

Endocrine disturbances include testicular atrophy, gynecomastia, and loss of axillary and pubic hair. These findings may relate to estrogen-androgen imbalance, although the testicular changes may be either primary or secondary to altered adenohypophyseal function. Patients in hepatic failure have altered tolerance for many therapeutic agents. Barbiturates are not normally detoxified, and their effects may be very prolonged. Other agents are less effective than normal if full activation requires hepatic action; thus, there is impaired 11β-hydroxylation of Compound E to Compound F.

Hepatic encephalopathy is a manifestation of severe hepatic failure. It is characterized by disturbances of consciousness, psychotic behavior, hyperactive reflexes, hyperventilation, and respiratory alkalosis. *Asterixis*, a flapping tremor of the hands, is frequently present, although not specific to this disorder. Although the pathogenesis of hepatic encephalopathy is complex and incompletely understood, it may be that elevated concentrations of ammonia in body fluids injure cerebral astrocytes, and these cells fail to regulate extracellular potassium and indirectly affect synaptic transmission. Other substances of possible import in hepatic encephalopathy include short chain fatty acids derived from diet or bacterial metabolism of carbohydrates, and octopamines, biogenic amines that may function as false neurotransmitters.

The *hepatorenal syndrome* is renal failure associated with severe liver disease. It appears to be a circulatory disturbance, with marked reduction in glomerular filtration rate because of corticomedullary shunting, oliguria, and azotemia. As a rule, no structural abnormalities are discernible in the kidneys; indeed, they can serve as excellent transplants.

Other findings in patients in hepatic failure frequently include spider telangiectases of the skin over the thorax and erythema of the ulnar aspect of the palms. Their pathogenesis is unknown.

Portal Hypertension

Portal hypertension is altered resistance to blood flow in the portal venous system and a pressure gradient between portal vein and inferior vena cava in excess of 10 to 12 mm mercury. The factors responsible for portal hypertension have already been noted (p. 259).

Ascites is a manifestation of portal hypertension. It is partly a consequence of increased lymph flow, but results primarily from excessive transudation from peritoneal capillaries, due to hypoalbuminemia and sodium retention. There is increased aldosterone secretion in response to an initial hypovolemia and failure of the liver to inactivate renin. The peritoneum is the major site of fluid accumulation because of the high hydrostatic pressure in the capillaries of the portal system. The ascitic fluid has a low protein content, 1 to 2 g per dl.

Collateral venous channels that bypass the liver are likely to develop when portal pressure exceeds 20 mm mercury. The most important are those between

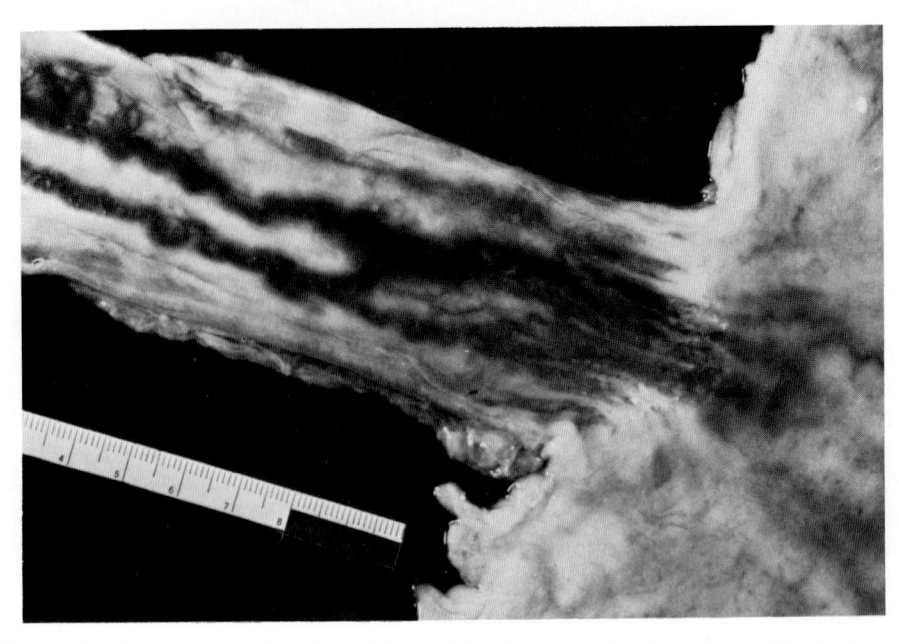

Figure 21.9. Esophageal varices. Several large, dilated esophageal veins are seen. Massive hemorrhage had taken place from an ulceration overlying one of these vessels at the junction of esophagus and stomach.

the lower esophagus and the azygous vein. The resulting esophageal varices are a frequent cause of hemorrhage, responsible for one-fourth of deaths among patients with cirrhosis (Fig. 21.9). Hemorrhage from esophageal varices can aggravate hepatic failure and induce hepatic encephalopathy.

Splenomegaly is an almost constant finding in patients with portal hypertension, and there may be evidence of hypersplenism: anemia, leukopenia, or thrombocytopenia. Gastric and duodenal peptic ulcers are increased in incidence. As pointed out earlier, an important consequence of portal hypertension and its collateral anastomoses is a high frequency of sepsis due to enteric organisms. Sepsis, furthermore, is likely to deepen the level of hepatic failure.

Attempts to alleviate the major hemodynamic consequences of portal hypertension involve establishing larger shunts between the portal vein and the inferior vena cava, or between the splenic and renal veins. These procedures, of course, increase the shunting of blood away from the liver and, if liver function is marginal, can be followed by deterioration of hepatocyte function, and encephalopathy.

Jaundice

Some degree of jaundice is virtually always present in hepatic failure, and it may be marked. It may result from an inability of the injured hepatocyte to conjugate bilirubin or from inability of the hepatocyte to force conjugated bilirubin through a canalicular and ductal system that may be partially obstructed by the abnormal architectural pattern of the parenchymal nodules and by fibrous septa. Thus, there may be elevated concentrations of both unconjugated and conjugated bilirubin. The hepatocyte, further, may be unable to reexcrete urobilinogen resorbed from the intestine.

Findings associated with jaundice may include severe itching, intestinal malabsorption of fats and fat-soluble vitamins due to impaired bile acid excretion, and hypercholesterolemia.

HEPATITIS

The term hepatitis is used here in the broad sense, and includes the several forms of viral hepatitis, alcoholic hepatitis, and drug-induced hepatic injury. Some of the causes of hepatic injury are outlined in Table 21.1. The regenerative capacity of the liver often permits a return to normal structure and function even after extensive injury. The integrity of the connective tissue framework of the liver lobule and of its limiting plate is a key factor in determining reconstitution of normal anatomy, or, in the case of chronic progressive injuries, an abnormal regenerative pattern that eventuates in cirrhosis.

Serum enzymes most useful in the detection of liver cell injury are the GOT (aspartate transaminase) and GPT (alanine transaminase). These enzymes are particularly indicative of acute injury. The GOT concentration is usually higher than the GPT, but the latter may be higher in acute viral hepatitis and in certain toxic injuries. Alkaline phosphatase is a normal constituent of bile, and the serum concentration is markedly elevated in any form of biliary obstruction. Since high alkaline phosphatase concentrations can also indicate bone disease, γ-glutamyl transferase (GGT) or 5'-nucleotidase concentrations are determined; they are elevated only in biliary obstruction.

Viral Hepatitis

This section deals with the hepatitis viruses, although such viruses as herpes simplex and cytomegalovirus may cause severe liver injury, particularly in immunologically compromised individuals.

Hepatitis A virus is an RNA virus. It is transmitted by the oral-fecal route, particularly among male homosexuals, and by contaminated shellfish. Transfusion or other parenteral transmission has not been demonstrated. The disease caused by this virus has an incubation period of 2 to 6 weeks, and is often mild; 90% of patients may be anicteric, and many are asymptomatic. The period of viremia is short. Complications are uncommon, and hepatitis A virus is not associated with chronic progressive liver disease. Some 50% of American adults have antibodies to the virus. Hepatitis A is decreasing in incidence, and may become a rarity in this country.

Hepatitis B virus is a DNA virus. It is transmitted by saliva and blood. Transmission by sexual intercourse accounts for some 40% of cases; other mechanisms include blood transfusion, medical and dental procedures, use of contaminated needles in the administration of street drugs, and transplacental transmission from mother to fetus. The incubation period of hepatitis B infection varies from 6 weeks to 6 months. The disease is generally more severe than hepatitis A, and viremia persists for months. Although the mortality is 0.5%, it may be as high as 12% in those infected by transfusion. Some 10 to 15% develop complications, particularly chronic persistent hepatitis and chronic active hepatitis, and about 1% progress to cirrhosis, most often macronodular. The hepatitis B surface antigen (HBsAg) is demonstrable in patients with this disorder and its complications, and its presence in many patients with primary carcinoma of the liver has strongly suggested that hepatitis B virus is an oncogenic virus in man. Antibodies to HBsAg and to the core antigen or Dane particle (HBcAg) are demonstrable in patients with acute or chronic disease.

Hepatitis C virus (preferably called non-A, non-B) now accounts for nearly 90% of post-transfusion hepatitis in this country. The incubation period in these patients varies between 3 weeks and 3 months. The acute disease is less severe than hepatitis B, and is not often fatal, but nearly one-third of patients show evidence of chronic infection and long term infectivity. Some may progress to cirrhosis and possibly to primary carcinoma of the liver. Hepatitis C is transmissible to chimpanzees.

Acute Viral Hepatitis

Acute viral hepatitis is characterized by a patchy degeneration and necrosis of liver cells. The hepatocytes may appear swollen (ballooning degeneration) because of loss of cellular glycogen, and their cytoplasm may have a ground glass appearance in hepatitis B infection, apparently a reflection of a high content of HBsAg. Necrosis of hepatocytes is often marked by extrusion of an "eosinophilic body" from the liver plate, representing the necrotic nucleus. Fatty change is usually not observed. There is inflammation of the entire lobule, composed principally of lymphocytes and mononuclear phagocytes, although a few polymorphonuclear leukocytes may be seen (Fig. 21.10). Kupffer cells are enlarged

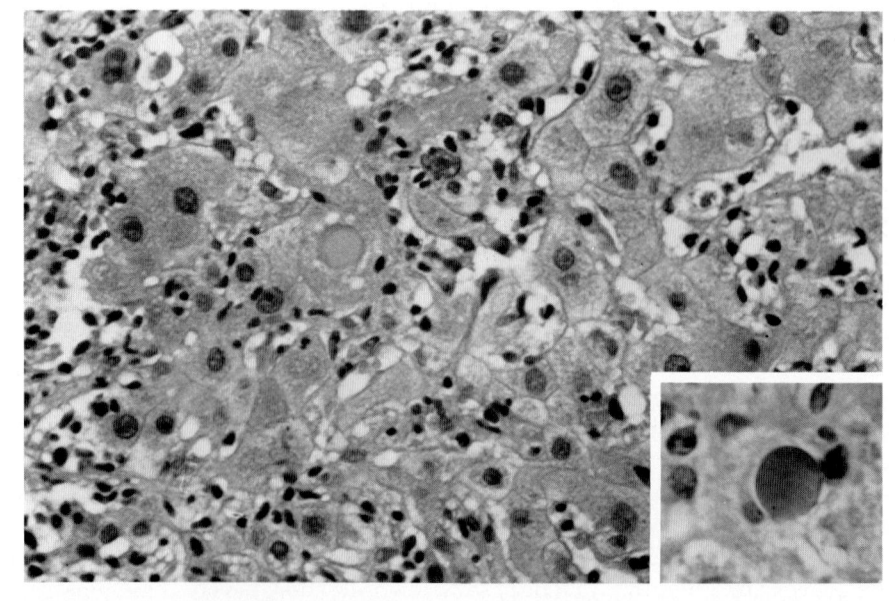

Figure 21.10. Acute viral hepatitis. There is moderate disarray of the liver plates, and several liver cells appear to be degenerating. There is considerable inflammatory cell infiltration, consisting predominately of lymphocytes and mononuclear phagocytes. The *inset*, at somewhat higher magnification, shows an eosinophilic body, representing an extruded necrotic liver cell.

and increased in numbers and contain lipofuscin pigment. The appearance of the liver is basically identical in hepatitis A, B, and C.

An occasional complication of acute viral hepatitis is *massive necrosis*, formerly called acute yellow atrophy. It can occur in all three types of hepatitis, and may also be seen in such chemical injuries to the liver as carbon tetrachloride poisoning and hypersensitivity to halothane anesthesia. There is almost total destruction of liver cells, leaving only the connective tissue framework of the lobules, Kupffer cells, bile ducts, and other portal triad structures. The liver cells appear to have been lysed, and there is little, if any, inflammation. The gross organ is shrunken and flabby, resembling a congested spleen. The mortality in massive necrosis is very high.

Chronic Persistent Hepatitis

Chronic persistent hepatitis occurs in hepatitis B and C, but not hepatitis A. It is characterized by persistent inflammation, often confined to the portal tracts, composed of lymphocytes. There may be minimal portal fibrosis. The lobular architecture is preserved, and the outlook for complete recovery is excellent. Evidence of disease usually subsides over a period of months.

Chronic Active Hepatitis

The liver in chronic active hepatitis shows extensive portal inflammation by lymphocytes and plasma cells. Prominent destruction of the limiting plate by "piecemeal necrosis" and "bridging necrosis" from portal triad to portal triad lead to distortion of the lobular architecture. These changes may be arrested or, in some, may progress to cirrhosis, usually of macronodular type.

Chronic active hepatitis may be a complication of hepatitis B, and, probably, hepatitis C. It also occurs as an autoimmune disorder, totally unrelated to viral hepatitis. This form of chronic active hepatitis is more likely to occur in women, and is associated with many immunologic phenomena, including elevated serum immunoglobulins, decreased serum complement, antibodies to smooth muscle, altered T cell function, rheumatoid factor, antinuclear antibodies, and LE cells. This disorder was formerly called *lupoid hepatitis.*

Alcoholic Hepatitis

The findings in alcoholic hepatitis differ dramatically from those in viral hepatitis. The liver cells usually show striking fatty change, and, most characteristically, large, waxy appearing eosinophilic cytoplasmic inclusions called Mallory bodies (Fig. 21.11). These inclusions appear fibrillar on electron microscopy and are composed of polypeptides and sugars. They are probably indicative of irreversible injury to the liver cell, a prelude to necrosis. Ballooning degeneration may also be prominent. There is variable polymorphonuclear leukocytic infiltration, often extending throughout the lobules. Strands of collagen may be deposited around the sinusoids.

These changes in the liver are thought to reflect a direct toxicity of alcohol, but nutritional deficiency may contribute to the injury.

Alcoholic hepatitis is preceded by extensive fatty change of the hepatocytes, a thoroughly reversible lesion. In most instances, alcoholic hepatitis is also reversible, but in some individuals, perhaps genetically predisposed, persistent injury

270   Pathology: Understanding Human Disease

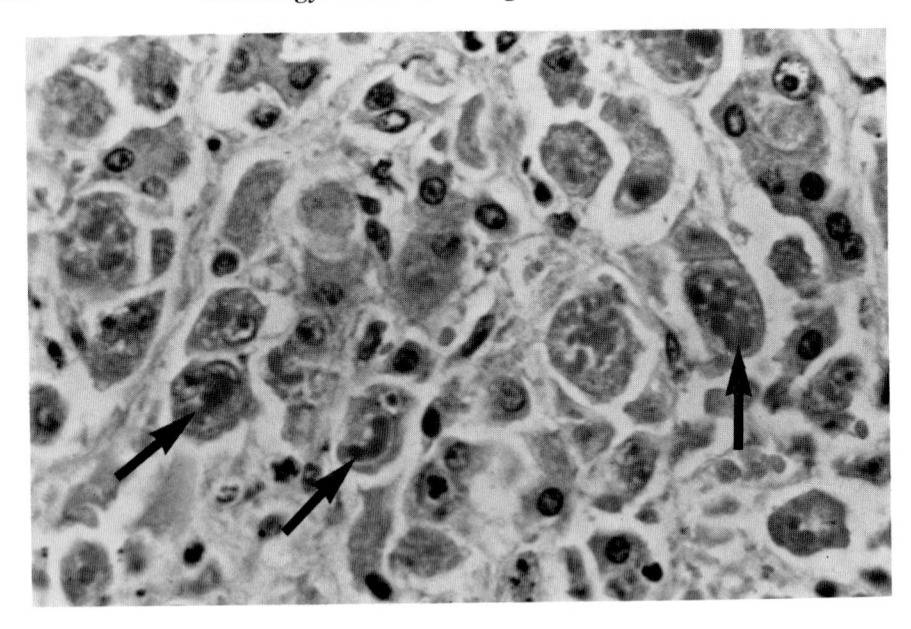

Figure 21.11. Mallory bodies. Many of the liver cells in this field show large amorphous cytoplasmic inclusions, a highly characteristic finding in alcoholic hepatitis.

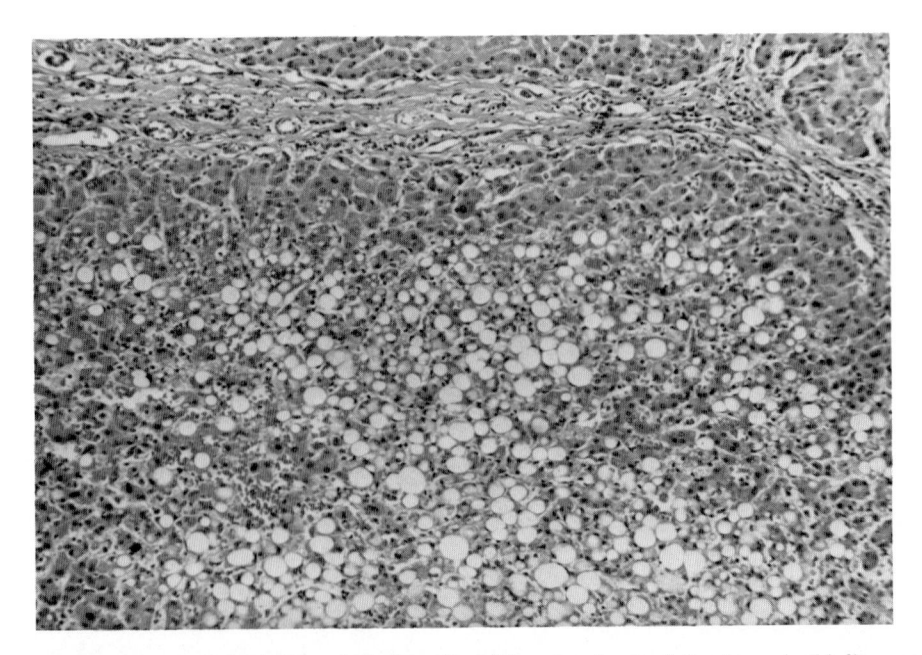

Figure 21.12. Early cirrhosis in an alcoholic patient. There is extensive fatty change in this liver, and patchy areas of acute inflammation, indicating areas of liver cell necrosis. There is moderate architectural distortion and an increase in fibrous septa (*above*).

from alcohol results in a micronodular cirrhosis (Fig. 21.12). Death may occur in hepatic failure from severe alcoholic hepatitis, often called *florid cirrhosis*.

Drug-induced Liver Injury

Some of the drugs that can cause liver injury are included in Table 21.1. They may be directly toxic to the liver, and injury may be dose-related, or they may induce hypersensitivity reactions.

Three patterns of injury are recognizable. Such drugs as methyl testosterone and the oral contraceptives produce cholestasis, with plugging of bile canaliculi and small ducts, but no liver cell necrosis and no inflammatory reaction. Others, including erythromycin and chlorpromazine, are associated with both cholestasis and liver cell necrosis. Both of these types of reactions usually subside with discontinuation of the offending agent, even, at times, with a reduction of dosage. Many agents, including methotrexate, halothane, and isoniazid, can produce changes in the liver indistinguishable from acute viral hepatitis, although some fatty change may be noted, and eosinophils may be prominent among the inflammatory cells. In the case of halothane, injury occurs on a second exposure to the agent. In this latter group of injuries, some may regress following withdrawal of the drug, but others can be progressive and terminate in cirrhosis with hepatic failure.

HEMOCHROMATOSIS

Hemochromatosis has, in part, been discussed in Chapter 10 (p. 102). It is a disorder of iron metabolism in which hemosiderin pigment is deposited in many organs, including the liver, pancreas, skin, heart, and endocrine glands. It may be an inherited disturbance of iron absorption from the gastrointestinal tract, but can also result from excessive breakdown of red blood cells and repeated blood transfusions.

Liver involvement is usually the most serious manifestation of disease, although diabetes may also present a threat to life. Hemosiderin pigment is seen in hepatocytes, Kupffer cells, and bile duct epithelium (Fig. 21.13). Liver cells are progressively injured, and there is gradual evolution of a micronodular cirrhosis and all of the manifestations of hepatic failure. There is a high incidence of complicating primary carcinoma of the liver, occurring in between 7 and 22% of all patients.

WILSON'S DISEASE

This disorder reflects an inherited error in copper metabolism. Copper accumulates in the lysosomes of hepatocytes and is responsible for the development of cirrhosis, usually micronodular, occasionally macronodular. The onset of disease is usually in late childhood. In addition to chronic liver disease, there is progressive brain damage. The characteristic green Kayser-Fleischer ring consists of copper deposits in the limbus of the cornea and Descemet's membrane.

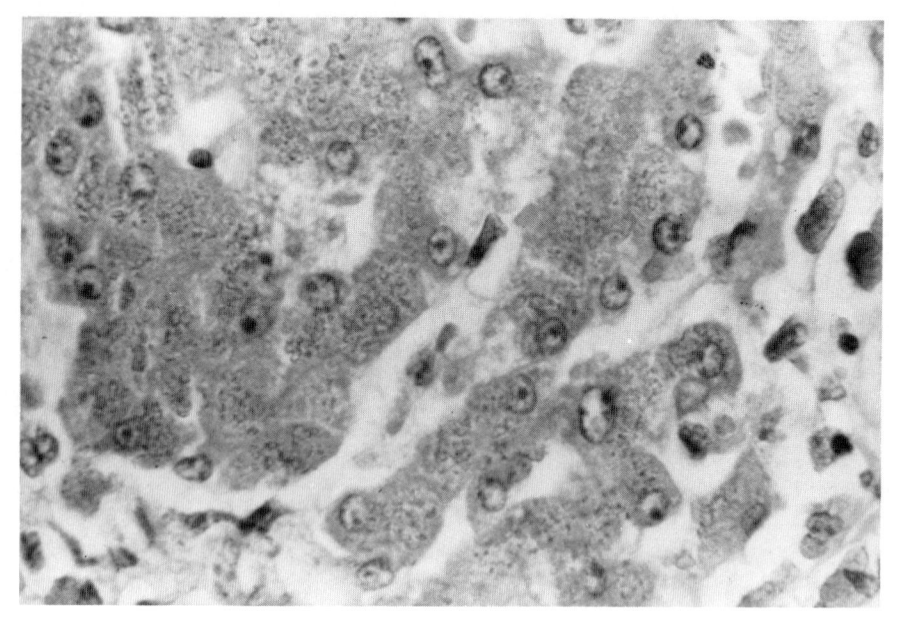

Figure 21.13. Hemochromatosis. The liver cells are filled with granular hemosiderin pigment. Hemochromatosis usually eventuates in a micronodular cirrhosis.

α-1-ANTITRYPSIN DEFICIENCY

α-1-Antitrypsin deficiency is a relatively uncommon cause of cirrhosis, but it is responsible for a significant proportion of childhood cirrhosis. Cirrhosis develops in some 15% of homozygotes and in an occasional heterozygote. The cirrhosis is micronodular.

There is usually evidence of cholestatic jaundice early in infancy, but cirrhosis and liver failure are not apparent till late childhood or adolescence. The liver cells contain cytoplasmic inclusion bodies that consist of α-1-antitrypsin. The fundamental defect in this disorder resides in the liver cells, and liver transplantation has been successful in correcting the deficiency.

BILIARY CIRRHOSIS

Biliary cirrhosis can be a complication of biliary atresia, or obstruction of the larger ducts by gall stones or by carcinoma of the pancreas, often with an ascending infection of the biliary tree. There is eventual hepatocyte necrosis and formation of bile lakes following rupture of canaliculi. The liver is grossly green in color, because of its bile content. The cirrhosis is micronodular, but there is somewhat less architectural distortion of the lobules, and ductal, canalicular, and cellular bile stasis is striking.

Primary biliary cirrhosis bears some resemblance to chronic active hepatitis. It affects especially middle-aged women and is often associated with immunologic disorders. Patients' sera contain antimitochondrial antibodies, and there may be elevated levels of serum cholesterol and lipid concentrations. The liver shows a micronodular cirrhosis, with an appearance of marked bile duct proliferation.

Damage to the ductal cells may cause a granulomatous reaction. Primary biliary cirrhosis is thought to be an autoimmune disorder.

HEREDITARY DISTURBANCES OF BILIRUBIN METABOLISM

There are several inherited disturbances of bilirubin metabolism that are manifested by jaundice. *Gilbert's disease*, inherited as an autosomal dominant, results from an inadequate uptake of bilirubin by hepatocytes. There is mild jaundice due to unconjugated bilirubin. The *Crigler-Najjar syndrome* manifests a deficiency of glucuronyl transferase. Complete absence of the enzyme (Type I) prevents any conjugation of bilirubin, and death in infancy is due to kernicterus. With partial deficiency (Type II), some conjugation takes place and survival is normal. In the *Dubin-Johnson syndrome* there is an increase in circulating conjugated bilirubin. The hepatocyte can conjugate bilirubin, but cannot excrete it into the bile canaliculi. The hepatocytes are heavily pigmented, the pigment having properties of both lipofuscin and melanin.

CIRCULATORY DISTURBANCES

The most important circulatory disturbance of the liver is *chronic passive congestion* (p. 145). Repeated episodes of severe congestion, with central lobular hemorrhage and necrosis, can cause some fibrosis and, rarely, a cirrhosis. *Infarction* of the liver is uncommon, but can follow obstruction or embolization of the hepatic artery or severe shock. The *Budd-Chiari syndrome* is the result of thrombosis of the hepatic vein. This may be caused by neoplastic invasion of the vessel or in such hypercoagulable states as polycythemia vera.

TUMORS OF THE LIVER

The most important tumors of the liver are primary and metastatic carcinomas. Adenomas are included because of current interest in their origin.

Adenoma

Hepatic adenomas are most frequently observed in women 20 to 40 years of age, and epidemiologic evidence strongly suggests a role of oral contraceptive agents in their genesis. The tumors are usually greater than 5 cm in diameter. Both grossly and microscopically, they appear as nodules of normal liver tissue, although bile ducts may be absent. Adenomas may present for the first time with massive intraperitoneal hemorrhage.

Primary Carcinoma

Most primary carcinomas of the liver are *hepatocellular carcinomas* (80%); the others are of bile duct origin (*cholangiocarcinomas*) or mixed. They occur predominantly in cirrhotic livers, particularly those with a macronodular pattern, but are also encountered in otherwise normal livers. The incidence of hepatocellular carcinoma in patients with cirrhosis varies from about 5% in micronodular cirrhosis to as great as 22% in some patients with macronodular disease. Primary carcinoma should be considered in any patient with cirrhosis whose liver enlarges rapidly or whose condition deteriorates despite adequate therapy.

274   *Pathology: Understanding Human Disease*

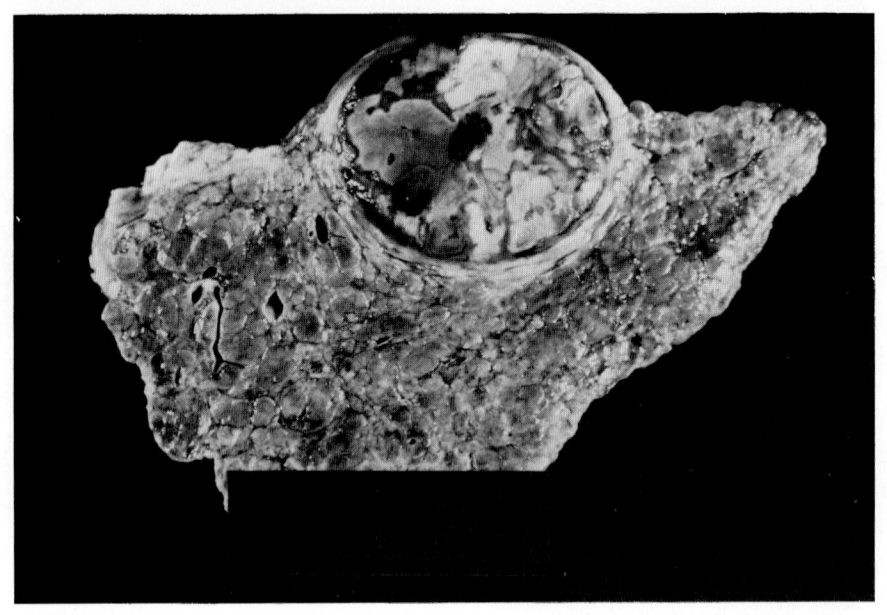

Figure 21.14. Hepatocellular carcinoma. This tumor, measuring 4 cm in diameter, appears sharply circumscribed from the surrounding cirrhotic liver. It shows several areas of hemorrhage and necrosis.

Grossly, hepatocellular carcinoma may be single or multiple; multiple masses often suggest multicentric origin. Tumor nodules may be distinguishable from the nodules of the cirrhotic process only by size, although hemorrhage and necrosis are frequent (Fig. 21.14). There is often gross vascular invasion and spread through the portal or hepatic veins. The histologic appearance may approximate normal liver and show bile secretion, or it may be quite pleomorphic and undifferentiated (Fig. 21.15). Cholangiocarcinomas are similar to carcinomas of the pancreas and biliary tree. They have a ductal pattern, and a prominent fibrous tissue stroma. Tumor masses are usually gray-white in color and hard in consistency. Only 30% of cholangiocarcinomas occur in cirrhotic livers as opposed to 80% of hepatocellular carcinomas.

Of great interest at present is the relationship between hepatocellular carcinoma and viral hepatitis, particularly hepatitis B. Considerable evidence has accumulated to indicate that, in this country, persistence of hepatitis B infection may be prerequisite to hepatocellular carcinoma. The majority of patients with this tumor are positive for HBsAg, and the incidence of carcinoma is higher among carriers of the antigen. Virus can be identified in liver cells around the tumors, and HBsAg has occasionally been identified in tumor cells themselves. It may well be that hepatitis B virus will be the first proven oncogenic virus in man.

Metastatic Carcinoma

Metastatic carcinomas of the liver are far more frequent than primary tumors. They are usually observed in otherwise normal livers and are less likely to occur in the presence of cirrhosis (Fig. 21.16). Many tumors may metastasize to the

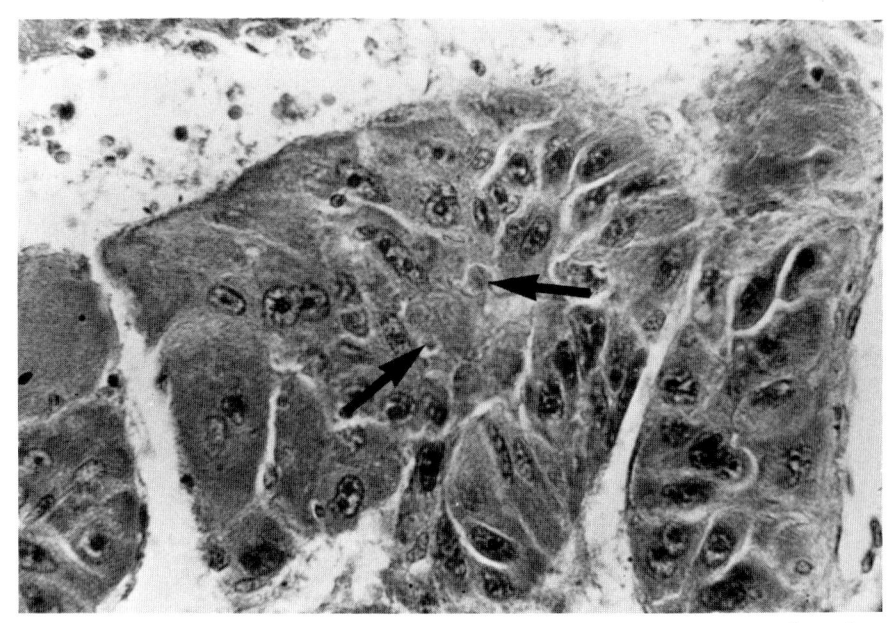

21.15. Hepatocellular carcinoma. The tumor cells retain a close resemblance to liver cells, and several droplets of bile secretion can be seen (*arrows*).

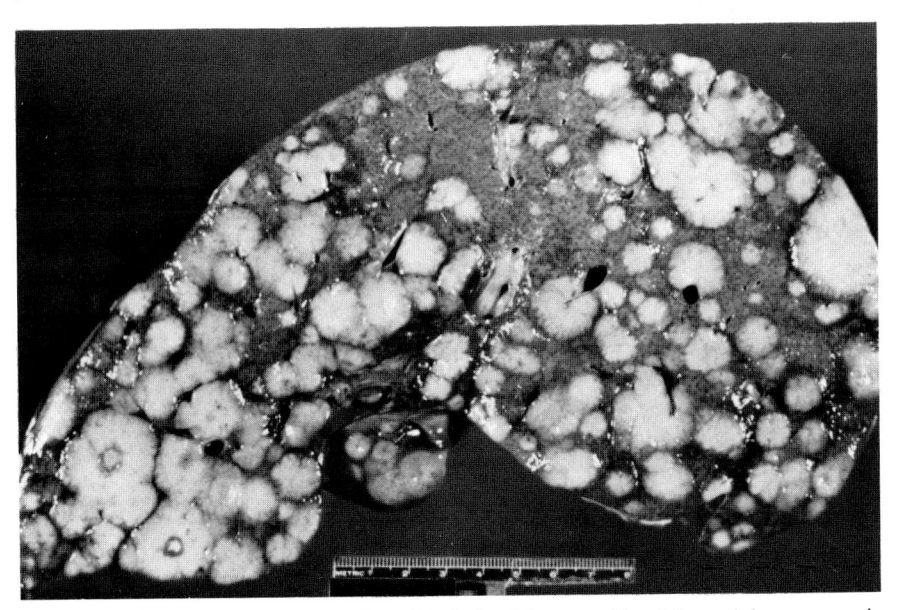

Figure 21.16. Metastatic carcinoma in liver. Myriads of firm grayish white nodules are seen in an otherwise normal liver. The primary tumor was in breast.

liver, particularly those from the gastrointestinal tract, breast, and lung. Metastases from gastrointestinal tumors are associated with very high serum levels of carcinoembryonic antigen. Seventy percent of hepatocellular carcinomas, on the other hand, secrete α-fetoprotein.

THE BILIARY SYSTEM

Brief consideration is given to cholelithiasis, cholecystitis, and carcinoma of the gall bladder and biliary ducts.

CHOLELITHIASIS

Stones are present in the gall bladder in nearly one in five adults, with a striking female predominance. They form in the gall bladder or major biliary ducts, and may be composed of bilirubin, cholesterol, or calcium carbonate.

The cause of stones is believed relatable to altered composition of bile. High concentrations of conjugated bilirubin in patients with hemolytic anemia lead to formation of biliary stones. Bile containing high concentrations of cholesterol, with decreased bile salts and lecithin, leads to cholesterol crystallization and stone formation. Gall stones are particularly likely to occur in the presence of obesity, ileal disease or bypass surgery, diabetes, and type IV hyperlipoproteinemia. Estrogen administration may also constitute a risk factor.

Most stones are mixed, containing cholesterol, calcium bilirubinate, and calcium carbonate. They are usually small and multiple, and occur in association with chronic cholecystitis (Fig. 21.17). Pure cholesterol stones are less frequent, and may be quite large. The principal complication of biliary stones is obstruction of the lower biliary ducts, particularly the common bile duct. If persistent, obstruction, often complicated by ascending infection, can lead to biliary cirrhosis. Obstruction of the cystic duct can cause *hydrops* of the gall bladder, or a small, scarred organ containing "white bile."

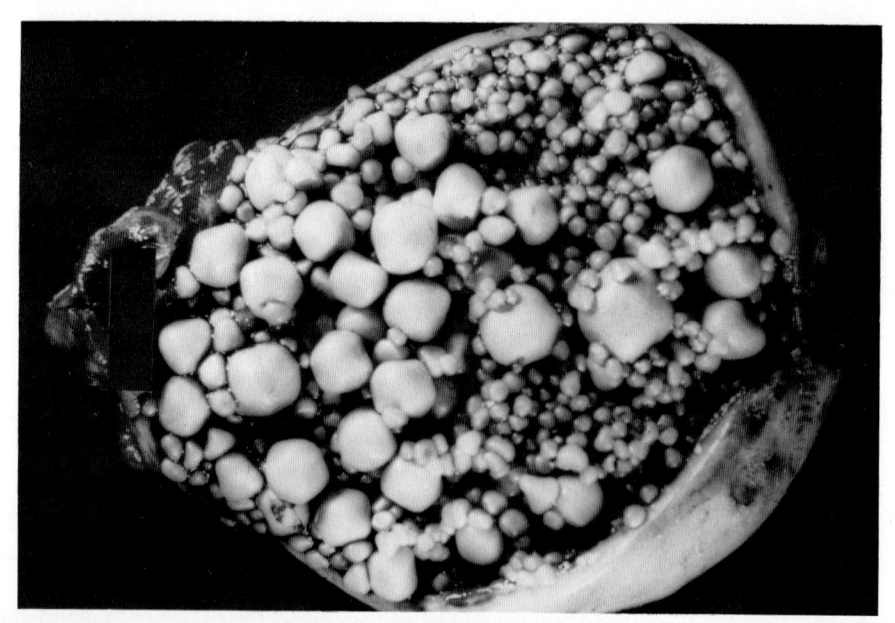

Figure 21.17. Chronic cholecystitis and cholelithiasis. The gall bladder wall is thickened and fibrotic. The organ is filled with mixed stones, varying in size from 1 mm to 1 cm.

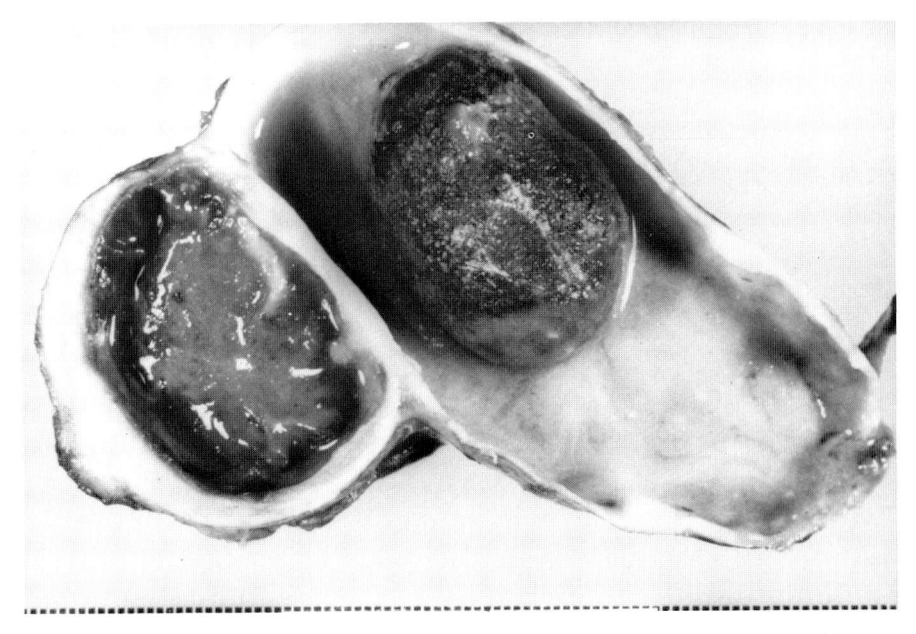

Figure 21.18. Chronic cholecystitis and cholelithiasis. This gall bladder, measuring only 4 cm in length, has a markedly scarred wall and contains a single mixed stone. The mucosa is flat and atrophic. A single diverticulum of the gall bladder is seen at the left.

CHOLECYSTITIS

Cholecystitis, acute or chronic, occurs mostly during middle age, again with a marked female predominance. Cholecystitis and cholelithiasis are closely related and usually concurrent; both processes appear related to alterations of bile constituents. Acute cholecystitis results from a chemical injury to the mucosa, often complicated by infection. The mucosa is ulcerated, the wall inflamed, and the contents purulent. Gangrene of the wall is not uncommon, called *empyema* of the gall bladder, and may result in perforation and peritonitis. Chronic cholecystitis is virtually always accompanied by cholelithiasis. The mucosa is flattened and the wall scarred.

TUMORS

The principal tumors of the biliary system are benign adenomas and papillomas of the gall bladder and adenocarcinomas of the gall bladder and biliary ducts. Carcinomas of the gall bladder constitute some 1 to 3% of all malignant tumors. They occur most often between ages 50 and 70, and 80% occur in women. Chronic cholecystitis and cholelithiasis are almost always present. The tumors arise in the neck or fundus of the gall bladder, and may infiltrate the wall or fill the lumen of the gland. Histologically, adenocarcinomas of the gall bladder are indistinguishable from cholangiocarcinomas. They metastasize early to the liver, either by direct spread or through the portal vessels. Mestastases to the porta hepatis lymph nodes and to the lungs are also frequent. The symptoms related to gall bladder carcinoma differ in no way from those of cholecystitis and cholelithiasis, making early diagnosis extremely difficult.

Carcinoma of the ampulla of Vater can obstruct the common bile duct and the pancreatic ducts while quite small (1 to 2 cm). They are likely to cause intermittent right upper quadrant pain, jaundice, and biliary colic, with acholic stools and other findings of complete biliary obstruction. Despite early recognition, the outlook for surgical cure is generally poor, and liver and lymph node metastases occur early.

Suggested Reading

Blumberg BS, London WT. Hepatitis B virus and the prevention of primary hepatocellular carcinoma. N. Engl. J. Med. *304:* 782, 1981.

Popper H. Pathologic aspects of cirrhosis. Am. J. Pathol. *87:* 227, 1977.

Redeker AG. Treatment of chronic active hepatitis. N. Engl. J. Med. *304:* 420, 1981 .

Rubin E. Acute and chronic viral hepatitis. Fed. Proc. *38:* 2665, 1979.

Tabor E, Seeff LB, Gerety RJ. Chronic non-A, non-B hepatitis carrier state. N. Engl. J. Med. *303:* 140, 1980.

Chapter 22

The Exocrine Pancreas

This chapter is confined to discussions of pancreatitis and pancreatic carcinoma. Cystic fibrosis is discussed in Chapter 34, and disorders of the islets of Langerhans are considered in chapters devoted to diabetes mellitus and the endocrine system.

PANCREATITIS

The term "pancreatitis" encompasses a group of inflammatory lesions of the pancreas that vary greatly in their severity. They may be recurrent, and can occasionally progress to a chronic destructive disorder with total atrophy of the exocrine gland. Abdominal or back pain is characteristic of all forms of pancreatitis, and intestinal malabsorption due to loss of pancreatic enzymes is frequent in severe and chronic disease.

Acute Pancreatitis

Mild acute pancreatitis is usually sudden in onset and manifested by pain, anorexia, nausea, and vomiting. The pancreas is congested and edematous, is focally infiltrated by polymorphonuclear leukocytes, and shows small, isolated areas of glandular necrosis. This form of pancreatitis appears to be self-limited, and is probably completely reversible, with reconstitution of an entirely normal architecture.

Acute pancreatitis of moderate severity shows, additionally, areas of interstitial hemorrhage and small foci of digestion of acinar and interstitial tissue (Fig. 22.1). Proteolytic enzymes released from injured acinar cells digest connective tissue and attack blood vessels. Lipase hydrolyzes interstitial pancreatic fat; glycerol is resorbed into the circulation, while free fatty acid forms soaps with calcium. Areas of fat necrosis consist of chalky yellow-white deposits, visible between pancreatic lobules (Fig. 22.2). Further spread of lipase can cause fat necrosis of mesenteric and omental fat, as well as retroperitoneal tissue (Fig. 22.3). Lipase traveling through the circulation can attack subcutaneous fat and the bone marrow. Acute pancreatitis of this type may be a recurrent disorder, associated with focal atrophy and fibrosis of the gland, and it may occasionally progress to chronic pancreatitis.

The most severe form of acute pancreatitis is hemorrhagic pancreatitis. It is likely to be associated with excessive food and alcohol intake. Pain is severe, there is hypovolemic shock, and death may occur within a few hours of onset. Virtually the entire pancreas together with surrounding tissue may be hemor-

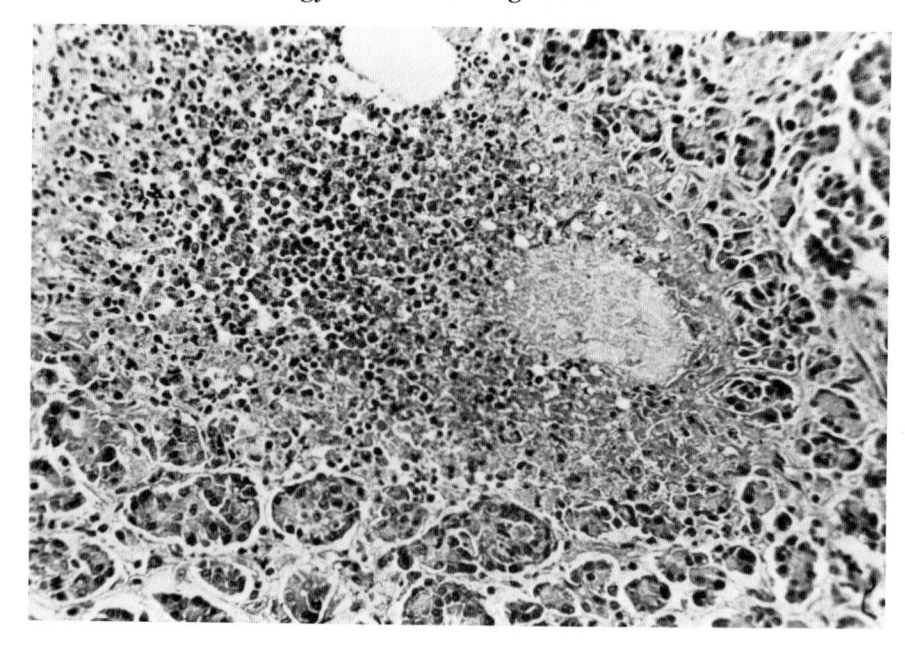

Figure 22.1. Acute pancreatitis. The *center* of the field shows extensive enzymatic digestion of acinar and interstitial tissue, and marked infiltration by polymorphonuclear leukocytes.

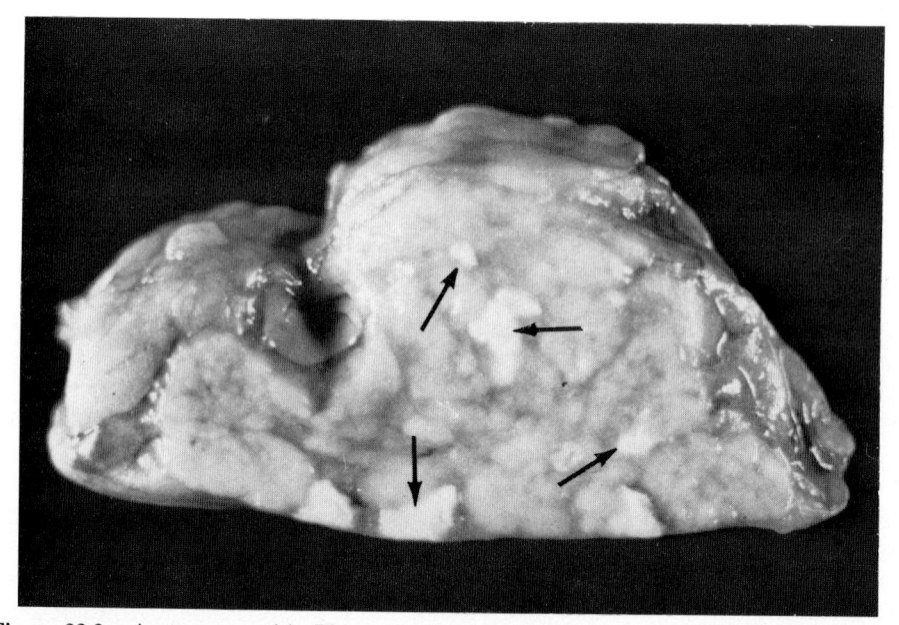

Figure 22.2. Acute pancreatitis. This cut section of pancreas shows multiple areas of fat necrosis between pancreatic lobules.

rhagic and liquefied (Fig. 22.4). There is massive fat necrosis of peritoneal and retroperitoneal fat. If the attack is survived, infection of the pancreatic bed with abscess formation is likely to occur, or fibrous tissue proliferation around the liquefied pancreas may form a *pseudocyst*.

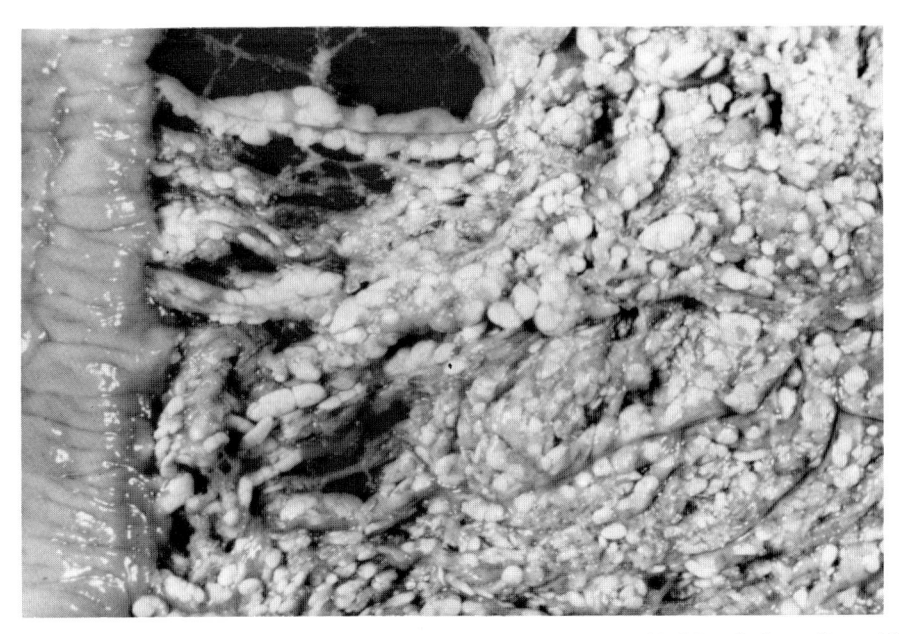

Figure 22.3. Acute pancreatitis. Shown here is the mesentery, studded by chalky yellow-white areas of fat necrosis.

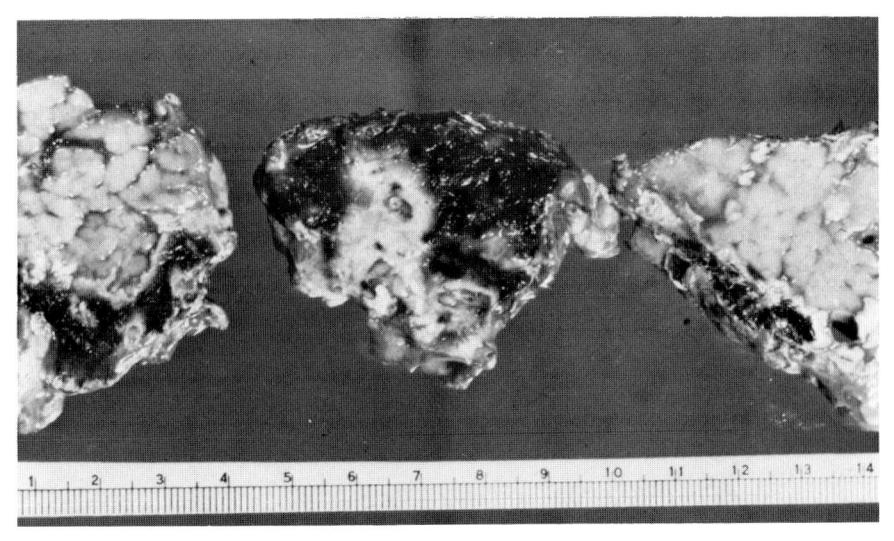

Figure 22.4. Hemorrhagic pancreatitis. The section of pancreas in the *center* shows extensive digestion and hemorrhage involving most of the parenchyma. Areas of hemorrhage are also noted in the other sections, as well as focal areas of fat necrosis.

Chronic Pancreatitis

Chronic pancreatitis is a progressive, often relapsing, disease that results in severe atrophy of the gland and loss of all pancreatic function. There is marked weight loss, generalized intestinal malabsorption with steatorrhea (Chapter 23),

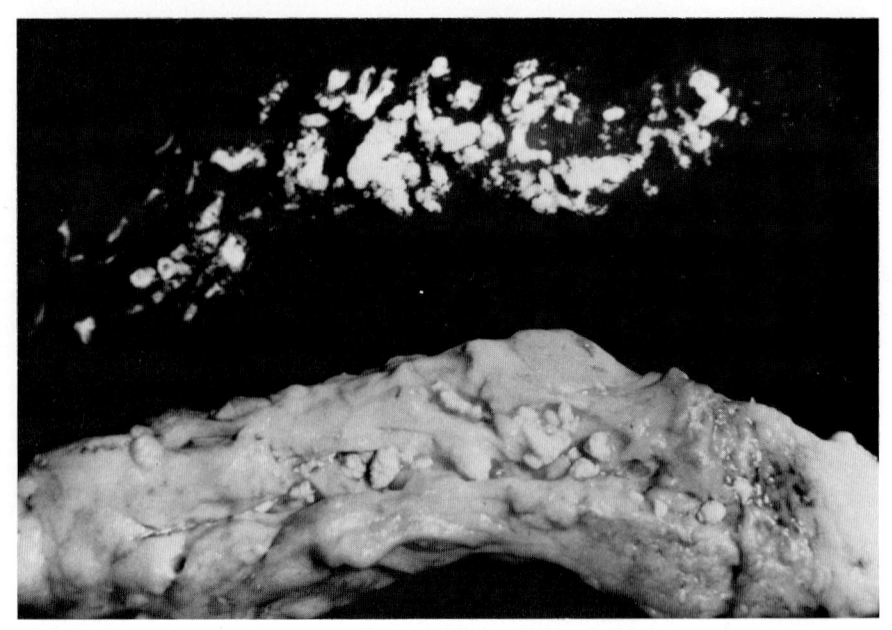

Figure 22.5. Chronic pancreatitis. There is extensive scarring of the pancreas. Many of the ducts are dilated and contain stones. The extensive calcification is emphasized by the x-ray of this specimen, shown *above*.

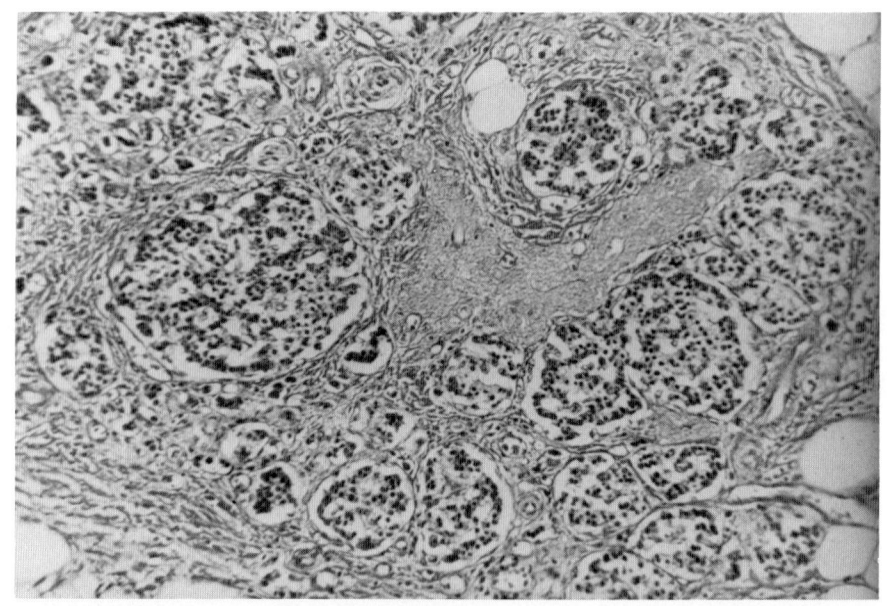

Figure 22.6. Chronic pancreatitis. Virtually all of the acinar tissue has been destroyed, and largely replaced by fibrous tissue. The islets have survived, however, and occupy most of this field.

diabetes mellitus, and edema due to hypoproteinemia. The severity and persistence of pain may lead to narcotic addiction. The pancreas is severely atrophic and fibrotic, often with areas of calcification (Fig. 22.5). Multiple stones are found in the pancreatic ducts, and squamous metaplasia of ductal epithelium may be striking. The islets, often spared until late in the course, are eventually destroyed (Fig. 22.6).

Pathogenesis of Acute and Chronic Pancreatitis

Although many mechanisms have been proposed to explain both acute and chronic pancreatitis, none has proved generally valid. Any explanation must account for some well established observations. One-third of patients with pancreatitis have coexisting biliary tract disease, usually cholecystitis and cholelithiasis, and another one-third are abusers of alcohol. There is a high incidence of pancreatitis in patients with hyperparathyroidism and other causes of elevated serum calcium concentration. There is also an increased incidence in patients with Cushing's syndrome, and an association with Types I and V hyperlipidemia. One hypothesis has implicated reflux of bile into the pancreatic duct via a common channel in the ampulla of Vater. Others propose that pancreatic duct obstruction results from spasm of the sphincter of Oddi, from squamous metaplasia of ductal epithelium, or from ductal inflammation and stone formation. A vascular basis is suggested by the occurrence of pancreatitis in patients with malignant hypertension and necrotizing arteriolitis, and several viruses, notably cytomegalovirus and mumps virus, are known to cause mild pancreatitis. There is no unifying concept, although it is likely that, regardless of mechanism, activation of intrapancreatic trypsinogen may trigger an attack.

Treatment of pancreatitis attempts to minimize stimulation of pancreatic enzyme synthesis and secretion. This is done by keeping the duodenum empty by continous suction until the attack has subsided.

Mild pancreatitis may not measurably alter pancreatic exocrine function, but recurrent episodes inevitably impair function. Early manifestations may be loss of normal pancreatic response to secretin or cholecystokinin. Any severe injury to the acinar epithelium results in release of enzymes into the bloodstream. Serum and urine amylase levels are helpful in the diagnosis of pancreatitis. Lipase determinations are more sensitive, and levels are elevated for a longer period, but the determination is more difficult to perform. Assessment of the amylase/creatinine clearance ratio and an immunoreactive trypsin assay have proven very valuable in the diagnosis of acute pancreatitis.

CARCINOMA OF THE PANCREAS

Carcinoma of the pancreas accounts for 5% of cancer deaths in both men and women. It is rare below the age of 40. Pancreatic carcinoma is associated with alcoholism, biliary disease, exposure to industrial chemicals, and, most recently, with ingestion of coffee. The incidence is at least doubled in cigarette smokers. The outlook for pancreatic carcinoma remains dismal; the diagnosis is but rarely made when the lesion is resectable, and the 5-year survival rate is only about 2%. Newer diagnostic techniques, including ultrasound, angiography, and retrograde pancreatic duct injection have not yet altered the prognosis.

Pancreatic carcinoma is an adenocarcinoma, basically identical with those of the gall bladder and biliary ducts. Virtually all arise in the pancreatic ducts, but they may vary in pattern; some are cystic, others mucinous, and others highly pleomorphic. All tend to have a prominent fibrous tissue stroma (Figs. 22.7 and 22.8).

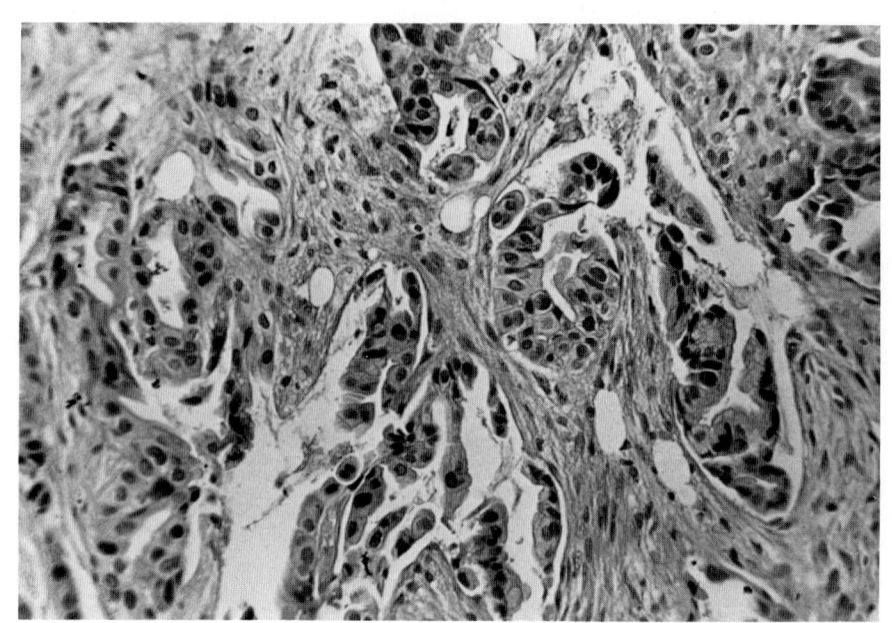

Figure 22.7. Adenocarcinoma of pancreas. The tumor shows a distinct ductal pattern and a rather marked proliferation of a fibrous stroma.

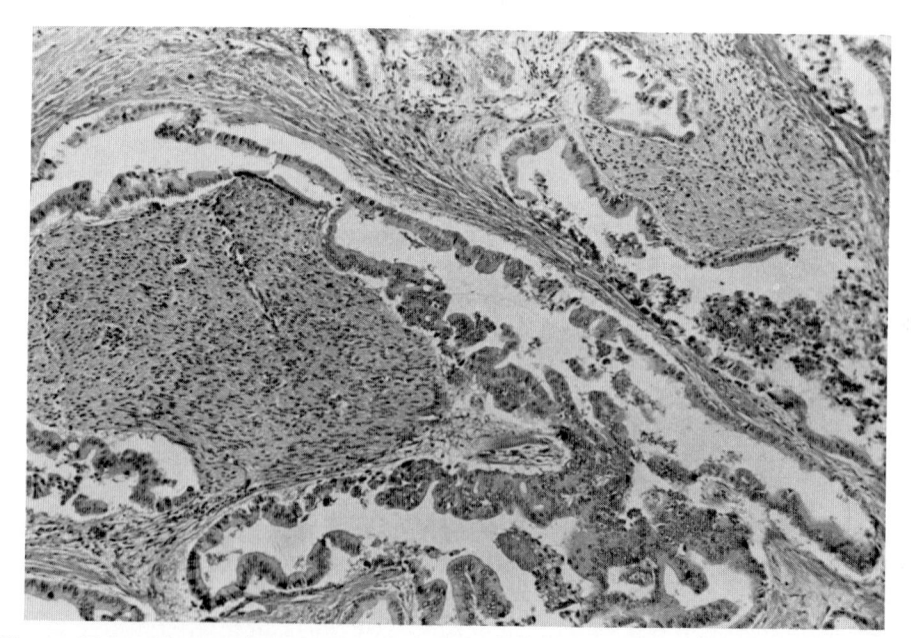

Figure 22.8. Adenocarcinoma of pancreas. This field shows rather well differentiated ductal carcinoma invading perineural lymphatics.

Some two-thirds of pancreatic carcinomas arise in the head, and tend to invade or compress the common bile duct (Fig. 22.9). Obstructive jaundice may be an early manifestation, although abdominal or back pain and loss of appetite usually appear first. Small liver metastases are often present when the diagnosis is first

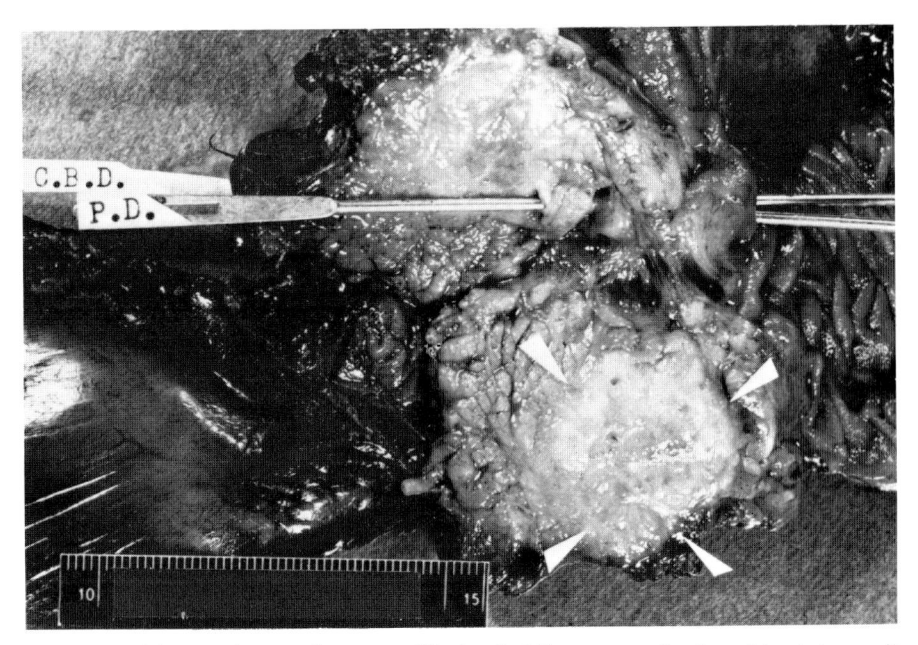

Figure 22.9. Adenocarcinoma of pancreas. The head of the pancreas has been bisected, revealing hard grayish white tumor tissue replacing and invading the normal pancreatic structure. The tumor is very poorly circumscribed. Probes are shown in the pancreatic duct and in the common bile duct. The opened duodenum is seen to the *right*.

made. An occasional early diagnosis can be made when a small lesion obstructs the main pancreatic duct and causes diarrhea and steatorrhea.

Carcinoma of the body and tail is likely to be larger in size when diagnosed. Aside from pain and weight loss, the earliest signs may be neuropathy, myopathy, diabetes mellitus, or a migratory thrombophlebitis due to hypercoagulability of the blood. At times, liver or peritoneal metastases may be the first evidence of disease.

Suggested Reading

Kalant H. Alcohol, pancreatic secretion and pancreatitis. Gastroenterology *56:* 380, 1969.
Sarles H. The exocrine pancreas. Int. Rev. Physiol. *12:* 173, 1977.

Chapter 23

The Digestive Tract

No attempt is made here to cover the multitude of digestive tract disorders. Relatively few topics are discussed in some detail, including gastritis, peptic ulcer disease, the malabsorption syndromes, Crohn's disease and ulcerative colitis, pseudomembranous enterocolitis, appendicitis, diverticulosis, and the important tumors.

GASTRITIS

Acute gastritis is a superficial injury to the gastric mucosa, often accompanied by erosions and brisk hemorrhage. It is particularly associated with alcohol or aspirin abuse, but is also seen with heavy smoking, uremia, and shock. It is a transient lesion, without permanent sequelae, although surgical intervention may be necessary to stop hemorrhage. Repeated episodes of acute gastritis may lead to a chronic inflammation of the superficial portion of the mucosa and some irregularity of the glands. It is not progressive, and is reversible.

Chronic Atrophic Gastritis

Chronic atrophic gastritis is characterized by lymphocytic and plasma cell infiltration of the entire thickness of gastric mucosa and the submucosa, with lymphoid follicle formation. There is gradual atrophy of the epithelium, atrophy of the glands, loss of chief and parietal cells, and replacement by an intestinal epithelium with many mucous cells (Fig. 23.1). In time, there is impairment of acid and pepsin secretion, and, eventually, achlorhydria.

One-fourth of patients with chronic atrophic gastritis have circulating autoantibodies against parietal cells, and there may also be a cell-mediated immune reaction against these cells. Intrinsic factor, secreted by the chief cells, becomes insufficient for vitamin B_{12} absorption in the small intestine and, when body stores are exhausted, pernicious anemia results. Virtually all patients with pernicious anemia have achlorhydria and antiparietal cell antibodies; some also have anti-intrinsic factor autoantibodies. There is frequent association with other autoimmune disorders, such as Hashimoto's thyroiditis, hypoparathyroidism, adrenal insufficiency, and diabetes mellitus. Most patients with chronic atrophic gastritis, however, do not appear to have an autoimmune process, and do not develop pernicious anemia.

Some 10% of patients with severe chronic atrophic gastritis eventually develop gastric carcinoma.

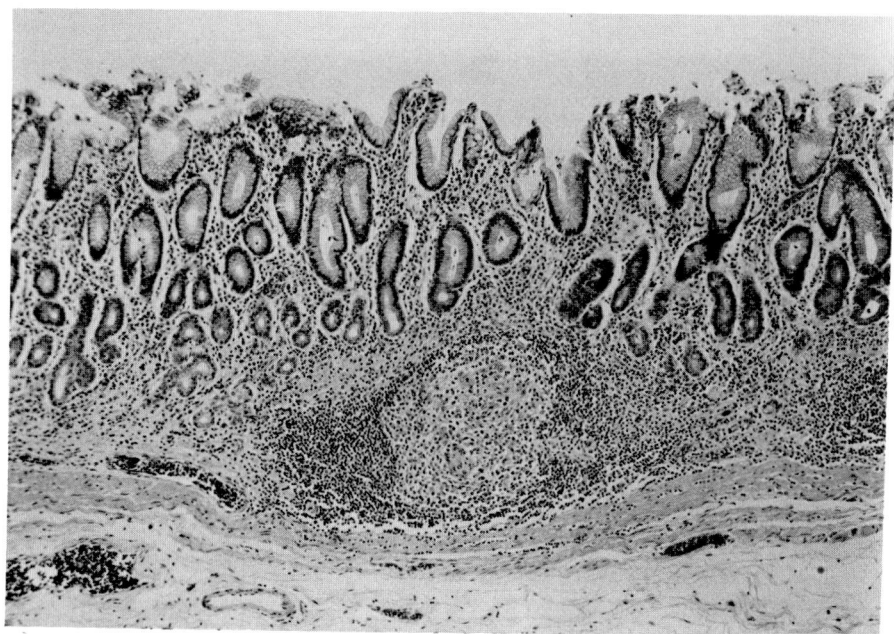

Figure 23.1. Chronic atrophic gastritis. The normal gastric epithelium has become atrophic and replaced by intestinal epithelium with many mucus-producing cells. There is extensive lymphocytic infiltration of the deeper layers of the mucosa.

Hypertrophic Gastritis

In hypertrophic gastritis, the folds of gastric mucosa are markedly thickened and covered with actively secreting epithelial cells. There may be hypersecretion, with loss of serum proteins and subsequent dependent edema (*Ménétrier's disease*), or simple hypersecretion, rich in acid, but without significant protein loss. Hypertrophic gastritis is also seen in the *Zollinger-Ellison syndrome*, due to constant stimulation by gastrin from a pancreatic islet or carcinoid tumor. The massive secretion of acid surpasses the neutralizing capacity of the duodenum, and multiple peptic ulcers are formed.

PEPTIC ULCER DISEASE

Acute Peptic Ulcer

Acute peptic ulcers are small, discrete, superficial lesions, usually multiple, and almost always gastric. They may occur with ingestion of alcohol, aspirin, or indomethacin, but are more often associated with severe stress, as in extensive burns, acute brain injury, the postoperative state, and shock. Although the ulcerations may, at times, reach several centimeters in diameter, complete healing is the usual result following alleviation of the cause.

Chronic Peptic Ulcer

The overall incidence of chronic peptic ulcer disease has, for unknown reasons, been declining slowly for several decades. Estimates of the current incidence in this country range from 6 to 14%, with a 3:1 male predominance. They are uncommon before the age 20, and the peak incidence is at about 50. There is distinct family clustering, and first degree relatives have a 3-fold risk of the disease. Blood Group O increases the risk of duodenal ulcer, Group A of gastric ulcers. Persons with the HLA B5 haplotype also appear at increased risk for ulcers.

Morphology

Chronic ulcers have a characteristic morphologic appearance. They are sharply punched out craters with perpendicular margins that are not elevated above the surrounding mucosa (Fig. 23.2). Radiating folds of normal mucosa, particularly in the stomach, help locate the ulcer (Fig. 23.3). The superficial portion of the crater is filled with necrotic debris and fibrin. Beneath this is a zone of inflammatory cell infiltration, predominantly polymorphonuclear leukocytes, surrounded by active granulation tissue (Fig. 23.4). The deepest portion is composed of scar; if the ulcer has penetrated deeply into the wall, the muscle coats may be completely replaced by scar tissue. Arteries and veins may be eroded and give rise to hemorrhage. Some one-third of patients with gastric ulcers will have episodes of massive bleeding. Other complications of chronic ulcers include obstruction and perforation. Gastric outlet obstruction is associated with severe vomiting, dehydration, alkalosis, and hypokalemia. Perforation may result in generalized peritonitis or peritonitis confined to the lesser omental sac. Perforation may be walled off by omental tissue. Posterior wall duodenal ulcers may perforate into the head of the pancreas.

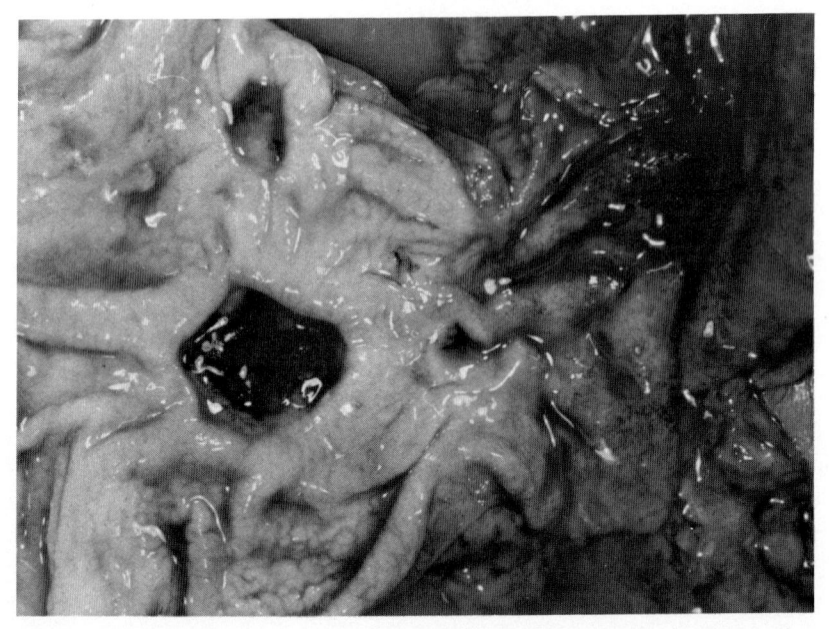

Figure 23.2 Chronic gastric peptic ulcer. This prepyloric ulcer consists of a sharply punched out crater. The base of the ulcer appears hemorrhagic. The margins of the ulcer are not elevated above the surrounding mucosa. A smaller chronic peptic ulcer is noted *above* this lesion.

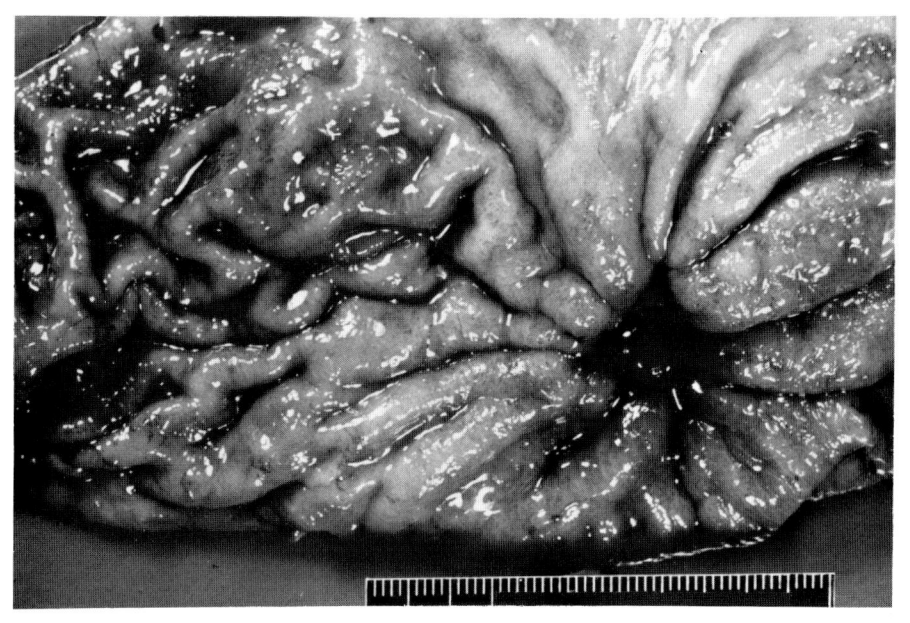

Figure 23.3. Chronic gastric peptic ulcer. Note the radiating folds of gastric mucosa starting at the ulcer margins.

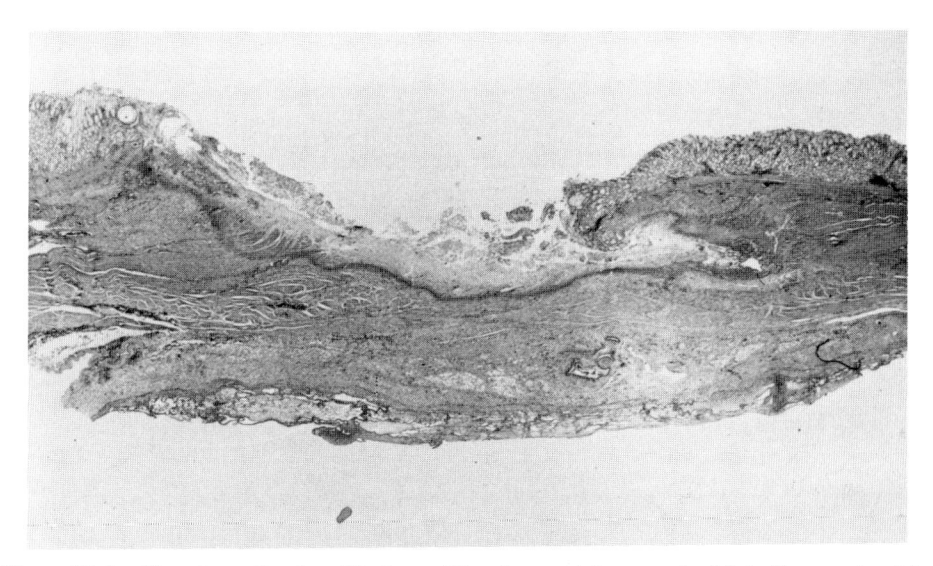

Figure 23.4. Chronic peptic ulcer. The base of the ulcer contains necrotic debris. Surrounding this is a dark staining zone of polymorphonuclear leukocytic infiltration. There is extensive surrounding fibrosis, which has replaced much of the musculature.

Pathogenesis

Peptic ulcers are observed only in digestive tract mucosa that is exposed to acid and pepsin secretions. They are focal lesions, usually solitary. Although the pathogenesis of ulcers is unresolved, most agree that peptic ulceration is related to an imbalance between the action of acid-pepsin secretions and the resistance of mucosa to acid and proteolytic digestion. In *duodenal ulcers*, there is an augmented capacity to secrete acid, often associated with an increased parietal cell mass in the stomach. There is rapid emptying of the stomach and a markedly lowered pH in the duodenum. Ninety per cent of these ulcers are found in the first portion of the duodenum. *Gastric ulcers* appear to result from impaired mucosal resistance to back-diffusion of hydrogen ions. The vast majority occur in the antrum. The secretion of acid and pepsin is frequently diminished, but there is markedly delayed gastric emptying. Gastric stasis distends the antrum and stimulates increased gastrin secretion. Reflux of bile from the duodenum might, at times, play a role. Bile salts and lysolecithin can injure the gastric mucosa, and interfere with its resistance to acid-peptic digestion.

MALABSORPTION

Malabsorption is a group of syndromes, not a disease. There may be impaired absorption of any or all constituents of the normal diet, including fat, protein, carbohydrate, vitamins, minerals, and water. It can relate to deficient digestion or abnormal absorption and transport. It can result from disease of the small bowel, pancreas, biliary system, or stomach, or it can follow surgical procedures or the administration of certain drugs.

The digestive and absorptive capacity of the digestive tract is in excess of normal need, and malabsorption is likely to be apparent only when extensive disease or abnormality is present. The malabsorption can be generalized, involving all dietary constituents, or it can involve impaired absorption of but one or several substances. Thus, loss of integrity of the distal ileum in Crohn's disease can result in malabsorption of vitamin B_{12}, bile salts, and phosphorus.

Manifestations of generalized malabsorption include changed bowel habits, with an increase in bulk or water content. Steatorrhea results from impaired fat absorption and is characterized by greasy, yellow, malodorous, voluminous stools. A high water content is expressed as diarrhea. Other manifestations may include weight loss, often despite a voracious appetite, abdominal cramps and distension, iron deficiency or macrocytic anemia, hypoproteinemia with edema, hypoglycemia, easy bruising due to hypoprothrombinemia, metabolic bone disease due to vitamin D_3 deficiency, kidney stones, and night blindness.

Some of the causes of malabsorption are shown in Table 23.1. The principal

Table 23.1
Some Causes of Malabsorption

Celiac sprue	Whipple's disease
Tropical sprue	Gastric resection
Crohn's disease	Dumping syndrome
Chronic pancreatic disease	Ileal resection or bypass
Pancreatitis	Blind loop syndrome
Cystic fibrosis	Lactase deficiency
Biliary tract disease	Abetalipoproteinemia
Bile duct obstruction	Zollinger-Ellison syndrome

causes in this country are celiac sprue (gluten-sensitive enteropathy), Crohn's disease, chronic pancreatitis, and surgical procedures on the digestive tract.

Water malabsorption can be due to substances that increase the osmotic pressure of the intestinal contents, excessive secretion of water, rapid intestinal transit, decreased intestinal surface area, and failure of active absorption. Causes of carbohydrate malabsorption include pancreatic disease, celiac sprue, lactase deficiency, and the stagnant loop syndrome (see below). Protein malabsorption may occur in pancreatic disease, in celiac sprue, following extensive resection, and in the stagnant loop syndrome. Malabsorption of fat is seen with pancreatic disease, biliary obstruction, and other causes of bile salt deficiency, celiac sprue, abetalipoproteinemia, and following surgical procedures. Bile salts are necessary to fat absorption; deficiency is manifested by failure of micelle formation. Any disorder that interferes with active bile resorption in the terminal ileum can exceed the capacity of the liver to synthesize bile salts and cause fat malabsorption.

Vitamin B_{12} is absorbed only in the terminal ileum. Malabsorption can result from lack of intrinsic factor or from ileal disease. Vitamin D_3 and calcium malabsorption can follow any disturbance of bile salt metabolism.

Steatorrhea may be associated with renal calcium oxalate stones. Oxalate is normally complexed with calcium in the intestine, limiting its absorption. In steatorrhea, calcium is bound to free fatty acid, and excessive oxalate is absorbed and excreted by the kidney. There is an increased incidence of cholesterol gall stones in patients with Crohn's disease or following ileal resection. This appears to be related to increased concentration of cholesterol in bile secondary to loss of bile salts.

Celiac Sprue

Celiac sprue, or gluten-sensitive enteropathy, is characterized by extensive loss of mucosal villi and microvilli of the entire small intestine, most marked in the proximal segments (Figs. 23.5 and 23.6). Its incidence is between 10 and 30 per 100,000 in this country. There is a familial incidence, although the genetic transmission is unclear. There is an increased incidence of HLA B8 in patients with celiac sprue.

The malabsorption syndrome of celiac sprue is a generalized malabsorption, usually becoming manifest in early childhood. The gluten-gliadin protein complex present in various grains binds to receptor sites of small intestine mucosa, stimulates the formation of antigluten antibodies and, perhaps, cell-mediated immunity which causes the injury to the mucosal cells. The disorder responds dramatically to withdrawal of gluten-containing foods from the diet, sometimes with complete return to normal of the intestine.

Whipple's Disease

Whipple's disease is a rare disorder manifested by generalized malabsorption, found most often in middle-aged patients and many times associated with arthritis and fever. There is distension of the intestinal villi by macrophages containing membrane-bound fragments of microorganisms believed to be the etiologic agent

292   *Pathology: Understanding Human Disease*

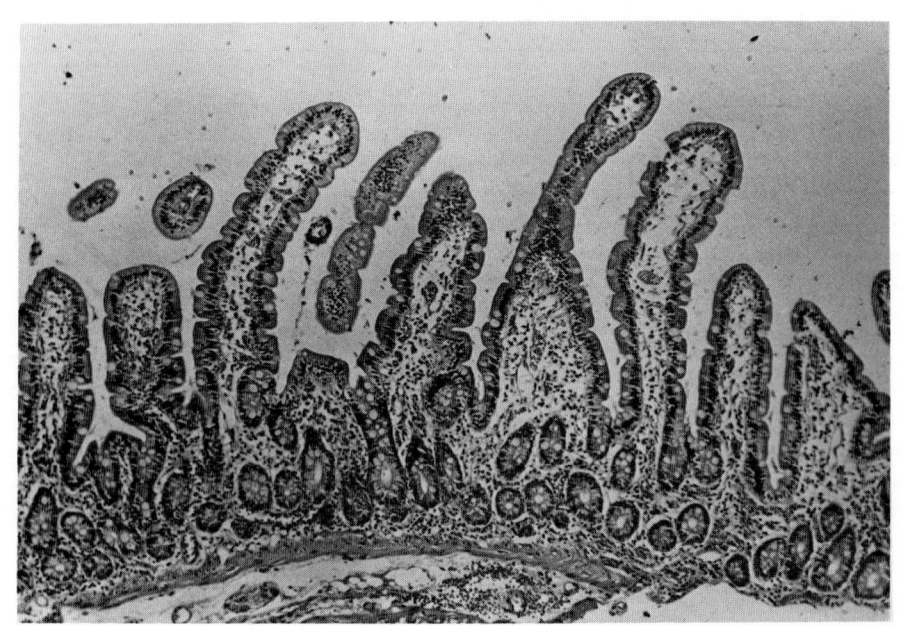

Figure 23.5. Normal small intestine mucosa.

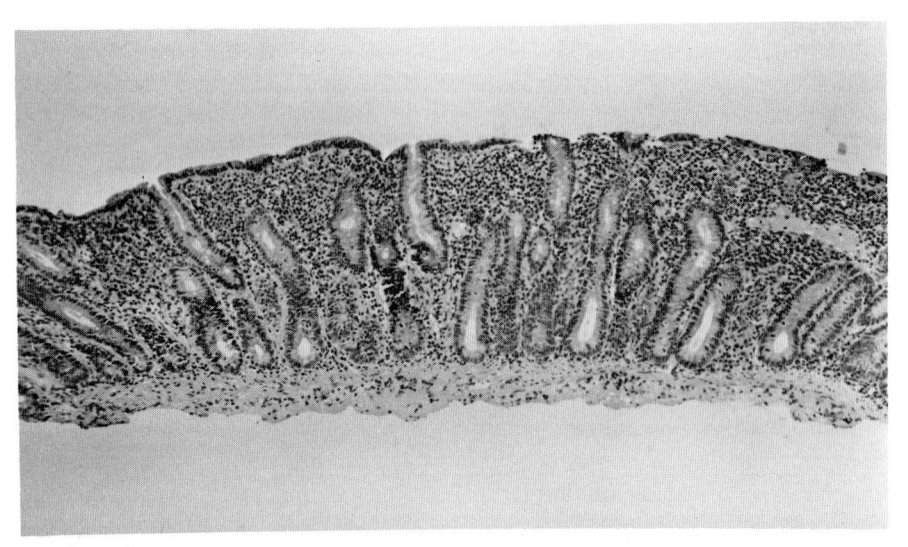

Figure 23.6. Celiac sprue. Compare with Figure 23.5. The mucosa is flat and atrophic. The normal villous structure of the mucosa is completely gone.

(Fig. 23.7). Although the organisms have not been cultured, the disease responds well to antibiotic therapy.

Postsurgical Syndromes

The *dumping syndrome* may be a sequel of gastrectomy or vagotomy performed for peptic ulcer disease. Food is not retained in the remaining stomach, and the

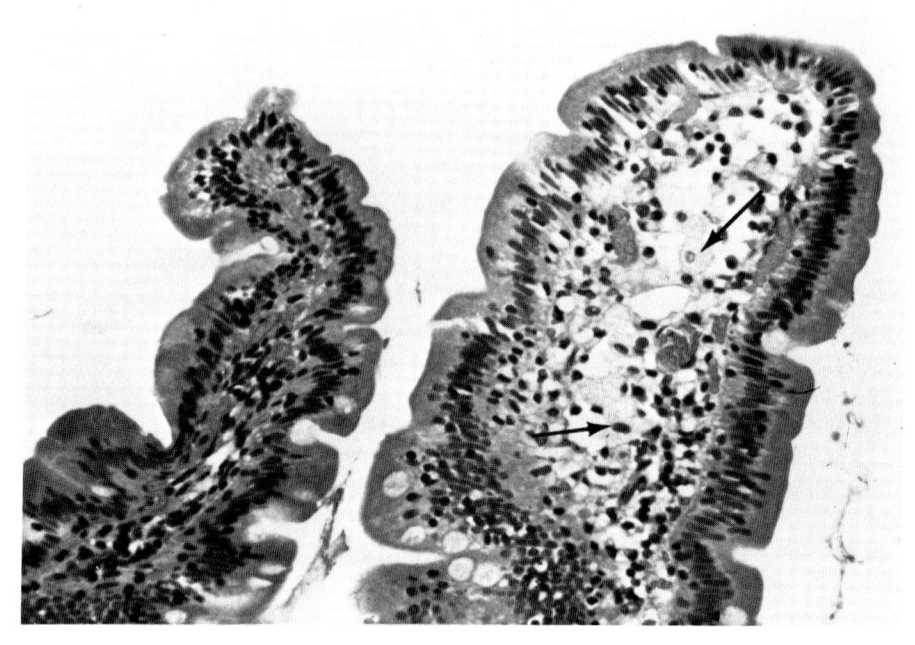

Figure 23.7. Whipple's disease. The intestinal villus to the *right* is distended by macrophages (*arrows*). The macrophages contain fragments of microorganisms.

small intestine is flooded with hyperosmolar chyme. Fluid is rapidly drawn into the gut, and the patient experiences postprandial fullness, weakness, and hypotension, and, since there is decreased secretion of bile and pancreatic enzymes, very partial digestion results in diarrhea. This syndrome is most severe following a high carbohydrate intake.

The *blind loop syndrome* can complicate gastroenterostomy, which leaves a blind proximal duodenal loop. Bile and food may reflux into this loop and become stagnant. There is mucosal injury and bacterial overgrowth, which, together with abnormal products of digestion, can evoke a severe diarrhea and malabsorption.

Severe generalized malabsorption can follow major small intestine resection, or jejunoileal bypass performed as treatment of morbid obesity. Colon resection has no important effects on absorption.

CROHN'S DISEASE

Crohn's disease is a disease of Western civilization. It occurs in all ethnic groups, but has a higher incidence among Jews and a lower incidence among blacks and Hispanics.

The clinical manifestations may include diarrhea, abdominal pain, fever, weight loss, iron loss or macrocytic anemia, peritoneal abscesses, fistulae, and perianal disease. Arthritis and uveal tract inflammation may also be seen. The disease characteristically occurs in recurring episodes, often with prolonged periods of remission.

Any part of the intestinal tract may be involved, most frequently the ileum.

294   *Pathology: Understanding Human Disease*

The lesions are characterized by transmural inflammation, often with "skip areas" of normal intestine. Early lesions are likely to show ulceration and acute inflammation, but the characteristic late changes consist of extensive ulceration, chronic inflammatory cell infiltration of the entire wall, with some 60% of patients showing noncaseating granulomas in the submucosa, muscularis, or serosa. The wall is greatly thickened and fibrotic, often with marked narrowing and partial obstruction of the lumen. Fissures extend into the wall, or to and through the serosa, accounting for fistulae and peritoneal abscesses (Fig. 23.8). Lymphatic dilatation is often a prominent feature. Perianal lesions are common in Crohn's disease and include anorectal fistulae, ischiorectal abscesses, and rectovaginal fistulae. These lesions are more likely to occur when the colon is involved.

Crohn's disease of the colon, often called granulomatous colitis, is a frequent involvement (Fig. 23.9). One-third of patients with Crohn's disease have involvement of ileum and colon, and 10 to 15% have disease limited to the colon. Table 23.2 differentiates between colonic Crohn's disease and ulcerative colitis.

The etiology of Crohn's disease is unknown; there has not been convincing evidence of the role of infections, immunologic disturbances, or emotional disorders. Genetic factors may play a role, but the disease is undoubtedly multifactorial in origin.

ULCERATIVE COLITIS

Ulcerative colitis is an inflammatory disease of the large intestine, manifested by bloody diarrhea. Its incidence in the United States is over 80 per 100,000

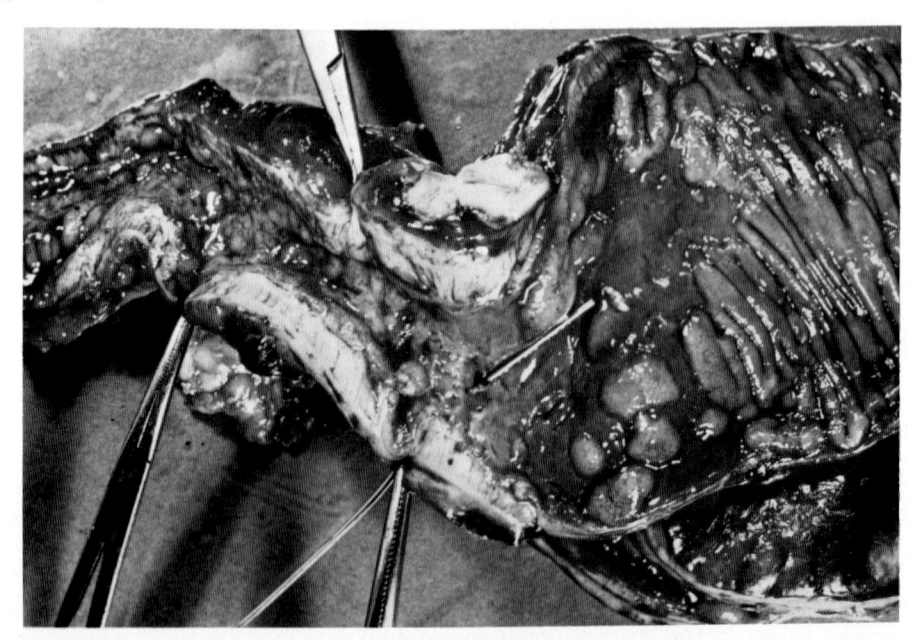

Figure 23.8. Crohn's disease. The segment of small intestine to the *left* shows marked constriction of its lumen, extensive scarring and thickening of its wall, and ulceration of the mucosa. A probe has been passed through a fistula at the *center*. To the *right of center*, there is extensive irregular ulceration of the intestinal mucosa.

The Digestive Tract 295

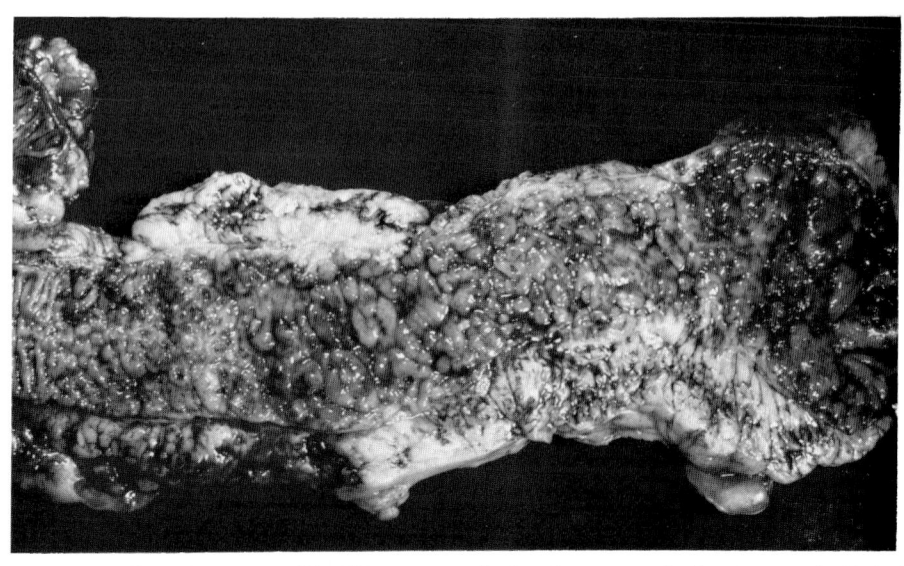

Figure 23.9. Granulomatous colitis. This segment of colon shows extensive involvement by Crohn's disease. The mucosa is irregular, showing many areas of ulceration and some hyperplasia. The marked thickening of the wall can be noted along the lower margin of the specimen.

Table 23.2
Differences between Crohn's Disease and Ulcerative Colitis

	Crohn's Disease	Ulcerative Colitis
Involvement		
Ileum	Usual	Never
Colon	50%	Always
Rectum	10–20%	Always
Anal and perianal	75%	25%
Pseudopolyposis	Slight	Marked
Depth of involvement	Transmural	Mucosa
Crypt abscesses	Occasional	Common
Loss of goblet cells	Occasional	Common
Granulomas	60%	Absent
Continuity of involvement	Frequent "skip areas"	Continuous
Fistula formation	10%	Rare
Carcinoma of colon	Uncommon	10-fold increase

population. Like Crohn's disease, it is more prevalent among Jews and less common in nonwhites. There is a slight female predominance. Ulcerative colitis can start at any age, although it is uncommon in infancy and childhood.

The lesions of uncomplicated ulcerative colitis are restricted to the mucosa or submucosa, and do not extend to the muscularis. The early changes include mucosal congestion and edema, infiltration of polymorphonuclear leukocytes, and the formation of abscesses at the base of mucosal crypts. This is followed by mucosal ulceration (Fig. 23.10). Repeated ulceration results in replacement of the mucosa by granulation tissue and superficial scarring. Pseudopolyps are frequent

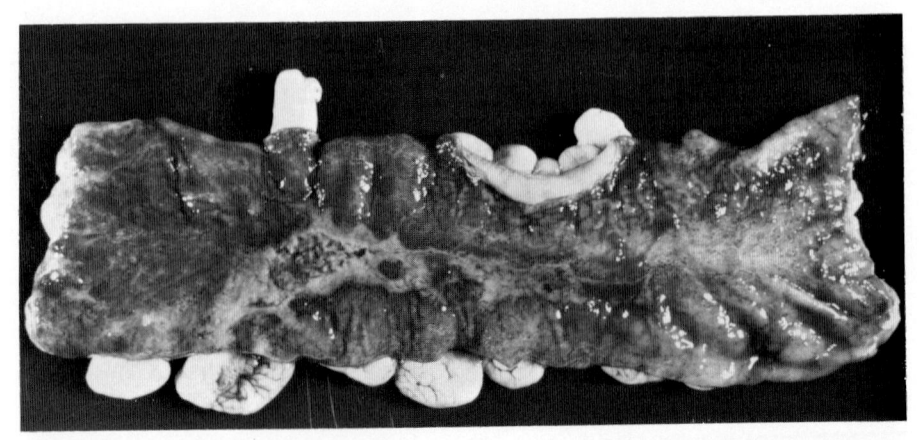

Figure 23.10. Acute colitis. The mucosa is deeply congested, and there is an irregular area of superficial ulceration to the *left of center*.

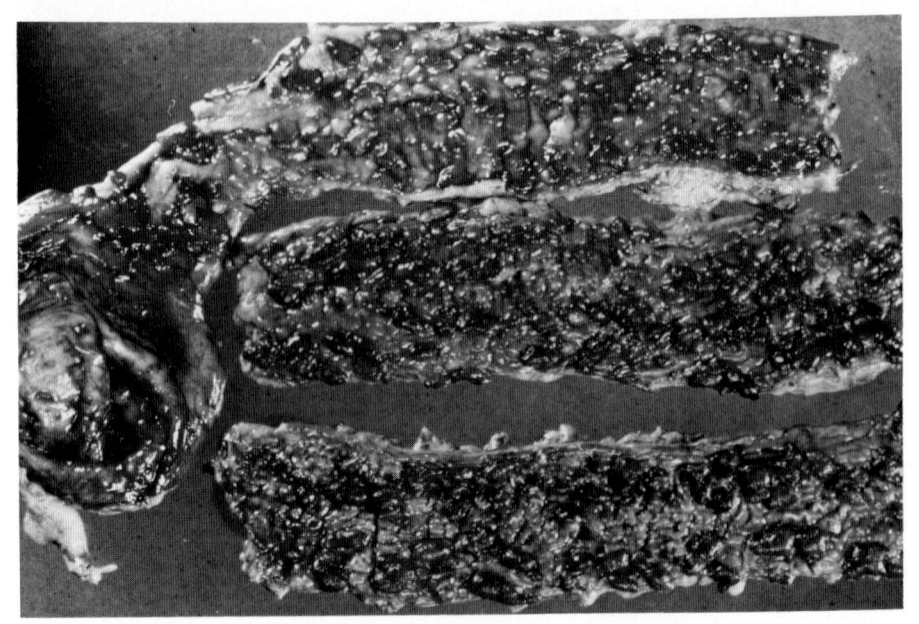

Figure 23.11. Chronic ulcerative colitis. There has been extensive ulceration of the mucosa and replacement by granulation tissue and superficial scarring. Many small polypoid areas of mucosal hyperplasia are noted.

and are composed of islands of hyperplastic epithelium surrounded by areas of ulceration (Figs. 23.11 and 23.12).

The etiology of ulcerative colitis remains unknown, although current thought favors a cell-mediated immunologic mechanism of injury.

Bloody diarrhea is the principal manifestation of disease. The total daily volume of stool may be normal or only slightly increased, and it may consist of no

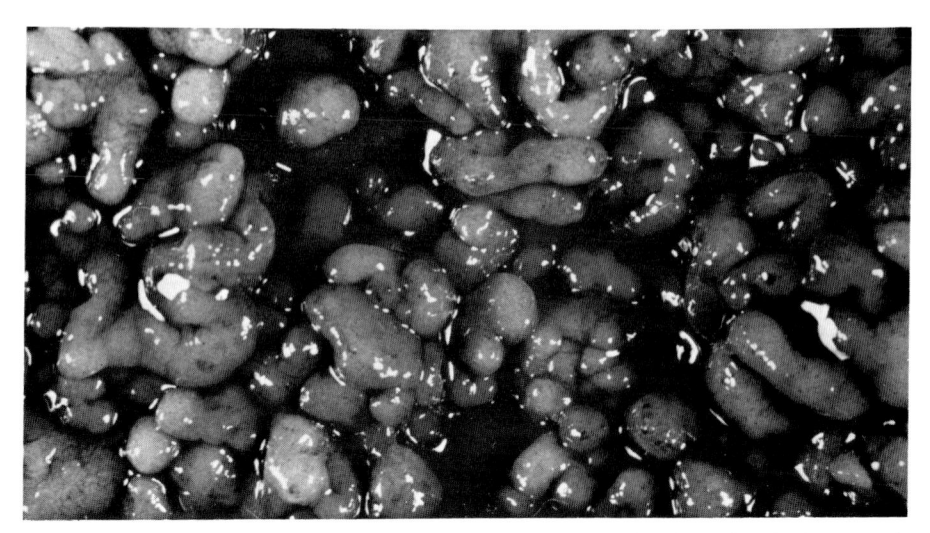

Figure 23.12. Chronic ulcerative colitis. Close-up view of mucosal surface, showing large numbers of pseudopolyps.

more than mixed blood and mucus. Other symptoms include tenesmus and the sensation of almost constant need to evacuate. This latter results from frequent propulsion of fecal material into the rectum.

There are three forms of ulcerative colitis. In *ulcerative proctitis*, disease is restricted to the rectum, and there are few systemic manifestations or complications. *Ordinary ulcerative colitis* begins in the rectum and extends in continuity to upper levels of the sigmoid and colon. This is usually a recurrent disease, but it may be continuous. Remissions may last for prolonged periods. The severity is determined by the extent of colon involved. *Acute fulminant ulcerative colitis* is a severe acute colitis involving the entire colonic wall, with constant diarrhea, and frequently complicated by peritonitis or by a dilated *toxic megacolon*. There are systemic manifestations of severe illness, and the mortality rate is high unless emergency surgery is performed.

Death can be caused by diffuse peritonitis or peritoneal abscesses, pylephlebitis, bacteremia, and disseminated intravascular coagulation.

The many complications of ulcerative colitis include perforation, hemorrhage, strictures, fissure *in ano*, and pararectal abscess. Carcinoma of the colon has a 10-fold higher incidence in patients with ulcerative colitis, and may occur in as many as 40% when the disease started in childhood and has continuously involved the entire colon. Carcinoma may be multicentric in origin.

Systemic complications or associations include fatty liver, macronodular or biliary cirrhosis, chronic active hepatitis, bile duct disorders, arthritis, clubbing of toes and fingers, and erythema nodosum (p. 455). *Pyoderma gangrenosum* is a purulent necrotizing and ulcerating lesion of the legs that occurs only in patients with ulcerative colitis or Crohn's disease.

Some of the differences between ulcerative colitis and Crohn's disease are summarized in Table 23.2.

DISORDERS CAUSED BY MICROORGANISMS

Comments on this subject are restricted to a few general principles.

Diarrhea can result entirely from the effects of toxins. The severe, often fatal, diarrhea of *cholera* is attributable to the ability of the toxin of the cholera vibrio to react with receptor sites of the intestinal mucosa and to activate adenylate cyclase. The mucosa is uninjured, but it pours out copious amounts of normal intestinal fluid, leading to severe dehydration and electrolyte depletion. The watery diarrhea associated with some strains of *Escherichia coli* has the same pathogenesis.

Staphylococcal food poisoning is caused by an endotoxin that produces superficial necrosis of the gastric and intestinal mucosa. The disorder evolves explosively and heals completely within 24 hr.

Some diarrhea-producing organisms invade the mucosa. These include the Shigella organisms that cause *bacillary dysentery*. The colon is edematous, heavily infiltrated by polymorphonuclear leukocytes, with focal hemorrhages and superficial ulceration. The small intestine is less involved.

Some Salmonella organisms, particularly *Salmonella typhosa*, invade the wall of the small intestine and its Peyer's patches, but become systemic infections, with extensive involvement of the reticuloendothelial system.

PSEUDOMEMBRANOUS ENTEROCOLITIS

Pseudomembranous enterocolitis can be a severe disorder, manifested by diarrhea, abdominal pain and distension, fever, hypovolemia, and shock. There is

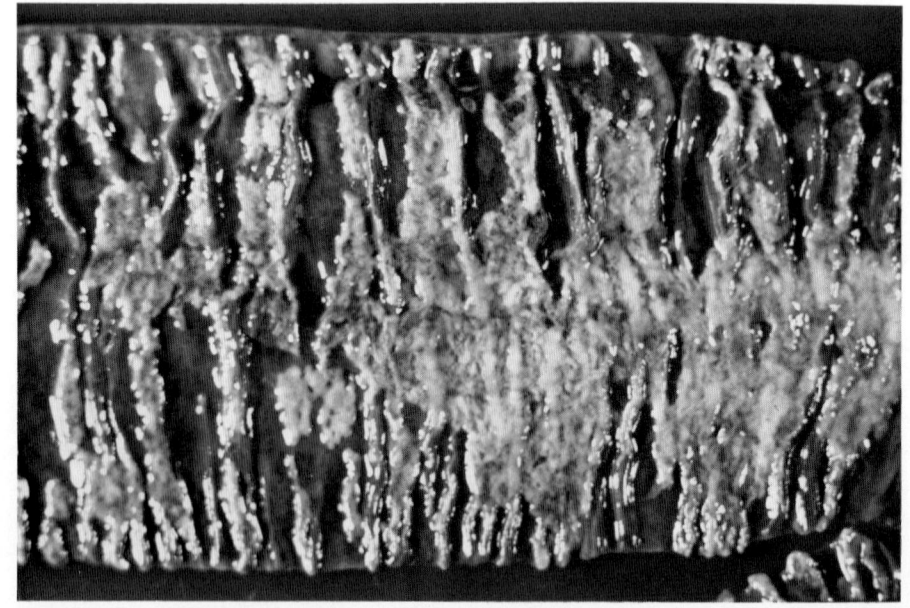

Figure 23.13. Pseudomembranous enterocolitis. This segment of ileum shows a shaggy pseudomembrane overlying areas of superficial necrosis.

extensive superficial necrosis of the mucosa of the colon and, occasionally, the small intestine, with formation of a shaggy yellowish or greenish pseudomembrane composed of necrotic debris, polymorphonuclear leukocytes, and fibrin (Fig. 23.13).

This disorder is now known to be caused by an exotoxin of *Clostridium difficile*. It can be a complication of major surgical procedures, debilitating disease, and broad spectrum antibiotic therapy. Pseudomembranous enterocolitis responds well to vancomycin therapy, but can relapse after therapy is stopped.

ACUTE APPENDICITIS

Acute appendicitis occurs most often between the ages of 10 and 30. It is heralded by nausea, vomiting, diarrhea, and periumbilical pain, later shifting to the right lower quadrant and becoming severe.

Appendicitis starts as an ulceration of the appendiceal mucosa, probably the result of ischemia following obstruction by spasm of the proximal musculature, fecaliths, or foreign bodies. Bacterial infection follows ulceration, and the process extends rapidly through the entire wall of the appendix. mesoappendix, and peritoneum (Fig. 23.14).

The complications of acute appendicitis include rupture of a gangrenous appendix, generalized peritonitis, or localized periappendiceal abscesses. Septic thrombophlebitis of the portal system (*pylephlebitis*) can spread infection to the liver.

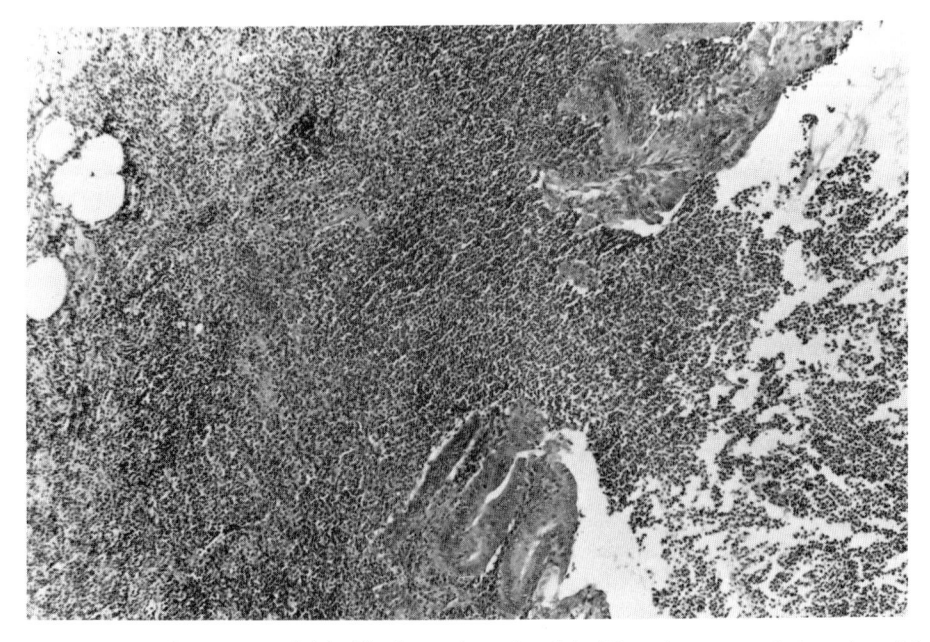

Figure 23.14. Acute appendicitis. The lumen is to the *right*. There is an area of ulceration of the mucosa, and massive polymorphonuclear leukocytic infiltration extends from this point throughout the wall of the appendix.

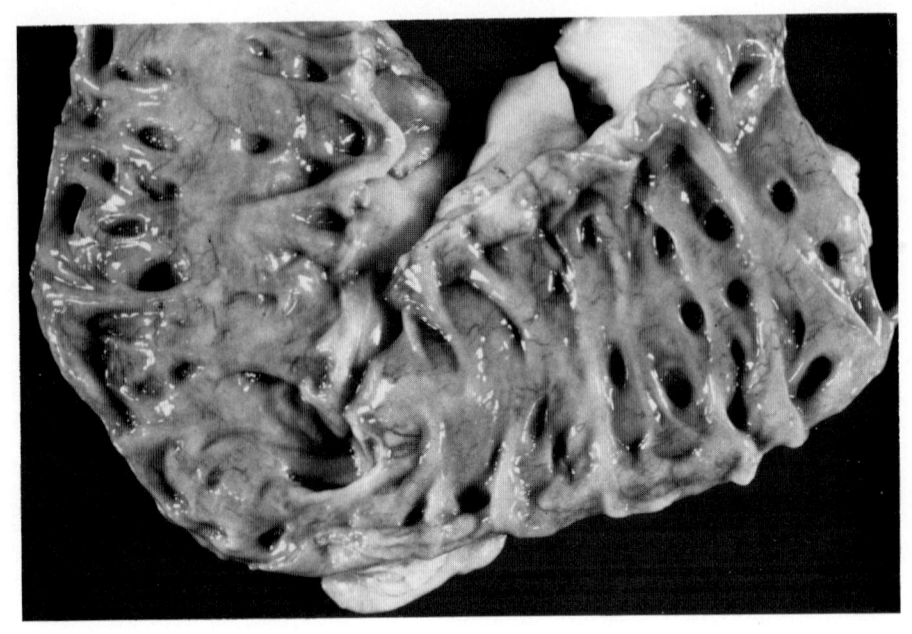

Figure 23.15. Diverticulosis of colon. Many diverticula are noted, arranged in rows at points corresponding to the teniae coli. These diverticula characteristically have small ostia, and obstruction of these openings frequently results in diverticulitis.

COLONIC DIVERTICULOSIS

Colonic diverticulosis is a common disorder affecting 50% of people over age 75. The diverticula are multiple, often arranged in rows beneath the teniae coli, at points of weakness where vessels penetrate the muscle coats (Fig. 23.15). The sigmoid is the area most involved, but diverticula can involve the entire colon.

Diverticulosis is common in the western world, rare in Africa, India, and the Orient. It is thought to result from lack of dietary fiber, causing prolonged intestinal transit time, and colonic segmental contractions that isolate small segments of bowel and subject them to very high intraluminal pressures.

Diverticula may become partially or totally obstructed, followed by ulceration and bacterial infection. Repeated episodes of diverticulitis can lead to extensive and encircling fibrosis and obstruction of the colon. The fibrotic mass may be confused with an infiltrating carcinoma of the colon.

TUMORS OF THE DIGESTIVE TRACT

Malignant tumors of the digestive tract are responsible for one-third of all cancer deaths in this country. There has been a gradual increase in the incidence of carcinoma of the colon, but a dramatic drop in gastric carcinoma.

Carcinoma of the Esophagus

Carcinoma of the esophagus is a disease of the elderly, and there is a 2:1 male predominance. The vast majority are squamous cell carcinomas, and they are

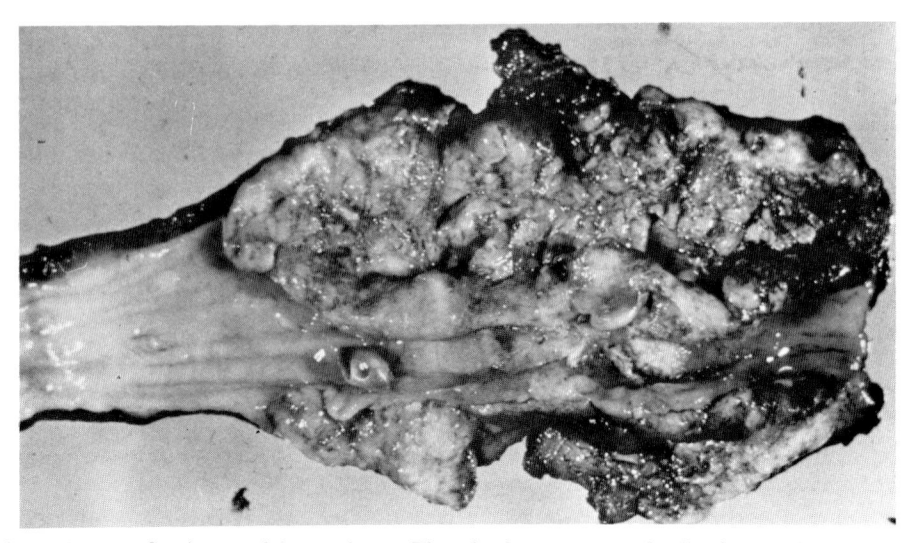

Figure 23.16. Carcinoma of the esophagus. There is a large tumor at the distal end of the esophagus showing a fungating growth into the lumen, but also extension through the wall to involve the surrounding tissues.

found in the middle and lower thirds of the organ. Although they may form fungating intraluminal masses, they are more likely to infiltrate the wall of the esophagus and show surface ulceration (Fig. 23.16). Dysphagia is the principal manifestation. Carcinomas of the esophagus tend to progress rapidly, and there may be early extension to the trachea, mediastinum, or pleura.

Adenocarcinoma of the Stomach

The incidence of gastric carcinoma in this country has dropped to one-third of the 1920 rate. In Japan, on the other hand, the incidence is 5 times that in this country; indeed, gastric carcinoma is the most common carcinoma. The incidence in Iceland and Finland is also unusually high.

Gastric carcinoma is an adenocarcinoma. It is most often located in the distal third of the stomach, in the antrum or pylorus, often along the greater curvature. The tumors may be cauliflower-like masses that protrude into the lumen, or they may diffusely infiltrate the stomach wall (*linitis plastica*) (Fig. 23.17). Infiltrating tumors often ulcerate and may be difficult to distinguish from chronic peptic ulcers (Fig. 23.18). Histologically, the adenocarcinomas may be well differentiated, forming glandular structures (Fig. 23.19), or anaplastic, composed of individually infiltrating mucus secreting cells, often having a signet ring appearance. Diffuse lymphocyte infiltration of the stroma is occasionally noted, and signals a somewhat better prognosis.

There is a distinct relationship between atrophic gastritis, particularly that associated with pernicious anemia, and the development of gastric carcinoma; indeed, half of patients with gastric carcinoma have achlorhydria. The intestinal metaplasia frequently observed in the gastric mucosa in atrophic gastritis is considered by some to be a premalignant change, containing the cells that

302   *Pathology: Understanding Human Disease*

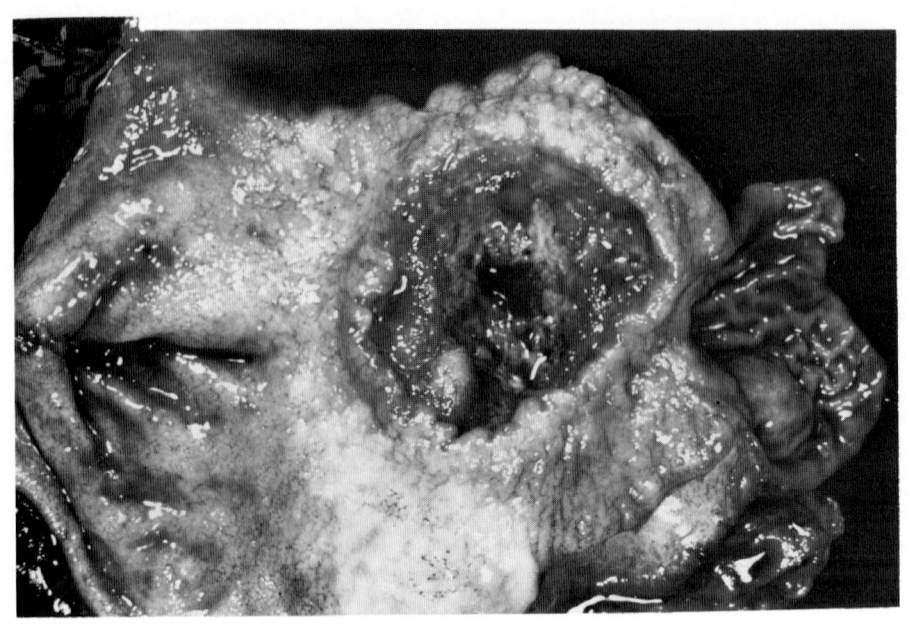

Figure 23.17. Gastric carcinoma. There is a large area of thickening of the mucosa and extensive central ulceration. The edges of the ulceration are markedly elevated.

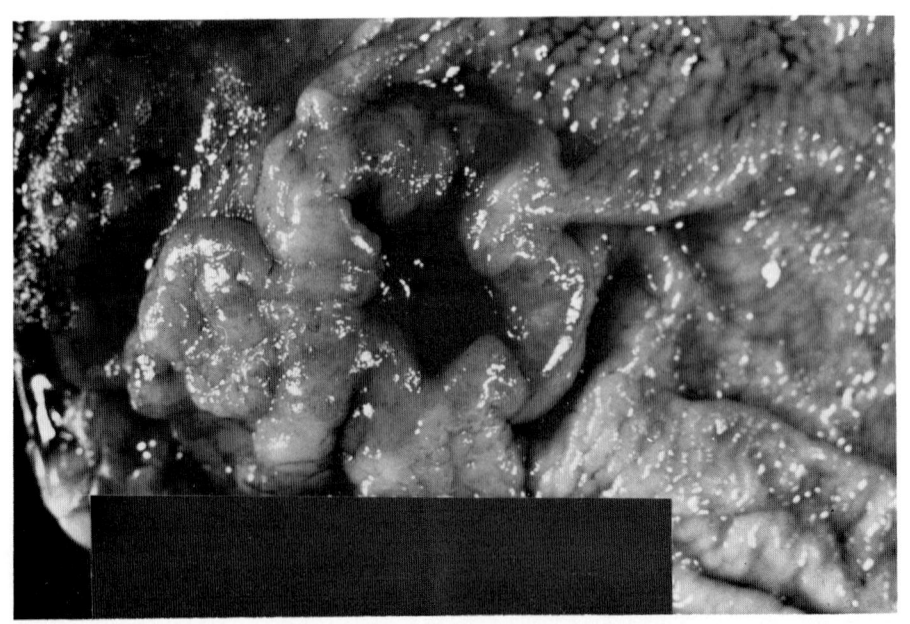

Figure 23.18. Gastric carcinoma. The central ulcerated area is surrounded by markedly elevated mucosal folds, diffusely infiltrated by tumor. Compare with Figure 23.2.

undergo malignant transformation. Adenomatous polyps of the mucosa may rarely become malignant, and perhaps 1 in 1000 gastric peptic ulcers undergoes malignant change. Individuals of Blood Group A are at slightly increased risk for gastric carcinoma.

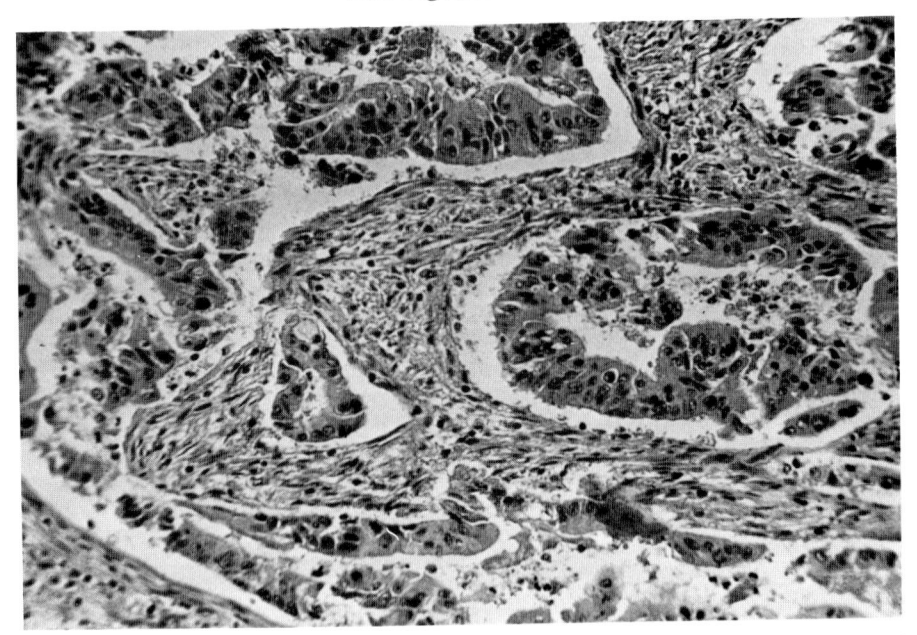

Figure 23.19. Gastric carcinoma. This is a well differentiated adenocarcinoma with an active fibrous stroma.

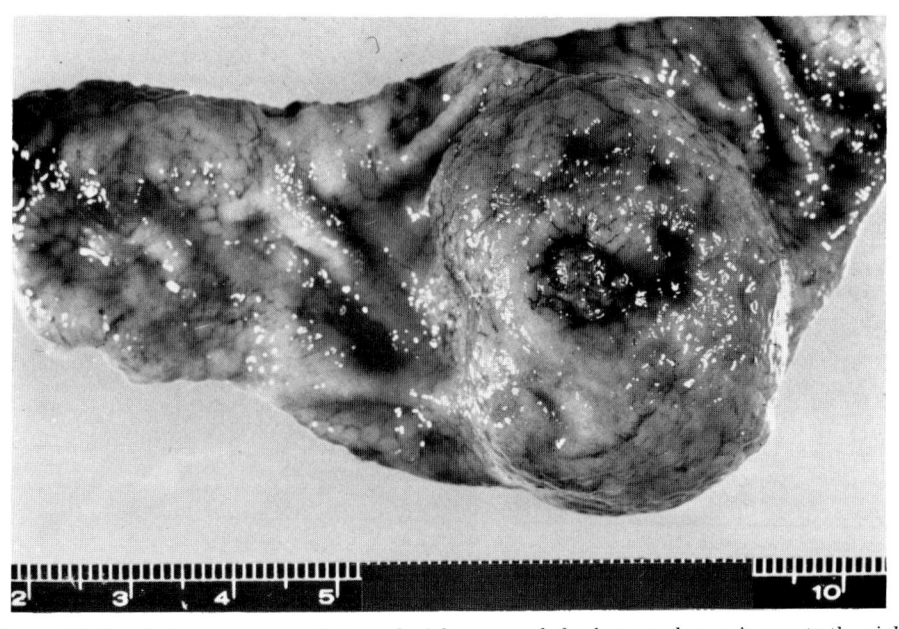

Figure 23.20. Leiomyosarcoma of stomach. A large rounded submucosal mass is seen to the *right*. This malignant smooth muscle tumor often arises in the muscularis mucosae and causes ulceration with bleeding of the overlying gastric mucosa.

The outlook for patients with gastric carcinoma is poor, with no better than a 20% 5-year survival after surgical excision. Metastasis to the left gastric lymph nodes or liver is often present at the time of diagnosis. An extensive screening program in Japan, using modern fiberoptic technique, has permitted the recognition of early lesions. Early diagnosis and surgical treatment have resulted in a 90% 5-year survival rate.

Tumors of the Small Bowel

Adenocarcinomas of the duodenum, jejunum, and ileum are uncommon, although their incidence is higher in patients with Crohn's disease. Carcinoid tumors (p. 351) are often observed, as are benign and malignant connective tissue tumors. Lymphomas may involve the small intestine, and appear to have a higher incidence in patients with celiac sprue.

Carcinoma of the Colon

Adenocarcinoma of the colon is the second most common form of cancer in the United States, involving some 75,000 persons each year. The incidence in this country is some 10 times greater than in Africa, India, or the Orient. In contrast to esophageal and gastric carcinomas, colon cancer shows a female predominance.

Half of colon carcinomas are located in the sigmoid or rectum, visible by sigmoidoscopy. In these locations, they are likely to infiltrate the wall, involving the entire circumference, forming a napkin ring-like constriction of the lumen (Fig. 23.21). Ulceration is usual. The manifestations are those of obstruction, bleeding, and sense of incomplete evacuation. Carcinomas of the cecum tend to be fungating masses that do not obstruct this larger caliber segment. Bleeding may be occult, and the presenting symptomatology may relate only to a progressive anemia.

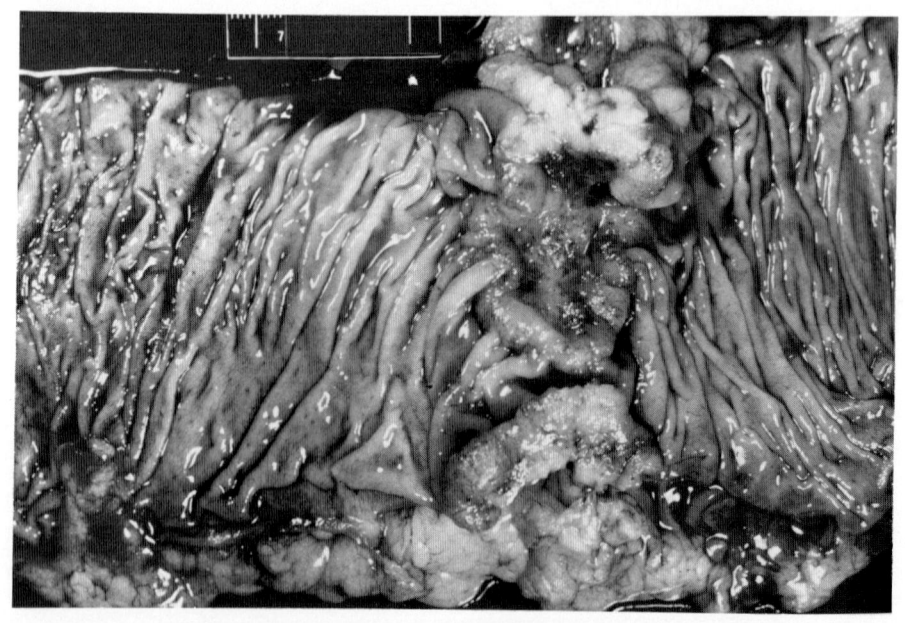

Figure 23.21. Carcinoma of colon. This tumor has infiltrated the wall of the colon and involved the entire circumference. This has resulted in a napkin ring-like obstruction of the lumen.

Prognosis

The prognosis of colon carcinoma correlates best with the depth of penetration through the intestinal wall. If the involvement extends to the muscle coats, but not to the serosa (Duke's Classification A), the outlook following surgery is excellent. If the serosa is involved, but lymph nodes are not (Class B), it is good. Lymph node metastasis (Class C) carries a more guarded prognosis. The overall 5-year survival rate approaches 60%.

Pathogenesis

The geographic incidence of adenocarcinoma of the colon parallels that of diverticulosis. Both are common in the United States and Western Europe, uncommon in Africa, India and the Orient. These observations have suggested that the high incidence of both lesions is related to low dietary fiber and retarded transit time in the digestive tract.

The evolution of carcinoma of the colon may also relate to intestinal polyps. *Adenomatous polyps* are frequent, often multiple lesions (Fig. 23.22). They have thin pedicles and are composed of irregularly arranged glandular structures in a delicate stroma (Fig. 23.23). Epithelial atypia is frequently marked, but these polyps are considered benign, unless their stalks are invaded (Fig. 23.24). Adenomatous polyps are frequently encountered near surgically removed colon carcinomas. How often these polyps become carcinoma and how many carcinomas started as adenomatous polyps cannot be answered at present. *Villous adenomas* are solitary lesions of the sigmoid and rectum. They have a broad base, and a

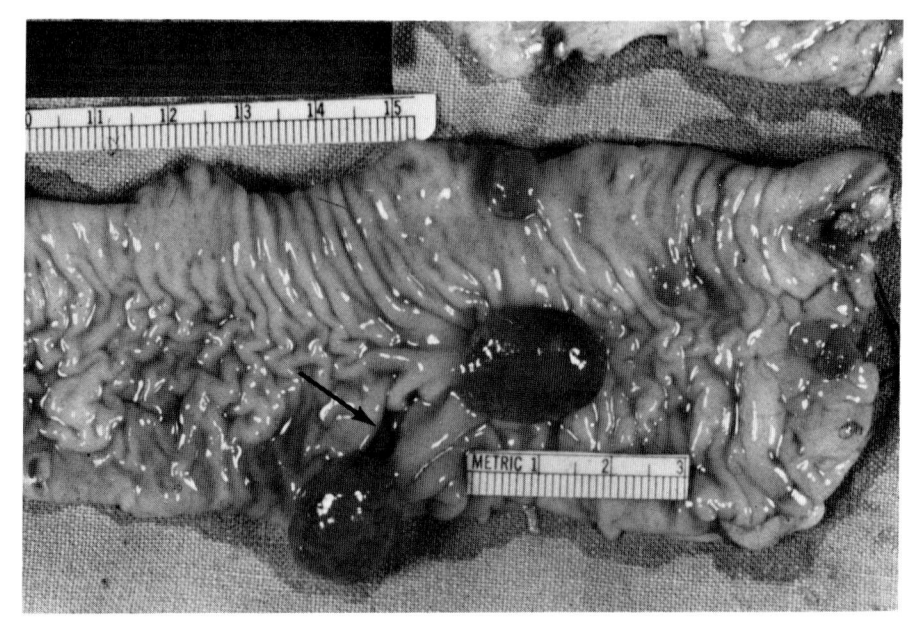

Figure 23.22. Multiple adenomatous polyps of colon. The thin pedicle of the lowermost polyp is visible (*arrow*). Although two of these lesions are quite large, they showed no evidence of malignancy.

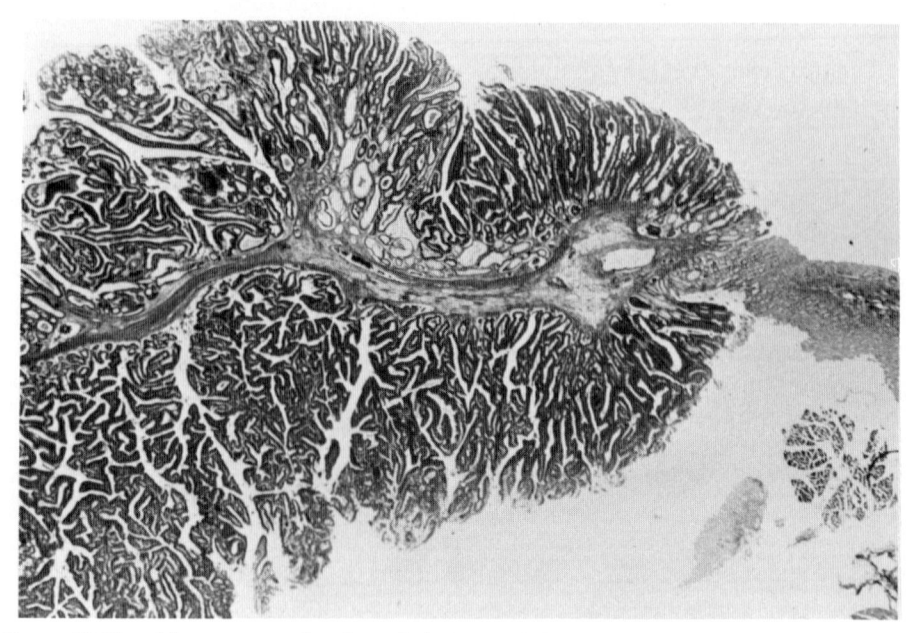

Figure 23.23. Adenomatous polyp. Irregularly arranged glands are attached to a delicate connective tissue framework. The pedicle of normal mucosa is seen to the *right*, and there is no evidence of invasion.

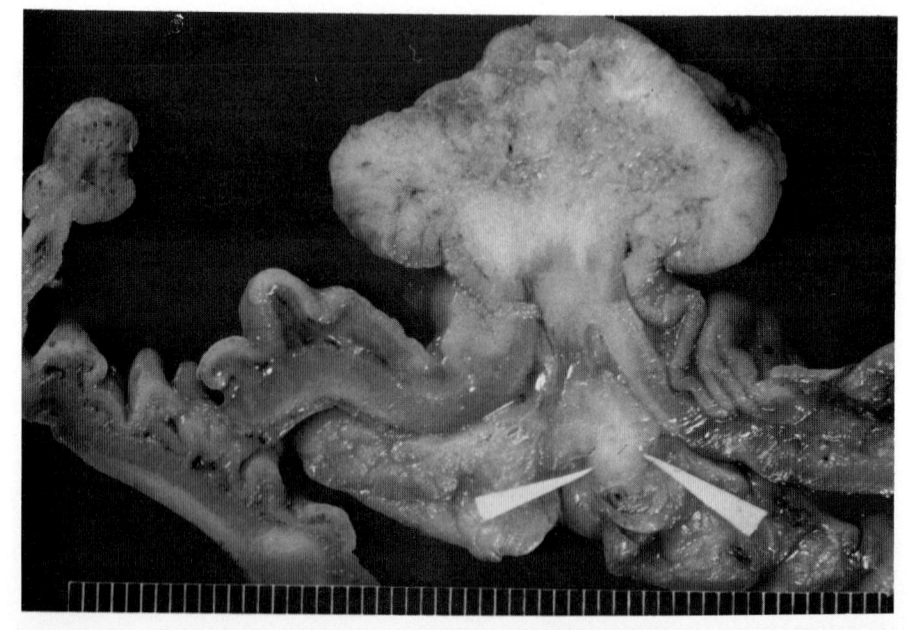

Figure 23.24. Polypoid carcinoma of colon. This cut section shows a polypoid lesion with a moderately broad base. This is a malignant lesion, and extension of tumor through the wall of the intestine is noted (*arrows*). A benign adenomatous polyp is seen at the *left-hand margin* of the photograph.

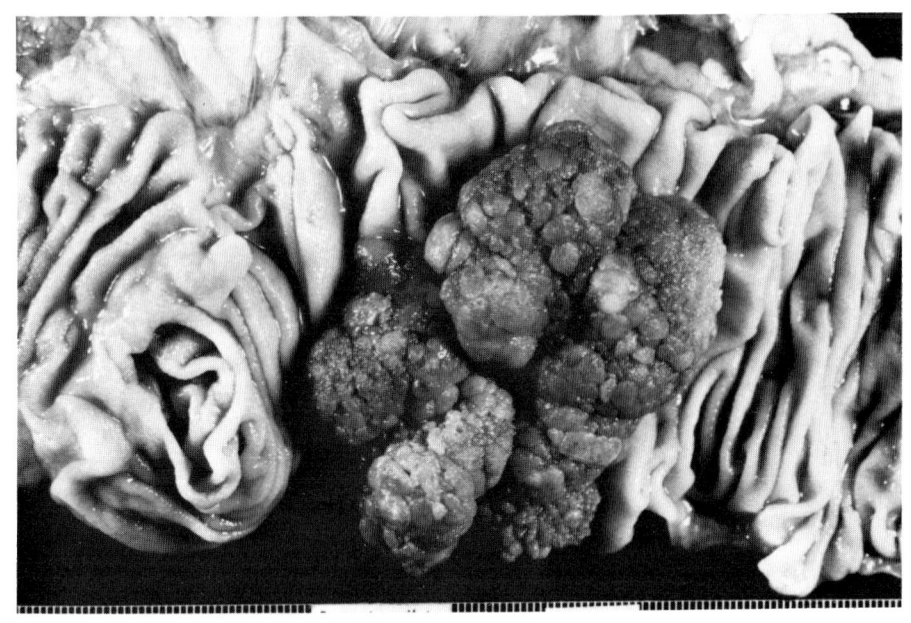

Figure 23.25. Villous adenoma. This polypoid lesion has a very broad base and a striking papillary structure that gives it a very large surface area.

striking frond-like papillary structure covered by a hyperplastic epithelium (Fig. 23.25). These lesions grow along the gut surface, and at least 25% become frank carcinomas. They are also noteworthy in secreting mucoid, watery fluid, rich in potassium, and can cause severe diarrhea and hypokalemia.

Familial polyposis is inherited as an autosomal dominant trait, in which hundreds or thousands of polyps cover the entire colonic mucosa. Carcinoma develops in virtually all with this disorder, often as early in life as the 10th to 15th year, and tends to follow an aggressive course

Carcinoembryonic Antigen

Carcinoembryonic antigen is a glycoprotein found in the glycocalyx of embryonal colonic tissue. It is normally almost absent in the adult, but is produced by colonic carcinomas, as well as carcinomas of the lung and pancreas. It is also detectable in patients with ulcerative colitis and with micronodular cirrhosis. If the circulating level of carcinoembryonic antigen is 7 to 10 times normal, invasive or metastatic carcinoma of the colon is the likely source.

Suggested Reading

Almy TP, Howell DA. Diverticular disease of the colon. N. Engl. J. Med. *302:* 324, 1980.
Buckwalter JA, Kent TH. Prognosis and surgical pathology of carcinoma of the colon. Surg. Gynecol. Obstet. *136:* 465, 1973.
Grossman MI. A new look at peptic ulcer. Ann. Intern. Med. *84:* 57, 1976.
Hill RB Jr, Kern FB. The gastrointestinal tract. Baltimore, Williams & Wilkins, 1977.
Price AB, Morson BC. Inflammatory bowel disease: the surgical pathology of Crohn's disease and ulcerative colitis. Human Pathol. *6:* 7, 1975.

Chapter 24

The Lymphoreticular and Hematopoietic Organs

The major emphasis of this chapter is on the lymphomas and leukemias. Other white blood cell disorders included are multiple myeloma and Waldenström's macroglobulinemia. A discussion of amyloidosis is inserted here, because of its frequent association with myeloma and other dyscrasias of immunoglobulin synthesis. Brief consideration is given to the myeloproliferative disorders, pernicious anemia, and the hemolytic anemias. Disturbances of coagulation have been discussed in earlier chapters.

LYMPHOMAS AND LEUKEMIAS

The principal disorders of white blood cell growth and function are the leukemias and the lymphomas, including Hodgkin's disease. These malignant tumors account for 10% of all cancer deaths in this country, and nearly half of cancer deaths before the age of 15.

Although the etiology and pathogenesis of any of the lymphomas or leukemias have not been proven, it is clear that multiple factors are involved, including genetic predisposition, deficiencies of the immune system, and such environmental influences as viral infections, cytotoxic drugs and other toxins, and ionizing radiation.

Hodgkin's disease occasionally has a familial pattern of incidence, and association with B18, B5, and A1 haplotypes. Genetically determined immunodeficiency states, such as ataxia telangiectasia and the Wiscott-Aldrich syndrome (p. 40), are accompanied by a markedly increased incidence of lymphoma and leukemia. There is a high incidence of myelogenous leukemia in patients with Down's syndrome, and evidence of chromosomal damage may be observed in several leukemias and in Burkitt's lymphoma. Immunosuppressed recipients of renal transplants have a 35 times greater chance of developing lymphoma or leukemia, while having only twice the normal incidence of other neoplasms. For unknown reasons, they are particularly likely to develop lymphoma involving the central nervous system.

There is strong evidence that viral infections play an important role in etiology. The Epstein-Barr virus, known to cause infectious mononucleosis, is close to being established as a cause of Burkitt's lymphoma. Many patients with Hodgkin's disease have high titers of antibodies to this virus, and the incidence of

Hodgkin's disease is 4 times higher than normal in individuals who have had mononucleosis. Reverse transcriptase, a marker of RNA viruses, has been identified in the tumor cells of many lymphoma and leukemia patients. A recent epidemiologic study has established that Hodgkin's disease is most likely to occur in individuals from economically privileged homes who have few siblings, a distribution closely paralleling that of poliomyelitis prior to the introduction of vaccines. This suggests that this lymphoma is an uncommon sequel to a common infection, with the likelihood of oncogenesis increasing with host age at time of infection. Other observations relating to known environmental factors include the high incidence of lymphoma and leukemia in victims of the atomic bomb attacks, although exposure to diagnostic and low dose therapeutic radiation (less than 300 rads) does not appear to increase measurably the risk of these disorders. There is an increased incidence in recipients of antineoplastic drugs, and some 10% of patients cured of Hodgkin's disease subsequently develop other lymphomas or leukemias. Industrial toxins such as benzene increase the attack rate of myelogenous leukemia.

The Non-Hodgkin's Lymphomas

These lymphomas are a heterogeneous group of disorders characterized by a neoplastic proliferation, usually monoclonal, of one or another type of lymphoreticular cell. Varying classifications that are difficult to reconcile with each other and frequent changes in concept of the nature of these diseases have made them difficult to understand.

The non-Hodgkin's lymphomas involve older individuals, 50 to 70, although there is a lesser peak in childhood. There is a slight male predominance. They often start as painless swelling of one or a few lymph nodes, most frequently in the cervical chains. There is spread to other nodes and, in time, to the liver, spleen, and bone marrow. As disease becomes more disseminated, systemic manifestations of fever, weight loss, and a hemolytic anemia may be noted. Abdominal pain is frequent, and symptoms referable to gastrointestinal or genitourinary tract involvement are frequent. Destructive lesions of bone can result in pathologic fractures. In some 5 to 10% of patients, there is a leukemic phase, with flooding of the blood by tumor cells. This is particularly likely to occur in lymphoblastic lymphoma, eventuating in acute lymphocytic leukemia. The meninges of the brain and spinal cord are infiltrated by tumor cells in some 12% of patients, sometimes an extension in continuity from paraspinal masses.

Involved lymph nodes are enlarged, sometimes discrete and other times forming matted masses. They may be firm or soft, and on cut surface show a loss of normal architecture and a homogeneous grayish white color.

The staging of the non-Hodgkin's lymphomas is very similar to that of Hodgkin's disease, described below.

Classification

The classification of lymphomas most used by pathologists and oncologists is essentially that introduced by Rappaport in 1956. It is based on the architectural pattern of the involved nodes (nodular or diffuse), and the cell type comprising the tumor (Figs. 24.1 to 24.4). Table 24.1 shows this classification, and the

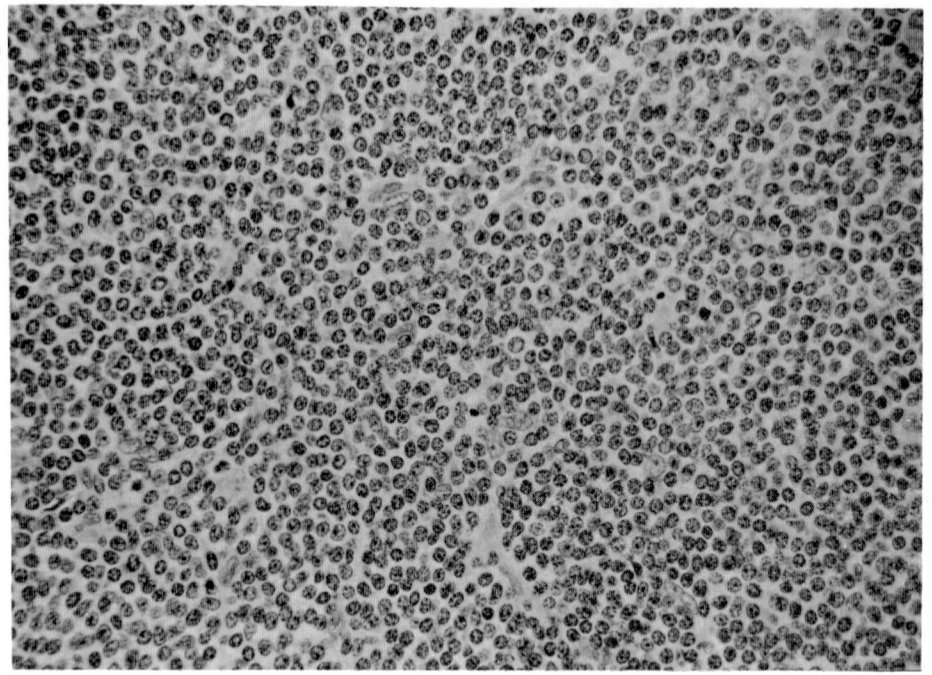

Figure 24.1. Diffuse well differentiated lymphocytic lymphoma. The normal lymph node architecture has been replaced by a diffuse pattern of normal appearing lymphocytes.

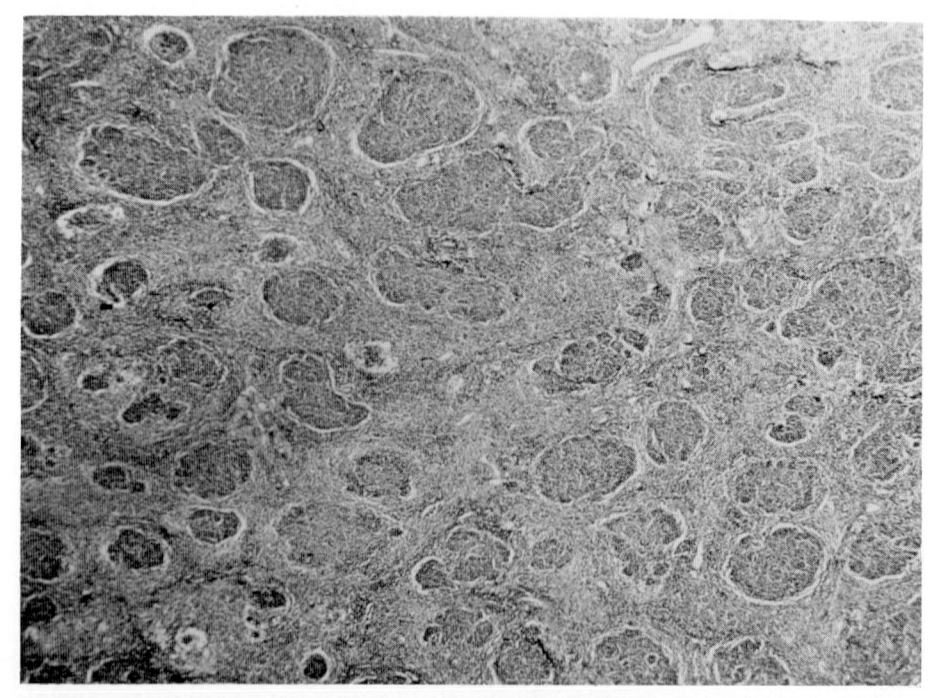

Figure 24.2. Nodular poorly differentiated lymphocytic lymphoma. This low power photomicrograph emphasizes the nodular configuration of the neoplastic process.

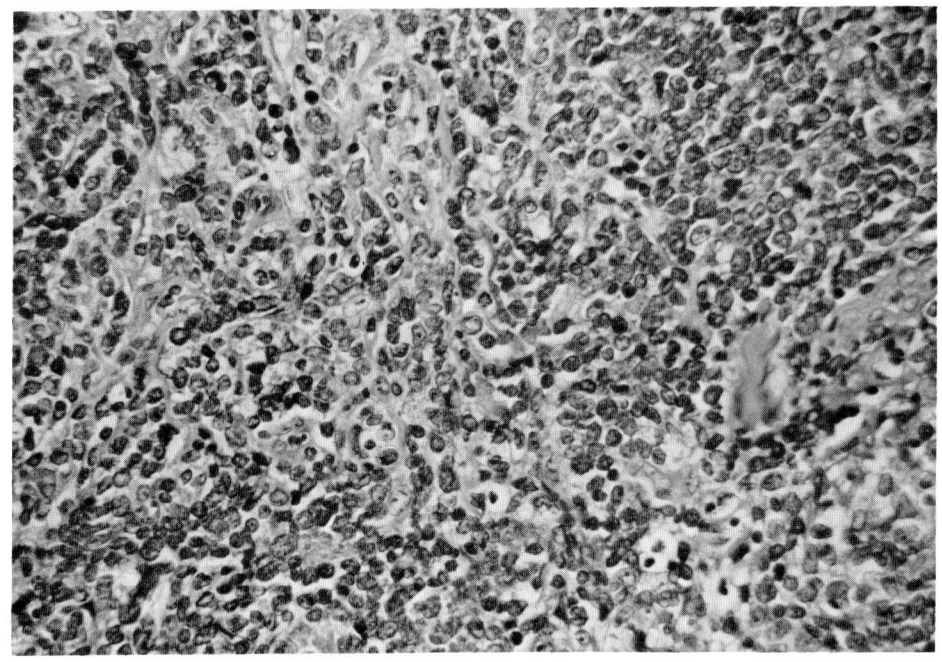

Figure 24.3. Lymphoblastic lymphoma. This lymphoma, formerly classified as poorly differentiated lymphocytic, consists of convoluted primitive T cells. The cells are identical with those of T cell acute lymphocytic leukemia.

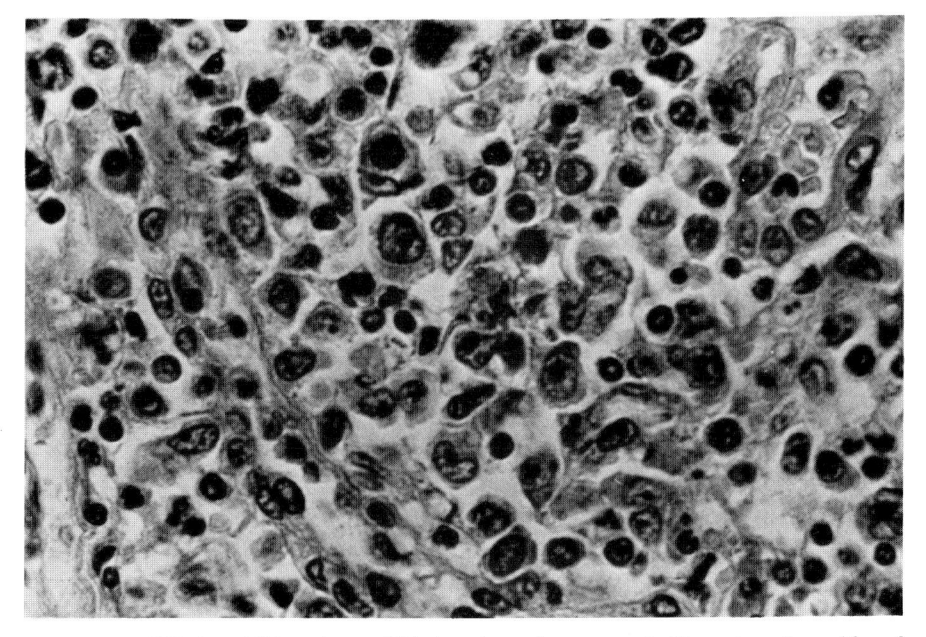

Figure 24.4. "Histiocytic" lymphoma. This lymphoma is composed of large transformed lymphocytes, rather than true histiocytes.

frequency and prognosis of nodular and diffuse forms. It is now clear that the neoplastic cells of almost all "histiocytic" lymphomas are in fact large transformed lymphocytes, and that the "mixed lymphocytic-histiocytic" group is not a tumor composed of two disparate cell types.

Table 24.1
Rappaport Classification of Non-Hodgkin's Lymphomas Based on Architecture and Cytology

	Nodular[a]	Diffuse[a]
Well differentiated lymphocytic	Rare	37% (50%)
Poorly differentiated lymphocytic	30% (72%)	13% (33%)
Mixed lymphocytic-histiocytic	13% (62%)	4% (20%)
Histiocytic	5% (30–60%)	29% (20%)
Undifferentiated, including Burkitt's lymphoma	0	3%

[a] First number is proportion of entire group. Number in parentheses is 5-year survival percentage.

A classification introduced by Lukes and Collins is considerably more complex, but is based on recent progress in understanding of the immune system. It may also prove more valuable in judging prognosis. The lymphomas are tumors of the immune system, composed primarily of T or B lymphocytes. In a series of 500 non-Hodgkin's lymphomas, 75% were of B cell origin, 20% T cell, and 5% undetermined or "null" cell, and only 0.2% was composed of true histiocytes. The lymphomas, according to Lukes and Collins, reflect an alteration of lymphocyte transformation, either a block in the sequence or a derepression, and the lymphoma types represent varying positions in the transformation sequence. Tumors of small lymphocytes, either T or B cells, represent a block in transformation, and are relatively nonaggressive in behavior. No transformed cells or plasma cells are seen, and patients with this pattern are poor antibody producers and may be hypogammaglobulinemic. Tumors of transformed cells result from derepression of the sequence and are highly aggressive. Since the follicle center is the site of B cell transformation, most B cell lymphomas, except those composed of small lymphocytes, are of follicle center cell origin. This includes all of the nodular lymphomas of the Rappaport classification as well as many diffuse lesions.

Table 24.2
Immunologic Classification of Non-Hodgkin's Lymphomas[a]

B Cell	T Cell
Small lymphocyte	Small lymphocyte
Plasmacytoid lymphocyte	Convoluted lymphocyte
Follicular center cell	Cerebriform cell of Sézary syndrome and mycosis fungoides
Small cleaved	
Large cleaved	Immunoblastic sarcoma
Small noncleaved	Histiocytic
Large noncleaved	U cell (unclassified)
Immunoblastic sarcoma	

[a] Modified from Lukes RJ. The immunologic approach to the pathology of malignant lymphomas. Am. J. Clin. Pathol. 72: 657, 1979.

Immunoblastic B cell sarcoma represents a derepression of the postfollicular stage of transformed B cells, as do the lymphoplasmacytic lymphomas, including Waldenström's macroglobulinemia. The essentials of the immunologic classification are shown in Table 24.2.

Lymphomas composed of convoluted T lymphocytes (lymphoblastic lymphoma) occur mostly in children and young adults. Half of the patients have mediastinal masses, including enlargement of the thymus, and more than half will evolve to acute lymphocytic leukemia.

Mycosis fungoides is a lymphoma of T cell origin that is primarily located in the skin, presenting as a psoriasis-like rash. It may remain confined to the skin for years, or disseminate as a leukemia, known as the Sézary syndrome.

Burkitt's lymphoma is a diffuse tumor of small noncleaved B lymphocytes. It is principally observed in the malaria belt of Africa, where it comprises the most common malignant tumor of children. It most frequently involves the mandible or maxilla, or occasionally the abdomen, but there is no generalized lymphadenopathy, and leukemic transformation is rare. The etiologic role of the Epstein-Barr virus is becoming convincing although not yet proven. All patients with African Burkitt's lymphoma have antibodies to the virus; the virus can be identified on tumor cell surfaces, and administration of virus to primates has evoked lymphomas. It is believed that malarial infection may serve as a cofactor in the etiology of Burkitt's lymphoma. Burkitt's lymphoma occurs sporadically in the United States, but the distribution of lesions and their behavior differ from the African form of disease.

Hodgkin's Disease

Hodgkin's disease is a malignant lymphoma in which a highly characteristic neoplastic cell type is seen, often together with apparently non-neoplastic inflammatory and reactive cells. Hodgkin's disease accounts for 40% of the lymphomas.

Many of the clinical manifestations of Hodgkin's disease, particularly early in the course of illness, are suggestive of an infection. There is fever, often remitting in character, night sweats, weakness, and weight loss. Other symptoms include an autoimmune anemia, pruritis, and a predilection to such virus infections as herpes zoster and certain bacterial and fungus infections that reflect an altered cell-mediated immune response. Painless enlargement of lymph nodes may be noted first in the cervical chains or the mediastinum, and occasionally in abdominal, axillary, or inguinal nodes (Fig. 24.5). The disease tends to follow a rather predictable pattern of progression. Mediastinal nodes are eventually involved in over half of patients, while bone marrow involvement is less common, except in the most aggressive forms of disease.

The peak incidence of Hodgkin's disease is between the ages of 20 and 40. It is uncommon in young children and in individuals over 60. There is a 4:3 male predominance.

The neoplastic cell in Hodgkin's disease is probably a bizarre histiocyte (macrophage), although some regard it as an atypical B cell. Most of the neoplastic cells are proliferating mononuclear cells, but the highly characteristic *Reed-Sternberg cell* has a bilobed or multilobed nucleus, with prominent eosinophilic

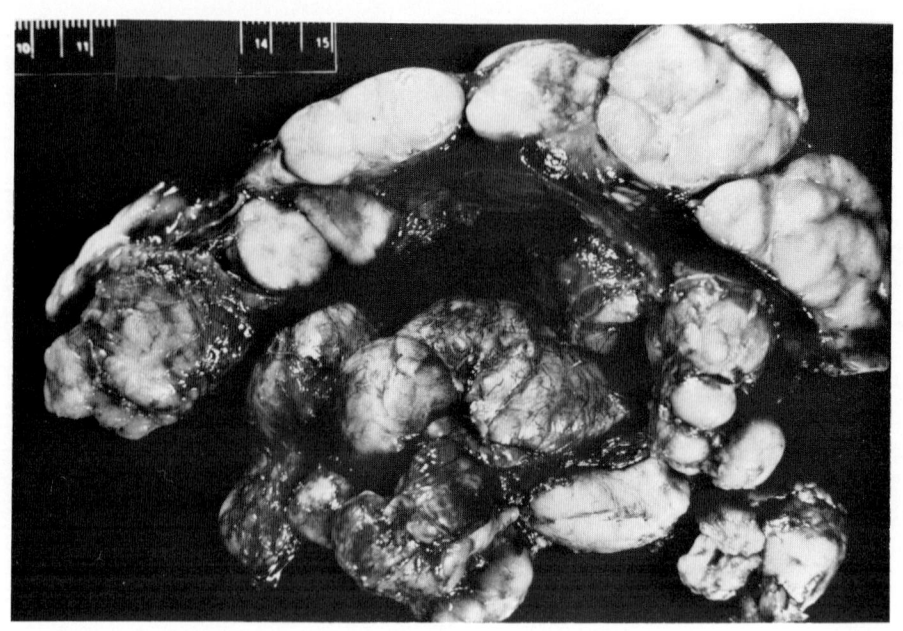

Figure 24.5. Hodgkin's disease. The group of lymph nodes shown here is hard and pale gray in color. Most are discrete, but several are matted together.

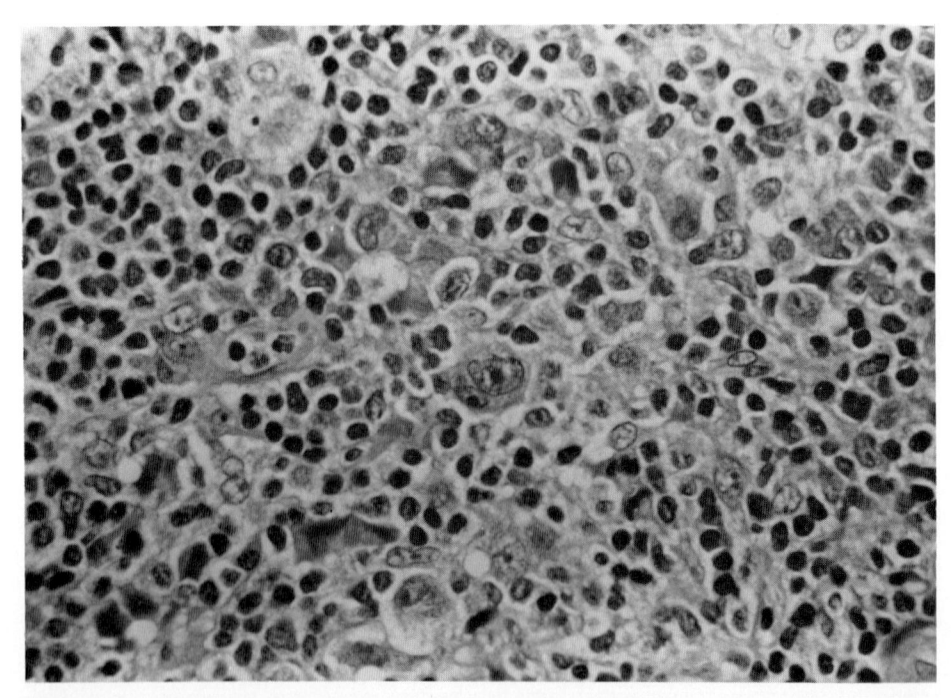

Figure 24.6. Mixed cellularity Hodgkin's disease. The large cell in the *center* is a Reed-Sternberg cell. The nucleus is bilobed, and there are prominent nucleoli surrounded by clear areas.

nucleoli that suggest "owl eyes." It varies in diameter from 15 to 45 μ, and does not appear to proliferate (Fig. 24.6).

Manifestations of impaired T cell function are prominent throughout the course of illness. There is anergy to skin tests that reflect cell-mediated immunity and a high incidence of complicating infections.

Four morphologic types of Hodgkin's disease are recognized. *Lymphocyte predominant Hodgkin's disease* is characterized by few Reed-Sternberg cells and large numbers of apparently mature lymphocytes. The involved nodes are most often cervical and are soft in consistency. Disease may be confined to a single node. The course of disease is often prolonged and relatively nonaggressive, and survival and cure rates are high.

Nodular sclerosing Hodgkin's disease may be a separate disease. There is a female predominance, and transitions between this and other forms of Hodgkin's disease are not observed. Nodules of tumor, containing variable numbers of Reed-Sternberg cells, are separated by bands of fibrous tissue (Fig. 24.7). Involved lymph nodes may be discrete or matted together, and are hard in consistency (Fig. 24.8). Mediastinal involvement is very common, as is involvement of scalene, supraclavicular, and lower cervical nodes. The prognosis is good.

Mixed cellularity Hodgkin's disease is characterized by nodes showing many Reed-Sternberg cells together with an admixture of plasma cells, eosinophils, polymorphonuclear leukocytes, and histiocytes, with areas of necrosis and fibrosis.

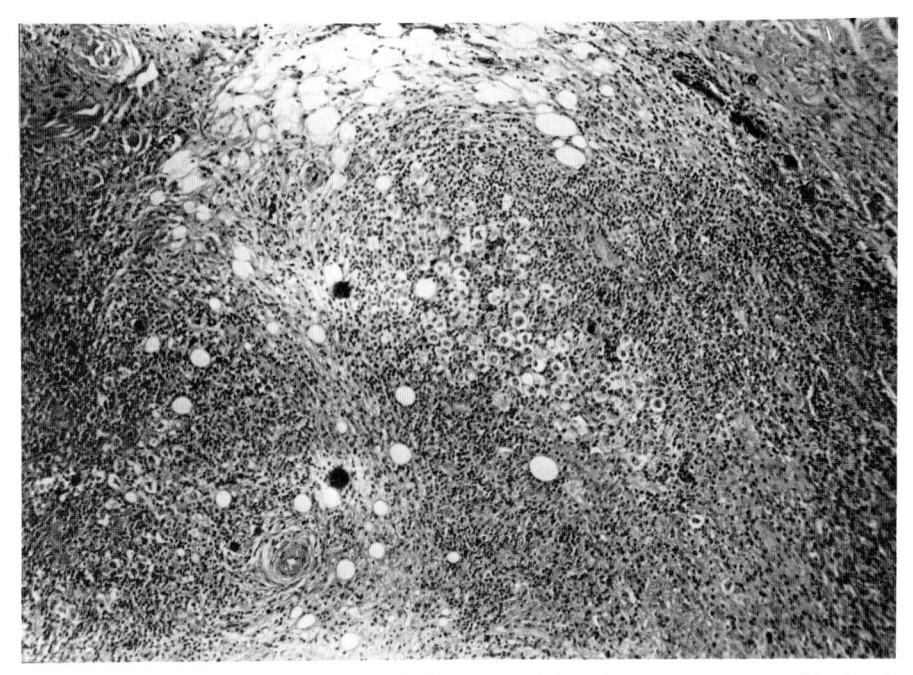

Figure 24.7. Nodular sclerosing Hodgkin's disease. Nodules of tumor are separated by bands of fibrous tissue. There are many Reed-Sternberg cells and tumor cells surrounded by clear spaces (lacunar cells).

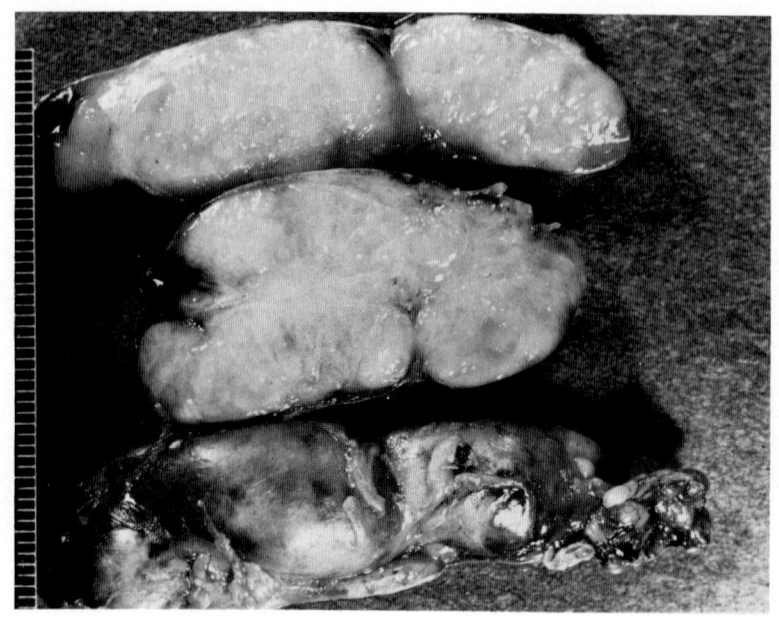

Figure 24.8. Nodular sclerosing Hodgkin's disease. These lymph nodes are hard in consistency and adherent to each other, and they show bands of fibrous tissue.

The involved nodes are hard and adherent one to another. The prognosis is guarded.

Lymphocyte depletion Hodgkin's disease is the most aggressive form of disease, seen particularly in older patients, and has a poor prognosis. Large numbers of Reed-Sternberg cells are seen, either in solid sheets or embedded in fibrous tissue. Few lymphocytes are seen.

Progression from lymphocyte predominant to mixed cellularity and from mixed cellularity to lymphocyte depletion is commonly observed.

The staging of Hodgkin's disease is a critical consideration in determining therapy. It often requires lymphangiography and sometimes laparotomy.

I. Involvement confined to single group of nodes
II. Two or more contiguous groups of nodes involved on one side of diaphragm, *e.g.*, cervical and mediastinal nodes
III. Involvement of nodes on both sides of diaphragm, and spleen
IV. Disseminated disease, involving liver, bone marrow, or multiple extranodal tissues

---

Each stage is further designated A or B. A denotes few systemic symptoms, while B indicates fever, weight loss, or night sweats, and a less favorable prognosis.

Tremendous progress has been made in the therapy of Hodgkin's disease. Aggressive combined therapy with modern radiotherapy and chemotherapeutic programs now achieves an over 80% 5-year survival. It is clear that many patients

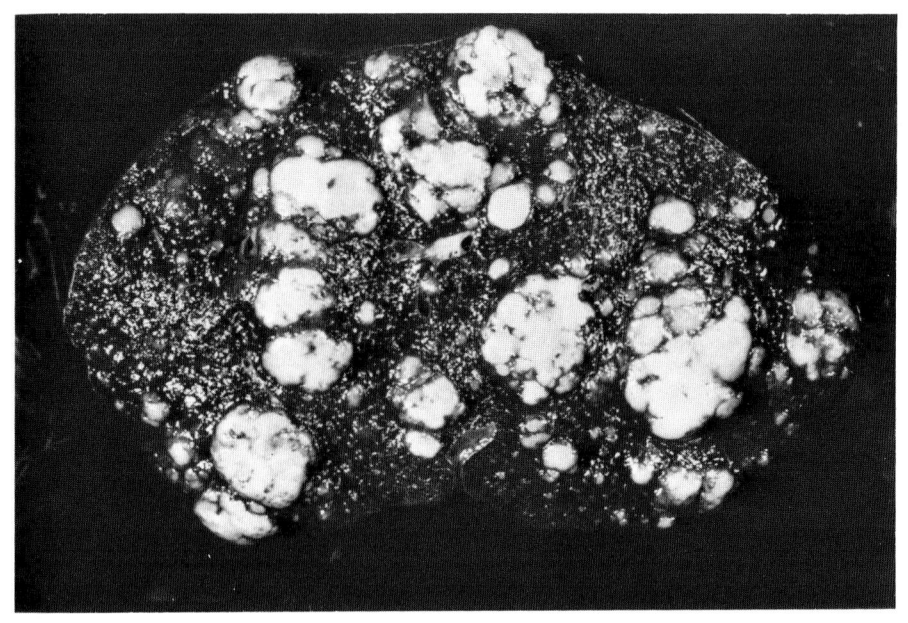

Figure 24.9. Cut surface of spleen showing multiple nodules of Hodgkin's lymphoma. This spleen weighed 450 g.

are now curable, although cured patients have an increased incidence of other lymphomas or leukemias.

Leukemia

The leukemias are a group of disorders in which there is uncontrolled proliferation of abnormal leukocytes in the bone marrow, usually spilling into the circulating blood. Involvement of the spleen is virtually constant, and the liver, lymph nodes, and other organs are frequently infiltrated by proliferating neoplastic cells.

The filling and replacement of bone marrow by abnormal cells results in anemia, thrombocytopenia, and a deficiency of functionally effective leukocytes. The manifestations of disease may include fever, weakness, bone pain, bleeding gums and generalized petechial or purpuric hemorrhages, severe, often systemic infections with Gram-negative bacilli, staphylococci, fungi, or pneumocystis, and hyperuricemia, due to massive breakdown of nucleic acids. Symptoms referable to infiltration of the meninges are frequent in the acute forms of disease.

The incidence of leukemia is between 4 and 7 per 100,000 population in this country. There is a slight male predominance in most forms of disease, a marked male predominance in others.

The leukemias are classified on the basis of cell type and the rapidity of the natural course of disease. Cell type is determined by cytologic markers associated with T or B lymphocytes, staining reactions with periodic acid and Sudan black, the presence of such enzymes as myeloperoxidase, several esterases, alkaline phosphatase, and terminal deoxynucleotidyl transferase (TDT), and identification of chromosomal abnormalities, including the *Philadelphia chromosome* (translocation between chromosomes 22 and 9). The acute leukemias are rapid in onset and usually fatal in months if untreated. The chronic leukemias are more gradual in onset, run their course over many months or years, usually accompanied by marked splenomegaly.

Acute Lymphocytic Leukemia (ALL)

This leukemia occurs predominantly in children and adolescents. It is the leading cause of cancer deaths in children under 15, and comprises 80% of childhood leukemia. The tumor cells are small or medium-sized lymphoblasts. Two-thirds of patients are classified as having the "common" form of disease, and their cells react with ALL antisera and are positive for TDT. Some 20% have T cell leukemia, and fewer are composed of B or null cells. The common cell type occurs predominantly in children, and has a favorable prognosis, about 50% of patients appearing to be cured by intensive therapy. T cell leukemia occurs in older children and young adults, is likely to involve the thymus gland, central nervous system, and testes, and has a poor prognosis.

Chronic Lymphocytic Leukemia (CLL)

CLL is the most common leukemia in this country. It occurs primarily in patients over 50, and there is a 2:1 male predominance. The disease is gradual in onset, characterized by variable enlargement of spleen, liver, and lymph nodes and often very high numbers of lymphocytes in the bloodstream. A complicating autoimmune hemolytic anemia is not uncommon.

The neoplastic cells are small lymphocytes; in at least 95% of patients they are

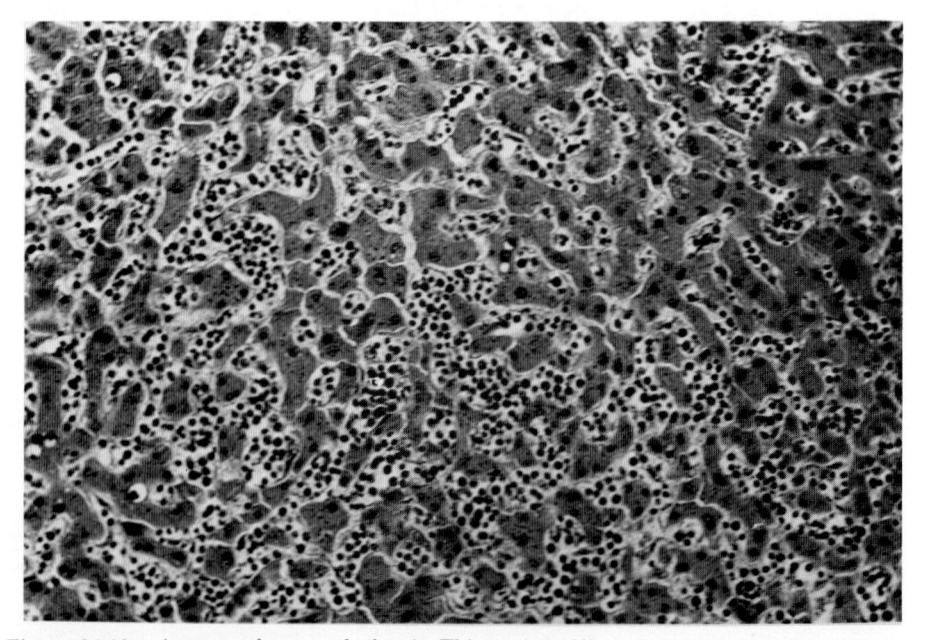

Figure 24.10. Acute myelogenous leukemia. This section of liver shows massive infiltration of the hepatic sinusoids by leukemic cells.

B cells. CLL appears to be the same disease as well differentiated lymphocytic lymphoma, the only difference being the dissemination of tumor cells in the blood.

CLL tends to run a course of years, particularly with therapy, and may be compatible with a normal life span in older patients.

Acute Myelogenous Leukemia (AML)

AML is the principal acute leukemia of adults, occurring at any time during adult life. It is the leukemia most noted in Japanese survivors of the atomic bomb explosions, and it is often the final expression of the myeloproliferative disorders (p. 321). The disease is rapid in onset, with variable enlargement of liver, spleen, and lymph nodes. Some 10% of patients are "aleukemic" when first seen; *i.e.*, leukemic cells are not present in the blood (Figs. 24.10 and 24.11).

AML in all likelihood encompasses several disorders of blast cell origin, including myeloblastic, promyelocytic, and myelomonocytic leukemias, as well as erythroleukemia. Patients with myelomonocytic or monocytic leukemia often have striking hyperplasia of gingival tissues, while disseminated intravascular coagu-

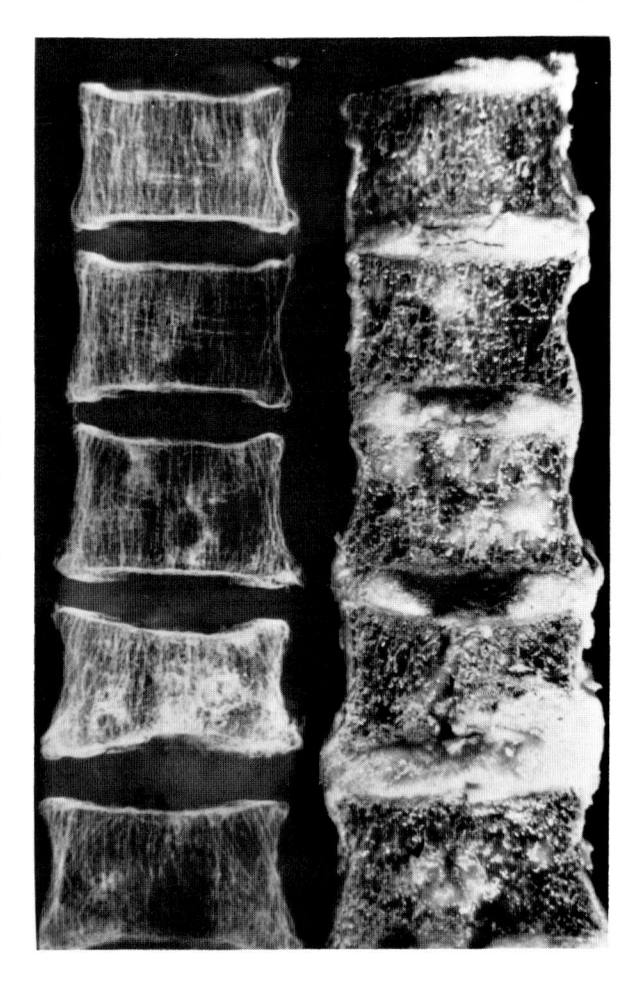

Figure 24.11. Acute myelogenous leukemia. The vertebrae at the *right* show multiple areas of bone destruction and replacement by leukemic cells. The x-ray at the *left* shows multiple areas of lucency and collapse of one of the vertebral bodies.

lation may be observed in those with promyelocytic disease. Auer rods are large eosinophilic granules that identify myelocytic and promyelocytic cells. The cells of AML are positive for peroxidase and their granules stain with Sudan black.

Intensive therapy leads to remission in 70% of patients, but there is usually a relapse in less than 1 year. Fewer than 5% are alive 5 years after diagnosis.

Chronic Myelogenous Leukemia (CML)

CML has a gradual onset. There is progressive enlargement of the spleen, often reaching 5000 g (Fig. 24.12). Bleeding and recurrent infections are late manifestations. Some 10 to 15% of patients die during the first year of illness, and most of the rest within 3 to 7 years. Death is usually preceded by a "blast crisis" in which 30% of patients have tumor cells that resemble lymphoblasts and are TDT-positive (Fig. 24.13).

The Philadelphia chromosome is identified in 90% of patients with CML; it is seen in all bone marrow elements. The cells tend to have very low levels of alkaline phosphatase.

Hairy Cell Leukemia

Hairy cell leukemia is an uncommon leukemia occurring in older patients, with a 4:1 male predominance. The neoplastic cells have nuclei that resemble lymphocytes and cytoplasm similar to monocytes. Some 10% of the cells seen on blood smear have hair-like projections, consisting of microvilli. The cells are phagocytic and have surface immunoglobulins. The total white blood cell count may be lower than normal and is rarely markedly elevated.

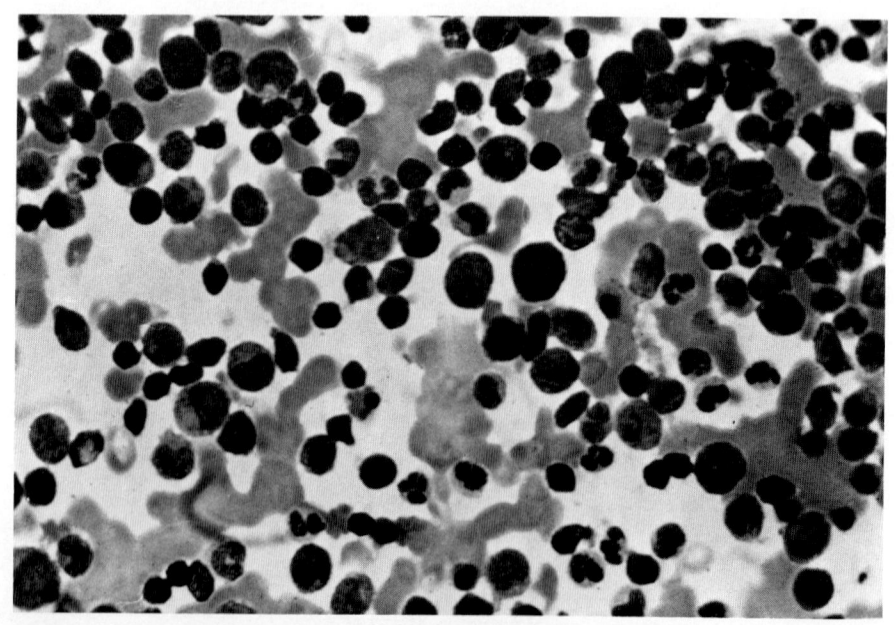

Figure 24.12. Chronic myelogenous leukemia. The bone marrow shows many blastic cells, but most are myelocytes and mature polymorphonuclear leukocytes.

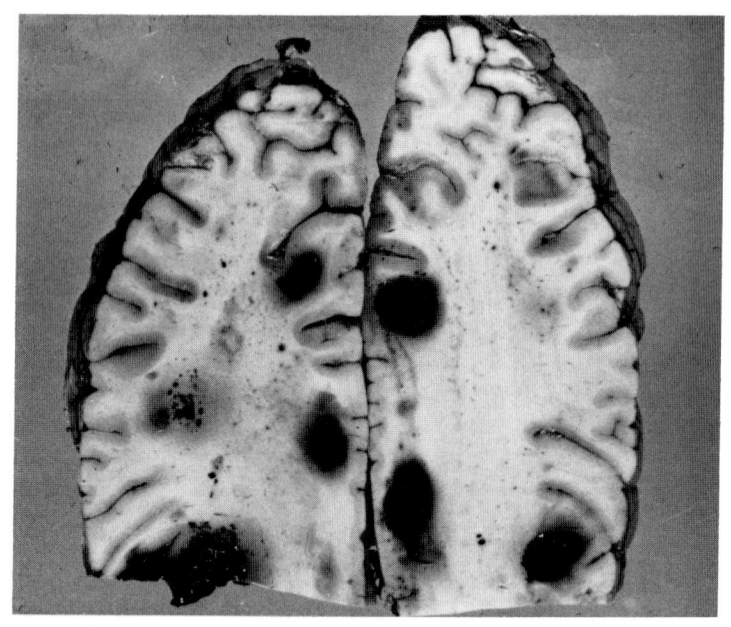

Figure 24.13. Multiple cerebral hemorrhages in a patient with chronic myelogenous leukemia in blast crisis.

The disease is gradual in onset and slowly progressive. There is massive splenomegaly and a striking predilection to infections, particularly by typical and atypical tubercle bacilli. With therapy, half of patients are alive after 10 years.

THE MYELOPROLIFERATIVE DISORDERS

These diseases are characterized by a proliferation of any of the marrow elements, usually more than one line in any given patient, frequently with associated fibrosis. The disorders included in this group are CML, *agnogenic myeloid metaplasia*, in which the marrow is largely replaced by fibrous tissue (*myelofibrosis*) and there is extensive extramedullary hematopoiesis of all blood elements, *polycythemia vera*, and *essential thrombocythemia*. All of these entities appear to be clonal disorders, even though more than one marrow component is involved. Each can terminate as acute myelogenous leukemia, although the likelihood of this happening varies considerably among them.

MULTIPLE MYELOMA

Multiple myeloma is the most important of the plasma cell dyscrasias. These disorders, called gammopathies, are characterized by a monoclonal neoplastic proliferation of plasma cells and the production of a specific immunoglobulin myeloma or M protein or one of its chains. Other monoclonal gammopathies include Waldenström's macroglobulinemia and heavy chain disease.

In multiple myeloma, there are multiple bone lesions composed of masses of mature or immature plasma cells, with destruction of cancellous and compact bone (Figs. 24.14 and 24.15). They are most notable in vertebral bodies, ribs,

322   *Pathology: Understanding Human Disease*

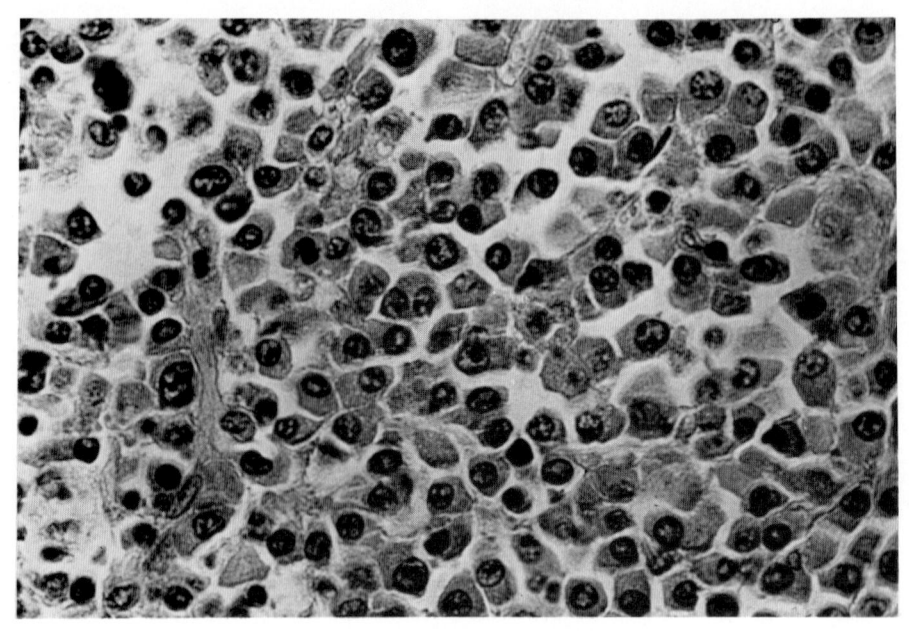

Figure 24.14. Multiple myeloma. Section of bone lesion showing a mass of mature and immature plasma cells.

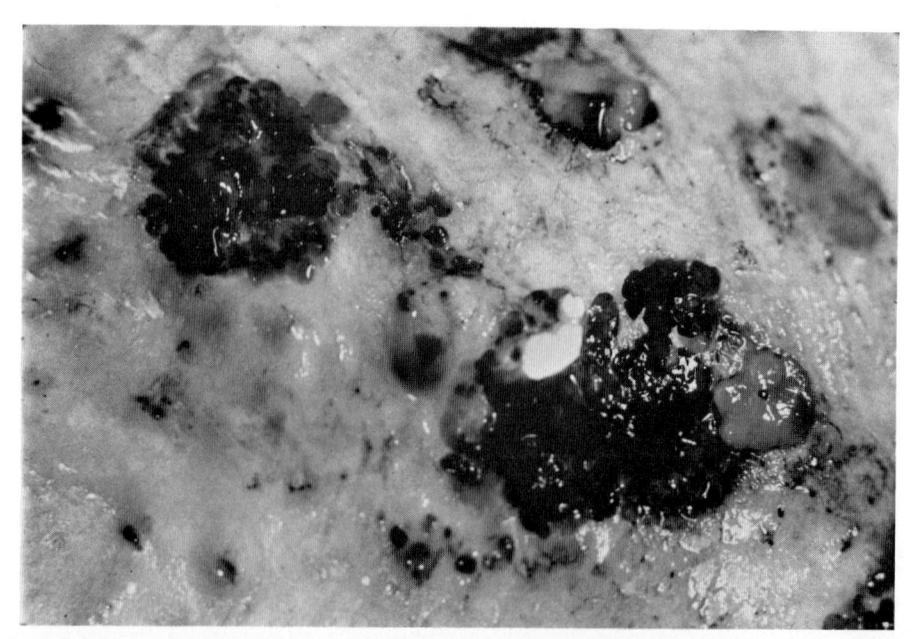

Figure 24.15. Multiple myeloma. This view of the inner aspect of the calvarium shows multiple areas of bone destruction by nodules of tumor.

pelvis, and skull, and appear radiographically as sharply punched out lucencies (Fig. 24.16). Other organs may be infiltrated by tumor cells, including the spleen, liver, and lymph nodes. Myeloma protein does not normally appear in the urine, but light chains of the specific immunoglobulin (Bence Jones protein) are filtered

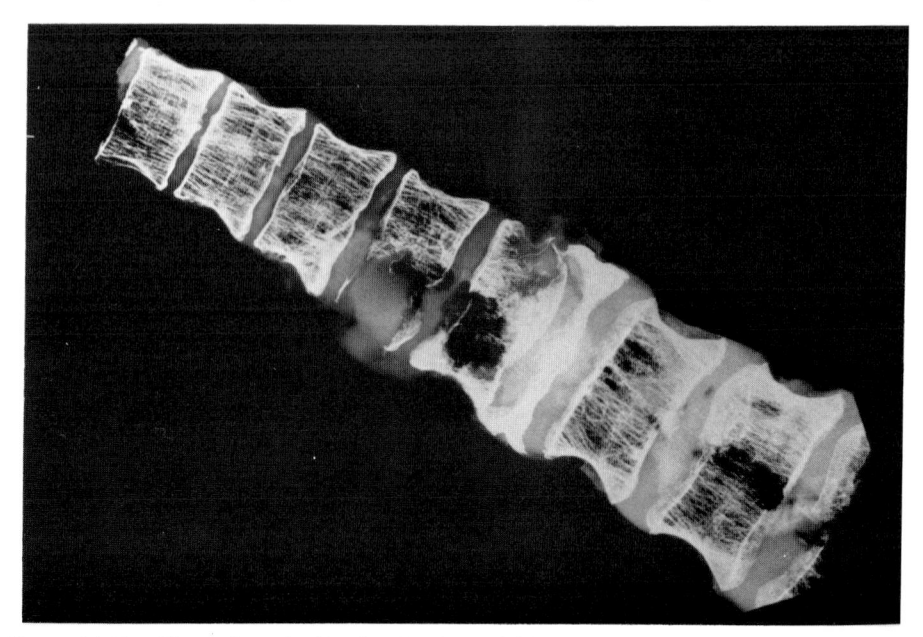

Figure 24.16. X-ray of vertebral bodies showing multiple punched out lesions of multiple myeloma. There is complete collapse of one vertebral body.

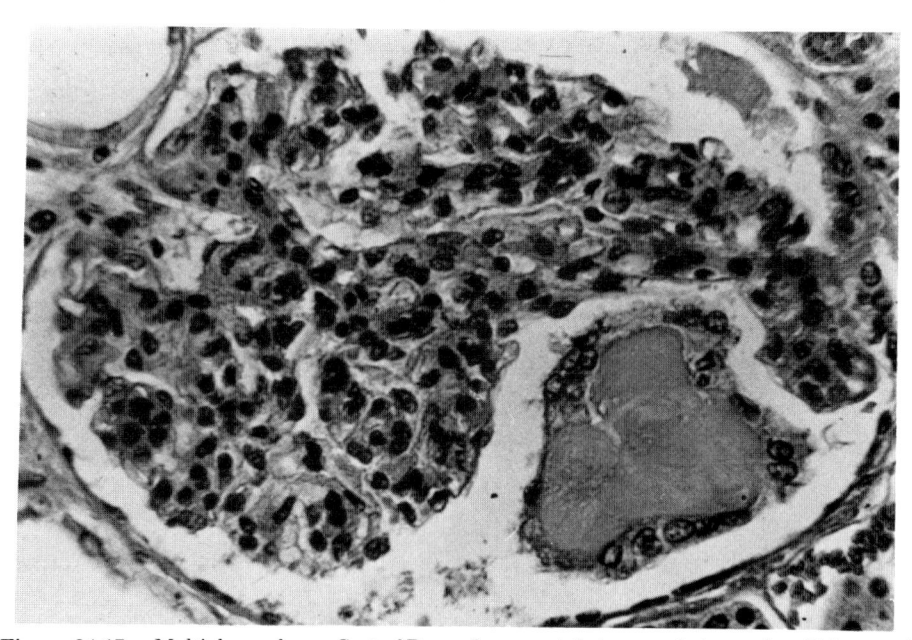

Figure 24.17. Multiple myeloma. Cast of Bence Jones protein in a renal glomerulus. This material has evoked a giant cell reaction.

by the glomeruli and tend to form casts, particularly in the collecting ducts (Fig. 24.17). These casts can evoke a giant cell reaction in the ducts. Together with diffuse infiltration of the kidney by neoplastic plasma cells, they can be responsible for renal failure. Bence Jones proteinuria occurs in some 70% of myeloma patients.

Multiple myeloma is a disease of older patients, with a peak incidence between 50 and 60. The presenting manifestations are usually weakness and anemia, often with neuropathy and proteinuria. Bone pain and fractures are late manifestations. Increased viscosity of the blood and a tendency to gel formation when exposed to cold temperatures may cause vascular insufficiency and gangrene of the extremities. There is impaired humoral immunity and increased susceptibility to infections. Most patients die of their disease in 1 or 2 years, although therapy may prolong life for several years.

In 60% of patients, the M protein is an IgG. IgA and IgM are less frequent. The M protein is identified as a prominent spike on plasma or urine electrophoresis. A few patients produce light chains only, and no complete immunoglobulin. Some 10% of patients with multiple myeloma are found to have systemic amyloidosis (see below).

WALDENSTRÖM'S MACROGLOBULINEMIA

This disease consists of infiltration of the bone marrow and often of spleen, liver, and lymph nodes by plasma cells, lymphocytes, and intermediate forms. The tumor cells produce an M protein, usually an IgM, but occasionally an IgG or IgA. Bence Jones protein is present in one-fourth of patients.

Waldenström's macroglobulinemia is a disease of the elderly. Its manifestations resemble those of a leukemia, since there is diffuse bone marrow replacement. Increased viscosity of the blood and cold agglutinins are prominent. A fatal outcome occurs in from 2 to 5 years.

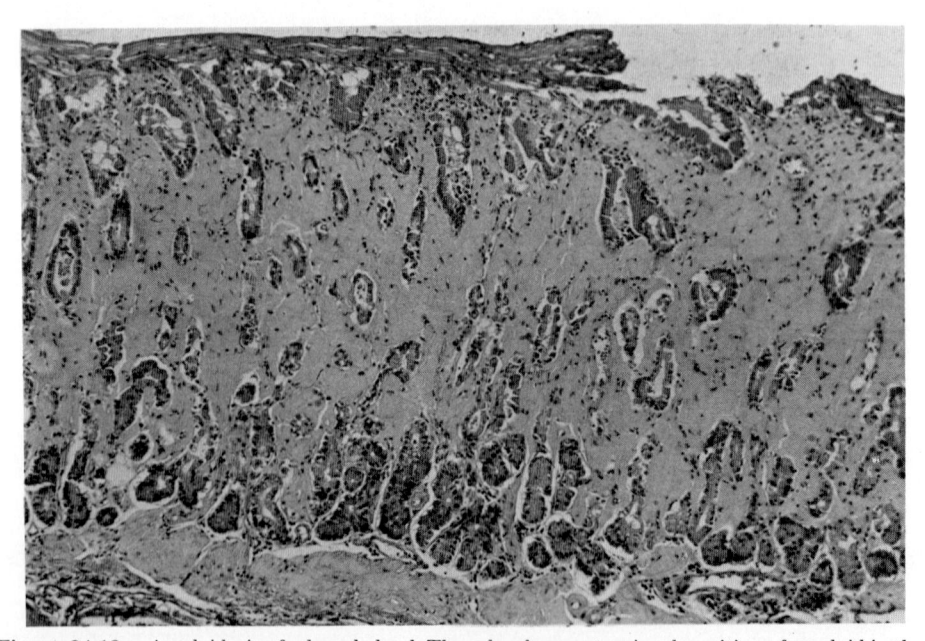

Figure 24.18. Amyloidosis of adrenal gland. There has been extensive deposition of amyloid in the adrenal cortex, with consequent atrophy and loss of cortical cells.

AMYLOIDOSIS

Amyloidosis has been referred to in many earlier chapters, but has not been discussed in any detail. It is included here because of the frequent association of one form of the disease with the monoclonal gammopathies.

Amyloidosis is not a single disease, but rather a group of disorders characterized by the extracellular deposition of hyaline eosinophilic material, often leading to atrophy of parenchymal cells (Fig. 24.18). Amyloid is seen as a fibrillar protein on electron microscopy (Fig. 24.19). It has a unique conformation that is responsible for its insolubility and the characteristic apple green birefringence seen when histologic sections stained with Congo red are viewed with polarized light.

There are at least two major chemical types of amyloid. In Type B amyloid, immunoglobulin light chains are the major protein component, while in Type A amyloid the principal protein is not an immunoglobulin. Other specific amyloids have been identified, particularly in relation to tumors of endocrine organs.

Amyloid B is encountered most often in patients with multiple myeloma or other plasma cells dyscrasias. Amyloid tends to be deposited in the heart, gastrointestinal tract, tongue, muscles, nerves, and skin (Pattern I).

Amyloid A is seen in association with such chronic infections as osteomyelitis, tuberculosis, or leprosy and in patients with rheumatoid arthritis, ankylosing spondylitis, Sjögren's syndrome, systemic lupus erythematosus, chronic ulcerative colitis, and Crohn's disease. The distribution of amyloid is predominately in liver, spleen, kidneys, and adrenals (Pattern II).

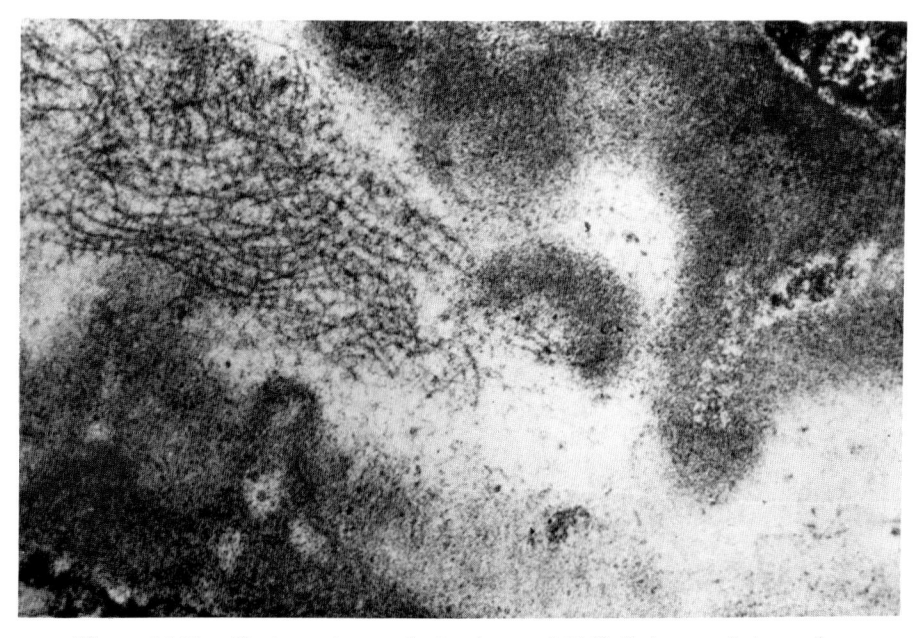

Figure 24.19. Electron micrograph showing amyloid fibrils in a renal glomerulus.

In many patients, the pattern of amyloid deposition is mixed. Monoclonal immunoglobulin spikes in most of these patients suggest an underlying plasma cell dyscrasia.

Some formation of amyloid may be associated with the aging process, noted in patients over 70. Deposits are not uncommon in the myocardium, spleen, islets of Langerhans, or brain.

The manifestations of amyloidosis depend on the sites of deposition. Cardiac involvement is reflected in congestive heart failure or arrhythmias, Diffuse gastrointestinal deposits can cause constipation or diarrhea and a generalized malabsorption syndrome. Involvement of liver and spleen results in marked enlargement of these organs. Amyloidosis affecting the renal glomeruli is often manifested by the nephrotic syndrome (Fig. 24.20). Some patients with Type B amyloid develop Factor X deficiency and may have hemorrhagic complications.

Arterioles are involved in virtually all instances of amyloidosis, and this permits morphologic diagnosis following biopsy, preferably of rectal mucosa.

ANEMIAS

Very brief consideration is given to the morphologic manifestations of a few anemias. Various aspects of these disorders have been discussed in earlier chapters.

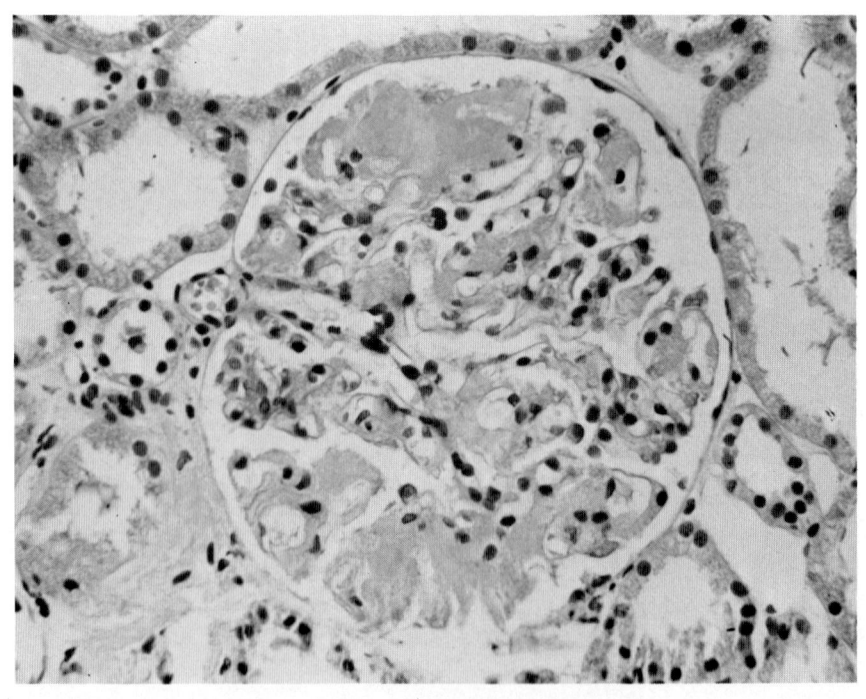

Figure 24.20. Amyloidosis. There is extensive deposition of homogeneous amyloid in this glomerulus. The patient had the manifestations of the nephrotic syndrome.

Pernicious Anemia

Pernicious anemia is a megaloblastic anemia that results from a deficiency of vitamin B_{12}. This is usually the result of atrophic gastritis (p. 286) and failure of intrinsic factor production, although, at other times, anti-intrinsic factor antibodies may be the mechanism of B_{12} deficiency. The disease is usually seen in middle-aged and elderly patients. Although many observations suggest an autoimmune mechanism (p. 84), this has not been firmly established. There is some association of pernicious anemia with several HLA haplotypes, but a clear genetic role in pathogenesis is lacking.

The bone marrow is markedly hyperplastic, with a predominance of large blastic cells, reflecting interference with DNA synthesis. All of the elements of the erythropoietic sequence are larger than normal, and the mature red blood cells in the circulating blood, although very variable in size, have an increased mean corpuscular volume, while maintaining a normal hemoglobin concentration. Nucleated red blood cells may also circulate. The red cells have a decreased life span, so that the anemia is partly the result of hemolysis. Polymorphonuclear leukocytes are also larger than normal, and their nuclei are hypersegmented.

Gastrointestinal changes include atrophy of the papillae of the tongue (atrophic glossitis) and atrophic gastritis. There is loss of both chief and parietal cells, and the normal mucosa is often replaced by intestinal type glands. Achlorhydria is constant and, in some 10% of patients, gastric carcinoma is the eventual outcome. Prominent central nervous system changes are noted, consisting of demyelination of the dorsal and lateral columns of the spinal cord (*combined system disease*). These are reflected in poor coordination and loss of vibratory sense. The myocardium shows striking fatty infiltration of its connective tissue, lending a "tigroid" appearance when viewed from the endocardial surface. The hemolytic component of the anemia results in mild icterus of the skin, and accumulation of hemosiderin pigment in the cells of the reticuloendothelial system.

The megaloblastic anemia of folate deficiency is entirely similar to pernicious anemia, except that the central nervous system is not involved.

Hemolytic Anemia

In the hemolytic anemias, there is a shortened life span of the red blood cells, and they are destroyed prematurely, at times in "hemolytic crises." The destruction of red blood cells may take place in the reticuloendothelial system, particularly in the spleen, or it may occur within the vascular system.

Extravascular destruction is the rule in the autoimmune hemolytic anemias, sickle cell (SS) disease, thalassemia, congenital spherocytosis, and glucose-6-phosphate dehydrogenase deficiency. Enlargement of the spleen is noted in these anemias, although repeated infarction in patients with sickle cell anemia often leads to fibrotic atrophy and a weight of but a few grams.

Destruction of red blood cells occurs within the vascular system in transfusion reactions, in disseminated intravascular coagulation, and in patients with certain types of prosthetic cardiac valves. The released hemoglobin is bound to haptoglobin, an α-2-globulin, and taken up by the reticuloendothelial system. This prevents its excretion by the kidney. If, however, the supply of haptoglobin is exhausted, hemoglobin and methemoglobin are found in the urine.

The bone marrow is hyperplastic in all hemolytic anemias, and foci of extramedullary erythropoiesis may be found. There are increased numbers of reticulocytes in the blood. There is jaundice due primarily to unconjugated bilirubin, and the increased conjugation and excretion of bilirubin by the liver often result in the formation of bilirubin stones in the gall bladder. Hemosiderin pigment accumulates in cells of the reticuloendothelial system. With severe marrow hyperplasia, there may be proliferation of new bone over the outer table of the flat bones, producing characteristic changes on x-ray, particularly of the skull. Persistent anemia results in myocardial hypertrophy, and, if severe, in high output congestive heart failure.

Suggested Reading

Aisenberg AC. Cell-surface markers in lymphoproliferative disease. N. Eng. J. Med. *304:* 331, 1981.

Berard CW, Greene MH, Jaffe ES, Magrath I, Ziegler J. A multidisciplinary approach to non-Hodgkin's lymphomas. Ann. Intern. Med. *94:* 218, 1981.

Glenner GG. Amyloid deposits and amyloidosis. N. Engl. J. Med. *302:* 1283, 1333, 1980.

Good RA, et al. Leukemias and lymphomas (symposium). Am. J. Pathol. *90:* 447, 1978.

Lukes RJ. The immunologic approach to the pathology of malignant lymphomas. Am. J. Clin. Pathol. *72:* 657, 1979.

Chapter 25

The Endocrine Glands

This chapter opens with some general considerations about the pathogenesis of endocrine disease and the biologic behavior of tumors of the endocrine glands. Presentation of the major disturbances of the hypothalamus, hypophysis, thyroid, parathyroid, and adrenal glands is followed by discussion of the multiple endocrine syndromes and the functional potential of tumors of neuroectodermal (APUD) origin.

GENERAL CONSIDERATIONS

Most endocrinopathies represent quantitative alterations of physiologic states. They can result from disease processes affecting the endocrine organs or from disturbances of feedback and other inhibitory or stimulatory mechanisms that control their hormone secretions. For each endocrine gland, we can anticipate destructive lesions, neoplastic lesions with varying degrees of autonomy of function, changes that reflect altered control mechanisms, and, perhaps, changes associated with the diversion of metabolic pathways.

The various endocrine systems vary greatly in their complexity. The control of serum ionized calcium concentration by the opposing effects of parathyroid hormone and calcitonin and the regulation of blood glucose concentration by insulin and glucagon are relatively simple systems. The control of circulating thyroid hormone or cortisol involves the hypothalamus, adenohypophysis, and the appropriate target organ, and altered function is likely to be reflected in structural changes in each component of the system. Disturbances of thyroid or adrenal cortical function are likely to require study of hypophyseal and hypothalamic function in order to determine the site of a causative lesion.

A decrease or loss of hormone secretion can result from genetically determined enzyme defects, as in some forms of cretinism and the adrenogenital syndromes. Destructive lesions decrease function, as in infections of endocrine glands, infarction, primary and metastatic tumors, and such autoimmune disorders as Hashimoto's thyroiditis, idiopathic hypothyroidism, and many instances of adrenal insufficiency. Finally, destructive lesions or impaired trophic functions of the hypothalamus or adenohypophysis will diminish target organ function.

Increased hormone secretion can be associated with autonomous tumors and hyperplasias of endocrine organs, autonomous secretion of hypothalamic and hypophyseal trophic hormones, or loss of hypothalamic inhibitory control, as in the case of prolactin secretion. Increased function can also result from the secretion of trophic hormones at abnormal, or "ectopic," sites and from autoimmune antibodies that act as trophic factors.

The concepts of primary, secondary, and tertiary hyperplasia were discussed in Chapter 13. These assume major importance in understanding the hyperplasias of the endocrine glands, the altered physiologic responses that follow prolonged stimulus for increased function, and the assumption of autonomy of function in a setting of physiologic hyperplasia.

Autoimmune phenomena play an important role in the pathogenesis of many endocrine disturbances. The resulting disorders tend to be familial and are associated with certain HLA haplotypes. There are several syndromes of *polyglandular failure* which may involve hypothyroidism, adrenal insufficiency, hypoparathyroidism, and hypogonadism, as well as myasthenia gravis, diabetes mellitus, pernicious anemia, and chronic active hepatitis.

Tumors of the Endocrine Glands

Tumors of the endocrine glands most often arise without obvious cause, but may develop, or dramatically change their growth patterns, in settings of prolonged stimulation from trophic or releasing hormones. Pituitary tumors producing prolactin appear to arise following loss of hypothalamic inhibition of prolactin secretion. Rapid growth of pituitary tumors producing adenocorticotrophic hormone (ACTH) may follow bilateral adrenalectomy in patients with Cushing's syndrome.

Most tumors of endocrine glands are either adenomas or adenocarcinomas. Many are endocrinologically functional; others are not. Although there is a general correlation between tumor size and degree of function, very small tumors may have critical endocrine function. This is particularly true of pituitary microadenomas, only a few millimeters in diameter, which can cause major endocrinopathies.

Some endocrine tumors produce more than one hormone, and some malignant tumors have broader function than their benign counterparts. Thus, while adrenal cortical adenomas are likely to produce the hormone of only one cortical zone, adrenal carcinomas may secrete hormones from two zones or from all three.

Autonomy of function of endocrine tumors is rarely complete. Benign tumors may respond reasonably well to normal control mechanisms, but even malignant tumors may alter their function if the stimulus is sufficient. Thus, parathyroid carcinomas will reduce their output of parathyroid hormone following a calcium load.

Primary hyperplasias are observed in the parathyroid glands, the adenohypophysis, the adrenal cortex, and the islets of Langerhans. These hyperplasias are biologically indistinguishable from neoplasms. Indeed, primary hyperplasia of the parathyroid glands can be a component of the multiple endocrine syndromes.

HYPOTHALAMIC DISORDERS

The endocrine functions of the hypothalamus follow two pathways. In the *tuberohypophyseal system,* nuclei in the medial basal hypothalamus secrete peptide hormones that stimulate or inhibit the release of adenohypophyseal trophic hormones. This system is regulated by neurotransmitters and by target organ hormones which exert a feedback effect on the hypothalamus. Blood glucose concentrations also affect this system. In the *neurohypophyseal system*, cells of the supraoptic and paraventricular nuclei secrete antidiuretic hormone and oxytocin, which migrate along axons in the pituitary stalk to the neurohypophysis where they are stored in perivascular nerve endings. Antidiuretic hormone secretion is responsive to volume receptors in the left atrium and pulmonary veins and to the renin-angiotensin system. It is also responsive to thirst and to emotional stimuli.

Interruption of the neurohypophyseal system by degenerative lesions of the hypothalamic nuclei, infections, primary or metastatic tumors, or trauma can result in diabetes insipidus, providing adrenal cortical function is maintained. Diabetes insipidus can also be nephrogenic, when the kidney is unresponsive to the effects of antidiuretic hormone on water resorption in the distal nephron, and it can follow disorders of the thirst center and compulsive water drinking.

Antidiuretic hormone secretion is "appropriate" when it is in response to hypovolemia or plasma hyperosmolality. "Inappropriate" antidiuretic hormone secretion can follow brain lesions that affect hypothalamic function or follow ingestion of certain drugs (chlorpropamide, narcotics) and in response to faulty signals from cardiac volume receptors after mitral valve surgery. Antidiuretic hormone may also be secreted by nonendocrine tumors, particularly bronchogenic carcinomas. The inappropriate antidiuretic hormone syndrome is characterized by a hypervolemia, hyponatremia, and hypo-osmolality. Edema is usually not present because compensatory mechanisms increase sodium excretion.

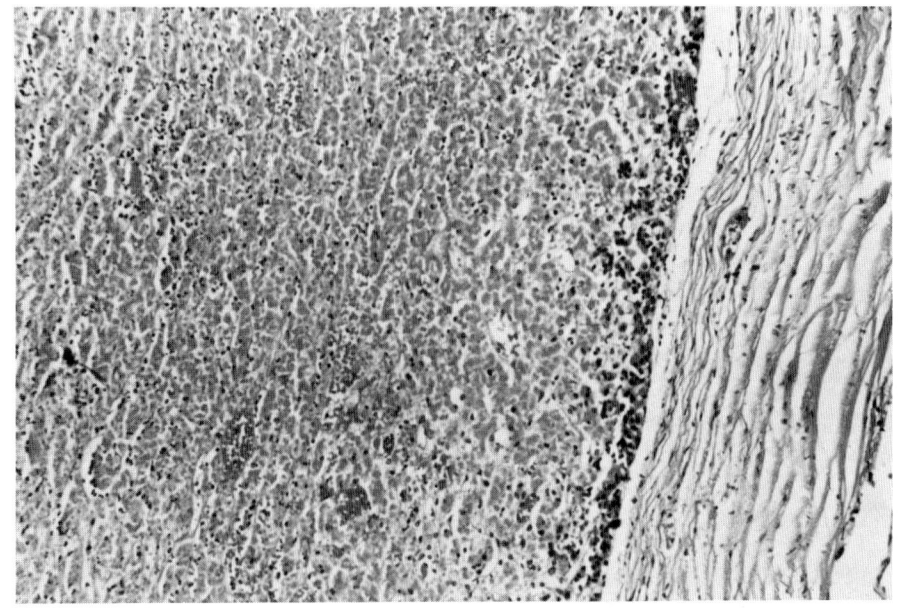

Figure 25.1. Infarction of pituitary. There is loss of all pituitary cells save a few just beneath the capsule. This infarction took place in association with hemorrhage and premature separation of the placenta.

DISORDERS OF THE ADENOHYPOPHYSIS

Hypopituitarism

Hypopituitarism usually involves loss of all anterior pituitary function. The causes include intrapartum infarction (Fig. 25.1), often in association with premature separation of the placenta (*Sheehan's syndrome*), infections, and neoplasms, primary or metastatic. Hypopituitarism often complicates the severe malnutrition of anorexia nervosa (p. 93). Isolated deficiencies of trophic hormones may also occur, as following failure of the hypothalamus to secrete thyrotrophin-releasing factor.

Hyperpituitarism

Hyperpituitarism almost always results from adenomas of the pituitary gland. The principal clinical syndromes of hyperpituitarism are hyperprolactinemia, Cushing's disease, and acromegaly. Pituitary adenomas have traditionally been classified on the basis of their staining characteristics, although it is now possible to determine the precise function of these lesions by immunohistologic methods. Tumors composed of cells that stain as chromophobes can become quite large, elevate the diaphragm of the sella, and compress the optic chiasm, the floor of the third ventricle, and, occasionally, other cranial nerves (Fig. 25.2). They can also invade the sphenoid sinuses, resulting in rhinorrhea. As they enlarge within the sella, they may cause pressure atrophy of the remaining adenohypophysis and hypopituitarism. Tumors composed of acidophil cells are smaller, but may enlarge the sella, while basophil adenomas usually remain small.

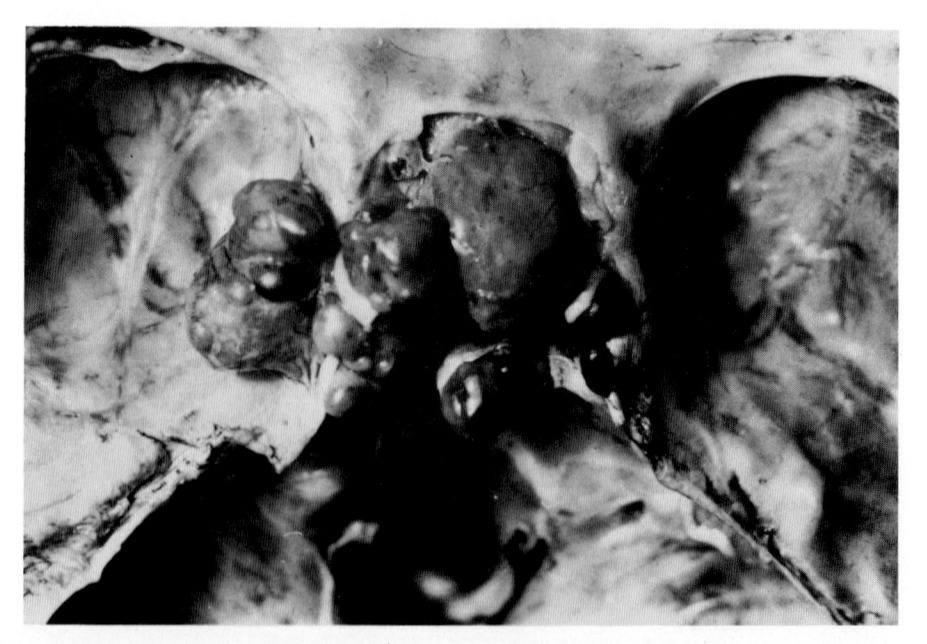

Figure 25.2. Pituitary adenoma. The sella turcica is seen just above *center*. A multinodular tumor mass has penetrated the diaphragm of the sella and is extending laterally into the temporal fossa. This tumor compressed the optic chiasm.

The Endocrine Glands

Pituitary adenomas are thought to comprise about 10% of all intracranial tumors. Recent recognition of the importance of small tumors has greatly changed the statistics, and one study of over 100 unselected autopies reported the incidence of microadenomas to be 27% (Fig. 25.3).

As many as 60% of adenomas secrete prolactin, and fewer produce somatotrophin or ACTH. Perhaps 15% are composed of "null" cells and are nonfunctional.

Hyperprolactinemia

Hyperprolactinemia is a recently recognized disorder which has manifestations of altered pituitary, gonadal, and adrenal cortical function. In women, it may be associated with amenorrhea, galactorrhea, hirsutism, and infertility. In men, there may be impotence, oligospermia, and, occasionally, galactorrhea. At least 80% of patients with hyperprolactinemia have pituitary adenomas, often microadenomas. The increased incidence of adenomas producing prolactin is thought to represent a true increase, probably related to prolonged use of oral contraceptive agents. Prolactin-producing adenomas can often be controlled medically with bromocriptine. They can, however, enlarge rapidly during pregnancy, and pose a serious threat to the patient's vision.

Cushing's Disease

Cushing's syndrome is discussed later in this chapter. It is noted here, however, that half of patients with the syndrome described by Cushing have ACTH-producing pituitary adenomas, usually microadenomas.

Nelson's syndrome occurs in some 40% of patients with Cushing's syndrome who have been treated for pituitary-dependent adrenal hyperplasia by bilateral

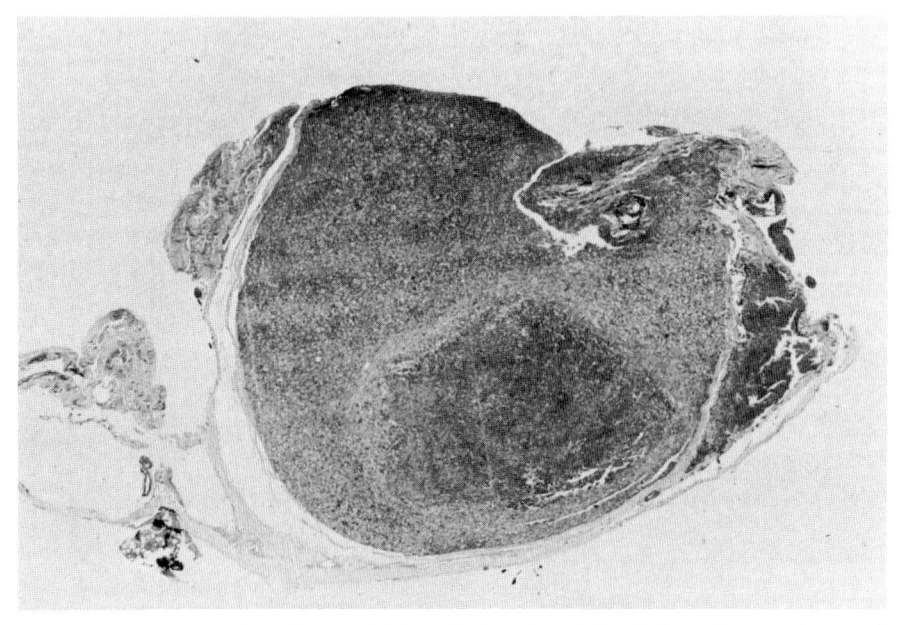

Figure 25.3. Pituitary microadenoma. This sagittal section of the pituitary shows a circumscribed adenoma measuring 3 mm in diameter.

adrenalectomy. Rapidly growing, locally aggressive ACTH-producing pituitary tumors appear in between 18 months and 12 years after surgery.

Craniopharyngioma

Craniopharyngiomas are benign tumors arising from remnants of Rathke's pouch. They are more often suprasellar than intrasellar, and may rarely be found within the sphenoid bone. They comprise between 1 and 3% of intracranial tumors. They may be solid or cystic and often contain sufficient dystrophic calcification to be visible on x-ray. Craniopharyngiomas can destroy the pituitary stalk or compress the base of the brain and optic chiasm. Histologically, the tumor is composed of squamous cells and epithelial cords, often closely resembling the adamantinoma, a tumor of the enamel-forming dental epithelium (Fig. 25.4).

The Empty Sella Syndrome

In this disorder, the sella turcica is enlarged, but contains either a normal or decreased amount of pituitary tissue. It is quite common, perhaps occurring in as many as 5% of adults. There are numerous causes, including intrasellar cysts, herniations of arachnoid tissue through the diaphragm of the sella, healed infarcts, and necrosis of adenomas. The empty sella syndrome occurs most often in obese middle-aged women who have had multiple pregnancies, and it may be accompanied by hyperprolactinema.

THYROID DISORDERS

Hyperthyroidism

Graves' disease is the most common cause of hyperthyroidism. It is an autoimmune disease in which autoantibodies against thyroid stimulating hormone

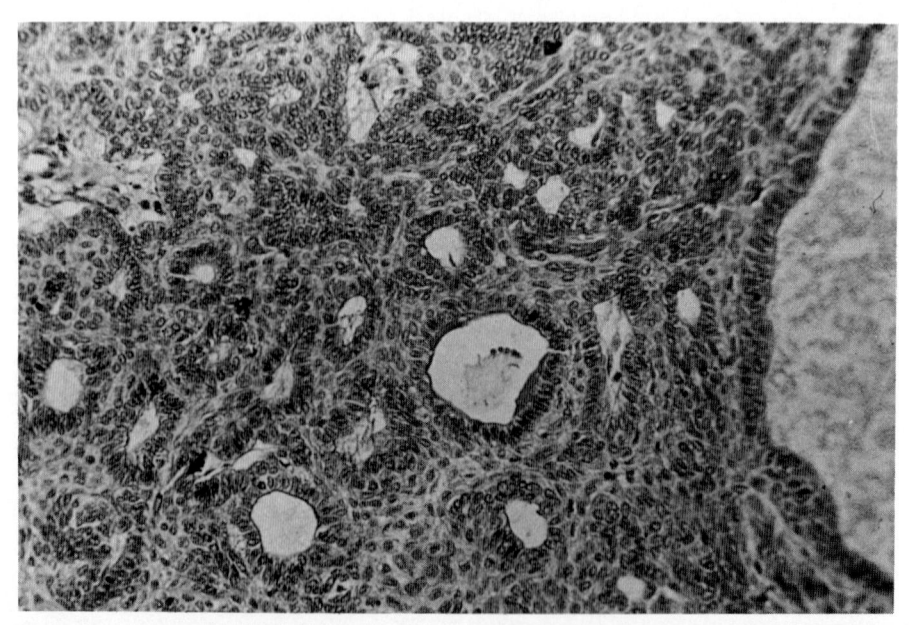

Figure 25.4. Craniopharyngioma. The tumor is composed of squamous cells and epithelial cords and tends to resemble the enamal-forming adamantinoma.

(TSH) receptor sites on the thyroid epithelium react with those sites in a way that stimulates thyroid function. Excessive secretion of T_4 and T_3 results in rapid pulse, palpitations, fatigability, heat intolerance, generalized muscular weakness, and fine tremors. The thyroid gland is enlarged and diffusely hyperplastic. The epithelial cells are tall columnar and often thrown into papillary folds (Fig. 25.5). Little colloid is seen in the follicles. There is increased vascularity and an increase in lymphocytes throughout the gland. There is a 5 to 1 female predominance.

Another feature of Graves' disease is ophthalmopathy, with exophthalmus and weakness of the occular muscles. The binding of an exophthalmus-producing factor, possibly related to thyrotrophin, may be aided by autoimmune globulins.

Hyperthyroidism may also occur in a multinodular gland (*Plummer's disease*). This could be an end result of prolonged stimulation of the gland by TSH and the assumption of functional autonomy by one or more hyperplastic nodules. Hyperthyroidism can also result from functioning ("hot") adenomas, occasionally thyroid carcinomas, early in the course of chronic thyroiditis, and, rarely, from TSH-producing pituitary adenomas. The ophthalmopathy of Graves' disease is not seen with any of these other causes of hyperthyroidism.

Hypothyroidism

Hypothyroidism present at birth is cretinism, and can be due to failure of TSH secretion, abnormal development of the thyroid gland, deficiency or absence of enzymes necessary to thyroglobulin synthesis, or profound iodine deficiency.

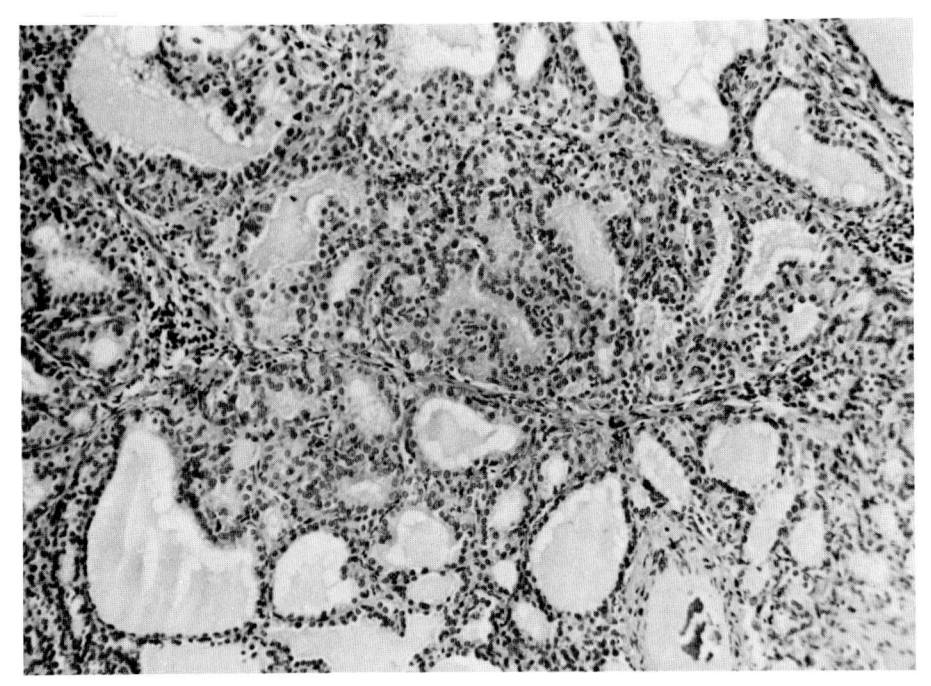

Figure 25.5. Graves' disease. There is diffuse hyperplasia of the thyroid gland. The follicular epithelium is tall and columnar. There is very little colloid, and that which is seen has a scalloped border. The epithelium often assumes a papillary configuration.

Hypothyroidism in adults is manifested by cold intolerance, amenorrhea in women, thickening of hair, thickening and dryness of the skin, lethargy and slow mental responses, and weakness. The term *myxedema* refers, additionally, to a diffuse subcutaneous edema, with high protein and mucopolysaccharide content. Hypothyroidism and myxedema show almost so great a female predominance as does Graves' disease.

Most patients with hypothyroidism have circulating antithyroid antibodies, and probably are manifesting late stages of chronic autoimmune thyroiditis, described below. Hypothyroidism can also be part of hypopituitarism, either involving all pituitary functions or reflecting a specific loss of thyrotrophin-releasing factor. It can follow ablation of the thyroid gland by surgery or by radioactive iodine administration.

Thyroiditis

The most important form of thyroiditis is *Hashimoto's thyroiditis*, an autoimmune disorder characterized by intense infiltration of plasma cells and lymphocytes, often forming lymphoid follicles (Fig. 25.6). The follicular epithelium shows involutional changes and undergoes progressive atrophy. There is a 10:1 female predominance. Although hyperthyroidism may be noted early in the course, the eventual result is hypothyroidism and myxedema.

Several autoantibodies are identifiable in patients with thyroiditis, including antibodies to thyroglobulin, T_3 and T_4, and a microsomal antigen. It is possible that Graves' disease, Hashimoto's thyroiditis (Fig. 25.7), and myxedema are

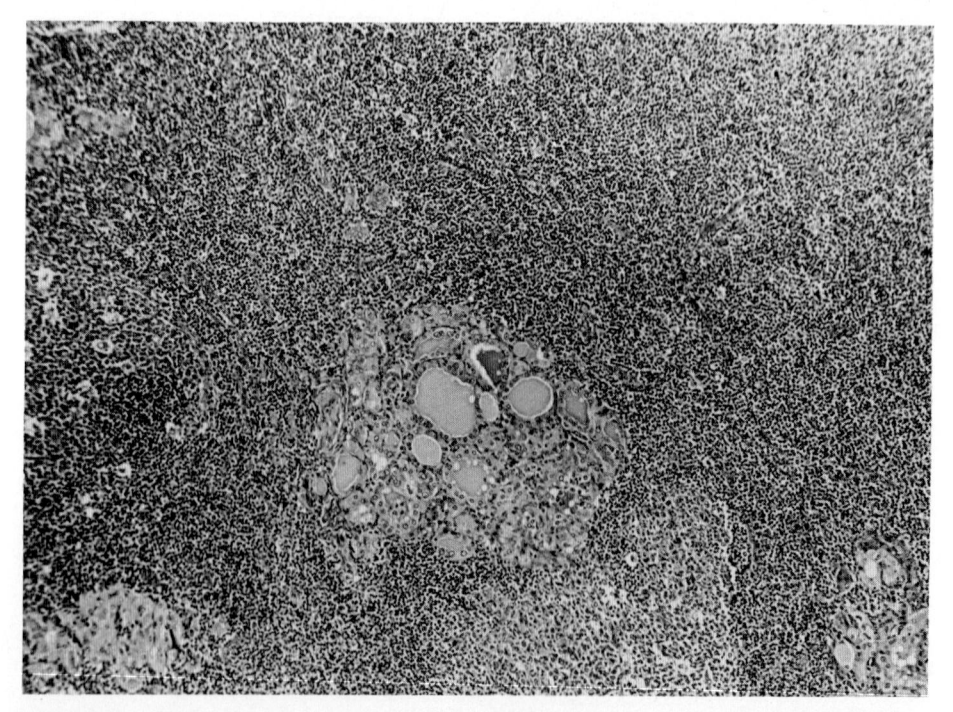

Figure 25.6. Hashimoto's thyroiditis. There is extensive infiltration of plasma cells and lymphocytes, forming lymphoid follicles. There is involution and atrophy of the follicular epithelium.

The Endocrine Glands

closely related autoimmune phenomena, and that they may represent different stages of a single disorder.

Subacute thyroiditis is a disorder manifested by acute swelling of the gland, sometimes with compression of the trachea, fever, and malaise. It is probably a

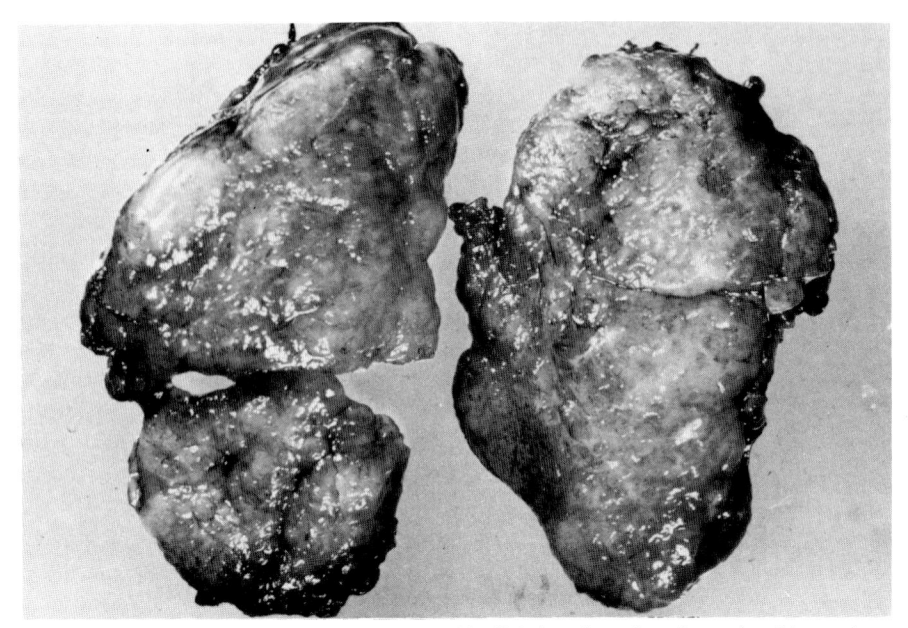

Figure 25.7. Hashimoto's thyroiditis. The gland is slightly enlarged, and very hard in consistency. The cut surfaces have a grayish white appearance.

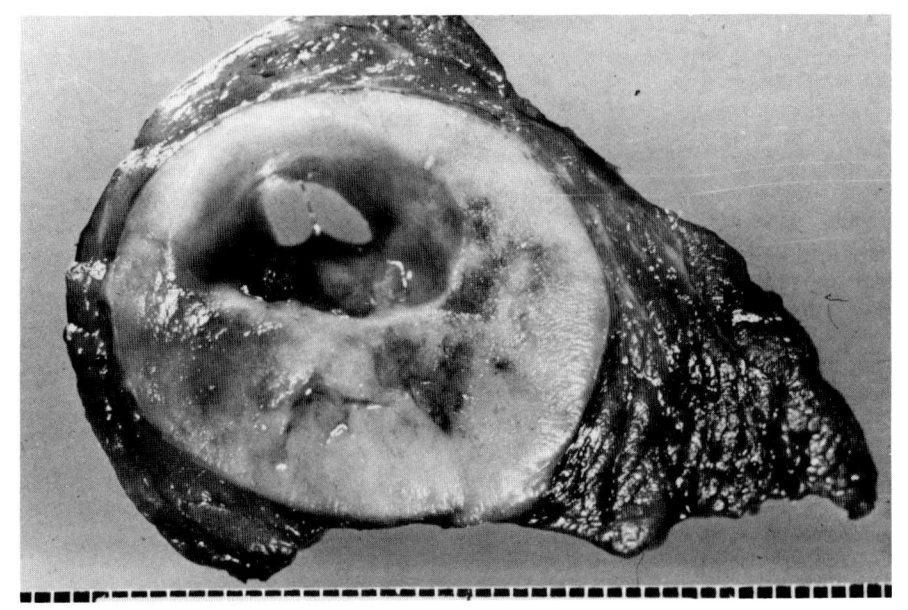

Figure 25.8. Thyroid adenoma. There is a well circumscribed nodule in apparently normal thyroid tissue.

virus infection. Histologically, there is injury to the follicular epithelium, and an inflammatory reaction, often granulomatous, with many large foreign body giant cells. Recovery is complete, although viral thyroiditis could lay the groundwork for an antoimmune thyroiditis.

Tumors of the Thyroid

Adenomas of the thyroid are common lesions. They are well circumscribed, usually solitary nodules up to several centimeters in diameter (Fig. 25.8), and maintain a follicular histologic pattern. Most adenomas take up radioactive iodine, but are not associated with hyperthyroidism.

Thyroid carcinomas account for 0.5% of all cancer deaths. The most frequent type is *papillary carcinoma*. It involves younger patients, usually under 40, and is characterized by slow growth and a relatively benign course, although half of patients have metastases to cervical lymph nodes (Fig. 25.9). Papillary carcinoma does not often cause death. It is TSH-dependent and can often be controlled with thyroxine administration. *Follicular carcinoma* is more aggressive, and tends to metastasize through the bloodstream to the lungs and bone (Figs. 25.10 and 25.11). If removed early, life expectancy is normal, but the overall 5-year survival rate is about 65%. *Undifferentiated carcinoma* occurs in elderly patients. It is a highly anaplastic, malignant tumor and shows extension to the structures of the neck, as weil as distant metastases.

Medullary carcinoma arises from the interstitial "C" cells of the thyroid, and may produce calcitonin and other peptide hormones. It closely resembles other tumors of neuroectodermal derivation and participates in the multiple endocrine

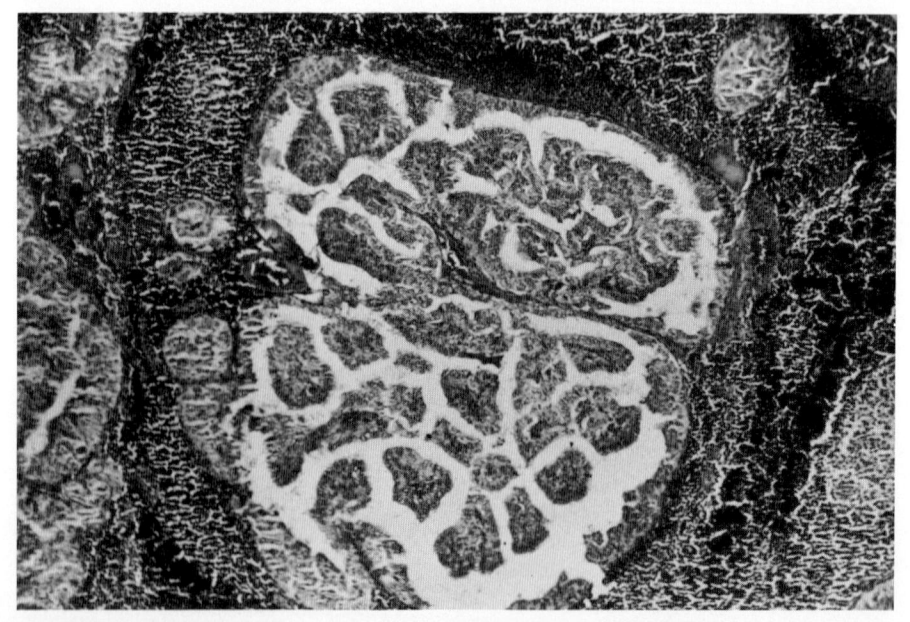

Figure 25.9. Papillary carcinoma of thyroid. This section shows a cervical lymph node metastasis. The papillary configuration of the tumor is apparent.

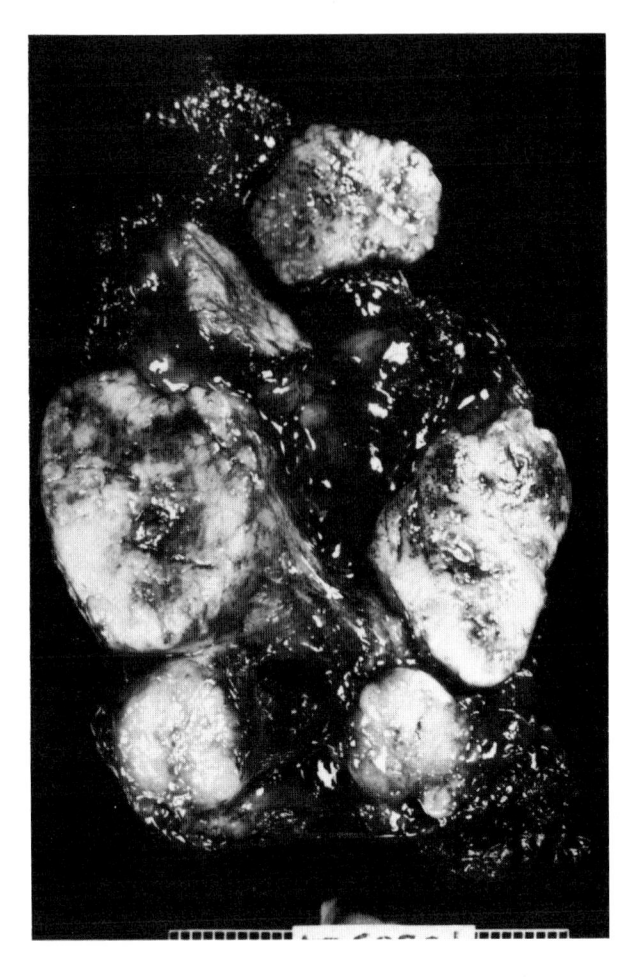

Figure 25.10. Follicular carcinoma of the thyroid. Several firm grayish white tumor nodules have been bisected in this thyroid lobe.

syndromes discussed below. A highly characteristic feature is the deposition of amyloid in the stroma (Fig. 25.12).

The suspected relationship between head and neck irradiation and the incidence of thyroid tumors has been questioned by recent epidemiologic studies (p. 119).

Other Thyroid Enlargements

Both diffuse and nodular nontoxic goiters (a goiter is any enlargement of the thyroid gland) may result from prolonged TSH stimulation of the gland. Such glands can be markedly enlarged and impinge upon the trachea and esophagus (Fig. 25.13). They are common findings in geographic areas of iodine deficiency, but can also be related to the ingestion of certain foods that inhibit thyroid hormone synthesis and to deficiencies of the various enzymes of the thyroid gland. Diffuse enlargement is probably the initial lesion with early diffuse hyperplasia and later involution (*colloid goiter*). Nodularity is probably a function of time and an uneven response of the gland to TSH. As noted earlier, individual

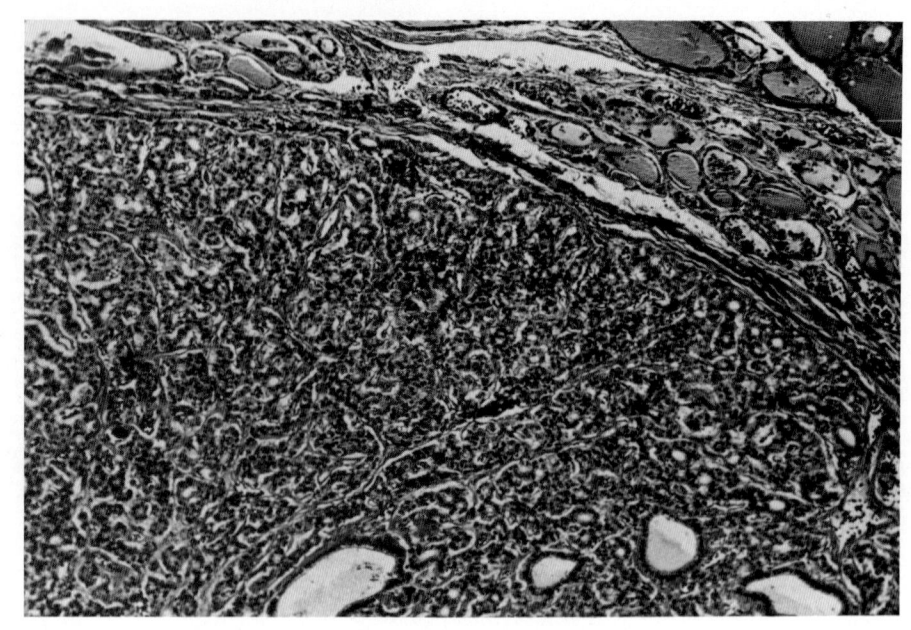

Figure 25.11. Follicular carcinoma. The tumor is quite well differentiated and maintains a follicular pattern. It appears to be well circumscribed and has a delicate capsule.

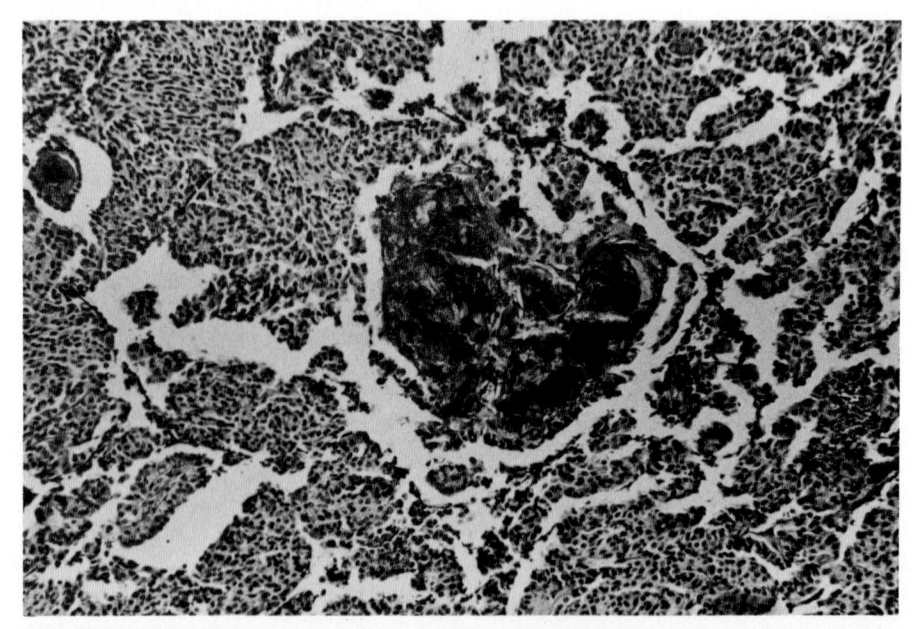

Figure 25.12. Medullary carcinoma of thyroid. The tumor cells are arranged in rather solid masses, separated by a delicate stroma. The material to the *right of center* is a deposit of amyloid, frequently seen in these tumors.

The Endocrine Glands 341

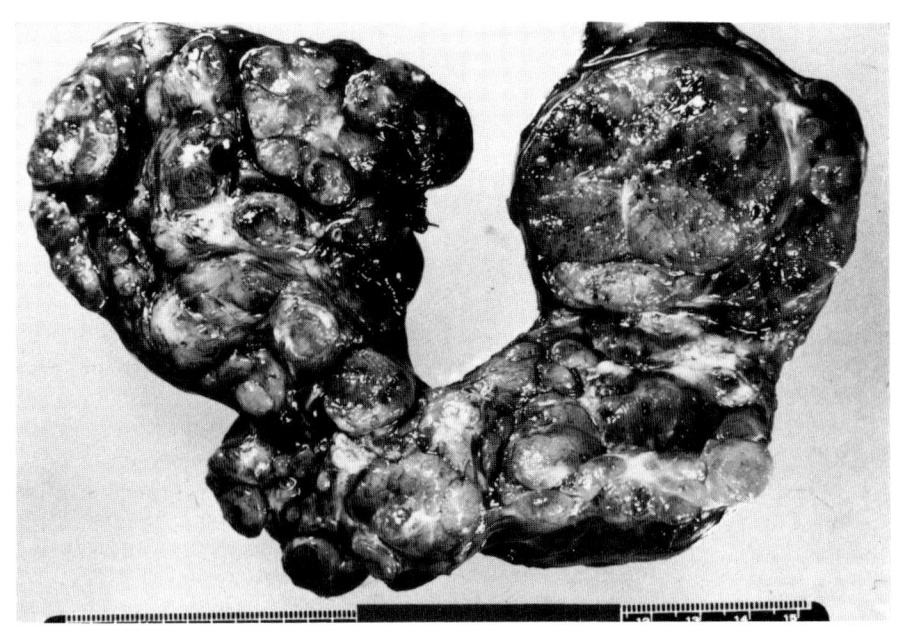

Figure 25.13. Nodular hyperplasia of thyroid. This markedly enlarged and nodular gland weighed 600 g.

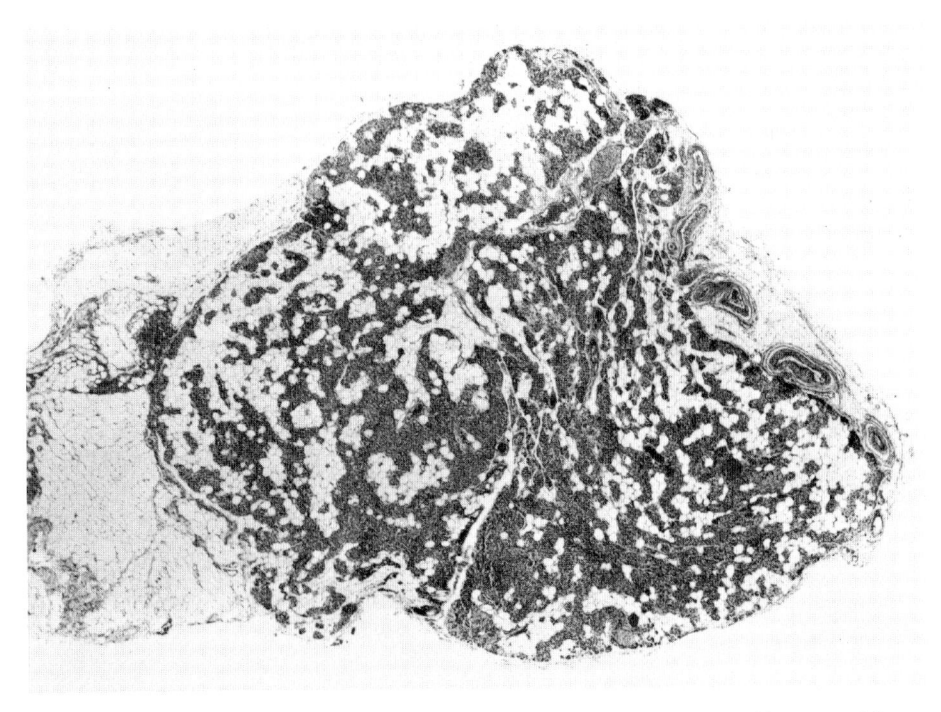

Figure 25.14. Normal parathyroid gland. Half of this structure is occupied by stromal fat.

nodules may occasionally assume autonomy of function and be responsible for hyperthyroidism.

THE PARATHYROID GLANDS

The significance of the parathyroid glands and their lesions relates entirely to disorders of calcium metabolism and to metabolic bone disease. These are discussed in Chapter 31.

Physiologic (secondary) hyperplasia is the most frequently encountered change in the parathyroid glands (Fig. 25.15). It is the expected finding in renal failure, but occurs also in response to intestinal malabsorption of calcium, in vitamin D_3 deficiency, and at times in patients receiving chlorothiazides or glucocorticoids. The glands are slightly or moderately enlarged and have lost their interstitial fat. If hyperplasia has been prolonged, there may be very slow return to normal structure and function when the cause of hyperplasia is corrected. Thus, parathyroid hormone secretion may remain inappropriately high for months or years following successful renal transplantation. At other times, permanent autonomy of function may arise in a setting of secondary hyperplasia (tertiary hyperplasia).

Primary hyperparathyroidism is characterized by persistent hypercalcemia, hypophosphatemia, and hypercalciuria. Patients may manifest the bone disease reflecting excessive osteoclastic and osteocytic bone resorption, *osteitis fibrosa* (p. 422), or they may present with renal stones. Severe hypercalcemia may cause disturbed central nervous system function, coma, and death. The principal cause of primary hyperparathyroidism is an adenoma of one of the parathyroid glands

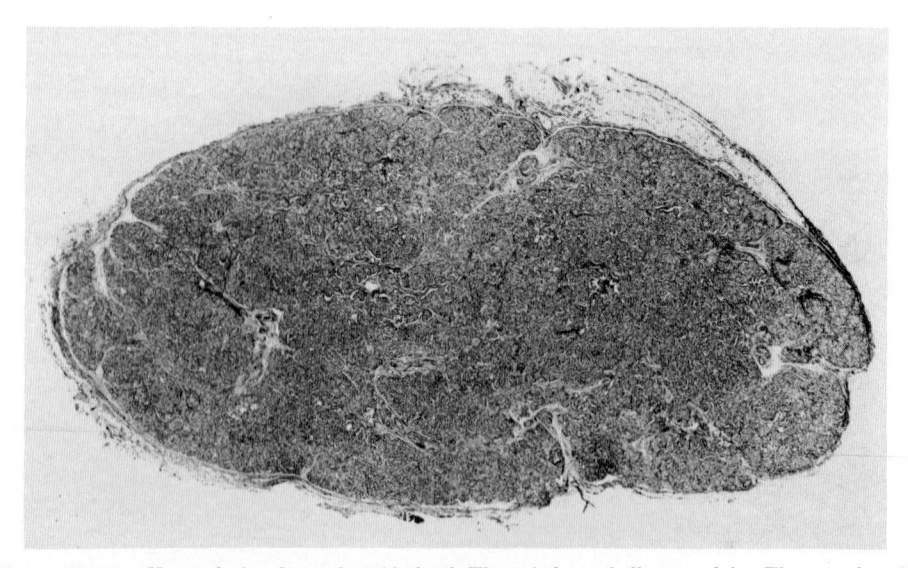

Figure 25.15. Hyperplasia of parathyroid gland. There is loss of all stromal fat. The parathyroid cells here are arranged in solid sheets and consist predominately of chief cells. Compare with Figure 25.14.

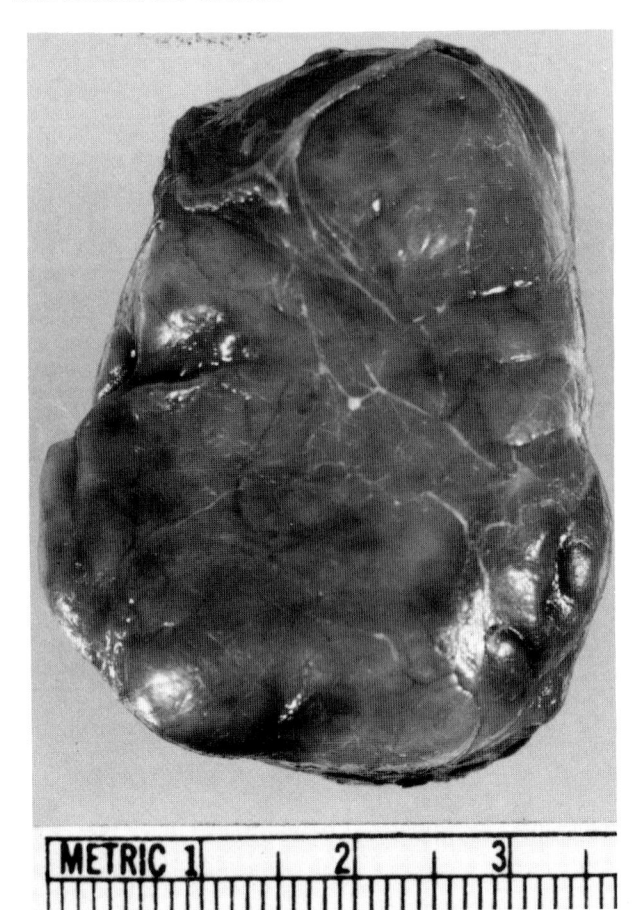

Figure 25.16. Parathyroid adenoma. This tumor was removed from a patient with primary hyperparathyroidism.

(Fig. 25.16). They vary in weight from 100 mg to over 50 g and are encapsulated tumors, composed most often of chief cells arranged in a variety of patterns (Fig. 25.17). They are rarely multiple. *Adenocarcinomas* are uncommon tumors, but also cause hyperparathyroidism. Perhaps 15% of patients with hyperparathyroidism show diffuse *primary hyperplasia*. Although the glands are morphologically indistinguishable from those of secondary hyperplasia, they should be regarded as in the gray zone between hyperplasia and neoplasia. Primary hyperplasia of the parathyroids is often associated with tumors of other endocrine glands (see below). Finally, parathyroid hormone is occasionally secreted by tumors of other endocrine glands or nonendocrine tissues.

Idiopathic hypoparathyroidism is characterized by tetany, thickening of the skull, hypoplasia of dental roots, fragility of fingernails, cataracts, and deposits of calcium in the basal ganglia. It may be an inherited or sporadic disorder, usually becoming apparent in childhood. There may be autoimmune antiparathyroid antibodies, and hypoparathyroidism may be associated with autoimmune disturbances of the thyroid and adrenal cortices and with diabetes mellitus.

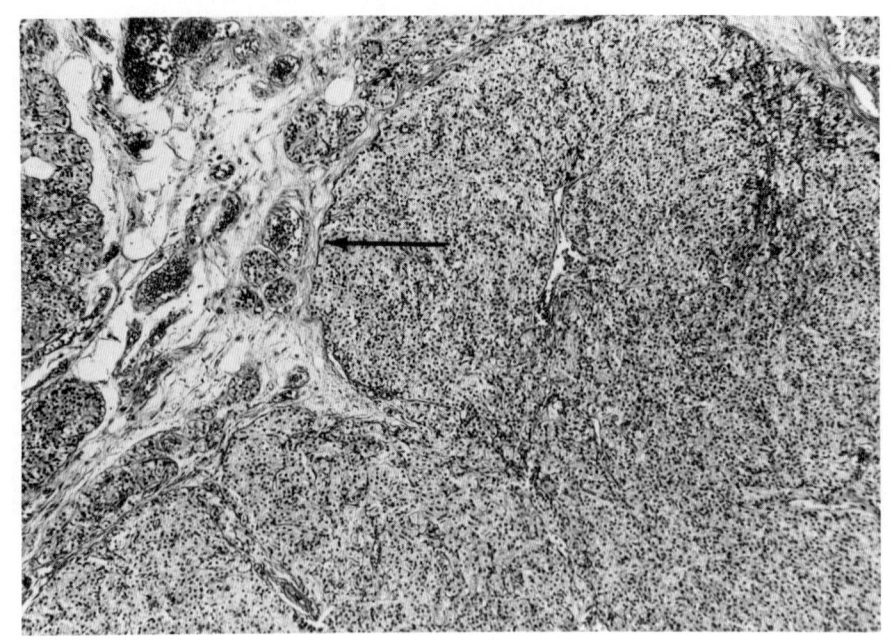

Figure 25.17. Parathyroid adenoma. The tumor is composed of light and dark chief cells. The *arrow* indicates a delicate capsule, separating the tumor from surrounding normal parathyroid tissue.

Pseudohypoparathyroidism results from failure of the peripheral organs to respond to parathyroid hormone. At times, this appears to be a disturbance of receptor sites. The parathyroid glands are enlarged and diffusely hyperplastic, and the concentration of circulating parathyroid hormone is markedly elevated. Patients with this syndrome have short stature, rounded facies, multiple defects in bone development, and mental retardation.

THE ADRENAL GLANDS

The adrenogenital syndromes were discussed briefly in Chapter 10. Emphasis here is placed on adrenal insufficiency, the syndromes associated with adenomas and adenocarcinomas of the adrenal cortex and the pheochromocytoma of the adrenal medulla.

Adrenal Cortical Insufficiency

Adrenal insufficiency, or *Addison's disease*, follows destruction of the adrenal cortex. Until recent years, the principal cause was bilateral adrenal tuberculosis, but this has become a rarity. Destruction of the glands by granulomatous inflammation also occurs in hematogenous dissemination of histoplasmosis (Fig. 25.18). By far the most frequent cause, however, is an autoimmune adrenalitis, in which loss of cortical cells is associated with lymphocyte and plasma cell infiltration (Fig. 25.19). There may be a concurrent Hashimoto's thyroiditis. Severe atrophy of the cortex may result from prolonged administration of glucocorticoids,

The Endocrine Glands 345

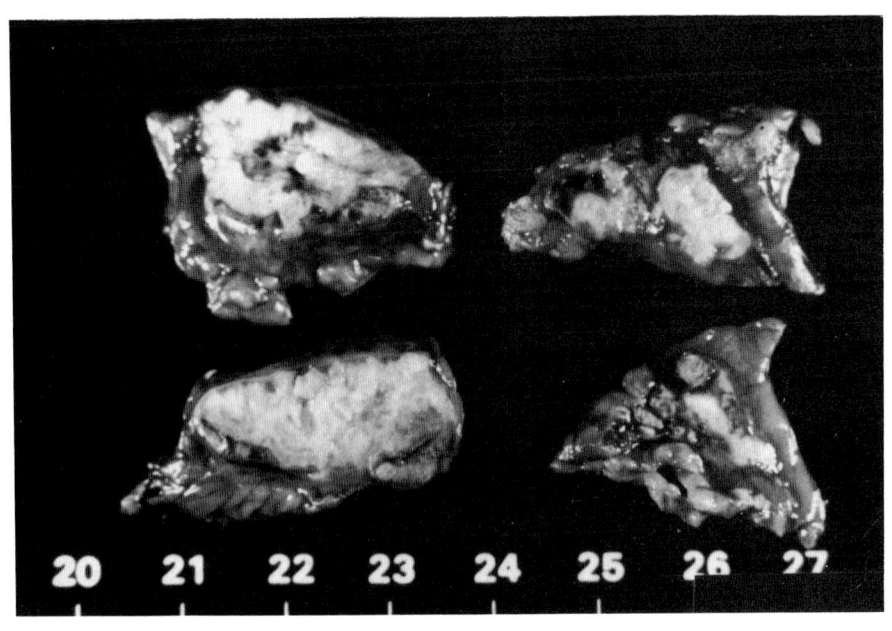

Figure 25.18. These bisected adrenal glands show extensive replacement of the parenchyma by the granulomatous lesions of histoplasmosis. (See also Fig. 4.13.)

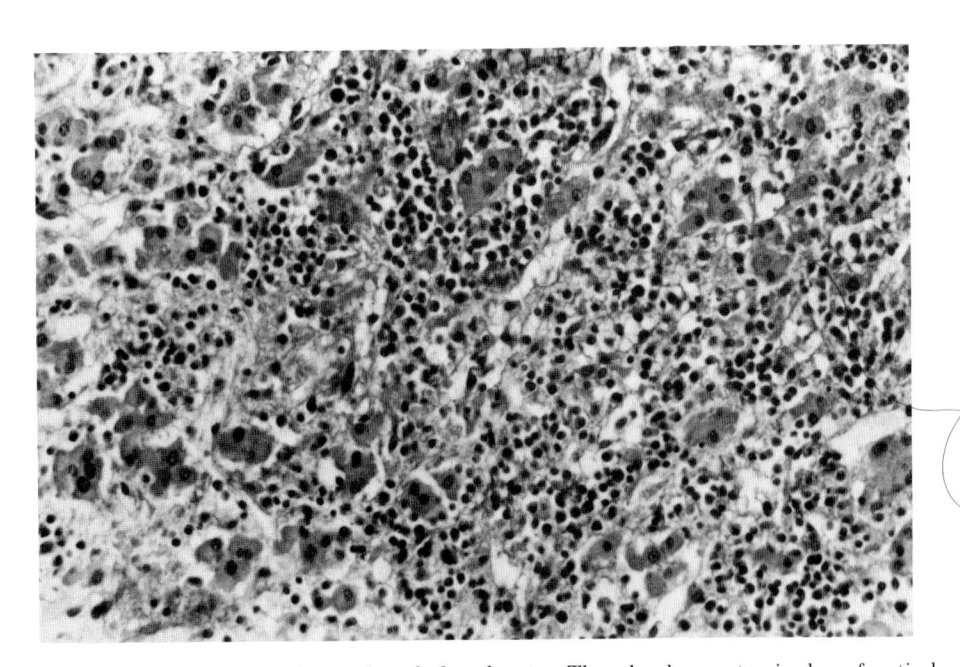

Figure 25.19. Autoimmune destruction of adrenal cortex. There has been extensive loss of cortical cells and striking infiltration of lymphocytes and plasma cells.

and care must be exercised in discontinuing therapy if adrenal insufficiency is to be avoided.

The manifestations of adrenal insufficiency include hyponatremia, hypoglycemia, and hyperkalemia. There is weakness, anorexia, weight loss, and increased pigmentation of skin and mucous membranes. Gastrointestinal disturbances are marked, and diarrhea may precipitate an Addisonian crisis, with severe dehydration and shock.

Adrenal Cortical Tumors

Adenomas of the cortex are common lesions. They vary in size from a few mm to 6 or 8 cm in diameter. They are sharply circumscribed from surrounding cortical tissue, although delicately encapsulated (Fig. 25.20). They generally appear bright yellow on cut surface because of their high lipid content. The tumor cells are well differentiated, difficult to distinguish from normal cortical cells. Adenomas may secrete aldosterone, glucocorticoids, or androgens. As a rule, only a single hormone is secreted. Other adenomas appear to be nonfunctional. The incidence of cortical adenomas is as high as 15% in women over 65.

Adenocarcinomas may be difficult to distinguish from adenomas, unless they have spread beyond the adrenal gland and metastasized to regional lymph nodes or distant structures. They may grow to very large size (Fig. 25.21). Adenocarcinomas may be well differentiated, or anaplastic, are often bright yellow in color, showing areas of hemorrhage and necrosis, and may appear to be well encapsulated. Adenocarcinomas may be associated with Cushing's syndrome, but are particularly likely to cause virilization in women. They may secrete hormones derived from two or all three of the cortical zones.

Primary hyperplasia is encountered in the adrenal cortex, and may be associated with excessive cortisol secretion or with hyperaldosteronism.

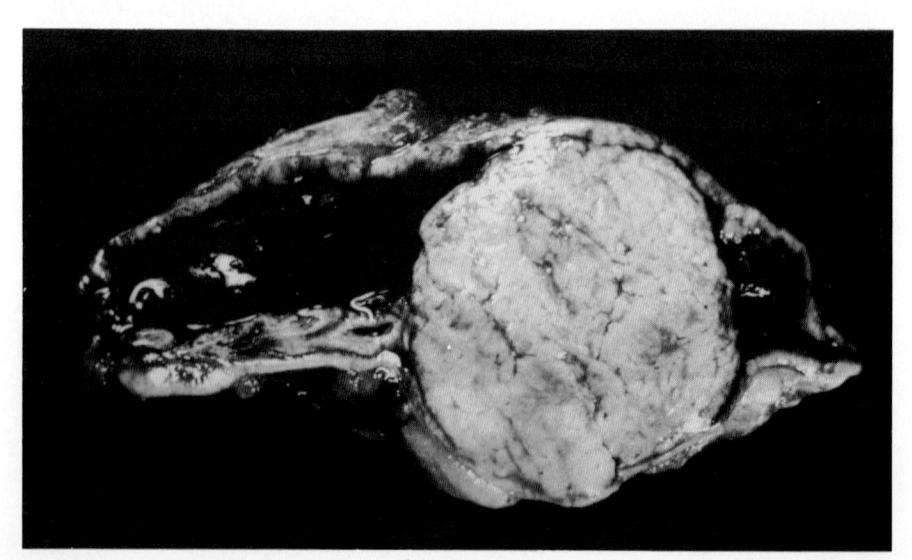

Figure 25.20. Adrenal cortical adenoma. The well circumscribed tumor nodule seen here appeared bright yellow in color, a result of the high lipid content of its cells. It measured 1.5 cm in diameter.

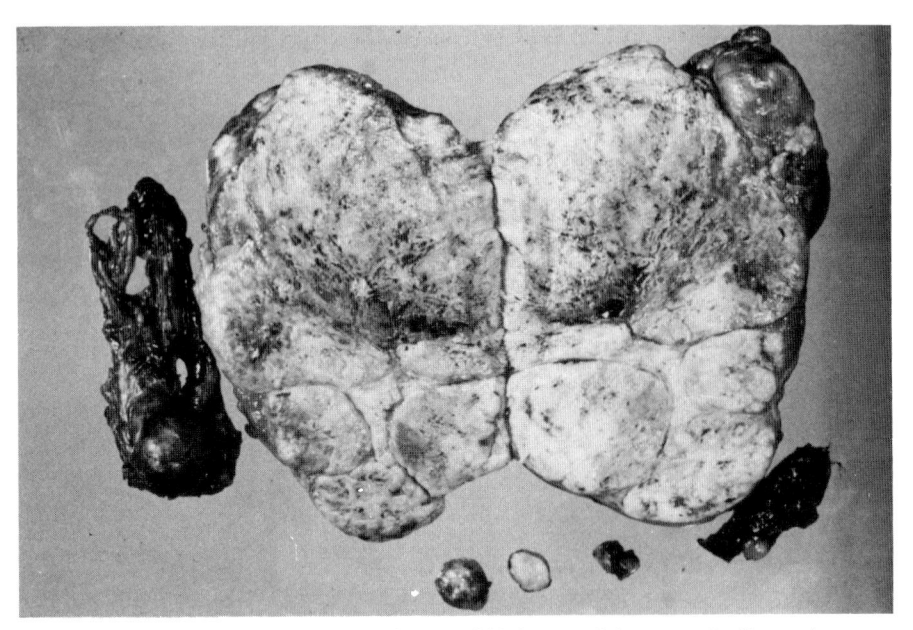

Figure 25.21. Adenocarcinoma of adrenal cortex. This large nodular mass of yellow and gray tumor tissue weighed over 400 g. Several involved lymph nodes are seen.

Cushing's Syndrome

Cushing's syndrome is the result of excessive cortisol secretion. It is characterized by truncal obesity, muscular wasting, moon facies, osteoporosis, hypertension, diabetes mellitus, a tendency to hypochloremic, hypokalemic alkalosis, hirsutism, acne, and predisposition to many types of infections. This syndrome was first described by Harvey Cushing in 1932, and was attributed to a pituitary adenoma composed of basophil cells. It soon became apparent that the syndrome could also reflect adrenal cortical disease, and, later, that it could be related to tumors of nonendocrine organs.

Recent progress in studying patients with the syndrome, including radioimmunoassay of plasma ACTH, the dexamethasone suppression test, refined x-ray polytomography of the sella turcica, and pituitary microsurgery through the sphenoid bone, has made it possible to determine accurately the basis of Cushing's syndrome in the individual patient. Although figures vary markedly, some 50% of patients with Cushing's syndrome have pituitary adenomas, often microadenomas, that secrete excessive ACTH. The adrenal glands respond with bilateral hyperplasia and increased cortisol secretion. This pituitary-dependent Cushing's syndrome is designated Cushing's disease, since it is the disorder originally described by Cushing. In one-fourth of patients, Cushing's syndrome is the result of autonomous cortisol secretion by adrenal adenomas, less frequently by adenocarcinomas, and rarely by primary hyperplasias. In the presence of a cortisol-secreting tumor, the normal adrenal cortical tissue becomes atrophic, and the pituitary basophils show *Crooke's hyaline change*, a cytoplasmic alteration that reflects suppression of ACTH secretion (Fig. 25.22). The remaining 25% of

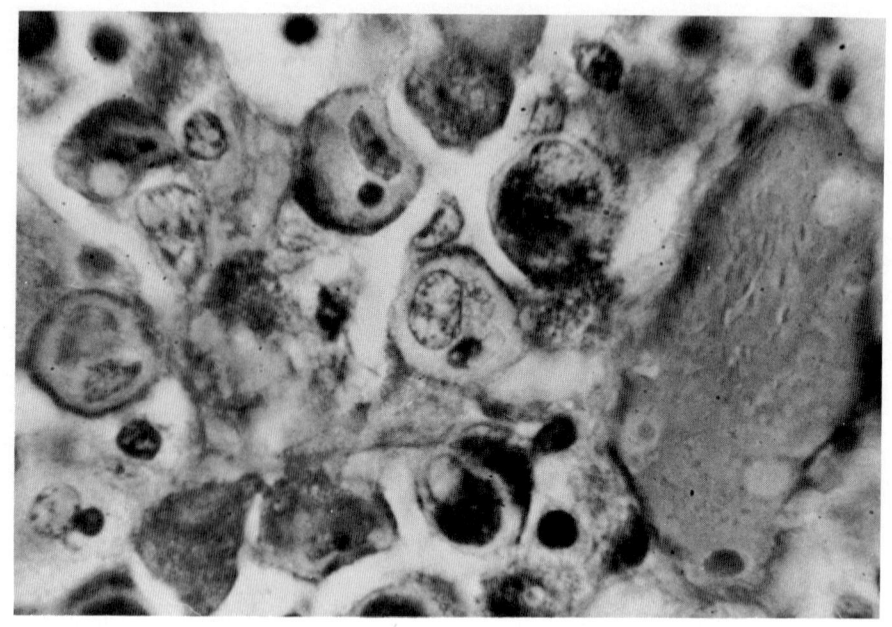

Figure 25.22. Crooke's hyaline change. The pituitary cell in the *center* and several others show loss of cytoplasmic granules and replacement by a pale hyaline appearance. This change in pituitary basophils is a reflection of suppression of pituitary ACTH secretion.

patients with Cushing's syndrome have tumors of the lung, carcinoid tumors, or other tumors composed of neuroectodermal cells that secrete ACTH. Here, again, there is bilateral adrenal hyperplasia. Cushing's syndrome may develop very rapidly in patients with these tumors. They tend to have very high plasma ACTH concentrations and high ketosteroid and corticosteroid levels. They may not show the typical facies and body configuration, but may have profound hypokalemic alkalosis.

Hyperaldosteronism

Primary hyperaldosteronism, or *Conn's syndrome*, is usually the result of a small adrenal cortical adenoma, occasionally a diffuse cortical hyperplasia. The manifestations include hypertension, weakness, metabolic alkalosis, and hypokalemia. Edema is characteristically absent. Secondary hyperaldosteronism is seen in congestive heart failure, in cirrhosis with portal hypertension, and in the nephrotic syndrome, predominately the effect of activity of the renin-angiotensin system.

The Adrenal Medulla

The only important lesions of the adrenal medulla are the tumors *pheochromocytoma* and *neuroblastoma*. Neuroblastoma is discussed in Chapter 35. Pheochromocytomas are catecholamine-producing tumors of pheochromocytes and are associated with sustained or episodic hypertension. They vary considerably in size, and have a brownish cut surface (Fig. 25.23). The cells are usually well

The Endocrine Glands

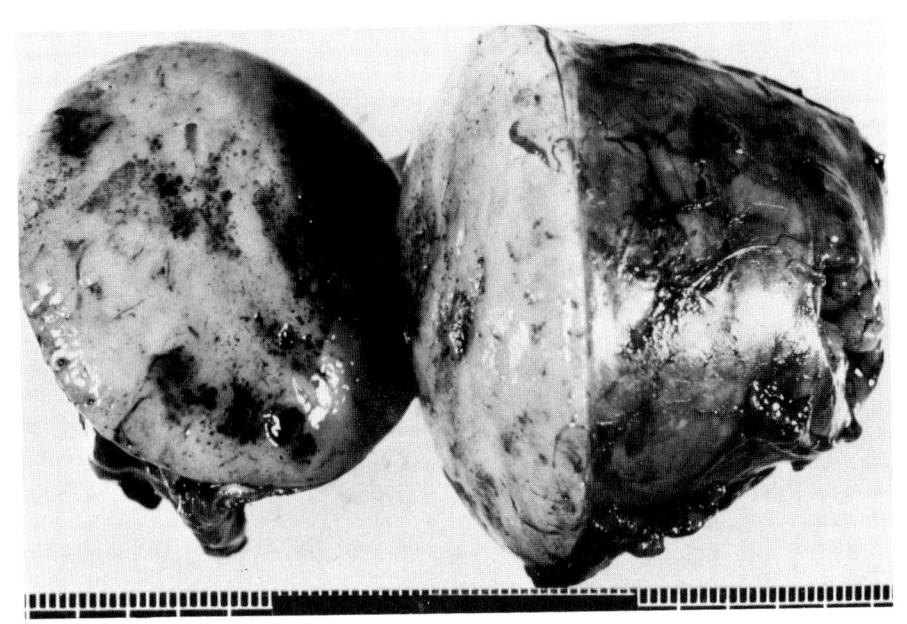

Figure 25.23. Pheochromocytoma. This adrenal medullary tumor had a deep brown color on cut surface.

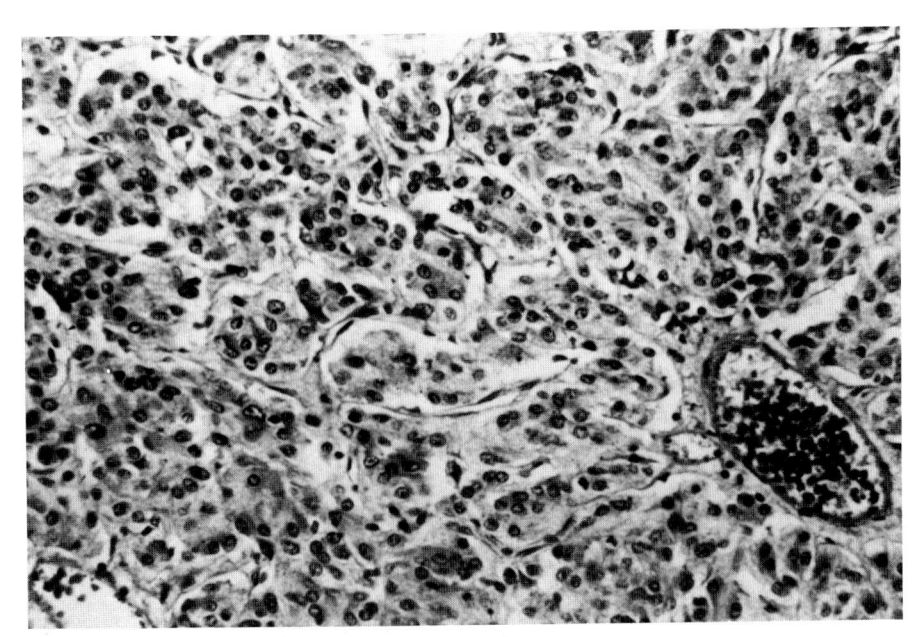

Figure 25.24. Pheochromocytoma. This tumor is well differentiated. The cells have uniform nuclei and abundant cytoplasm, often appearing granular.

differentiated, but some tumors show pleomorphism (Fig. 25.24). Pheochromocytomas are most o′ten benign, but some 10% behave as malignant tumors. Malignant pheochromocytomas are likely to be bilateral, and are often seen as a component of one of the inherited multiple endocrine syndromes.

THE THYMUS

The important lesions of the thymus are hyperplasia and neoplastic thymomas. They are of principal interest because of their association with myasthenia gravis, discussed in Chapter 33.

THE MULTIPLE ENDOCRINE SYNDROMES AND TUMORS OF THE APUD SYSTEM

There are two syndromes consisting of neoplastic lesions of several endocrine glands, both transmitted as autosomal dominants.

Wermer's syndrome (Type I) consists of a pituitary adenoma, a pancreatic islet cell adenoma or adenocarcinoma, and a parathyroid adenoma or primary hyperplasia. The pituitary tumor is most likely to produce growth hormone and result in acromegaly. The parathyroid lesion is usually functional, and the islet cell tumor may produce insulin, glucagon, or gastrin (Figs. 25.25 and 25.26). Excessive gastrin secretion may result in multiple recurrent duodenal peptic ulcers, gastric hypersecretion, and diarrhea (*Zollinger-Ellison syndrome*). Carcinoid tumors are occasionally seen in association with Wermer's syndrome, as may be adrenal cortical and thyroid tumors.

Sipple's syndrome (Type II) consists of medullary (interstitial cell) carcinoma of the thyroid and pheochromocytoma of the adrenal medulla. The adrenal lesions are often bilateral and malignant. Parathyroid adenoma or hyperplasia is a frequent component of this syndrome, and other associated lesions include multiple mucosal neuromas, megacolon, and carcinoid tumors.

These two syndromes, composed of lesions that are morphologically remarkably alike, and the observations relating to the secretion of peptide hormones by

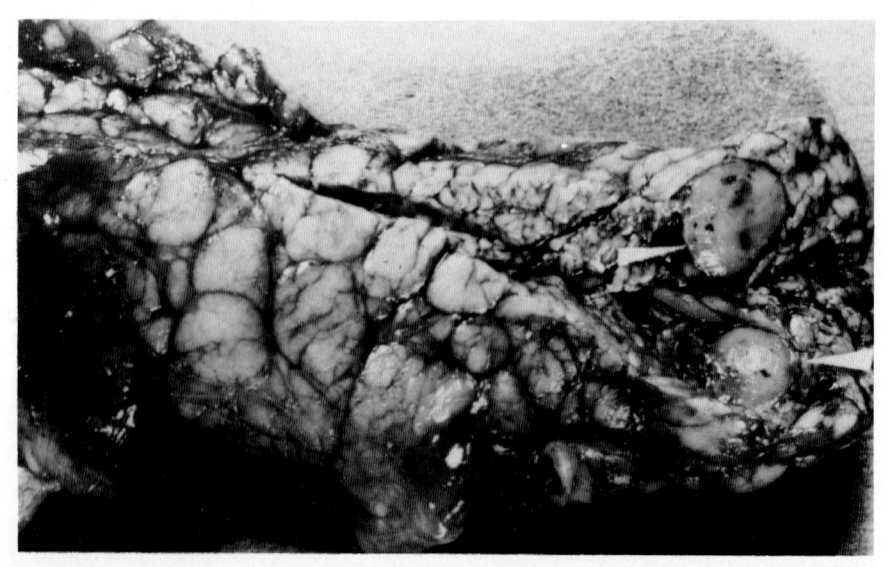

Figure 25.25. Pancreatic islet cell adenoma. The *arrows* point to a bisected adenoma. These lesions are well circumscribed, and appear pinkish gray in color. They are most frequently encountered in the tail of the pancreas.

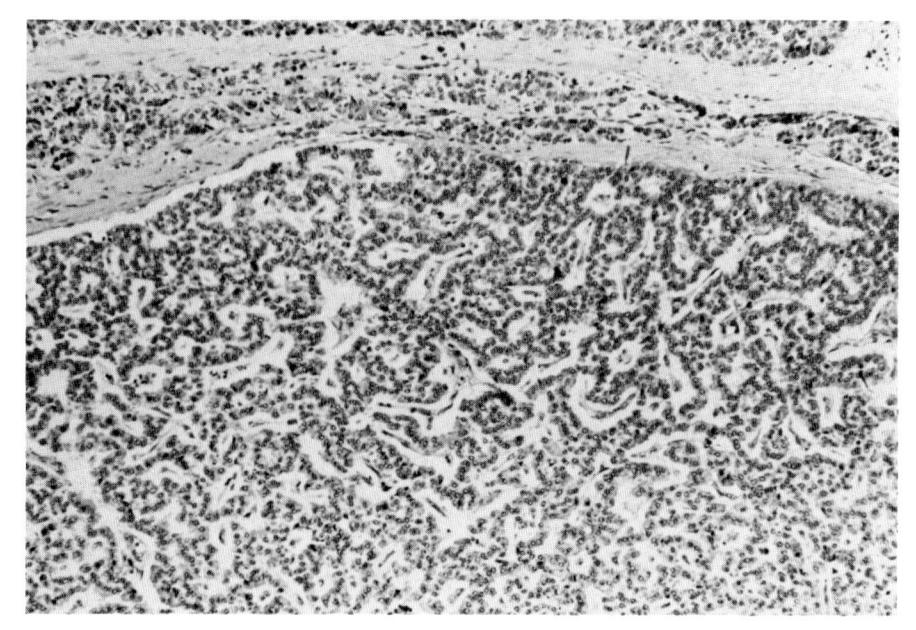

Figure 25.26. Islet cell adenoma. The large tumor nodule resembles normal islet tissue. There is also a striking resemblence to may other tumors of neuroendocrine origin, including carcinoids.

tumors of nonendocrine tissues are best explained by the neuroectodermal origin of their cells. Neuroectodermal cells migrate to the primitive gut and form the adrenal medulla, paraganglia, and the carotid body. From the gut, cells migrate with the buds that form the peptide-producing endocrine glands: hypothalamus, hypophysis, intersitital cells of the thyroid, parathyroids, and islets of Langerhans. Some cells remain in the gastrointestinal tract; others become part of the bronchial mucosa, pancreatic ducts, biliary ducts, or salivary glands. The migrant neuroectodermal cells are APUD cells, for **a**mino **p**recursor **u**ptake and **d**ecarboxylation, and their derivatives produce, or have the capacity to produce, low molecular weight peptide hormones.

Carcinoid tumors are observed throughout the gastrointestinal tract and in the bronchi. Nearly half are in the appendix, and some 15% occur in the ileum. They are all low grade malignant tumors, metastasizing to the liver and to regional lymph nodes. Most carcinoids produce serotonin, which is normally inactivated by the liver. When liver metastases are present, the release of serotonin to the general circulation produces the *carcinoid syndrome*, consisting of diarrhea, vasomotor flushing, asthma, and right-sided endocardial and valvular fibrosis. Carcinoid tumors, which are morphologically indistinguishable from many of the tumors observed in the peptide-producing endocrine glands, can also produce ACTH, antidiuretic hormone, catecholamines, insulin, glucagon, or gastrin.

The capacity of APUD cells to produce any of the peptide hormones is reflected in the hormone secretions of many bronchogenic and pancreatic carcinomas, and the multiple hormones produced by some endocrine tumors, *e.g.*, secretion of ACTH as well as catecholamines by some pheochromocytomas.

Suggested Reading

Abboud CF, Laws ER. Clinical endocrinological approach to hypothalamic-pituitary disease. J. Neurosurg. *51:* 271, 1979.

Bolande, RP. The neurocristopathies. Human Pathol. *5:* 409, 1974.

Heath H III, Hodgson SF, Kennedy MA. Primary hyperparathyroidism. N. Engl. J. Med. *302:* 189, 1980.

Kirby RW, Kotchen TA, Rees ED. Hyperprolactinemia—a review of recent clinical advances. Arch. Intern. Med. *139:* 1415, 1979.

Trindall GT, Hoffman JC Jr. Evaluation of the abnormal sella turcica. Arch. Intern. Med. *140:* 78, 1980.

Zervas NT, Martin JB. Management of hormone-secreting pituitary adenomas. N. Engl. J. Med. *302:* 210, 1980.

Chapter 26

Diabetes Mellitus

Diabetes mellitus and its complications comprise the third leading cause of death in the United States. There are some 10 million diabetics in this country. The incidence of disease doubles with each decade of life, and with every 20% increment of excessive weight. The occurrence of blindness is 25 times that of the general population, and renal disease shows a 15-fold increase. The incidence of atherosclerotic gangrene of the extremities is 5 times as common in diabetics, that of heart disease is doubled.

Diabetes mellitus is not a single disease, but rather a group of disorders that share the common end result of impaired carbohydrate metabolism with secondary effects on protein and fat metabolism. This metabolic disturbance can reflect either altered insulin production or utilization and usually results from complex interactions of genetic and specific environmental factors. Some of these have been discussed in Chapters 9 and 10.

There are major differences between juvenile onset, or insulin-dependent, diabetes and maturity onset, or non-insulin-dependent, diabetes.

JUVENILE ONSET DIABETES

Ten per cent of diabetics fall into this category. The onset of disease is usually before age 25, and is often abrupt. The course of illness is usually severe, and renal failure from complicating diabetic nephropathy is the major cause of death. Patients with juvenile onset disease almost always have decreased insulin secretion, and insulin replacement is essential in treatment.

Juvenile onset diabetes has a strong association with certain HLA haplotypes, particularly B8, B15, Dw3, and Dw4, and individuals with two disease-related alleles have a 10 times greater likelihood of developing overt disease. Despite strong genetic influences, the concordance of this type of diabetes in identical twins is only 50%, indicating that other factors are of major import.

The pancreas in juvenile onset diabetics shows a striking reduction in β-cells of the islets of Langerhans to some 10% of normal. Most patients have cytotoxic autoantibodies to β-cells demonstrable in their sera, particularly early after the onset of disease. Of particular significance are islet cell surface antibodies that, in the presence of complement, can lyse rat β-cells maintained in culture. It is of interest that juvenile onset diabetes may be associated with such other autoimmune disorders as Graves' disease, Hashimoto's disease, Addison's disease, hypoparathyroidism, pernicious anemia, and myasthenia gravis.

The induction of autoimmunity is thought to result from virus infections. There is good evidence that juvenile onset diabetes can follow infection by Coxsackie B and mumps viruses, and cytomegalovirus, Epstein-Barr virus, and varicella and rubella viruses have also been implicated. The time interval between infection and onset of diabetes may be very short (Coxsackie B infections) or might be as long as 15 to 20 years in the case of intrauterine rubella infection.

Juvenile onset diabetes, then, would appear to result from genetic factors that predispose to an altered immunologic response to certain virus infections. Autoimmunity might also follow exposure to environmental chemicals that can injure the β-cells.

MATURITY ONSET DIABETES

Maturity onset diabetes is usually diagnosed after the age of 40. Its onset tends to be gradual and it runs a prolonged course, with death most often relatable to severe vascular disease. Maturity onset diabetes accounts for 90% of all diabetes.

Although maturity onset diabetes is not associated with known HLA alleles, there is a strong genetic influence in the disorder, and concordance of disease in identical twins approaches 100%. In most patients, nutritional factors are highly significant, and the disorder becomes overt in the presence of obesity.

Obesity-related diabetes is a disease of insulin receptors. Although insulin secretion may be normal or increased, the enlargement of fat cells is accompanied by a decrease in the number of insulin receptor sites on the cell membrane. Receptor sites are also reduced in number in muscle cells. Reduction of caloric intake and weight loss tend to return the numbers of receptor sites to normal. Most patients with maturity onset diabetes related to obesity do not require insulin therapy, but can be maintained well with weight reduction and oral hypoglycemic agents. Nutrition also plays an important role in the severity of the atherosclerosis that frequently complicates maturity onset diabetes. Atherosclerosis in these patients correlates well with obesity and saturated fat consumption. It is rare in diabetics in undernourished populations.

Other mechanisms may also result in maturity onset diabetes. These include the production of abnormal insulins or proinsulins, circulating insulin antagonists, mutations of the receptor binding sites of the insulin molecule, and the formation of antibodies to the insulin receptor sites.

THE PATHOLOGY OF DIABETES MELLITUS

Most of the morphologic findings in patients with diabetes reflect its complications; very few are inherent to the disease.

The pancreas may appear completely normal in both juvenile onset diabetes and maturity onset diabetes, but the islets of Langerhans are frequently abnormal in juvenile onset diabetes. They tend to be small and decreased in number, and contain few if any β-cells. Early in the disease, lymphocytic infiltration may be prominent, suggesting that cell-mediated immunity plays a role in the autoimmune destruction of β-cells. The islets are completely normal in most patients with maturity onset diabetes. Some show hyalinization of the islets, and the hyaline material often has the tinctorial characteristics of amyloid (p. 325).

The microangiopathy of diabetes is fundamental to the disease. It consists of a striking thickening of all capillary basement membranes, often observable long before there is chemical or clinical evidence of disease. The basement membrane thickening is striking in the capillaries of skin and skeletal muscle, and leads to characteristic changes in the renal glomerulus and the retina.

Capillary *microaneurysms*, although not pathognomonic of diabetes, occur in many tissues, including the retina, the renal glomerulus, and the myocardium.

The important complications of diabetes involve the blood vessels, kidneys, eyes, and peripheral nerves. They occur in both juvenile onset and maturity onset diabetes. Renal complications tend to be more severe in the former, atherosclerosis more severe in the latter. It is of interest that many of the late complications occur in tissues that do not require insulin for glucose uptake.

Several mechanisms are involved in the late complicatons, including an unexplained premature aging of body cells. Accumulations of sugar alcohols, especially sorbitol, a metabolic intermediate of glucose, can change intracellular osmotic pressure and lead to swelling and injury. This mechanism is important in the development of cataracts, in diabetic neuropathy, and possibly in some of the vascular lesions. Glycosolation of amino groups of cellular proteins may also contribute to altered cell functions.

Vascular Disease

Atherosclerosis tends to be more severe in the diabetic, to have an earlier onset and a more rapid course, and to involve both large and small arteries. Ischemic heart disease and a high incidence of occlusive peripheral vascular disease are the principal consequences. It should be noted that the severity of atherosclerosis may not correlate well with the duration of clinically overt diabetes.

Arteriolar hyalinization and hypertrophy also tend to be marked, particularly in the kidney, in part, at least, related to the high incidence of hypertension. It is possible, however, that arteriolar sclerosis in diabetes may be a primary change, and contribute to hypertension, rather than only a reflection of existing hypertension.

Diabetic Nephropathy

The kidneys may be involved in several ways in diabetes. The high incidence of hypertension is, of course, reflected in nephrosclerosis. A pathognomonic feature of this nephrosclerosis, however, is that efferent as well as afferent arterioles show hyalinization of their walls.

There is an increased incidence of pyelonephritis in diabetes, not infrequently accompanied by papillary necrosis. This latter may be related to thickening of the vasa recta, making the papillae highly subject to ischemic injury.

The most characteristic renal lesion in diabetes is intercapillary glomerulosclerosis, or Kimmelstiel-Wilson disease. This consists of an increase in mesangial matrix and cellularity, either diffuse in distribution or accompanied by striking mesangial nodules (Fig. 26.1). Intercapillary glomerulosclerosis is one of the principal causes of the nephrotic syndrome, but also leads to progressive renal failure. The glomeruli in diabetic patients tend to be much larger than normal, and, early in disease, the glomerular filtration rate may be considerably elevated.

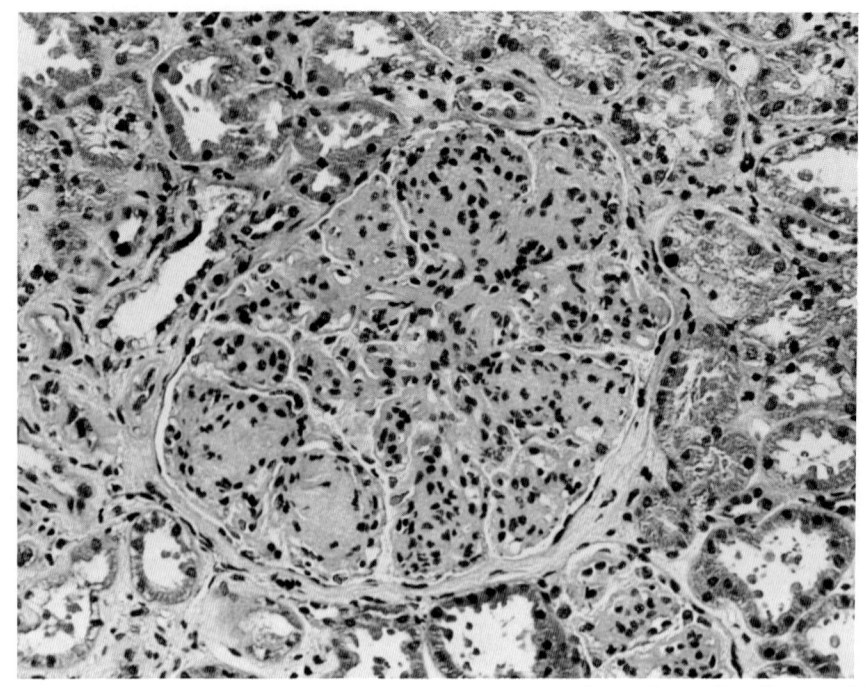

Figure 26.1. Nodular intercapillary glomerulosclerosis. This large glomerulus shows multiple nodules composed of mesangial matrix and incorporated cellular elements. The mesangium is generally increased and, where visible, the capillary walls are thickened.

Manifestations of intercapillary glomerulosclerosis usually appear some 10 to 15 years after diabetes is diagnosed, but they may occasionally occur much earlier. More than 50% of juvenile onset diabetics die of this complication.

Eye Changes

Diabetic retinopathy is related to the duration of diabetes and consists of capillary aneurysms (Fig. 26.2), beading of vessels at the nerve head, exudates due to leakage of proteins through diseased capillary walls, hemorrhages, microinfarcts, and proliferative retinitis. The latter results from hemorrhage into the vitreous, with organization and scar formation that can result in retinal detachment and blindness. *Cytoid bodies*, seen in microinfarcts, are degenerated nerve endings.

There is a close association between diabetic retinopathy and nephropathy, often referred to as the diabetic renal-retinal syndrome. By the 20th year of illness, most juvenile onset diabetics manifest both renal failure and loss of vision. The incidence of retinopathy has been recorded to be as high as 97% in uremic diabetics.

Cataracts are thought to be the result of sorbitol accumulation in the lens fibers. They are often described as "snowflake" cataracts, and are seen most in juvenile onset diabetes.

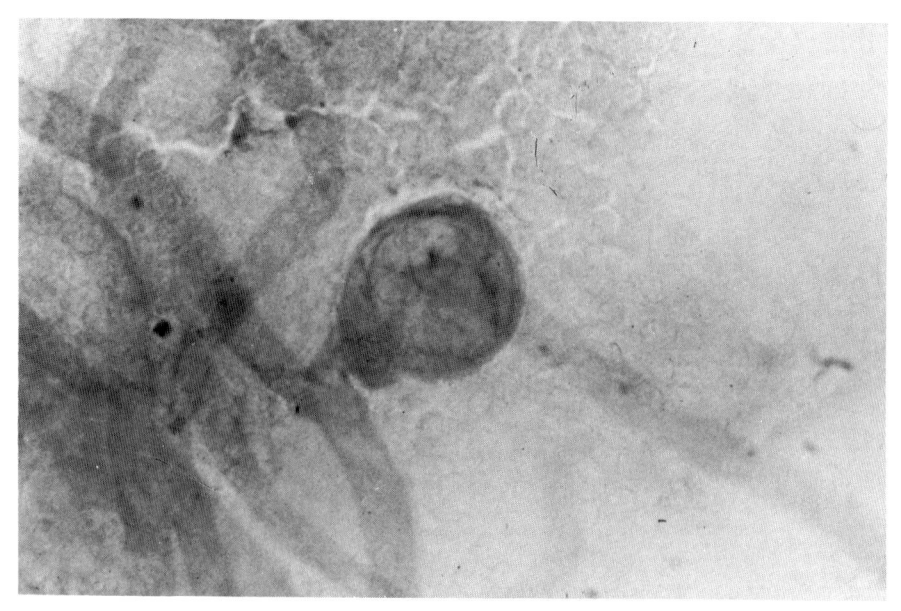

Figure 26.2. Retinal microaneurysm. An aneurysm arising from the wall of a capillary is seen in the *center* of the field. These lesions, characteristic but not pathognomonic of diabetes, are observed also in glomeruli and the myocardium.

Diabetic Neuropathy

Diabetic neuropathy consists of segmental demyelination of peripheral nerves, thought to be metabolic, rather than vascular, in origin. There is symmetrical sensory and, to a lesser extent, motor loss, most marked in the lower extremities. Loss of pain sensation is responsible for repeated injuries and ulceration of the legs. Postural hypotension may be a manifestation of diabetic neuropathy.

Metabolic Control and the Complications of Diabetes

It has long been debated whether the severity of the complications of diabetes can be influenced by careful metabolic control of the disorder. Although there is currently no answer, new techniques of controlling diabetes may clarify the question. These include islet transplantation, and sophisticated automated mechanical devices to control insulin administration. Of particular interest is the effect on vascular disease. There are no known diabetes-linked genetic determinants of atherosclerotic vascular disease, and it is hoped that good metabolic control will decrease the risk factors for atherosclerosis.

Suggested Reading

Drash AL. The etiology of diabetes mellitus. N. Engl. J. Med. *300:* 1211, 1979.
Factor SM, Okun EM, Minase T. Capillary microaneurysms in the human diabetic heart. N. Engl. J. Med. *302:* 384, 1980.
Friedman EA. Diabetic renal-retinal syndrome. Arch. Intern. Med. *140:* 1149, 1980.
Gabbay KH. The insulinopathies. N. Engl. J. Med. *302:* 165, 1980.
Williamson JR, Kilo C. Vascular complications in diabetes mellitus. N. Engl. J. Med. *302:* 399, 1980.

Chapter 27

The Female Genital Tract

DEBORAH E. POWELL, M.D.

This chapter discusses the pathology and pathophysiology of some of the diseases affecting organs of the female genital tract. The female genital tract is a system of interrelated organs, including the vulva, vagina, cervix and uterus, Fallopian tubes, and ovaries. Since the number of organs in this system is large, the number of diseases affecting them is great. Thus, only a few of the major diseases are covered in this chapter which is not in any way intended to be comprehensive. The organs of the female genital system are discussed in an ascending fashion beginning with the vulva and ending with the ovaries.

VULVA

Vulvar Carcinoma

The most common type of cancer affecting the vulva is squamous cell carcinoma. It is more common in older patients, although it may be seen in young individuals. Like most squamous cell carcinomas it metastasizes first to regional lymph nodes. The prognosis of this type of squamous cancer is dependent on the degree of differentiation of the lesion, its size, and the presence or absence of metastatic spread. *Bowen's disease* is a type of intraepithelial squamous cell carcinoma which may be seen in the area of the vulva (Fig. 27.1).

VAGINA

Vaginitis

Inflammation of the vagina may be due to infections or to chronic irritation or hormonal imbalances. Common infectious causes of vaginitis include trichomonas and candida. *Trichomonas* organisms may be seen in secretions as well as in Pap smears taken from the vagina and cervix. This organism also inhabits the male urethra, where it may be asymptomatic. Fungal infection, caused most commonly by *Candida albicans*, is especially prevalent in pregnant and diabetic patients and produces severe itching and a thick cheesy yellowish white discharge. Another relatively common form of vaginitis is *atrophic vaginitis* seen in the postmenopausal patient or in younger individuals who have been castrated. It is felt to result from low levels of estrogens and lack of maturation of the vaginal epithelium.

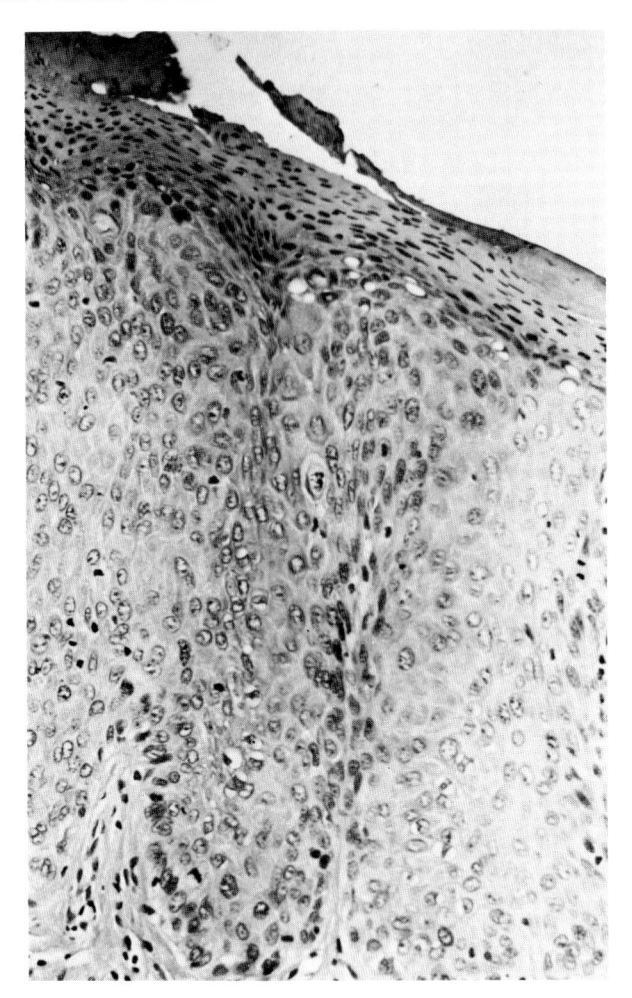

Figure 27.1. Bowen's disease is a form of *in situ* squamous carcinoma of the vulva. The malignant cells extend through the entire thickness of the epidermis and there are nuclei present in the keratin layer (parakeratosis).

Vaginal Adenosis and Clear Cell Carcinoma

Vaginal adenosis is the presence of glands and glandular epithelium within the squamous epithelium or superficial submucosal tissues of the vagina. This lesion has received special prominence because of its association in a large number of patients with maternal diethylstilbestrol ingestion during pregnancy. Its occurrence is, however, not restricted to patients whose mothers received this drug. The glandular epithelium within the vaginal wall may resemble epithelium of Fallopian tube, endocervix (Fig. 27.2), or endometrium and may undergo squamous metaplasia. *Clear cell adenocarcinoma* of the vagina is an unusual type of malignancy which has also been identified in young women whose mothers received diethylstilbestrol during pregnancy. It should be emphasized, however, that less than 1% of exposed women will develop this tumor. Histologically, the tumor resembles the clear cell carcinomas seen in the ovary and other sites in the female genital tract and is characterized by varying cystic and papillary patterns, clear cells, and "hobnail" cells (Fig. 27.3). Although uncommon, the prognosis for this tumor is quite poor.

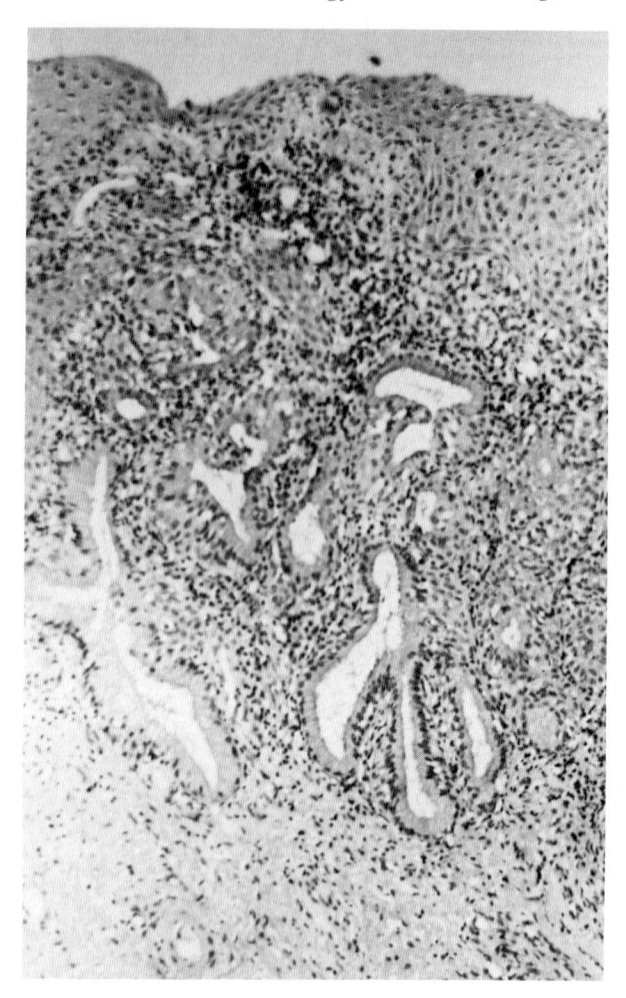

Figure 27.2. Vaginal adenosis. Endocervical type glands are present beneath the squamous mucosa of the vagina.

CERVIX

Cervicitis

Acute cervicitis is frequently due to pyogenic bacteria, and is likely to occur after childbirth or in association with gonococcal infections. Acute cervicitis may also be due to other infectious agents, notably herpes virus II. *Chronic cervicitis* can be seen in a high percentage of adult females and may be symptomatic or asymptomatic. In most instances, the etiologic agent is not known. The chronic inflammatory cell infiltrate and subsequent episodes of inflammation and repair may cause obstruction of the endocervical glands, with trapping of mucous secretion within these glands and ultimate formation of large *Nabothian cysts* which may be seen on the surface of the cervix.

Cervical Intraepithelial Neoplasia and Invasive Carcinoma

In response to repeated episodes of chronic inflammation and irritation, the cervical epithelium may undergo morphologic changes. These are most likely to

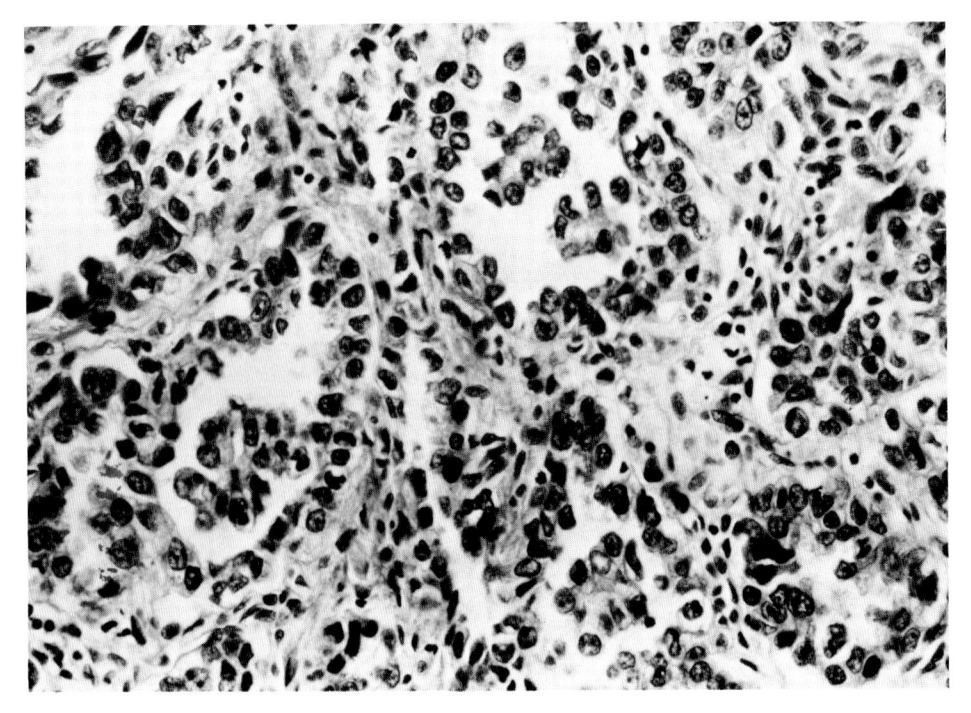

Figure 27.3. Clear cell adenocarcinoma of the vagina. The tumor forms cystic spaces lined by "hobnail" cells with a large nucleus protruding into the cyst lumen.

occur in the transformation zone or squamocolumnar junction of the cervix. The epithelial abnormalities that may occur are squamous metaplasia, epithelial dysplasia, and carcinoma *in situ*. The latter two epithelial abnormalities have been referred to collectively as cervical intraepithelial neoplasia and are felt to represent precursor lesions for invasive carcinoma of the cervix. *Squamous metaplasia* is felt to represent a protective mechanism whereby the easily damaged ciliated mucin-producing epithelium of the endocervical canal and glands is replaced by a thicker stratified squamous epithelium (see Fig. 13.5). While squamous metaplasia is not considered to be a premalignant epithelial alteration, *dysplasia* with its attendant alterations in individual cell morphology and cellular maturation patterns is felt to represent one of the first stages of neoplastic transformation. Dysplasia is characterized as mild, moderate, or marked, based on the extent of the morphologic and maturation alterations in the epithelium (Fig. 27.4). *Carcinoma in situ* represents a full thickness alteration of the cervical epithelium and represents the stage of cervical neoplasia immediately preceding invasive carcinoma (Fig. 27.5). While not all cases of carcinoma *in situ* progress to invasive squamous carcinoma, most of them have this potential, although the time interval necessary for the invasive process to occur may be as long as 10 to 20 years. The varying degrees of dysplasia are considered to have a lesser chance of developing into invasive malignancy, although they, too, are

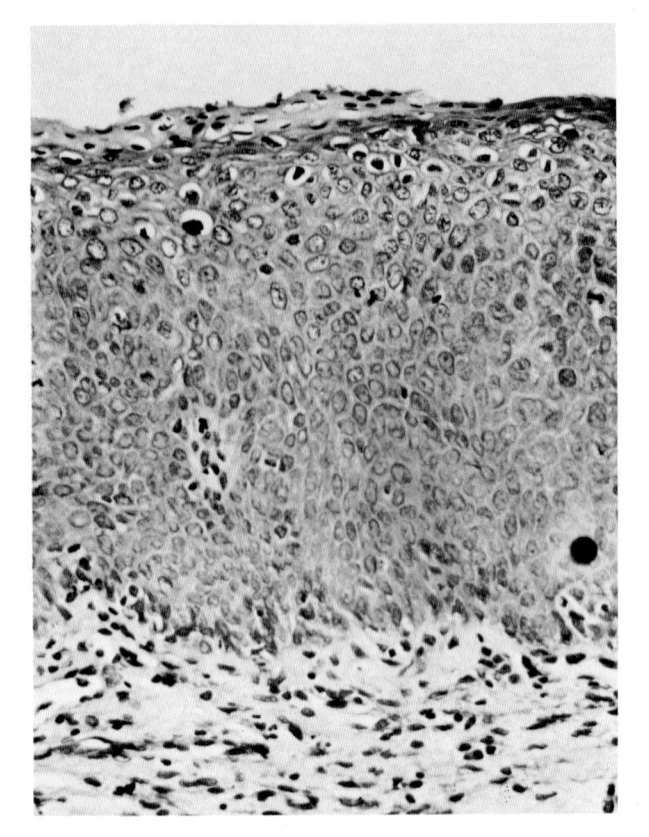

Figure 27.4. Marked cervical epithelial dysplasia. The maturation pattern of the cells is abnormal as well as the cell morphology, and the abnormal proliferation extends through most of the thickness of the epithelium. Only the most superficial layers show evidence of maturation.

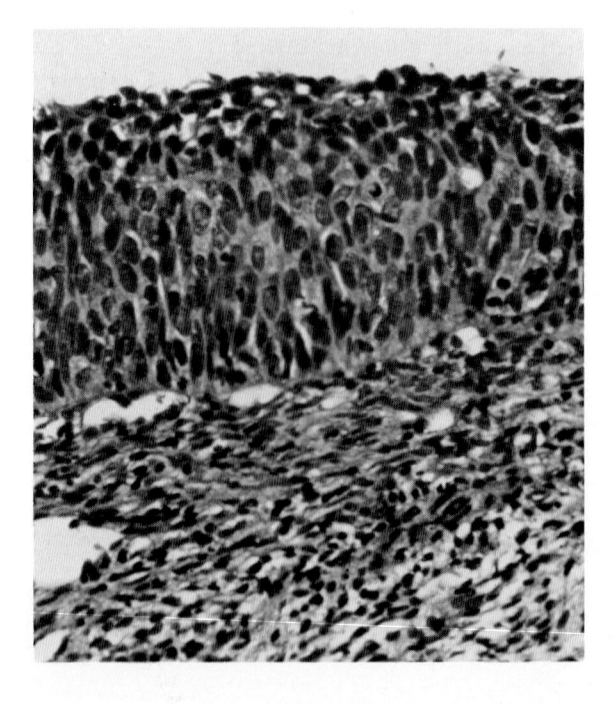

Figure 27.5. Carcinoma *in situ* of the cervix. The neoplastic cells involve the full thickness of the epithelium but do not extend beneath the basement membrane.

capable of progressing in this fashion. It is because the possibility of invasive malignant transformation exists in all of these preneoplastic lesions that dysplastic changes in the cervix are treated early and aggressively.

The next change in the transition to frankly invasive squamous carcinoma is the development of *microinvasion*. Microinvasive carcinoma is cervical cancer which has extended no more than 3 mm beneath the basement membrane of the overlying cervical epithelium or its glands (Fig. 27.6). This is an early stage of invasive cancer which is usually treated differently than the more deeply invasive forms. *Invasive squamous cell carcinoma* is divided into three types, based on morphologic patterns (Fig. 27.7). These are *large cell nonkeratinizing, large cell keratinizing,* and *small cell carcinoma.* These histologic types vary in their frequency of occurrence, their prognosis, and their response to therapy. *Adenocarcinoma* of the cervix is much less common, and, like squamous cell carcinoma, exists in an *in situ* and an invasive form.

Cervical carcinoma spreads to regional lymph nodes, including those of the internal and external iliac chain and obturator groups. It may also spread laterally, as well as anteriorly and posteriorly, to involve the pelvic walls, compress and

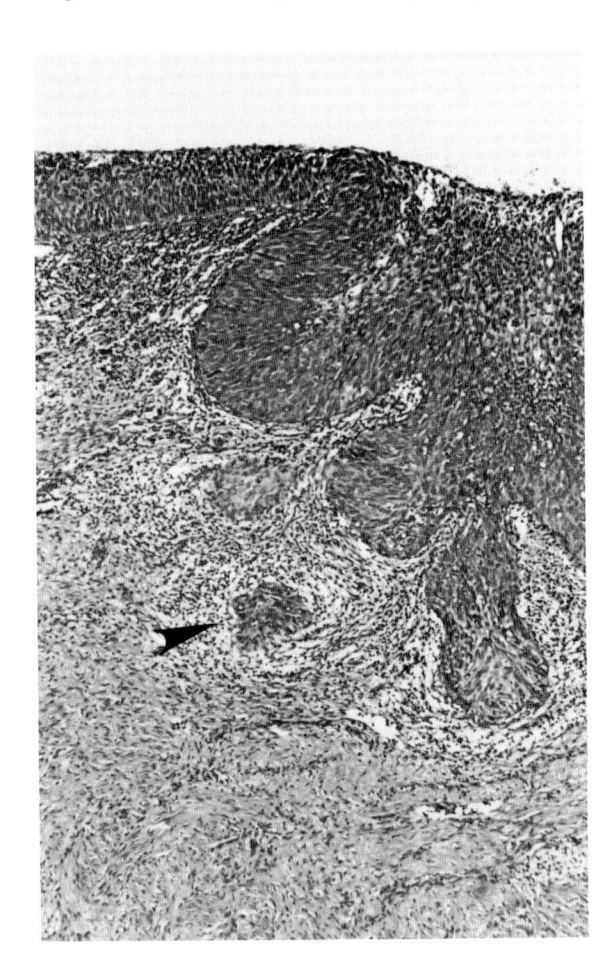

Figure 27.6. Microinvasive carcinoma of the cervix. Detached nests of tumor cells invade the cervical stroma (*arrow*) to a depth of no more than 3 mm beneath the epithelial basement membrane.

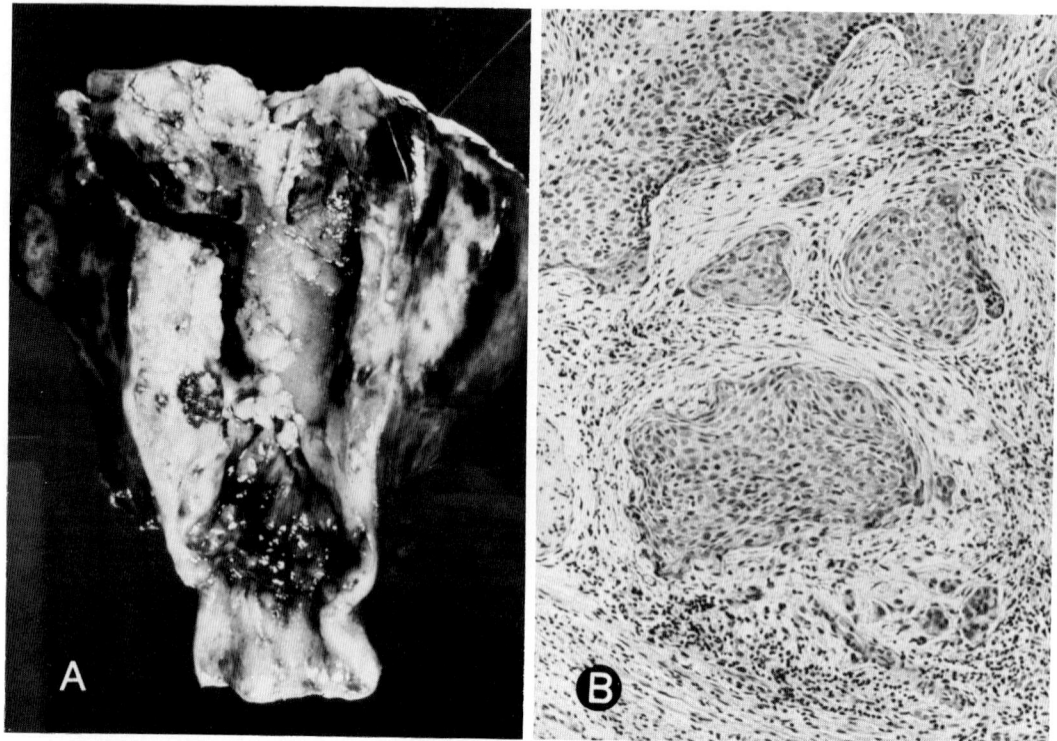

Figure 27.7. *A*, invasive squamous carcinoma of the cervix may present as a large ulcerating tumor mass involving the endocervical canal. *B*, the most common histologic pattern of invasive squamous carcinoma of the cervix is large cell nonkeratinizing. The tumor cells have abundant cytoplasm but do not form keratin pearls.

invade the ureters, or invade the wall and mucosa of the bladder and rectum. Ureteral obstruction with attendant pyelonephritis may be seen in far advanced carcinoma

Exfoliative Cytology and Cervical Intraepithelial Neoplasia

Exfoliative cytology is a technique for examining cells which are shed or collected from various epithelial surfaces in the body. Use of this technique as a means of detecting carcinoma and premalignant lesions has been most effective in the area of the uterine cervix. Characteristic cell changes of dysplasia, carcinoma *in situ*, and invasive carcinoma, as well as squamous metaplasia and varying hormonal and inflammatory changes, may be seen in cells removed by scraping the uterine cervix and endocervical canal (Fig. 27.8). Examination of these cells in the classic Pap smear has probably been responsible for the decreasing incidence of cervical cancer in the United States. When used as a screening procedure in conjunction with colposcopy (direct microscopic visualization of the cervix) and colposcopically directed biopsy (Fig. 27.9), a definitive diagnosis of preinvasive cervical cancer can be made.

The Female Genital Tract 365

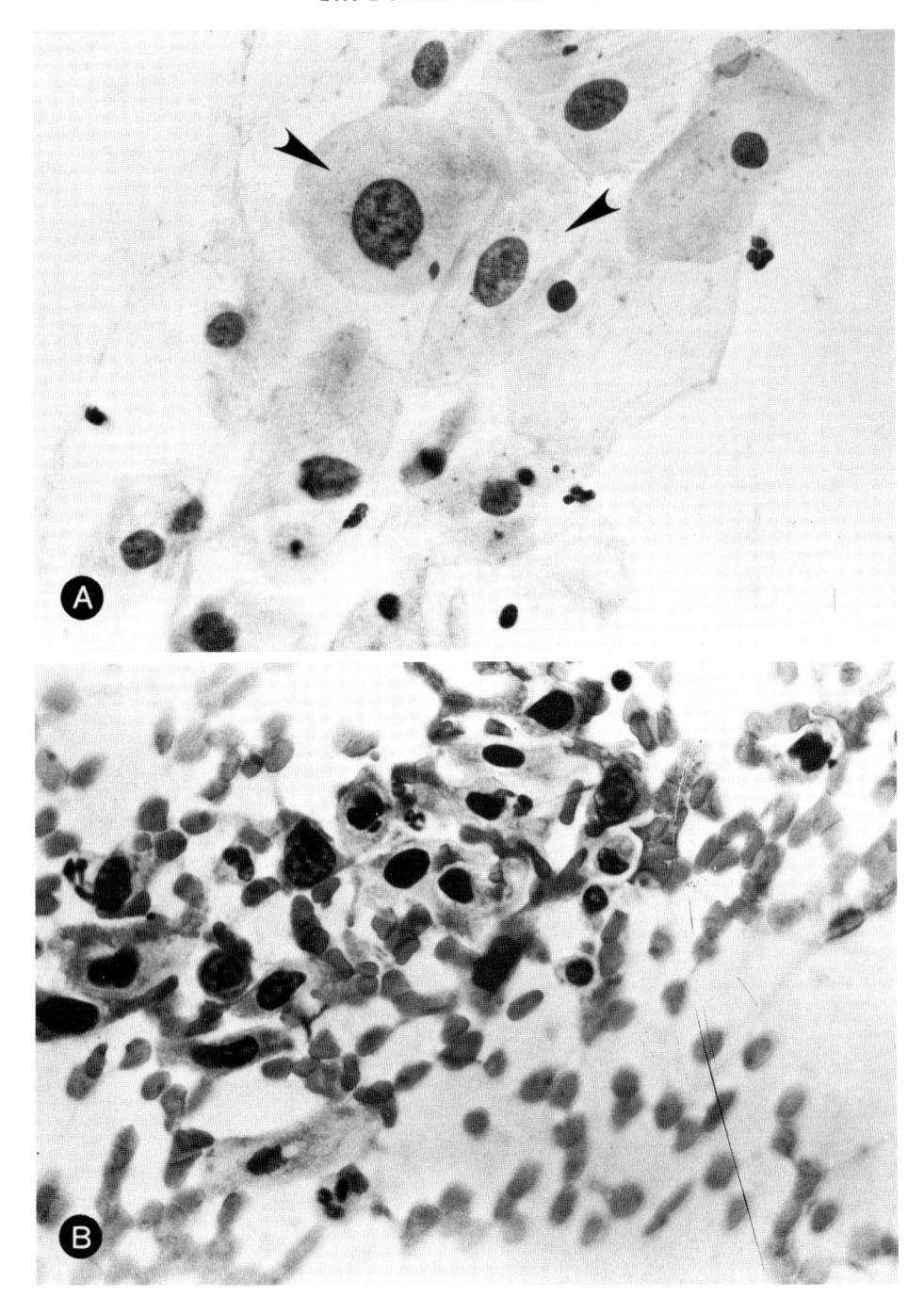

Figure 27.8. Cytology of cervical neoplasia. *A*, dysplastic cells (*arrows*) show nuclear enlargment with clumping of nuclear chromatin. *B*, cells from squamous carcinoma show more marked nuclear enlargement with increased nuclear/cytoplasmic ratio and dark staining or hyperchromatic nuclei.

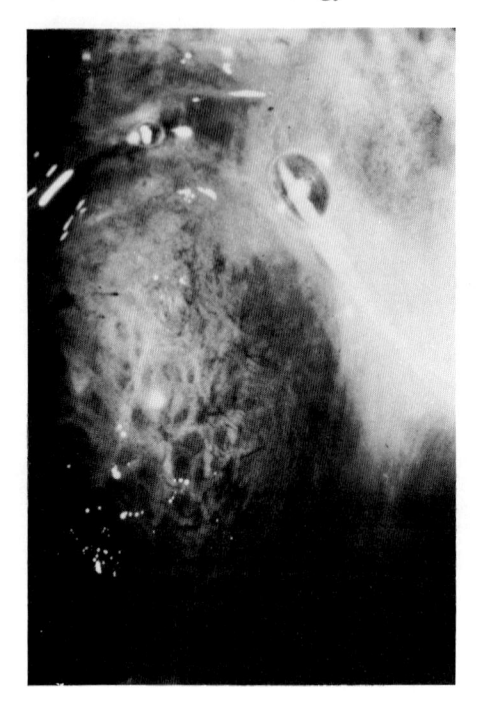

Figure 27.9. Colposcopy of the cervix. Examination of the cervix with the colpomicroscope reveals an abnormal pattern of epithelium and blood vessels in the *lower left*. The cervical os with white IUD string is in the *upper right*.

Epidemiology of Cervical Neoplasia

Carcinoma of the cervix is decreasing in frequency in the United States and is less common than some other types of cancer involving the female genital tract. There are approximately 16,000 new cases of invasive cervical cancer in the United States every year and some 7,500 deaths from cervical cancer. The disease affects primarily premenopausal women, with the peak incidence of invasive disease at ages 35 to 45. Certain risk factors are associated with an increased chance of developing cervical cancer. These include the early onset of sexual activity as well as large numbers of sexual partners. The association of cervical neoplasia with genital herpes infection (herpes virus II) is well known. More recently, a possible role of human papilloma virus in the etiology of cervical cancer has been suggested and this association is the object of current studies.

UTERUS

Endometritis

Endometritis is inflammation of the endometrium. The most common infectious causes include pyogenic bacteria causing postpartum inflammation, and tuberculosis, which may cause a granulomatous endometritis. Inflammation of the endometrium is also seen in conjunction with intrauterine contraceptive devices, and may represent their mechanism of effectiveness. The endometritis seen with intrauterine devices is usually not of infectious origin.

Endometrial Polyps

Endometrial polyps represent one of the hyperplastic lesions of the endometrium (Fig. 27.10). They are seen in women of all ages and may be single or multiple. They are composed of glands and stroma which often do not reflect the cyclic changes seen in the normal portions of the endometrium. The stroma of these lesions may have a compact fibrous tissue element with increased numbers of prominent vascular channels. While presumably reflecting abnormalities in estrogen, these endometrial polyps are considered to be benign and do not represent premalignant lesions.

Endometrial Hyperplasia

Hyperplasias of the endometrium occur in response to abnormalities of estrogens. Estrogen abnormalities are also felt to be etiologically important in the development of endometrial carcinoma, and some of the hyperplastic lesions of the endometrium appear closely tied to the evolution of endometrial cancer.

The abnormalities of estrogens may be of three major types: abnormal amounts of circulating estrogen, abnormal types of estrogens, or abnormal patterns of estrogen production. An example of an abnormal amount of estrogen is the production of abnormally high estrogen levels by a functioning ovarian tumor, such as a thecoma. Examples of abnormal patterns of steroid hormone production,

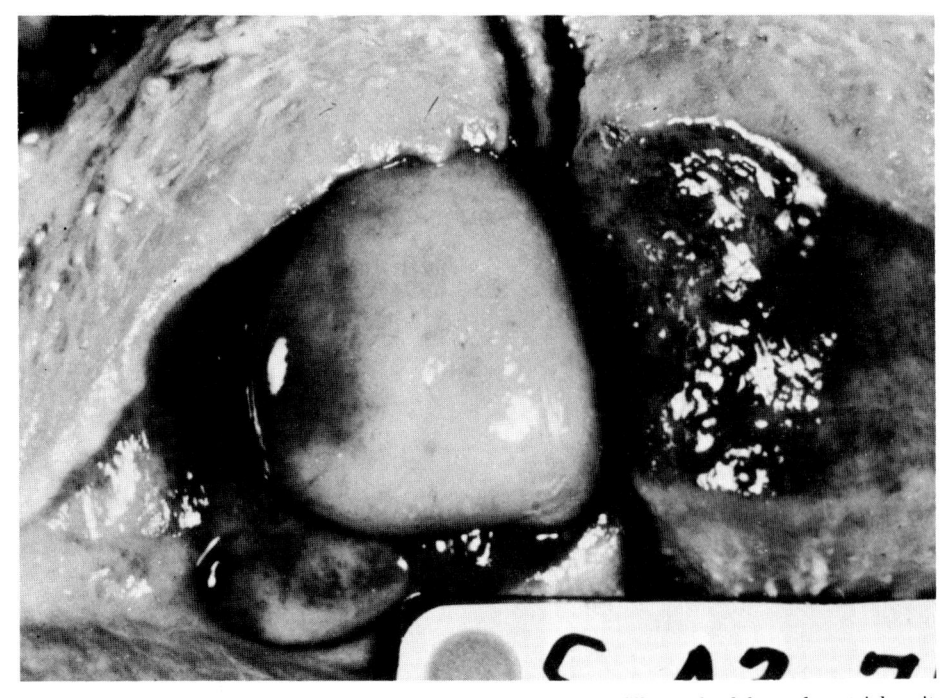

Figure 27.10. Endometrial polyp. The large white fleshy polyp fills much of the endometrial cavity which is seen opened as the dark area to the *right* in the photograph.

including estrogen production, may be seen in patients with the polycystic ovarian syndrome. These patients are frequently anovulatory, and therefore the normal interruption of estrogen stimulation of the endometrium by cyclic progesterone stimulation is not present. An example of abnormal estrogen production is offered by the *estrone hypothesis*. In the female, particularly in the premenopausal female, the most common circulating estrogen is estradiol. Postmenopausally, estradiol production by the ovary is decreased, but androstenedione is still produced by the adrenal cortex as well as by the ovarian stroma. Conversion of the androstenedione to estrogens may occur in several sites, including peripheral fat. The estrogen produced in these sites is most often estrone rather than estradiol. Estrone production in peripheral fat is an example of an abnormal type of estrogen and is particularly interesting, considering that obesity is one of the prime risk factors for the development of endometrial carcinoma.

There are two common patterns of endometrial hyperplasia. *Cystic hyperplasia*, also known as "Swiss cheese" hyperplasia, is a pattern characterized by an increase in both the numbers and size of endometrial glands and in the amount of endometrial stroma. This concurrent overgrowth of both glands and stroma means that the endometrial glands are still widely separated from each other. The glands are characteristically dilated and can be recognized grossly and microscopically, giving the resemblance to Swiss cheese (Fig. 27.11). Like the glands in other patterns of hyperplasia, the lining epithelium shows the nuclear

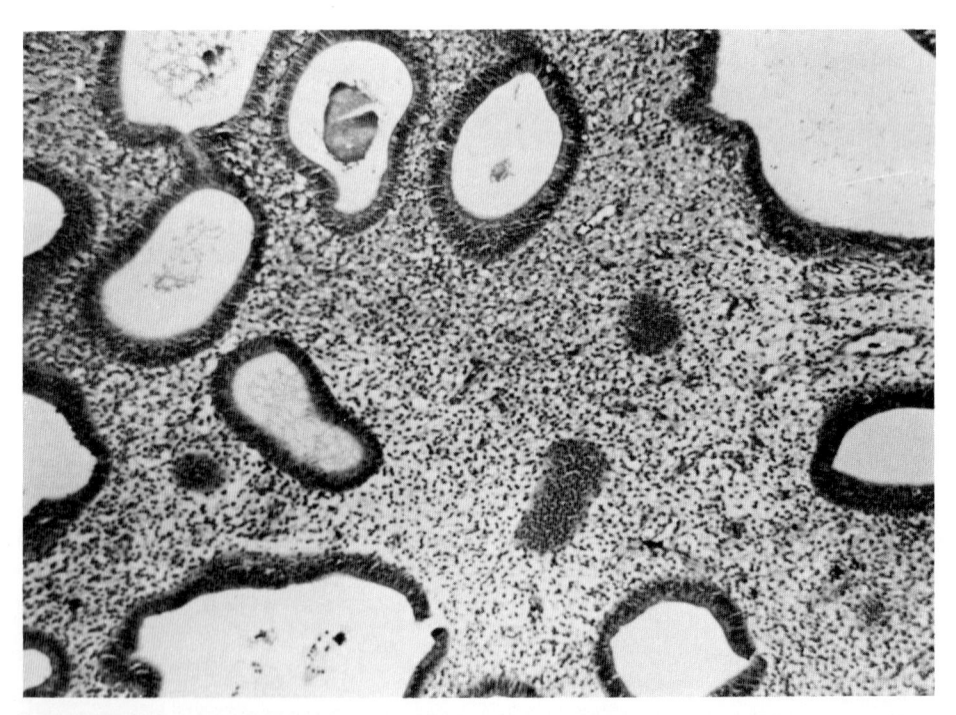

Figure 27.11. Cystic hyperplasia of the endometrium is characterized by a proliferation of both endometrial stroma and glands. The glands are cystically dilated giving a "holey" or Swiss cheese appearance to the endometrium.

pseudostratification and lack of vacuolization characteristic of the estrogen phase of the endometrial cycle. Cystic hyperplasia is most commonly seen in postmenopausal women, and is not felt to be a premalignant lesion.

A second type of endometrial hyperplasia is *adenomatous hyperplasia.* There is overgrowth and increase in number of the endometrial glands with a relatively slight or absent proliferation of stroma, which results in a characteristic close crowding of the endometrial glands with a back-to-back appearance. The glands of adenomatous hyperplasia may exhibit varying degrees of nuclear atypia. When the glands show considerable close crowding and nuclear atypia as well as pale staining and abundant cytoplasm, the lesion is called atypical adenomatous hyperplasia (Fig. 27.12), believed to represent a transition between hyperplasia and frank carcinoma. It is estimated that approximately 3 to 25% of patients with adenomatous hyperplasia will develop endometrial carcinoma if left untreated.

Adenocarcinoma of the Endometrium

Excluding the breast, endometrial adenocarcinoma is the most frequently occurring carcinoma in the female genital tract. It is, however, not the most frequent cause of death. Approximately 37,000 new cases of endometrial carcinoma are diagnosed in the United States each year, but less than 3,500 deaths are reported. In general, endometrial carcinoma is a disease of postmenopausal women, most frequently diagnosed in the sixth decade of life. Risk factors include

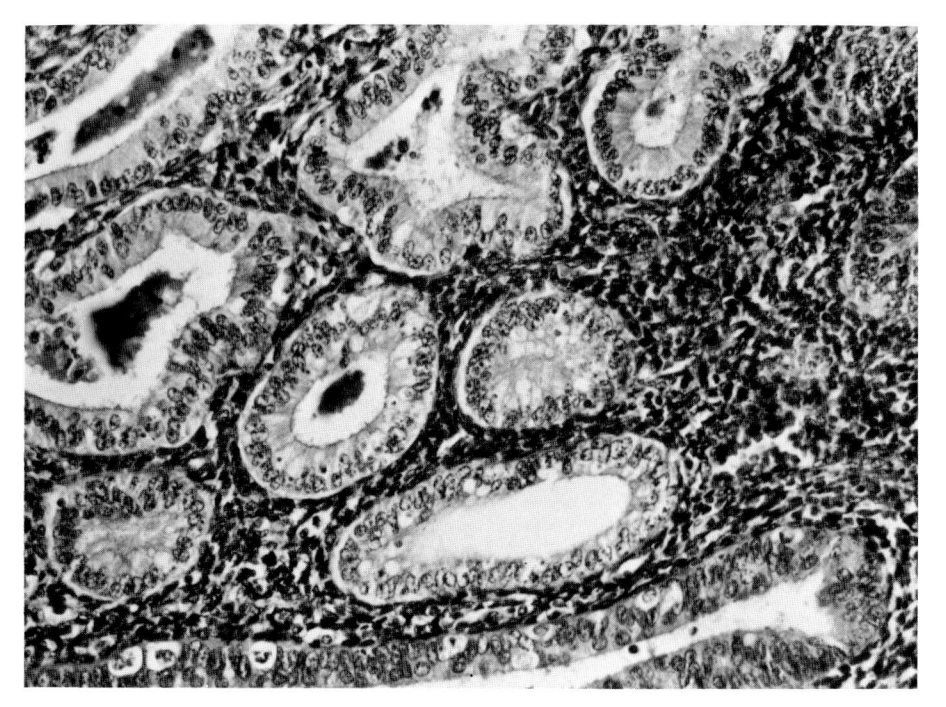

Figure 27.12. Atypical adenomatous hyperplasia. The glands are paler staining than normal endometrial glands and there is atypia of gland nuclei. This type of hyperplasia may progress to endometrial adenocarcinoma.

obesity, hypertension, and diabetes. Endometrial carcinoma is felt to be associated with abnormal estrogen stimulation of the endometrium. Patients with this type of cancer tend to have few children, an early menarche, and a late menopause. More recently, the development of endometrial adenocarcinoma has been associated with exogenous estrogen therapy. This is felt to increase the risk of

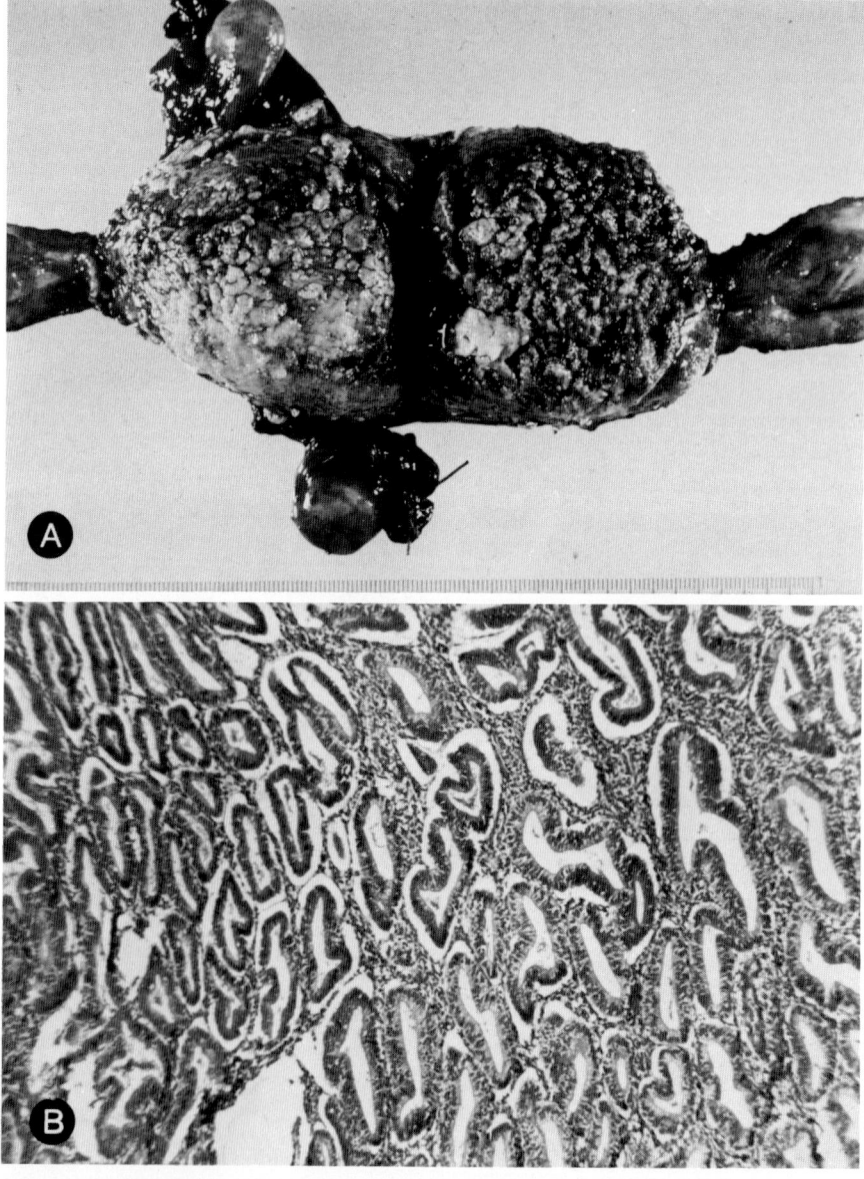

Figure 27.13. Endometrial adenocarcinoma. *A*, the opened uterus shows masses of friable tumor filling the endometrial cavity. *B*, well differentiated adenocarcinoma shows closely packed proliferating tumor glands.

developing endometrial cancer to 4 to 5 times that of the untreated population. The risk appears to be related to the duration of estrogen therapy, and may be minimized by treating patients with a combination of estrogen and progestational compounds.

Endometrial adenocarcinoma is a malignancy of the endometrial glands and is histologically graded by the degree of glandular differentiation (Fig. 27.13). Squamous epithelium may also be seen in endometrial adenocarcinoma; this may result from the occurrence of squamous metaplasia in non-neoplastic endometrial tissue. An endometrial adenocarcinoma which contains benign metaplastic squamous epithelium is termed an *adenocanthoma* (Fig. 27.14). These tumors tend to be rather well differentiated adenocarcinomas and their prognosis is quite good. When malignant squamous elements are identified, the tumor is termed an *adenosquamous carcinoma*. Usually, the glandular component of these tumors is less well differentiated and their prognosis is poor. Other prognostic factors include the depth of invasion into the uterine wall; tumors that are deeply invasive into the myometrium carry a poorer prognosis than those that are confined to the endometrium itself. Endometrial carcinoma is not usually diagnosed by Pap smear as is cervical cancer. Fortunately, these lesions present relatively early in their course as abnormal uterine bleeding.

Nonepithelial Tumors of the Uterus

Nonepithelial tumors of the uterus are derived either from the endometrial stroma or from the myometrium. The most common of these are the benign *leiomyomas* of the myometrium, commonly and incorrectly called "fibroids." They are frequently asymptomatic, but they may produce a wide variety of

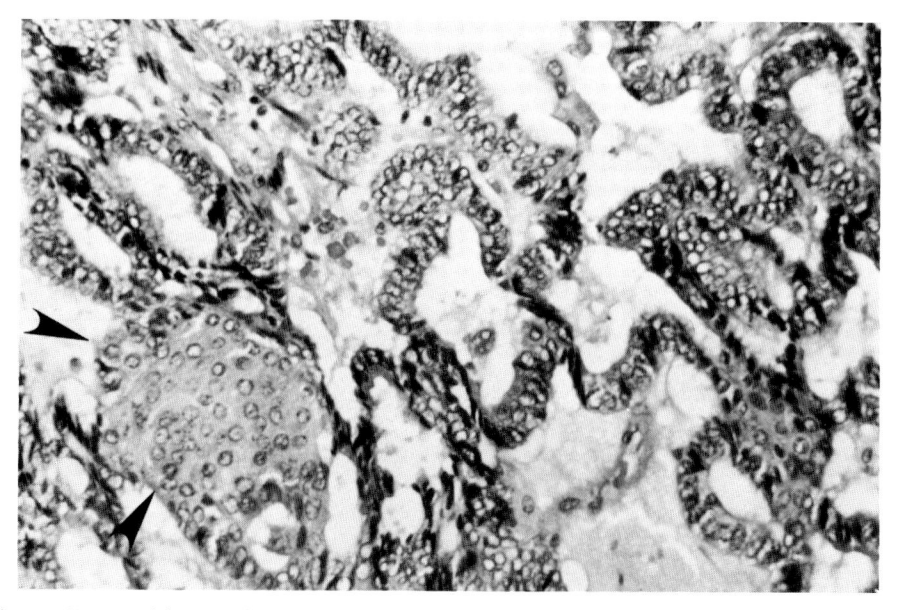

Figure 27.14. Adenocanthoma of the endometrium is characterized by malignant glands and intermingled nests of benign metaplastic squamous epithelium (*arrows*).

symptoms, including abnormal uterine bleeding, pain, a pelvic mass, or difficulties with pregnancy and delivery. Leiomyomas may occur at any age and vary greatly in size (Fig. 27.15). These tumors may undergo varying degrees of change, including degeneration, necrosis and hemorrhage, fibrosis, and dystrophic calcification. In general, they are benign tumors, and are not felt to undergo malignant degeneration.

The nonepithelial malignant tumors of the uterus are, like their benign counterparts, derived from the endometrial stroma or from the myometrium. The sarcomas are classified as those consisting of one cell type (pure tumors) and those consisting of multiple cell types (mixed tumors). These tumors may consist either of elements which are native to the uterus or of those which are normally not found in the uterus. Tumors composed of elements native to the normal uterus are referred to as homologous tumors while those containing some foreign elements are referred to as heterologous tumors. An example of a pure sarcoma is the *leiomyosarcoma*, or malignant tumor of smooth muscle. This tumor most frequently arises *de novo* and is not derived from a previously existing benign smooth muscle tumor. Leiomyosarcomas are characterized by rapid growth and varying degrees of cellular atypia, but the most reliable criterion of malignancy is the presence of more than 10 mitotic figures in 10 high power microscopic fields. Tumors containing less than 5 mitotic figures per 10 high power fields are felt to be benign, while those with mitotic activity in the range of 5 to 10 have an intermediate behavior.

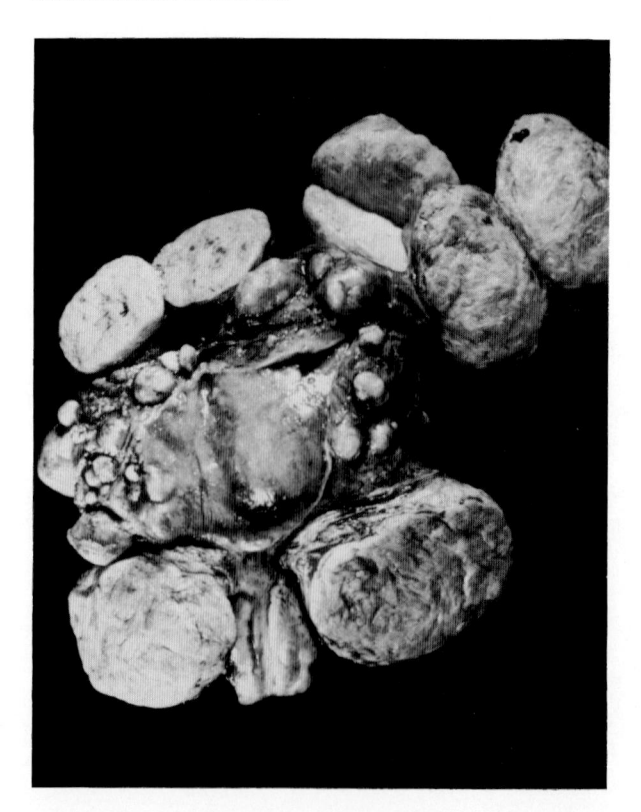

Figure 27.15. Uterus with multiple benign leiomyomas which are located beside the cervix, beneath the endometrium and serosa, and within the myometrium. The tumors vary greatly in size.

Sarcomas of the endometrium are derived from endometrial stroma. The endometrial stroma is an interesting tissue since it can change its morphology. Examples of this change are seen in the formation of decidua under the influence of progesterone and chorionic gonadotrophin. Endometrial stromal cells can undergo malignant change and maintain their characteristic morphology. These tumors are referred to as endometrial stromal sarcomas and are examples of pure homologous sarcomas of the uterus. When there is malignant transformation of the endometrial stromal cells into a variety of different tissues such as cartilage or smooth muscle, the tumors are referred to as mixed mesodermal or mixed Müllerian tumors.

Sarcomas of the uterus are usually found in postmenopausal women. The mixed mesodermal tumors often present with abnormal bleeding and are large polypoid masses which frequently undergo considerable necrosis (Fig. 27.16) They fill the endometrial cavity and may protrude into the endocervix and apex of the vagina.

Endometriosis

Endometriosis is the presence of endometrial tissue in sites other than its normal location in the endometrial cavity. There are two types of endometriosis: *internal endometriosis*, or *adenomyosis*, and *external endometriosis*. Internal endometriosis is the presence of endometrial glands and stroma within the myometrium. The cause of this condition is felt to be a downgrowth of the basalis layer of the endometrium into the myometrium. Since the basalis portion of the endometrium is noncycling, these downgrowths usually do not have the capacity

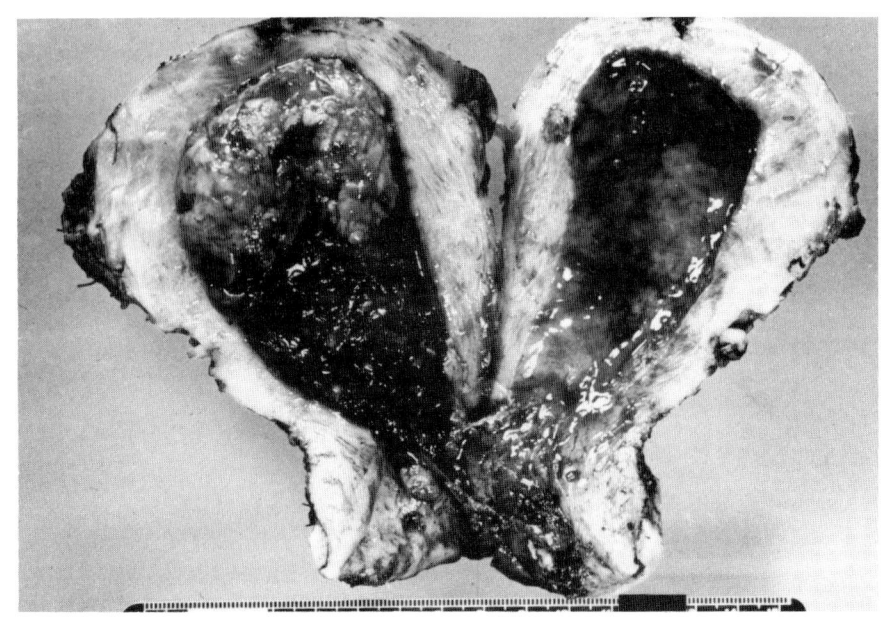

Figure 27.16. Malignant mixed Müllerian tumor of the uterus characteristically arises in the endometrium and fills the endometrial cavity as a large mass as well as invading the uterine wall.

to respond to cyclic hormone stimulation and therefore are not usually associated with bleeding and ensuing pain.

External endometriosis consists of implants of functioning endometrial tissue in sites distant from the uterus. The most common areas of involvement include the ovaries, broad ligaments, rectovaginal septum, and sites in the peritoneal cavity, including the appendix, bowel, and umbilicus. Endometrial implants may also be seen in abdominal scars. The etiology of external endometriosis is uncertain. Theories have included a regurgitation of endometrial fragments in a retrograde fashion through the Fallopian tubes at the time of menses, with implantation of these fragments onto various structures in the peritoneal cavity, as well as the metaplastic theory which recalls the embryologic origin of the endometrium from the coelomic epithelium of the primitive peritoneal cavity. According to this latter theory, any sites in the adult covered by peritoneum, such as the covering of the ovary and the serosa of the colon and the bladder, have the embryologic capacity to undergo metaplastic transformation or differentiation into endometrial glands and stroma. The etiology of external endometriosis probably is a combination of these different theories. Unlike internal endometriosis, the explants of endometrium on other pelvic organs are functional and can undergo cyclic maturation and bleeding under the influence of endogenous or exogenous hormones. These lesions form areas of old and recent hemorrhage and may undergo cyst formation with scarring. Many symptoms are associated with external endometriosis which are at least in part related to the sites of endometrial deposits. These may include pain, abnormal bleeding from other organ sites, and infertility.

Abnormal Uterine Bleeding

Many of the diseases of the uterus which have been discussed are associated with the symptom of abnormal bleeding. This may occur during the normal menstrual cycle or at times other than the menstrual cycle. Some of the causes of abnormal uterine bleeding have been mentioned in this section and include pelvic lesions such as endometriosis, tumors of the uterus, endometrial polyps and hyperplasias, and cervical and vaginal carcinoma. Other causes of abnormal uterine bleeding include complications of pregnancy. Functional and dysfunctional uterine bleeding represent abnormalities or alterations of the delicately balanced pituitary-ovarian-endometrial axis. Systemic diseases may also cause abnormal bleeding from the uterus. These include blood disorders, such as leukemias, various coagulopathies, and bleeding diatheses.

FALLOPIAN TUBE

Pelvic Inflammatory Disease

Pelvic inflammatory disease is the symptom complex produced by inflammation of varying pelvic structures in association with acute and chronic inflammation of the Fallopian tube, or *salpingitis*. Pelvic inflammatory disease often presents as pelvic pain, sometimes as an acute abdomen and peritonitis. Pelvic inflammatory disease, especially if chronic, can also produce the symptoms of a pelvic mass. There are multiple infectious causes of acute salpingitis. Postpartum bacterial salpingitis is often caused by *Escherichia coli* or pyogenic bacteria and usually originates from a uterine source, spreading to the Fallopian tube via lymphatics of the broad ligament. Tuberculosis is also associated with acute salpingitis, usually by hematogenous spread from a pulmonary focus. Patients with intrauterine contraceptive devices have up to a 3 times increased incidence of acute salpingitis compared to the general population.

The classical cause of salpingitis is gonococcal infection. Infection spreads from the cervix through the endometrial cavity immediately after the menstrual period to a focus in the Fallopian tube or periovarian tissue. There is acute inflammation of the tubal epithelium and submucosa. As a result, the fimbriated ends of the tube may form adhesions. The Fallopian tube becomes distended and filled with pus and is referred to as a *pyosalpinx*. After the acute inflammatory phase subsides, the polymorphonuclear leukocytes and necrotic debris are resorbed and removed by macrophages and a sterile fluid remains in the distended sealed off and scarred Fallopian tube. This is called a *hydrosalpinx*. The scarring of the Fallopian tube and the multiple adhesions between fimbria and ovary may be a cause of infertility and may also lead to ectopic pregnancy. Acute salpingitis and pelvic inflammatory disease are usually bilateral, but may present symptomatically as unilateral involvement.

Ectopic Pregnancy

Ectopic pregnancy is a pregnancy implanting in some site other than the endometrial cavity. The most common site is within the Fallopian tube (Fig. 27.17), but ectopic pregnancies also occur on the ovary and at other points within the abdominal cavity. Factors predisposing to ectopic pregnancy include pelvic

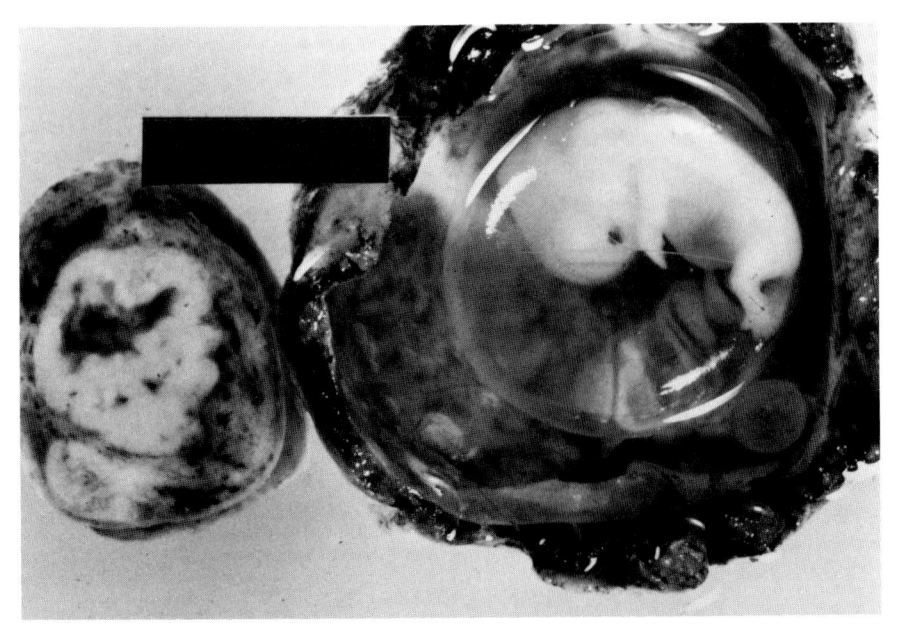

Figure 27.17. Ectopic pregnancy in the Fallopian tube. The gestational sac with a small fetus distends the lumen of the tube. The ovarian corpus luteum of pregnancy is seen at the *left*.

inflammatory disease, tubal endometriosis, extratubal tumors, and intrauterine contraceptive devices. Since the pregnancy has implanted and is developing at a site not normally adapted to nurture a developing conceptus, the pregnancy is less likely to survive in these locations. Complications of ectopic pregnancy include tubal rupture with abdominal hemorrhage, hematosalpinx, and shock. In ectopic pregnancy, the endometrium undergoes decidual change under the influence of chorionic gonadotrophin produced by the developing conceptus. However, the abnormally located pregnancy usually does not produce normal levels of chorionic gonadotrophin and the decidua is frequently expelled with bleeding, often perceived as a normal, if slightly late, menstrual period. The pregnancy, however, may continue in its ectopic site and present with bleeding and signs of an intra-abdominal catastrophe at some later time.

DISEASES OF PREGNANCY

There are many disorders of pregnancy and the placenta which cannot be covered in this section. This discussion is limited to trophoblastic disease and spontaneous abortion.

Trophoblastic Disease

Trophoblastic disease refers to abnormalities in the growth of the trophoblast. Trophoblast is tissue which is formed by the developing embryo as a means of anchoring the fetus to the endometrium, and, as such, is tissue that is foreign to the maternal host but is generally tolerated. There are two types of trophoblastic cells which make up the epithelium covering the connective tissue of the chorionic villi, designated cytotrophoblast and syncytiotrophoblast. The syncytiotrophoblasts are multinucleated giant cells and are associated with the major production

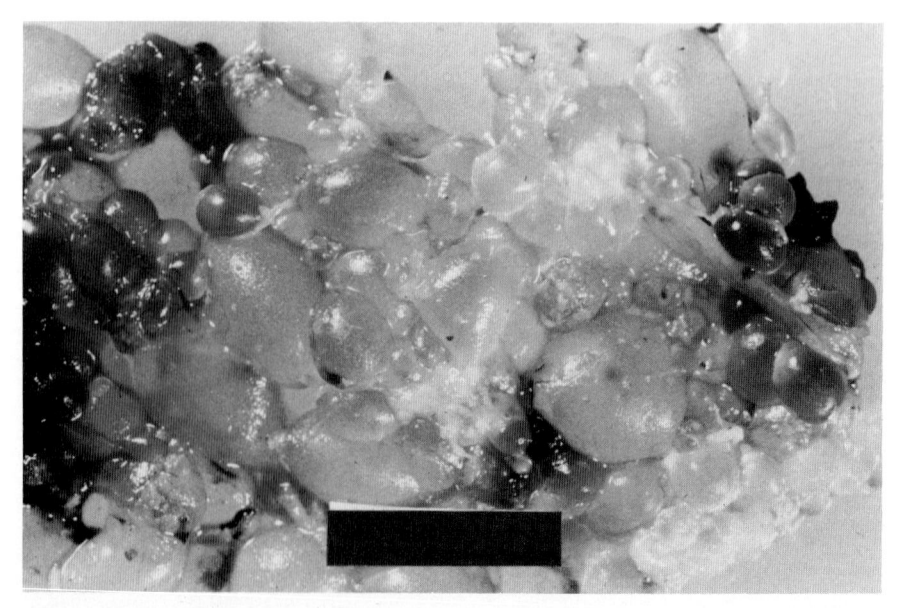

Figure 27.18. Hydatidiform mole. Each large vesicle represents a swollen chorionic villus.

of chorionic gonadotrophin (HCG). Three histologic entities are included in the term trophoblastic disease. These are hydatidiform mole, chorioadenoma destruens, and choriocarcinoma. All three entities have in common an overgrowth or proliferation of the trophoblast.

Hydatidiform mole is considered to be an abnormal pregnancy and not a true neoplasm. In a molar pregnancy there is usually no fetal development, probably because of early failure of formation of a fetal cardiovascular system. Instead of being aborted, however, the trophoblast remains intact and continues to grow. Hydatidiform mole has been compared to a bunch of grapes, because of the gross appearance of large masses of swollen watery placental villi (Fig. 27.18). Histologically there are three criteria which need to be present for the diagnosis of molar pregnancy, including hydropic degeneration and swelling of the villi, active proliferation of the trophoblast with varying degrees of atypia, and few to totally absent blood vessels within the hydropic stroma of the villi. *Chorioadenoma destruens* has the same histology as hydatidiform mole, but the molar tissue has extended into the uterine myometrium (Fig. 27.19).

Choriocarcinoma is a biologic and histologic malignancy of the trophoblast. This tumor most frequently arises in the uterus following an abnormal or normal pregnancy, but can arise from primitive germ cells in the ovary or testis or in teratomas of the retroperitoneum, mediastinum, pineal gland and other sites. These malignant tumors recapitulate the growth patterns of the placenta, with malignant cytotrophoblast and syncytiotrophoblast (Fig. 27.20). The malignant syncytiotrophoblast continues to produce chorionic gonadotrophin.

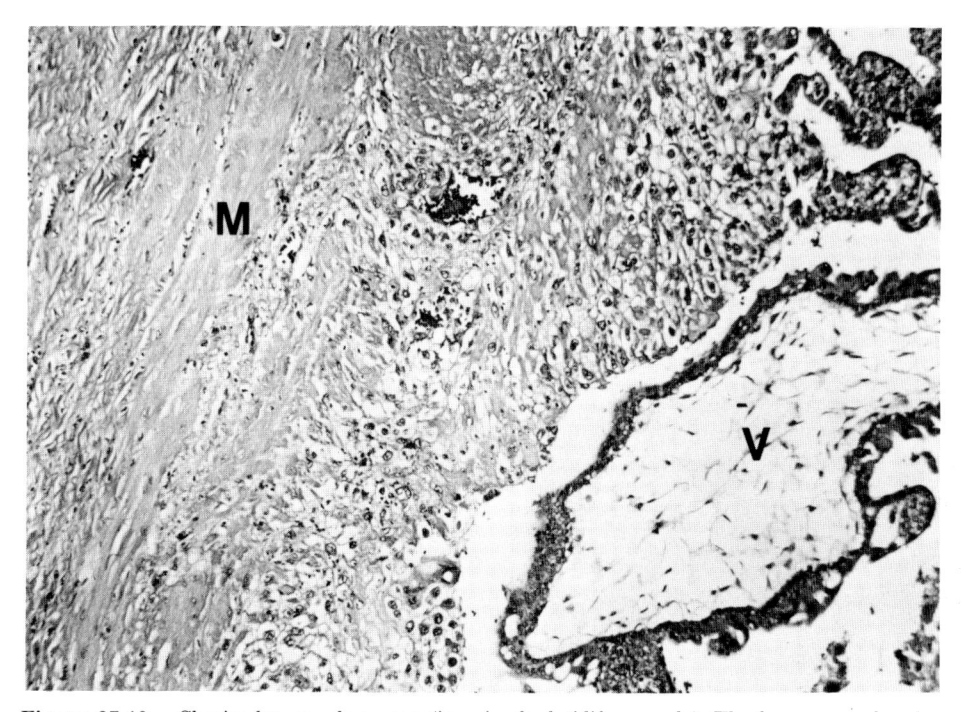

Figure 27.19. Chorioadenoma destruens (invasive hydatidiform mole). The large avascular chorionic villus (*V*) surrounded by proliferating trophoblast is seen invading myometrial fibers (*M*).

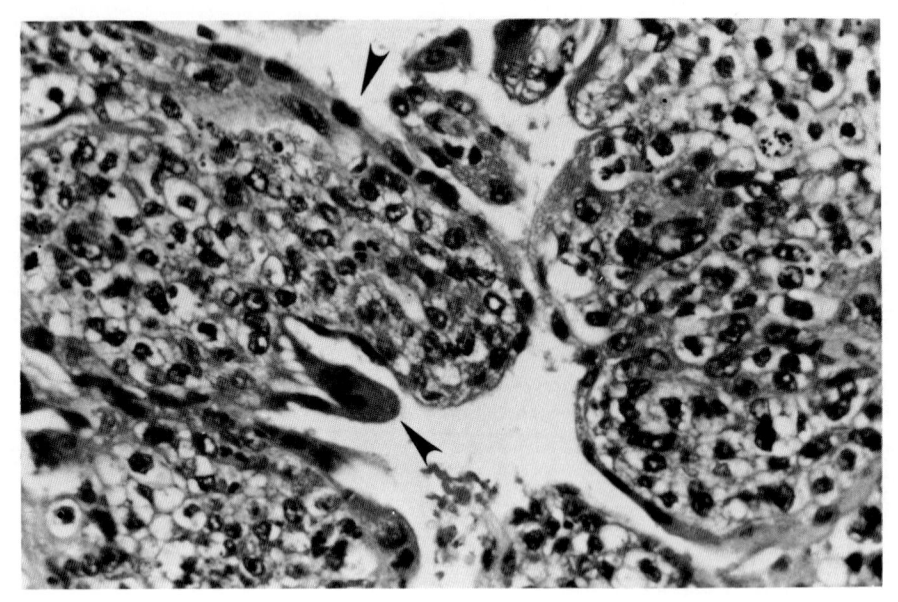

Figure 27.20. Choriocarcinoma is characterized by two types of malignant cells. The large multinucleated syncytiotrophoblasts (*arrows*) cover or "cap" the sheets of singly nucleate cytotrophoblasts.

The different histologic types of trophoblastic disease are seen with varying degrees of frequency. In the United States, hydatidiform mole occurs in approximately 1 in every 2000 to 2500 pregnancies. This incidence is much higher in the Far East. Choriocarcinoma is a very rare tumor, occurring in only 1 of every 100,000 pregnancies. Although only about 1% of hydatidiform moles subsequently develop choriocarcinoma, choriocarcinoma is more likely to develop after a molar pregnancy than after an abortion or a normal full term pregnancy.

Clinical signs of trophoblastic disease include vaginal bleeding in the first or second trimester, uterine enlargement beyond the gestational age, early development of pre-eclampsia or toxemia of pregnancy, hyperemesis gravidarum, hyperthyroidism, and congestive heart failure.

Trophoblastic tissue can spread or metastasize to other organs in any of the three diseases of trophoblast. Benign hydatidiform mole may disseminate to many tissues, most commonly lung, liver, and brain. Complicated trophoblastic disease defines those lesions which have spread to other organs, and noncomplicated disease refers to lesions which are removed with the initial uterine evacuation. It is impossible to tell on histologic grounds alone which lesions will spread outside the uterus.

The most important marker in trophoblastic disease is the serum determination of chorionic gonadotrophin, usually by radioimmunoassay of the β-subunit of this polypeptide hormone. The hormone and each of its two polypeptide chains have biologic and immunologic activity, and antibodies can be made to the whole molecule and to each of the polypeptide chains. Therefore, both the whole molecule and the polypeptide subunits can be assayed by radioimmunoassay. Whole molecule HCG is very similar to human luteinizing hormone and both hormones have the same α-subunits. Therefore, biologic tests and tests with antibodies directed toward the whole molecule will measure levels of both hormones. Radioimmunoassays with antibodies directed specifically to the β-chain of HCG are more accurate, since only HCG will be detected.

Patients with all forms of trophoblastic disease produce HCG. After the evacuation of a molar pregnancy or other type of trophoblastic disease, the levels of HCG in serum fall. If the disease has been totally removed from the uterus, the levels of HCG will return to normal. If, however, the patient develops complicated trophoblastic disease and the trophoblastic tissue spreads to other organ sites, the levels of HCG will remain elevated or rise. Patients with metastatic or complicated trophoblastic disease are further subdivided into low risk and high risk categories. High risk trophoblastic disease includes patients with metastases demonstrated in brain or liver and with high levels of serum HCG. These patients are treated more aggressively than the low risk group, which has lower levels of serum HCG and metastases limited to sites other than the brain or liver.

Spontaneous Abortion

More than 10% of all pregnancies end in spontaneous abortion, usually in the first trimester. Spontaneous abortion represents the most common abnormality of the developing pregnancy. The cause of these early first trimester abortions is usually not known, but in many instances is felt to be due to an abnormal development of the fertilized ovum. In spontaneous abortion specimens, the trophoblast appears normal, with relatively limited trophoblastic proliferation. Varying degrees of degeneration, including hydropic degeneration of placental villi, may be seen.

OVARY

Ovarian Tumors

Although ovarian carcinomas are uncommon, there are now more cases diagnosed yearly in the United States than cases of invasive cervical cancer, and there are 1.5 times as many deaths from ovarian tumors as there are from cervical cancer. After carcinoma of the breast, ovarian cancer is the leading cause of death in the group of gynecologic malignancies. Part of the reason for this relatively high death rate is that ovarian cancer is usually diagnosed late, when patients are already clinically Stage III or IV.

It is often confusing and difficult for students of pathology to try to differentiate among the different ovarian neoplasms. Because there are so many different tumors arising from the different portions of the ovaries, it is important to devise some kind of classification system to separate these tumors into more manageable subtypes. The classification established by the World Health Organization separates tumors into major categories based on the presumptive histogenic origin of their tumor cells. These major categories are the epithelial tumors, germ cell tumors, stromal tumors, and metastatic tumors involving the ovary.

Epithelial Tumors of the Ovary

The most common of the ovarian tumors are those with a presumed histogenic origin from the surface epithelium (germinal epithelium or mesothelium) that covers the ovary. Normally, this epithelium is one cell layer thick and is sometimes difficult to see in histologic sections. The epithelium is in reality a mesothelium, similar to the layer covering most of the organs within the peritoneal cavity. Embryologically, it is derived from the coelomic epithelium and thus has similar embryologic origin to much of the epithelium lining various organs of the female genital tract. Because of its embryologic relationship to Müllerian epithelium, the germinal epithelium, when undergoing neoplastic transformation, can recapitulate the epithelium lining Fallopian tubes, endometrium, or cervix. This capacity for transformation into different epithelial types produces the different histologic appearances of the epithelial tumors of the ovary.

Each of the epithelial tumors of the ovary exists in three forms: a benign, a malignant, and an intermediate form which is termed a borderline tumor or tumor of low malignant potential. These latter tumors are important to subclassify, because patients with these tumors exhibit a very high survival rate, greater than 90 to 95% at 10 years (Fig. 27.21).

The most common of the epithelial tumors of the ovary are the *serous cystadenomas* and *cystadenocarcinomas*. These tumors are lined by a columnar

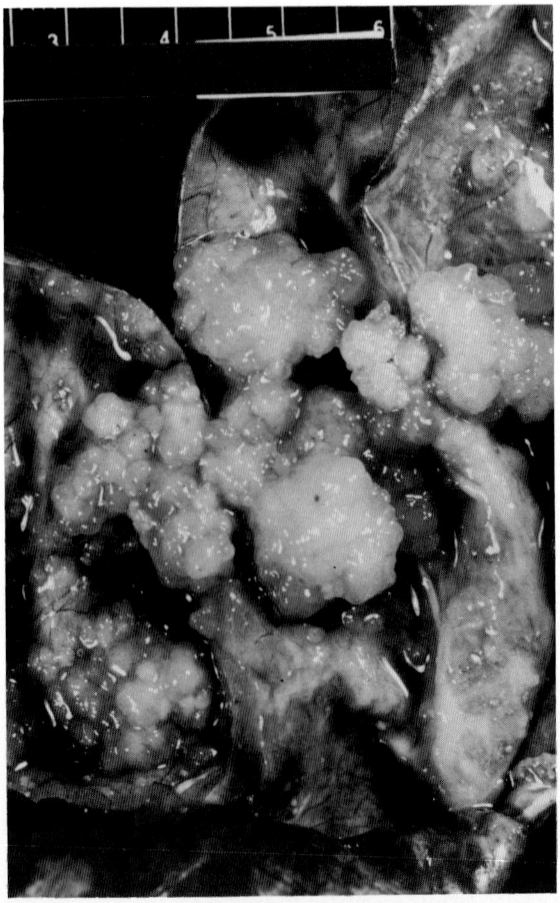

Figure 27.21. The inner surface of a borderline serous tumor of the ovary shows papillary epithelial projections protruding into the lumen of the cystic tumor.

epithelium which resembles the lining of the Fallopian tube. The serous cystadenomas consist of single or multiple cystic structures, lined by a single layer of columnar epithelium, while the cystadenocarcinomas show areas of solid tumor growth and papillary proliferation of the epithelium within cyst structures as well as considerable nuclear atypia and mitotic activity. The borderline serous tumors of the ovary show no invasion of the stroma. The serous tumors, like other papillary tumors, may contain small spherical calcified *psammoma* bodies (Fig. 27.22). *Mucinous cystadenomas* and *cystadenocarcinomas* are lined by a goblet cell type of epithelium resembling the endocervix or epithelium of the gastrointestinal tract. They are characteristically multilocular, with microscopic as well as grossly visible cysts. The benign tumors are lined by a single layered epithelium, while malignant lesions are lined by hyperchromatic cells, often with little cytoplasmic mucin, and closely resemble adenocarcinomas of the colon. The borderline varieties show some epithelial proliferation within the lumens of the cysts and mild nuclear atypia.

Endometrioid cystadenomas and *cystadenocarcinomas* are tumors which resemble endometrial adenocarcinomas, but are located within the ovary. Interestingly, they may also be associated with primary adenocarcinomas of the endometrium. They are thought to derive from foci of endometriosis within the ovary, although previously existing endometriosis can be identified histologically in fewer than half of cases. *Clear cell carcinomas* of the ovary are usually seen in their malignant form, although, rarely, benign clear cell cystadenomas are identified. These tumors contain both cystic and solid areas, with two distinct cell types. The characteristic clear cells have a vacuolated cytoplasm with a small,

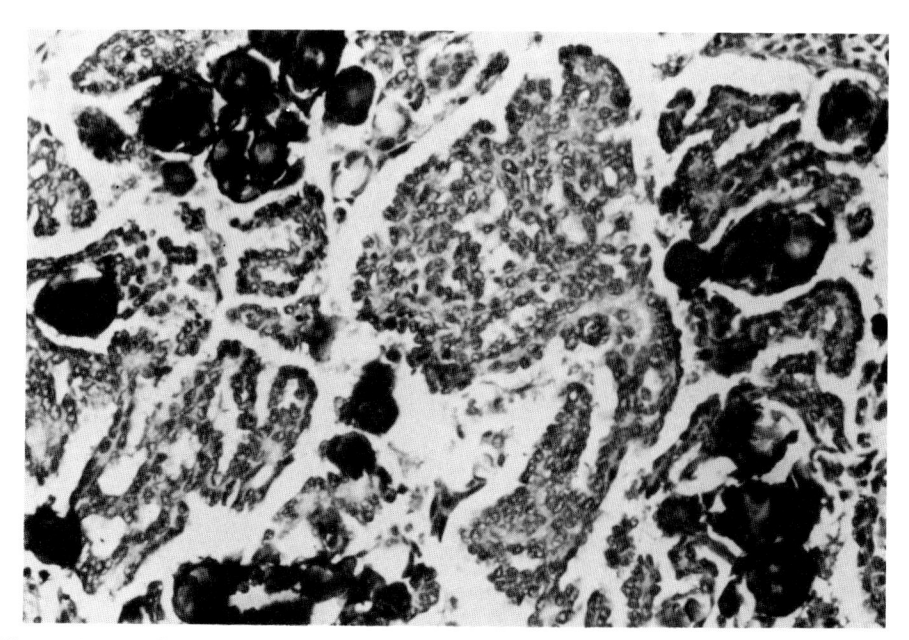

Figure 27.22. Serous cystadenocarcinoma of the ovary often forms papillary structures lined by tumor cells. Masses of dark staining calcified "psammoma" bodies are seen in this tumor.

somewhat atypical nucleus. The hobnail cell, which lines cystic spaces, has a large nucleus which protrudes from one end of the cell into the lumen of the cyst. *Brenner tumors* are the fifth variety of epithelial tumor. They are most often benign, although borderline and malignant counterparts exist. They consist of masses of fibrous stroma different from the normal ovarian stroma, in which small epithelial nests resembling transitional type epithelium are identified.

Germ Cell Tumors of the Ovary

Most of the germ cell tumors occur in premenopausal patients, with the large majority occurring in children and young adults. Benign cystic teratoma or dermoid cyst, however, may be found in patients of all ages. Germ cell tumors are felt to be derived from primitive undifferentiated germ cells which have not differentiated fully into oocytes. Many of the germ cell tumors have histologic counterparts in the primary germ cell tumors of the testis. The *dysgerminoma* is the ovarian counterpart of the testicular *seminoma* (see Fig. 30.7). The dysgerminoma is a malignant tumor of children and young women, composed of large cells with ground glass or clear cytoplasm, arranged in sheets interspersed with clusters of normal appearing lymphocytes. These tumors may occasionally be found in patients with abnormal ovarian development, but are more often seen in totally normal individuals. Ovarian dysgerminomas have a fairly good prognosis because of their extreme radiosensitivity and their relatively infrequent bilateral occurrence. Some dysgerminomas have recently been shown to produce very low

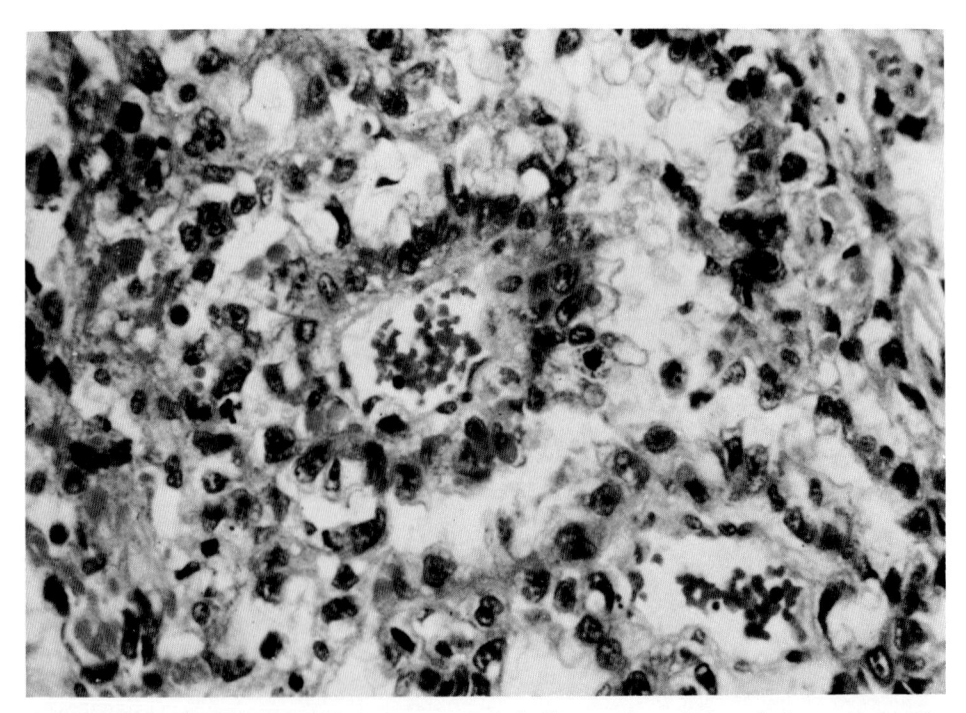

Figure 27.23. Schiller-Duvall body is characteristically seen in endodermal sinus tumors. The central blood-filled vascular space is surrounded by a rosette of tumor cells.

levels of chorionic gonadotrophin. *Endodermal sinus tumors* of the ovary are rare tumors which are very vascular in appearance. They were so named because they were felt to recapitulate the growth of the rat placenta and have characteristic Schiller-Duvall bodies (Fig. 27.23). The primitive cells of the endodermal sinus tumor often contain intra- and extracytoplasmic eosinophilic globules which contain α-fetoprotein (Fig. 27.24). This tumor production of α-fetoprotein can be used as a marker for monitoring recurrence after therapy. *Embryonal carcinoma* of the ovary is the counterpart of embryonal carcinoma of the testis. It is a germ cell tumor showing areas resembling endodermal sinus tumor as well as primitive cells arranged in sheets and gland formations. Multinucleated tumor giant cells can also be seen. Embryonal carcinomas of the ovary are associated with the production of chorionic gonadotrophin as well as α-fetoprotein. *Choriocarcinoma* can rarely present as a primary germ cell tumor of the ovary. This diagnosis is usually made in premenarchal girls, since in postmenarchal patients choriocarcinoma is much more frequent as a gestational uterine tumor. Choriocarcinoma of the ovary is associated with the production of chorionic gonadotrophin, and contains two identifiable cell types, syncytiotrophoblasts and cytotrophoblasts (Fig. 27.20).

Teratomas are the most common germ cell tumors of the ovary. They are most frequently cystic tumors composed of many different types of mature adult

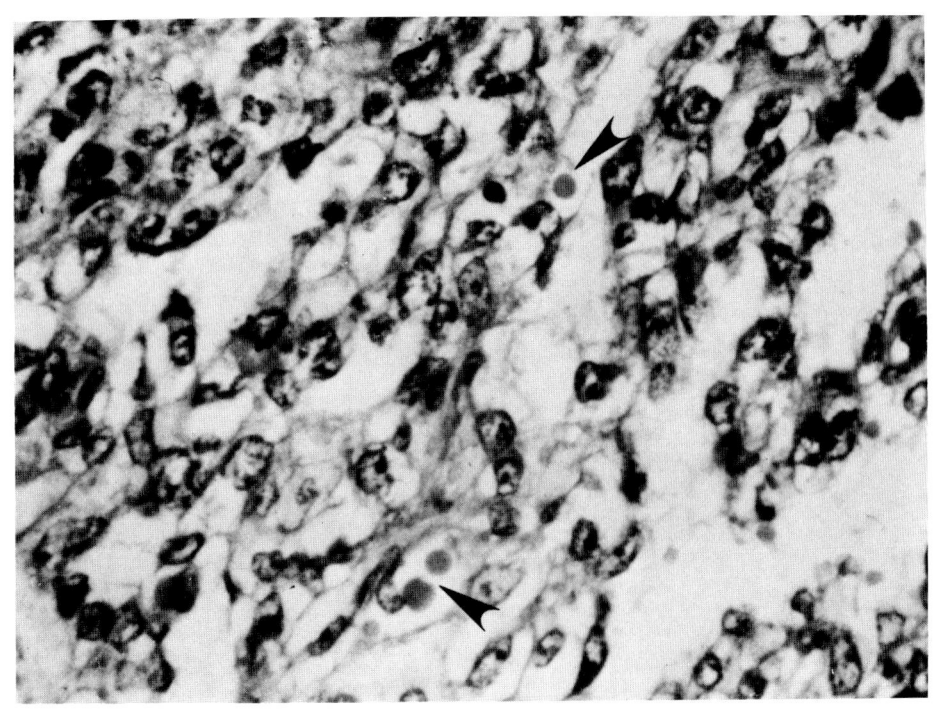

Figure 27.24. α-Fetoprotein production by endodermal sinus tumor. The rounded globules (*arrows*), present both within tumor cell cytoplasm and extracellularly, represent α-fetoprotein produced by the tumor.

appearing tissues, the most common being skin and skin appendages. In this form they are referred to as dermoid cysts (Fig. 27.25). Teratomas, however, may also be solid as well as cystic, and may contain varying proportions of immature or embryonal tissues. The malignancy of teratomas increases with the amount of embryonal tissue in the tumor (Fig. 27.26). Pure teratomas have not been associated with increased serum α-fetoprotein or chorionic gonadotrophin, but teratomas may occur as part of mixed germ cell tumors in which embryonal carcinoma, endodermal sinus tumor, or even choriocarcinoma may be present and be responsible for the production of marker proteins.

Stromal Tumors

The stromal tumors of the ovary are generally either benign or of relatively low grade malignancy. They are considered to be derived from the specialized stroma of the ovary which has the capacity for hormone production. Because of the similar embryologic origin of the ovary and testis the specialized mesenchyme from which these tumors are derived also has the capacity for differentiating into the specialized sexcord and stromal elements of the testis, the Sertoli and Leydig cells. The stromal tumors are divided into two major types depending on whether the differentiation of the tumors is masculine or feminine. *Granulosa cell tumors* are tumors of low malignant potential. They consist of small, darkly staining cells resembling the cells at the periphery of the developing ovarian follicle. The cells are often arranged in rosette-like structures with central eosinophilic material (Call-Exner bodies) (Fig. 27.27). These tumors often are nonfunctional, but may be estrogen-producing, and they may be either pure or intermixed with varying amounts of thecal cells.

Thecomas are benign tumors of the ovary which are derived from primitive

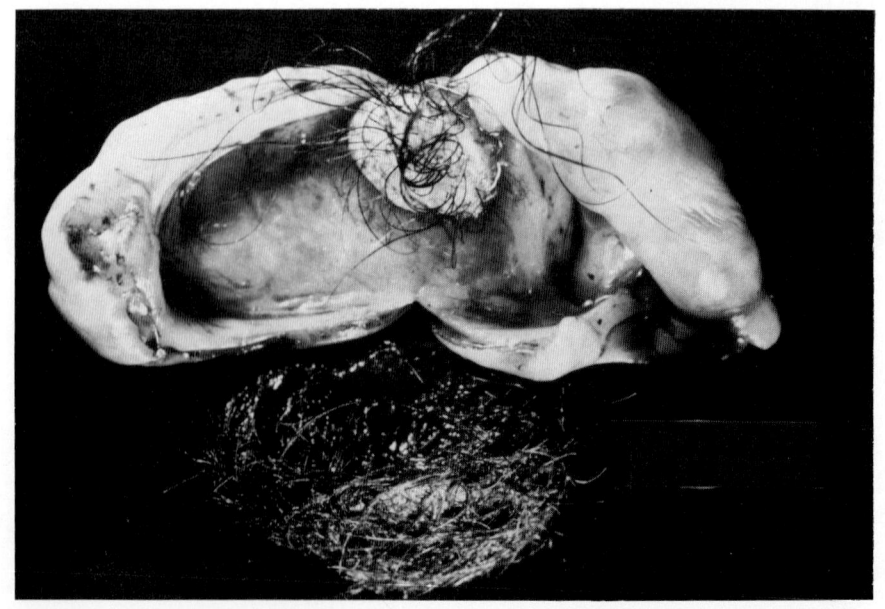

Figure 27.25. Dermoid cyst of the ovary is a benign cystic teratoma frequently lined by skin and often containing hair, keratin, and even teeth.

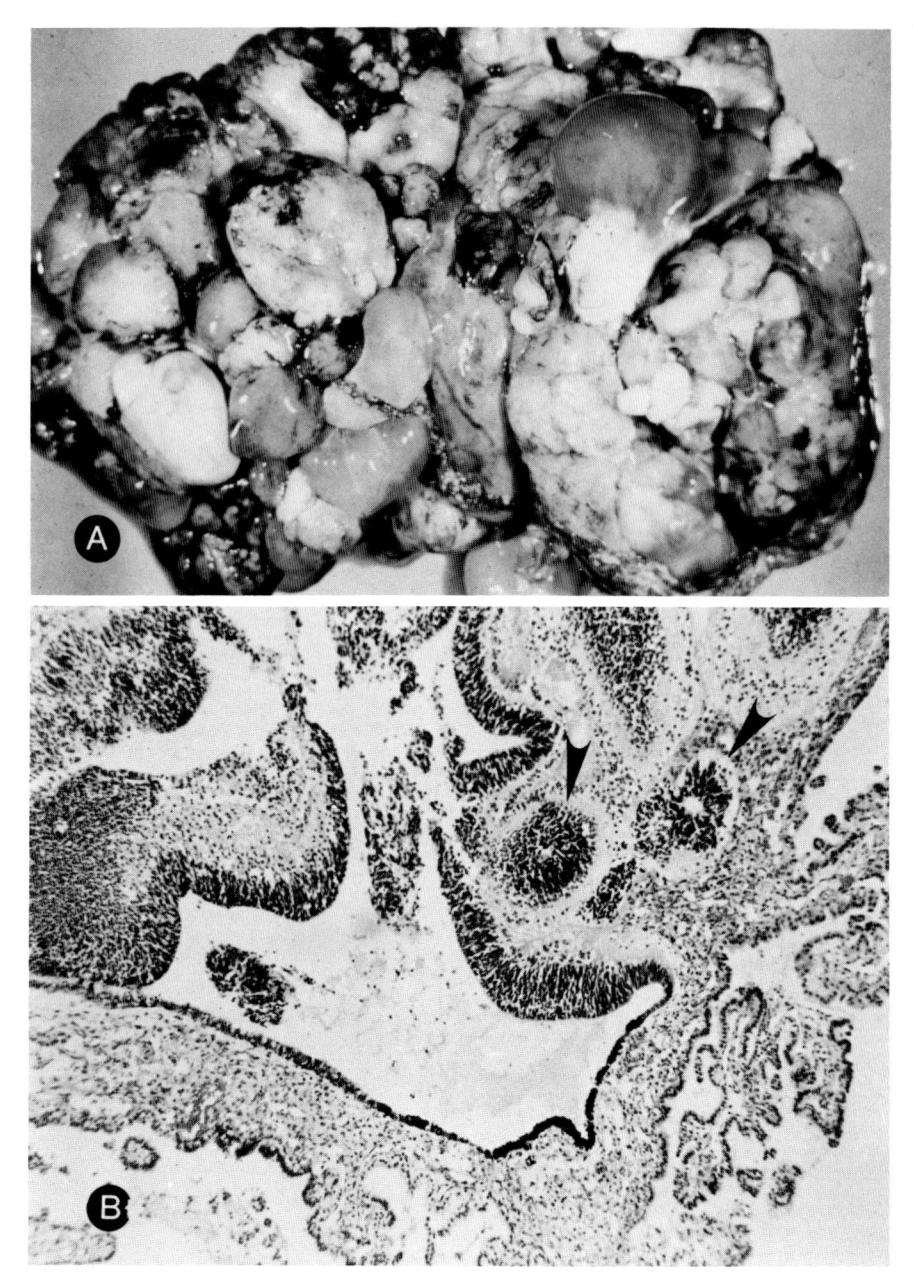

Figure 27.26. Malignant teratoma of ovary. Teratomas, with the exception of dermoid cysts, usually have both solid and cystic areas (*A*). Histologically, the degree of malignancy is determined by the amount of immature tissue present. Immature neurotubular structures are seen in this tumor in *B* (*arrows*).

mesenchyme differentiating as theca cells. In the normal ovary, the thecal cells are responsible for steroid hormone production, and these tumors are often feminizing. Thus, the patient may present with postmenopausal or abnormal uterine bleeding, or even carcinoma of the endometrium. The cells are elongate

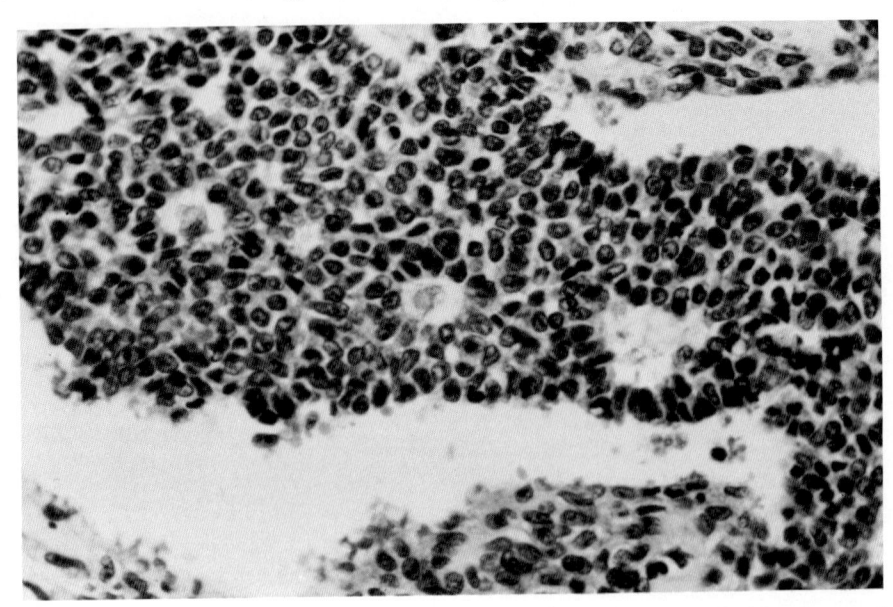

Figure 27.27. Granulosa cell tumors are composed of small dark staining cells. The characteristic Call-Exner bodies are seen here as cystic spaces with central pale staining material.

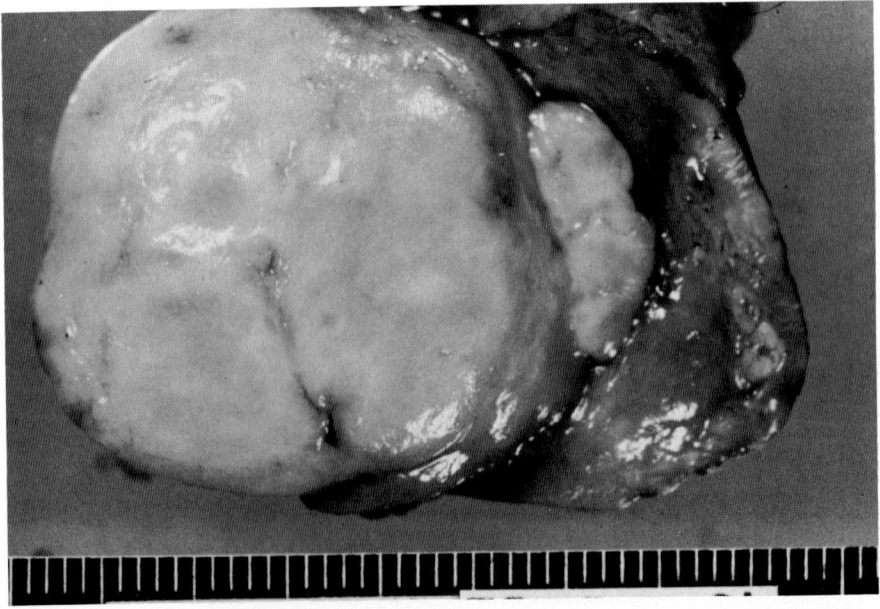

Figure 27.28. Thecoma. Thecomas are solid tumors which grossly are often distinctly yellow in color, a result of the presence of lipid within tumor cells.

and eosinophilic, often with foamy cytoplasm, and fat stains on frozen sections of the tumor often are strongly positive. Thecomas and granulosa cell tumors are characteristically solid tumors (Fig. 27.28). The *fibroma* is a less common tumor of the ovary which is also composed of eosinophilic spindle cells producing large amounts of collagen. *Sertoli-Leydig cell* tumors of the ovary or *androblastomas* are stromal tumors which show differentiation along male cell lines. Most commonly, they are androgen-producing and are responsible for either hirsutism or frank virilization in the patient.

Metastatic Ovarian Tumors

Metastatic carcinoma is fairly common in the ovary. One of the most common tumors to metastasize to the ovary is breast carcinoma. A metastatic tumor of characteristic appearance is the Krukenberg tumor, a metastatic adenocarcinoma which, in the ovary, shows numerous signet ring cells. A component of the tumor is an atypical proliferation of the benign ovarian stroma around the tumor-like nests.

Polycystic Ovarian Syndrome and Hyperthecosis

Polycystic ovarian syndrome is a name given to a spectrum of histologic changes in the ovary with accompanying clinical manifestations, such as the *Stein-Leventhal syndrome*. Patients with polycystic ovary disease usually present with secondary amenorrhea or oligomenorrhea, often characterized by infertility and anovulation. They may have associated hirsutism and obesity. The classic ovary of polycystic ovarian syndrome is enlarged, with a thickened, fibrotic, white appearing capsule. Beneath the capsule are multiple cystic follicles which present as large cysts (Fig. 27.29). Histologically, there is an increase in ovarian stroma and, particularly, a hyperplasia of the theca layer surrounding the dilated follicles. Usually, there is no evidence of recent ovulation. These patients exhibit a number of endocrine abnormalities. They usually have elevated serum testosterone levels. They may also have decreased or low normal levels of follicle-stimulating hormone (FSH) and increased levels of luteinizing hormone (LH) in the face of

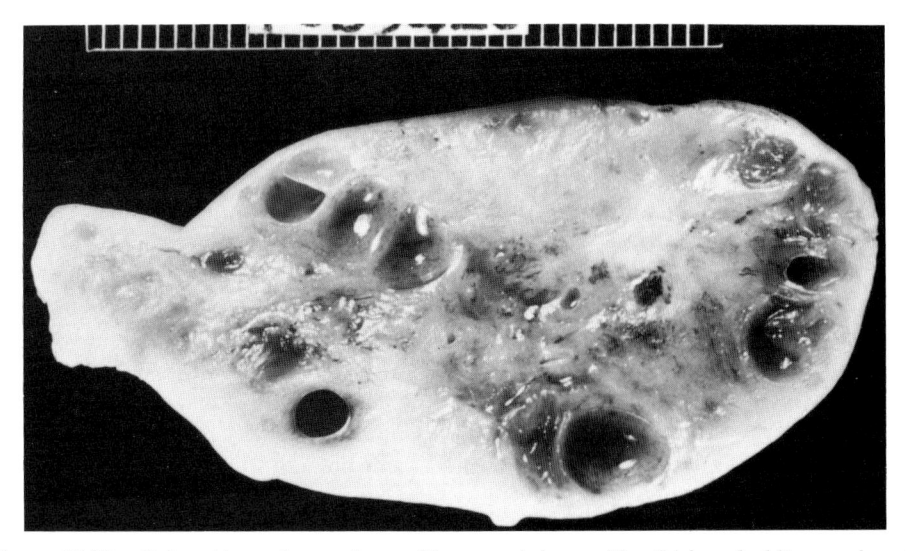

Figure 27.29. Polycystic ovarian syndrome. The ovary is large with a thickened white capsule and multiple subcapsular cystic follicles.

anovulation. The disorder represents an abnormality of the hypothalamic-pituitary-ovarian axis, although the primary site of abnormality is not clear. There may be an abnormally increased luteinizing hormone production and an increased functioning ovarian stroma which leads to production of the precursor hormone, androstenedione. This, in turn, is converted to androgen, particularly testosterone, and some also may be converted in peripheral fat depots of obese patients to estrogens, primarily estrone. The increased estrogen production further suppresses FSH and increases LH production, leading to perpetuation of the disturbance. Because of the increased estrogen levels, the patients may develop endometrial hyperplasia and, on occasion, endometrial carcinoma. *Hyperthecosis* of the ovary is considered to be at one end of the spectrum of polycystic ovarian disease. This condition may be seen in the postmenopausal patient whereas polycystic ovary disease is usually seen in the premenopausal younger woman. Hyperthecosis is a condition of increased ovarian stroma, usually without cystic follicle development.

Differential Diagnosis of Pelvic Masses

Patients with disease of the ovaries often present clinically with a pelvic mass. In consideration of the differential diagnosis of pelvic masses the physician must think in a logical fashion, first considering the *structures* that are present in the female pelvis, the *diseases* of those structures that can produce masses, those diseases that are common *versus* those that are rare, and, finally, those diseases that are appropriate for the *age* of the patient. Although ovarian tumors, particularly ovarian cancer, are the first consideration of many gynecologists, benign and malignant tumors of the uterus, tubal disease, including salpingitis and ectopic pregnancy, abnormalities of pregnancy, and diseases involving the bladder and bowel can also present as pelvic masses in the female patient.

PATHOLOGY OF ORAL CONTRACEPTIVE PILLS

Oral contraceptive preparations are widely used not only for contraception but also for treatment of menstrual irregularities, endometriosis, and many other diseases. Although these hormonal preparations are extremely effective, they are associated with significant pathologic changes. In the female genital tract, oral contraceptive pills are associated with a benign microglandular hyperplasia in the endocervix which is important to distinguish from adenocarcinoma. There is as yet no evidence of an increased incidence of cervical neoplasia in oral contraceptive pill users. The endometrium in patients who are receiving oral contraceptive medication shows the effect of exogenous hormones. There is decrease in gland development, with an altered stroma to gland ratio. The stroma frequently undergoes decidual change relatively early in the menstrual cycle.

Some of the most serious complications of oral contraceptive medication include vascular changes. Intimal hyperplasia and fibrosis occur in both arteries and veins in the pulmonary and systemic circulations in some users of contraceptive pills. These lesions may be produced experimentally with steroid hormones in animals, and are sometimes found in pregnant and postpartum patients as well. They appear to be associated with an increased incidence of thrombosis and embolization in patients on oral contraceptive pills and are related to the amount

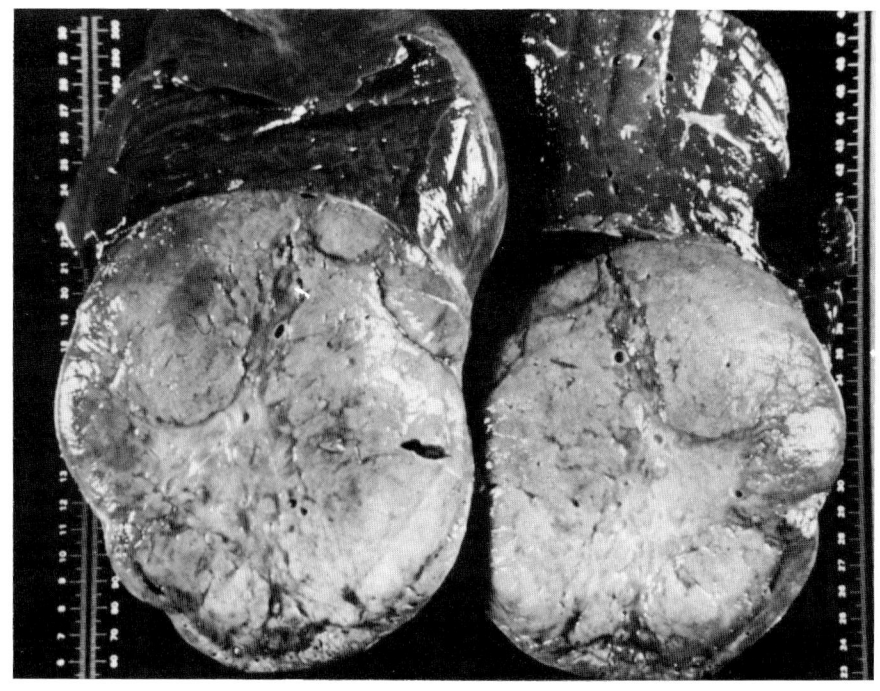

Figure 27.30. Hepatic adenoma. This large benign liver tumor was removed from a 17-year-old woman who had been on oral contraceptive pills for 6 months.

of estrogen in the pill. Patients over 40 years of age taking oral contraceptive pills have been found to have an increased risk of myocardial infarction, which is accentuated if they have other risk factors, including hypertension and smoking.

Many patients on oral contraceptive pills develop intrahepatic cholestasis, with some abnormalities detectable in liver function tests. Recently, benign hepatic tumor-like lesions termed focal nodular hyperplasia and hepatic adenoma have been reported in young women on oral contraceptive pills. These lesions frequently present with intra-abdominal hemorrhage and shock. Grossly, they are multinodular tumor masses which may involve much of the liver parenchyma (Fig. 27.30). Histologically, there is a benign proliferation of irregularly structured hepatocytes, with varying degrees of fibrosis and vascular change. Areas of infarction and organizing thrombi may be seen within these nodular lesions. Rare instances of hepatocellular carcinoma have been reported in patients receiving oral contraceptive pills.

Suggested Reading

Christopherson WM. Dysplasia, carcinoma *in situ*, and microinvasive carcinoma of the uterine cervix. Human Pathol. *8:* 489, 1977.

Dehner LP. Gestational and nongestational trophoblastic neoplasia: a historic and pathobiologic survey. Am. J. Surg. Pathol. *4:* 43, 1980.

Fechner RE. Benign hepatic lesions and orally administered contraceptives. Human Pathol. *8:* 255, 1977.

Kempson RL, Bari W. Uterine sarcomas: classification, diagnosis, and prognosis. Human Pathol. *1:* 331, 1970.

Robboy SJ, et al. Intrauterine diethylstilbestrol (DES) exposure and its consequences. Pathologic characteristics of vaginal adenosis, clear cell adenocarcinoma, and related lesions. Arch. Pathol. *101:* 1, 1977.

Scully RE. Recent progress in ovarian cancer. Human Pathol. *1:* 73, 1970.

Vellios F. Endometrial hyperplasias, precursors of endometrial carcinoma. In: Sommers SC, ed. Pathology annual. New York, Appleton-Century-Crofts, 1972.

Chapter 28

The Breast

DEBORAH E. POWELL, M.D.

This chapter emphasizes some of the more common diseases of the female breast, although there is brief consideration of gynecomastia and carcinoma in the male breast. Carcinoma of the female breast now affects 1 in every 11 American women and is the leading cause of cancer deaths in women in the United States. Because diseases of the breast are so common, understanding them and their symptoms and diagnosis is extremely important for the practicing physician.

PATHOPHYSIOLOGY OF THE BREAST

The lobule or acinus is the secretory unit of the breast. It consists of small glandular groups which actively secrete during late pregnancy. The secretory glands of the lobule are surrounded by a loose periductular stroma. Both stroma and the epithelium lining the lobules and smaller ducts of the breast are affected by hormones, notably estrogen, progesterone, and prolactin. During pregnancy, the lobular units of the breast undergo a striking degree of hyperplasia so that the lobules occupy most of the breast parenchyma. During this physiologic hyperplasia, the epithelial cells also increase in size and become modified for secretory activity, developing an abundant, foamy, and frequently vacuolated cytoplasm. Similar secretory changes can be seen in patients on oral contraceptive pills and other forms of hormonal manipulation. In the postmenopausal breast, the lobular units atrophy and the surrounding parenchyma becomes replaced by fibrofatty tissue.

FIBROCYSTIC DISEASE

Fibrocystic disease, or cystic mastopathy, is the most common disease of the female breast. Up to 50% of women may show some form of this disease. Fibrocystic disease is most frequently found in women in the reproductive age groups and frequently regresses in severity after the menopause. However, it may persist in the postmenopausal patient. Fibrocystic disease is usually bilateral, although the changes may be more pronounced in one breast. The disease frequently presents as multiple lumps or nodules within the breast (Fig. 28.1), less commonly as a solitary mass. Characteristically, the multiple lumps or

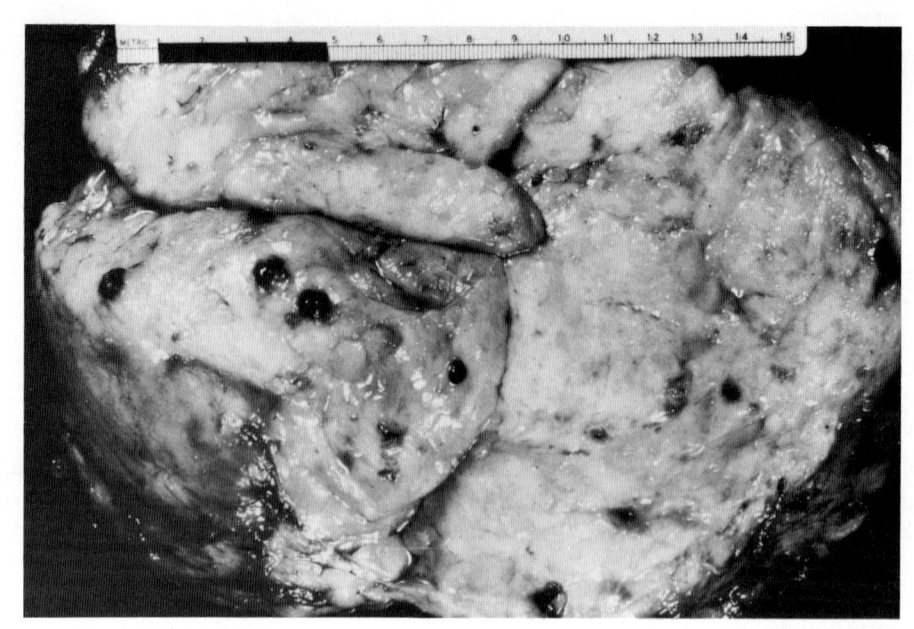

Figure 28.1. Fibrocystic disease. Numerous cysts are interspersed with white fibrotic stroma. Many of the cysts are dark because of the presence of old blood within them.

nodules are painful, and frequently increase in size and discomfort immediately before the menstrual period. The masses will often regress and become less tender immediately after menses.

Fibrocystic disease encompasses a wide variety of pathologic changes, and the large number of synonyms used for this disorder reflects its complexity. Because fibrocystic disease has many different morphologic patterns which may not all be present in the same breast, it is important to understand which of the morphologic changes may place the patient at increased risk for the subsequent development of breast cancer and which changes are prognostically, as well as pathologically, benign. It is convenient to divide fibrocystic disease into two types, proliferative and nonproliferative.

Nonproliferative Fibrocystic Disease

Nonproliferative patterns of fibrocystic disease are not associated with an increased risk of subsequent development of breast cancer. Much of the nodularity is due to *cyst* formation. The cysts may contain lipid-laden macrophages which may be seen in cytologic specimens from needle aspirations or nipple discharge. Areas of thickening or induration may be caused by *stromal fibrosis* or *sclerosing adenosis*. Sclerosing adenosis produces a characteristic whorled pattern of small epithelial ducts. The outline of the lobule can still be observed, but the internal structure is totally disorganized, with small ducts surrounded by proliferating fibrous tissue (Fig. 28.2).

Proliferative Fibrocystic Disease

Proliferative fibrocystic disease is proliferation or increased growth of the epithelial cells lining the ducts and lobules of the breast. *Atypical lobular*

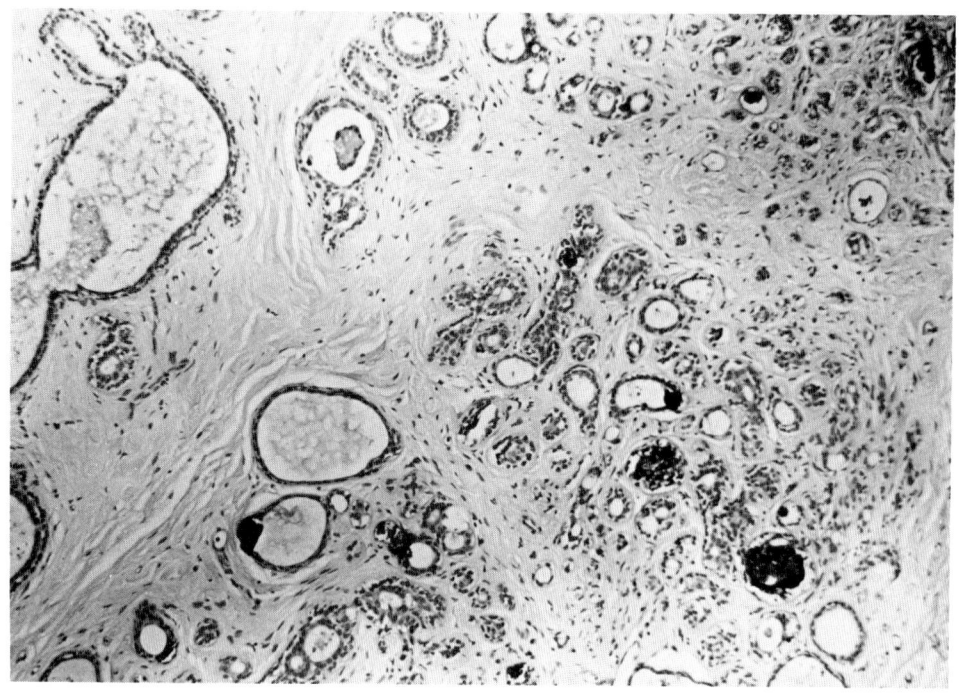

Figure 28.2. Nonproliferative fibrocystic disease. There is cystic dilatation of ducts and fibrosis of stroma. Sclerosing adenosis with dark areas of calcification within the ducts is seen at the *lower right*.

hyperplasia is a relatively rare lesion but, when present, is associated with an increased risk of subsequent development of carcinoma approximately 6 times that of the normal population. *Ductal hyperplasia*, in contrast, is rather common (Fig. 28.3). The epithelium may form papillary projections or bridging tufts across the lumen of the ducts, called *papillomatosis*. Duct hyperplasia may be associated with considerable nuclear atypia. When nuclear atypia is marked, or the intraductal growth pattern is quite advanced, the lesion is called *atypical hyperplasia*. This lesion, when present in the postmenopausal patient, is associated with an increased risk of breast cancer approximately 3 times that of the normal population. It does not appear to present an increased risk to the premenopausal patient. Calcification can occur within the ducts, within the epithelium lining the ducts, and within the stroma in fibrocystic disease. Calcification within ducts and stroma does not of itself appear to be associated with an increased cancer risk, although it may be detected on mammography and be the cause of biopsy for the patient.

FAT NECROSIS

Fat necrosis usually presents in the breast as a solitary mass. It is important mainly because, clinically and pathologically, it may mimic an infiltrating carcinoma. The lesion is frequently seen in older patients, although it can occur at any age and is often not associated with a history of prior trauma. Grossly, the lesion

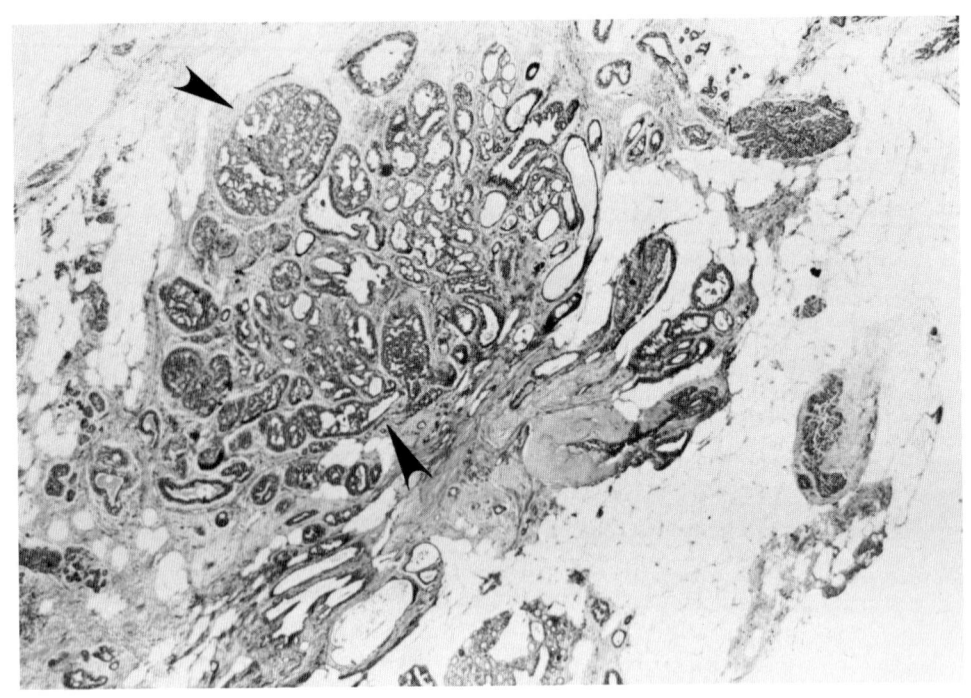

Figure 28.3. Proliferative fibrocystic disease. The distended ducts show a proliferation of the lining epithelium into the duct lumens (*arrows*). This is sometimes called papillomatosis.

is poorly circumscribed and firm, with areas of hemorrhage. Microscopically, the lesion may show characteristic fat necrosis mixed with fibrosis, granulation tissue, old and recent hemorrhage, and varying amounts of inflammation. Breast ducts may be trapped within the lesion, but no infiltrative pattern of glands is identified.

BENIGN BREAST TUMORS

Fibroadenoma

Fibroadenomas are the most common benign tumors of the breast and are most frequently found in young women in the third decade of life, but may occur at any age. The lesion is usually a solitary discrete nodule, appearing well circumscribed. Fibroadenomas vary in size from less than 1 cm to many centimeters and many hundreds of grams. The largest are called giant fibroadenomas. Grossly, fibroadenomas are usually white to tan in color. Microscopically, as the name implies, they are composed of varying proportions of glands and stroma (Fig. 28.4). The epithelium of the glands may show proliferative changes as well as apocrine metaplasia. Fibroadenomas may become active and increase in size in women who are on birth control pills or during pregnancy. Such lesions have been termed lactating adenomas. These are usually tan in color, owing to the large number of glands within them. The glands show well developed secretory activity, with foamy cytoplasm of the individual gland lining cells and secretory activity within their lumina.

Large fibroadenomas and fibroadenomas with very active stroma are referred

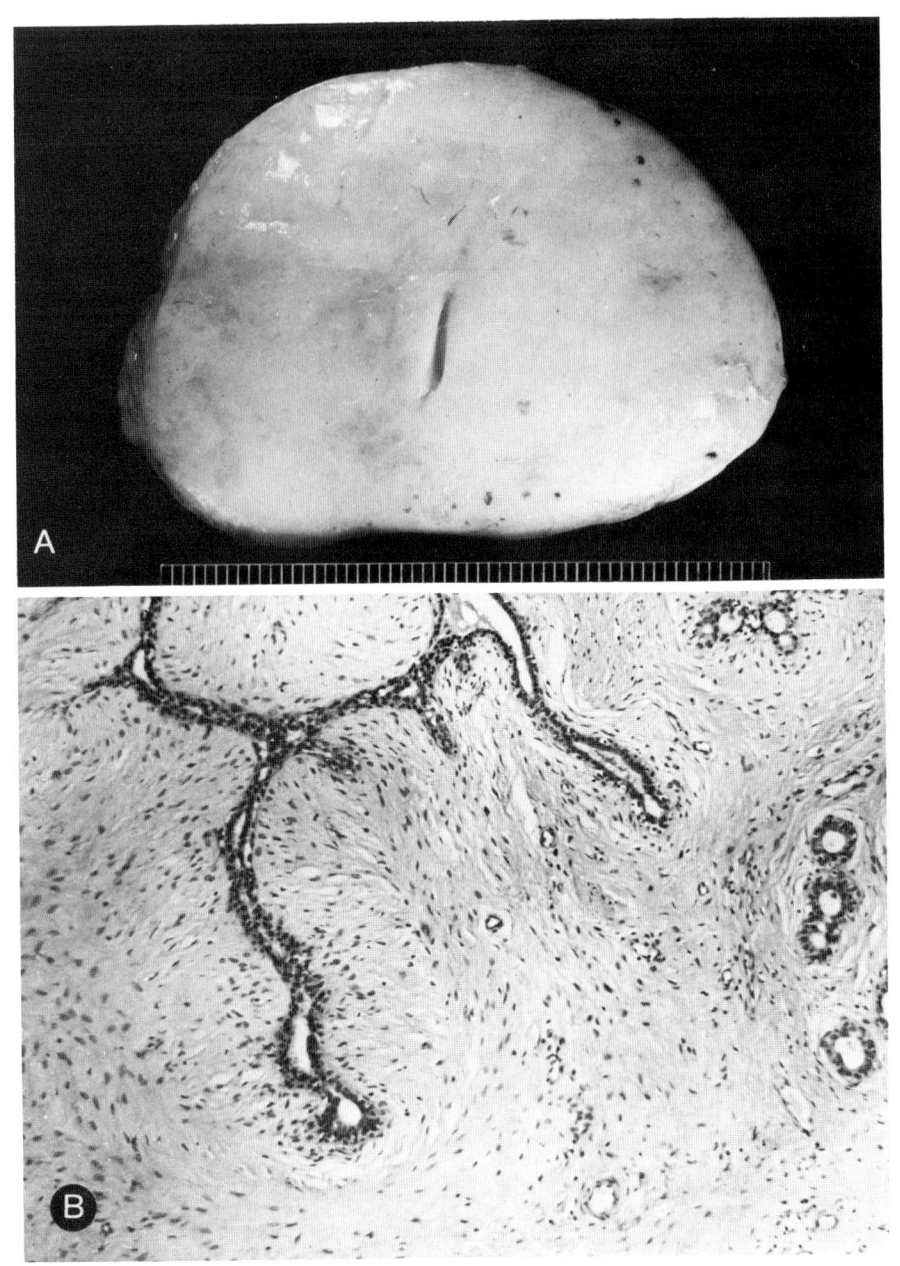

Figure 28.4. Fibroadenoma. *A*, the gross appearance of these tumors is white, firm, and well demarcated from the surrounding breast parenchyma. *B*, the tumor microscopically is formed by compressed glands and young fibrous stroma.

to as *cystosarcoma phyllodes*. In both the benign and rarer malignant varieties, the glandular elements are unremarkable and do not undergo malignant change. The benign cystosarcoma phyllodes has a more densely cellular stroma than that of the typical fibroadenoma. In the malignant variety, the stromal cells show considerable nuclear pleomorphism and the tumor resembles a fibrosarcoma with trapped glandular elements; it is best differentiated from its benign counterpart by the presence of numerous mitotic figures, more than 10 per 10 high power fields. Because they are sarcomas, these tumors do not tend to metastasize to regional lymph nodes. Cystosarcoma phyllodes may recur many times at the original site before metastasizing via the bloodstream.

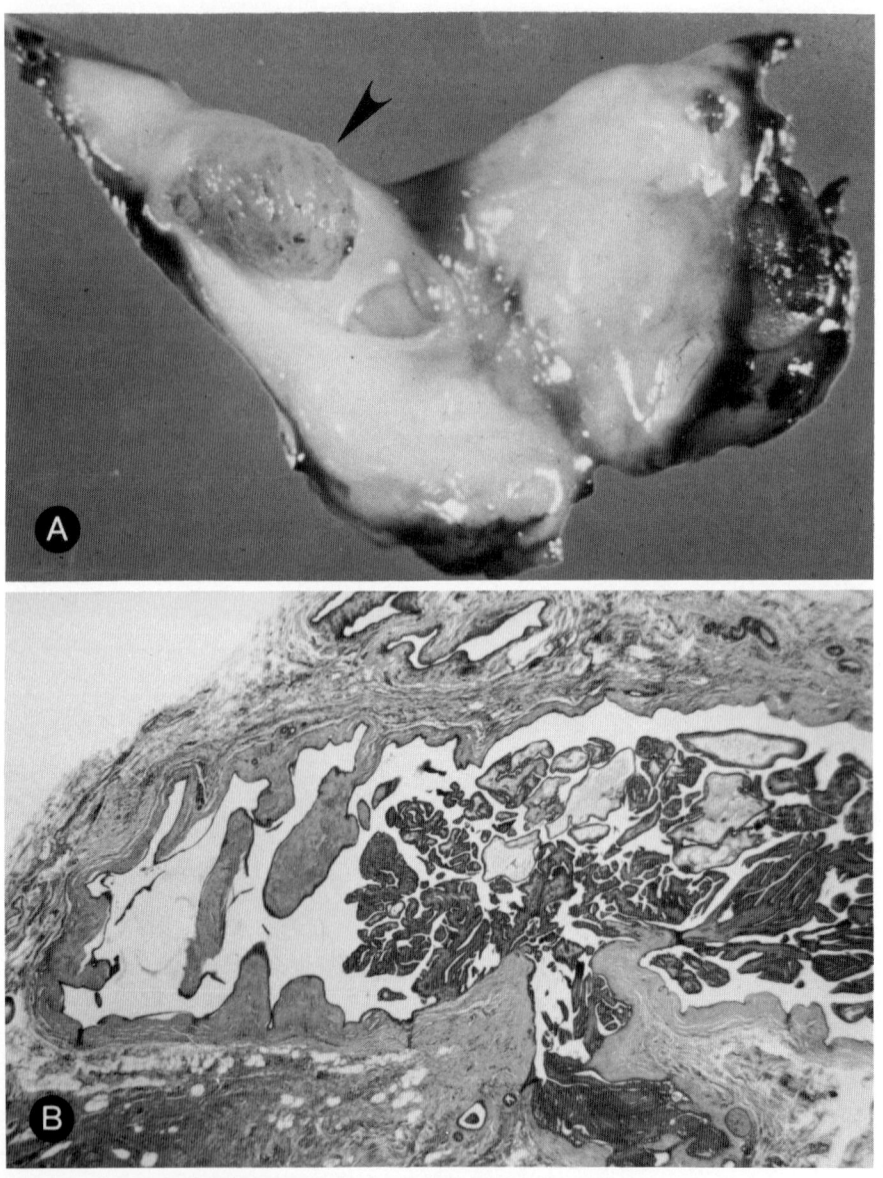

Figure 28.5. Intraductal papilloma. *A*, the papilloma (*arrow*) is a fleshy polypoid structure growing into the lumen of the opened duct. *B*, the dark staining papillary fronds of the papilloma are seen within the greatly dilated duct.

Intraductal Papilloma

Intraductal papillomas are lesions of clinical importance because they are frequently nonpalpable and often present with the symptom of nipple bleeding or discharge. The lesion is usually solitary, and thus differs from intraductal papillomatosis, which is a form of proliferative fibrocystic disease. Intraductal papilloma is a polyp-like growth, usually arising from the wall of one of the larger ducts of the breast (Fig. 28.5). It is frequently found in the duct system immediately beneath the nipple and the areola. They can range from a few millimeters to several centimeters in size. Histologically, they consist of fibrovascular stalks covered by columnar epithelial cells which can show varying degrees of nuclear atypia. These lesions only rarely undergo malignant change.

CARCINOMA OF THE BREAST

Carcinoma of the breast is an adenocarcinoma derived from the epithelial cells lining the ducts and lobules. Although experimental studies have nicely demonstrated that all breast cancer probably originates in the ducts, for convenience sake and because of interesting clinical differences, the major types of breast cancer are subdivided into lobular and ductal adenocarcinoma. Each of these two major subdivisions has a noninvasive or *in situ* form as well as an infiltrative form. Like *in situ* carcinomas in other locations, carcinoma *in situ* of the breast has a very good prognosis, since the tumor, being entirely intraepithelial, has no

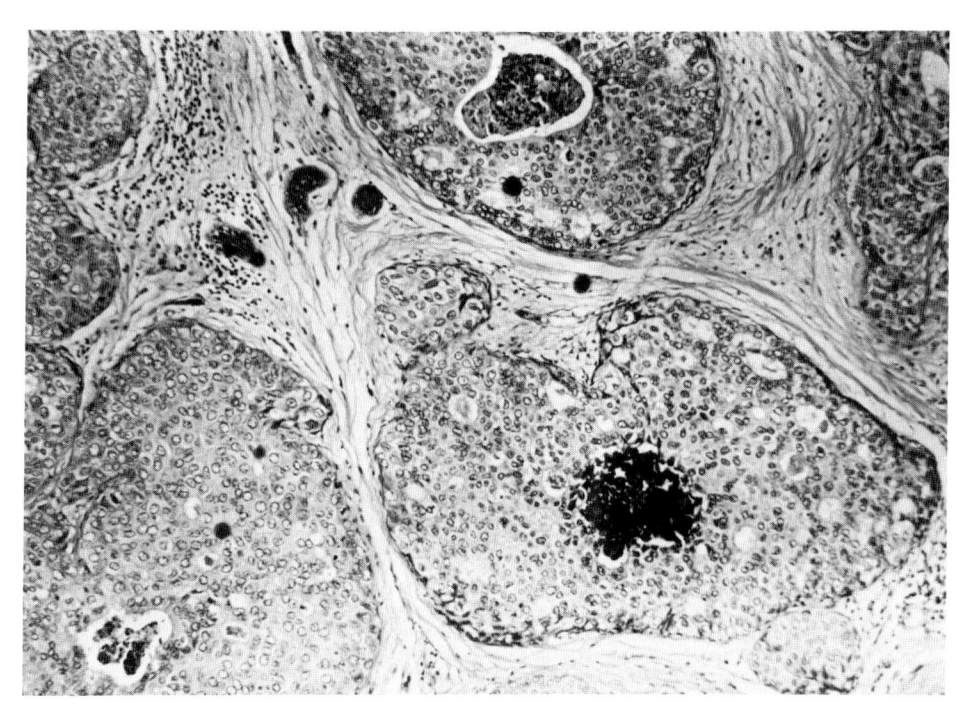

Figure 28.6. Intraductal carcinoma. The comedo pattern of intraductal carcinoma shows central necrosis which is calcified and dark staining in this photomicrograph. The tumor cells distend the ducts.

access to vascular and lymphatic spaces and should have an extremely low incidence of metastasis.

Ductal Carcinoma

Carcinoma of duct origin is the most common type of carcinoma of the breast and comprises approximately 85% of all breast cancers. The noninvasive form of ductal carcinoma is *intraductal carcinoma* of the breast. There are different patterns of noninvasive ductal carcinoma, termed comedo and cribriform carcinoma (Fig. 28.6). Recent studies have shown that if intraductal carcinoma is diagnosed by biopsy and no further definitive treatment, such as mastectomy, is performed, 40 to 50% of patients will develop invasive carcinoma within 10 years in the same breast.

The most common type of breast cancer is invasive ductal adenocarcinoma. This is a tumor composed of infiltrating masses of small glands or sheets of cells (Fig. 28.7). Depending on the degree of ductal or glandular differentiation, the tumors are considered to be well differentiated, moderately differentiated, or poorly differentiated. The degree of differentiation is important in the prognosis of the tumor. Ductal carcinoma may also be associated with small calcifications within tumor glands or stroma which may be detected by mammography (Fig. 28.8). Infiltrating ductal carcinoma may be associated with a fibrous connective tissue response apparently stimulated by the tumor cells. In the older literature, such tumors were called *scirrhous carcinoma*.

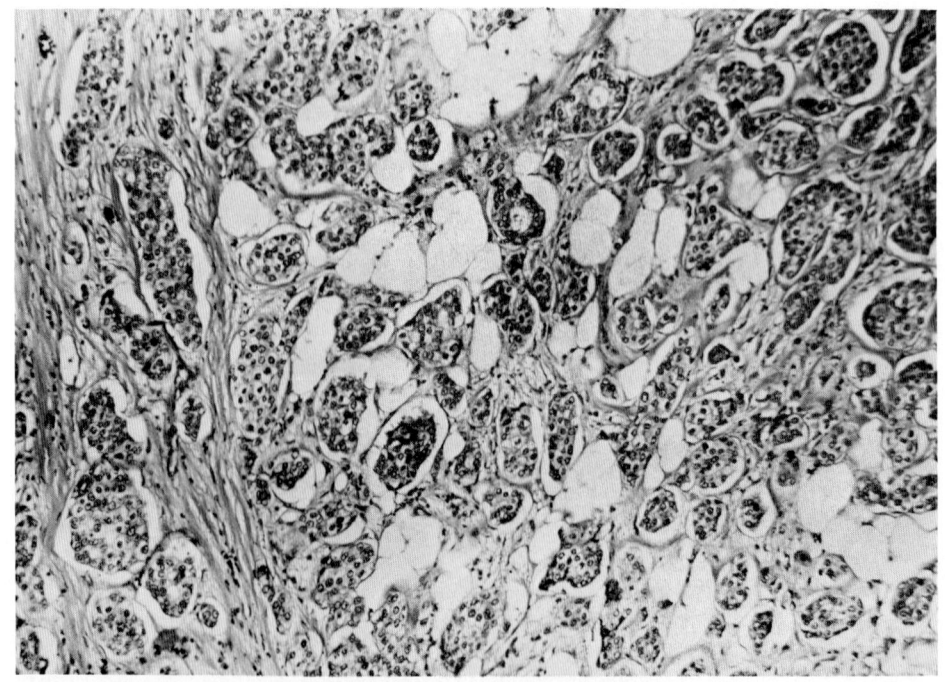

Figure 28.7. Invasive ductal adenocarcinoma. This well differentiated adenocarcinoma shows invasion of fat by clusters and gland-like formations of tumor cells.

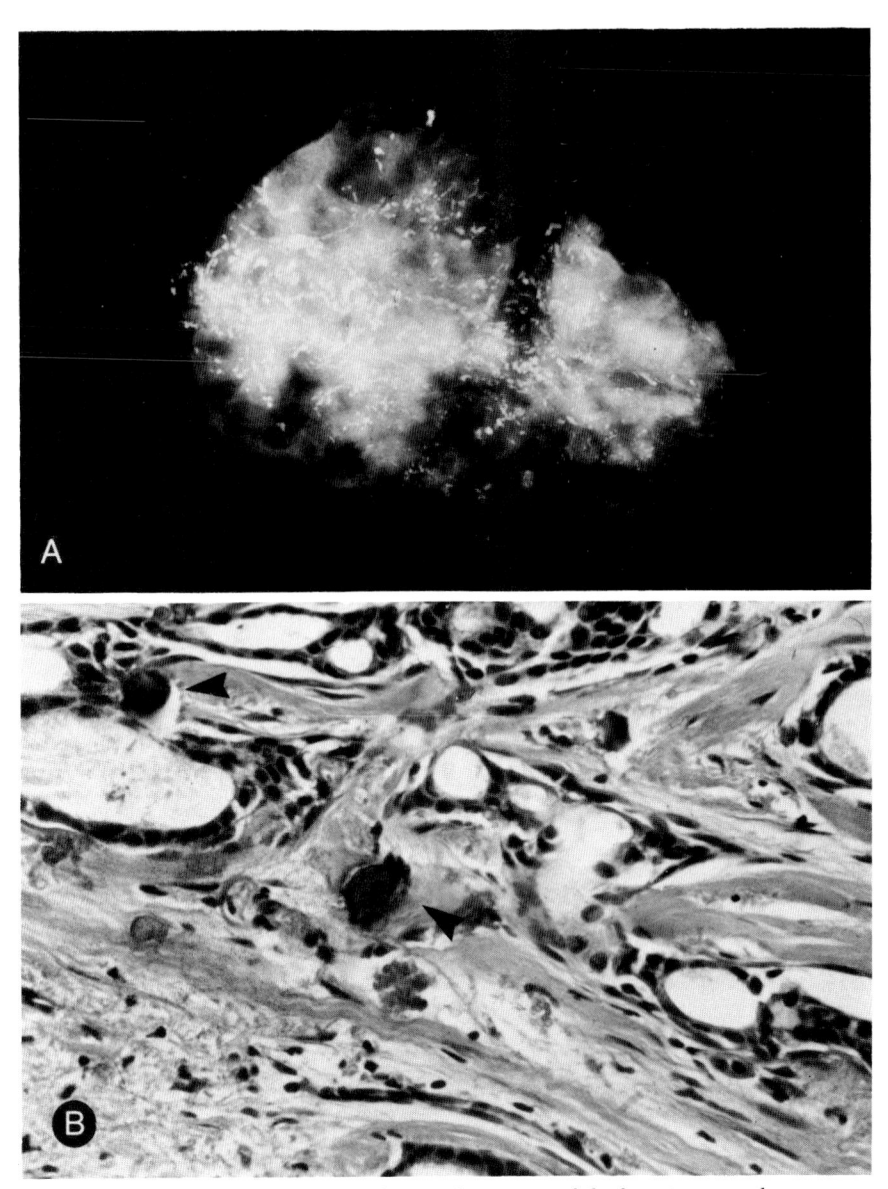

Figure 28.8. Calcification in breast carcinoma. *A*, an x-ray of the breast cancer shows numerous areas of white calcifications within the tumor. *B*, histology of the infiltrating duct carcinoma shows dense black calcifications (*arrows*).

Other less common types of infiltrating carcinoma of duct origin are also recognized. *Medullary carcinoma* is composed of large cells with vesicular nuclei and prominent nucleoli. The tumors often form large bulky masses, and histologically their cells form sheets rather than well defined ductal structures. They are frequently associated with a prominent infiltrate of lymphocytes and plasma cells. Despite their large size, and the ominous cytologic appearance of these tumors, the prognosis is somewhat better than in the more usual type of infiltrative ductal carcinoma. *Colloid* or *mucinous carcinoma* has a gelatinous, slimy appearance and, histologically, the tumor consists of large lakes of mucin in which tumor cells float as isolated cell clusters (Fig. 28.9). *Papillary carcinoma* assumes the pattern of papillary projections or cribriform nests of tumor cells which infiltrate the stroma of the breast. *Tubular carcinoma* is an extremely well differentiated form of infiltrating ductal carcinoma. The tumor cells form well defined glands and tubules which, however, are lined by a single epithelial cell layer instead of the double layer of epithelial and myoepithelial cells seen in normal breast ducts. The lesion can be confused with sclerosing adenosis, but the single cell layer lining helps to differentiate it. Tubular carcinoma very infrequently metastasizes to regional lymph nodes and is associated with an extremely favorable prognosis for the patient. Another unusual type of ductal carcinoma of the breast is *Paget's disease*. In Paget's disease, the nipple is invaded by large tumor cells which cluster along the epidermal basement membrane. Grossly, the nipple often appears ulcerated or reddened. In virtually all cases, an underlying noninvasive or infiltrating carcinoma is found. Frequently the lesion may be an intraductal carcinoma involving one of the major duct systems of the breast.

Lobular Carcinoma

Lobular carcinoma is less common than carcinoma of duct origin. Like ductal carcinoma, lobular carcinoma exists in *in situ* and infiltrative forms. Lobular carcinoma *in situ* is a lesion which has been much discussed recently. The entire lobule is involved by a proliferation of small regular tumor cells. These cells, although cytologically unimpressive, fill and distend the small units of the lobule, obliterating the lumen (Fig. 28.10). Lobular carcinoma *in situ* is less clearly

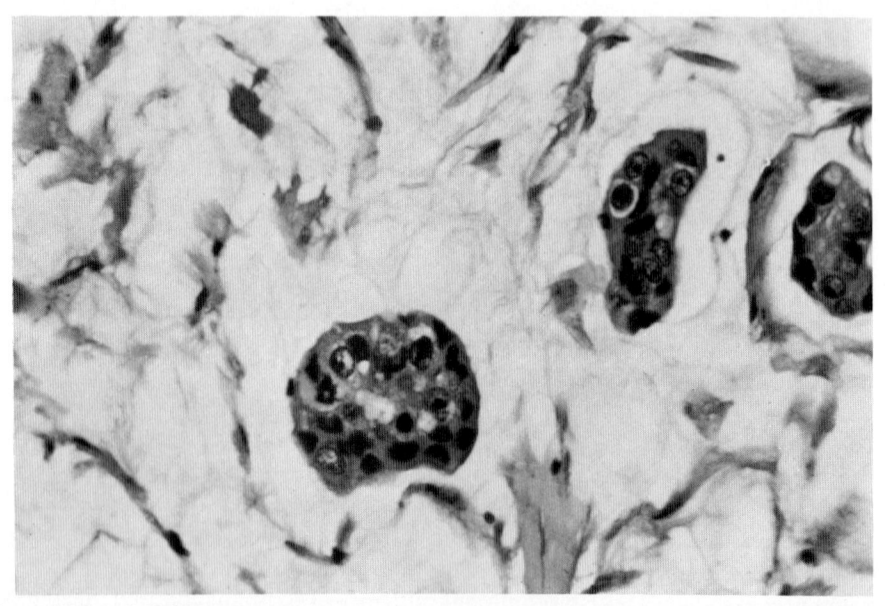

Figure 28.9. Colloid carcinoma of the breast. Nests of tumor cells appear detached and float in lakes of pale staining mucin. These tumors are a special type of invasive ductal carcinoma.

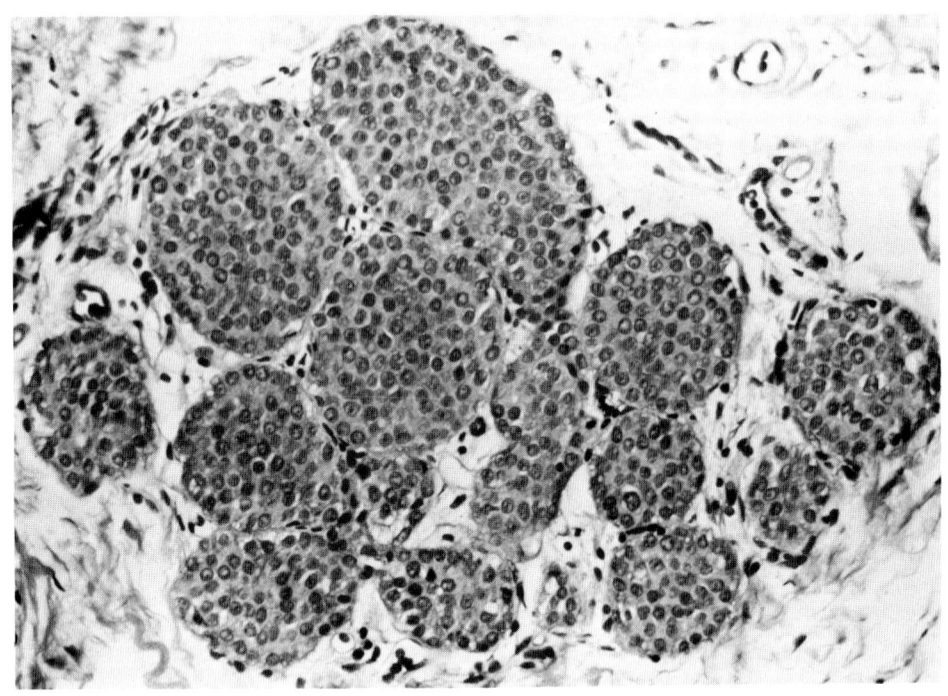

Figure 28.10. Lobular carcinoma *in situ*. The small ducts of the breast lobule are filled and distended by a proliferation of small tumor cells.

premalignant than intraductal carcinoma. Patients who have had lobular carcinoma *in situ* diagnosed by breast biopsy have an approximately 20% risk of subsequently developing infiltrating carcinoma of the breast. However, these subsequent carcinomas are frequently in the opposite breast. Lobular carcinoma is characterized by a high incidence of simultaneous bilateral cancers. When lobular carcinoma, either *in situ* or infiltrative, is found in one breast, there is up to a 25% chance of finding a simultaneous lobular cancer in the opposite breast. Infiltrating lobular carcinoma characteristically appears as small regular cells similar to those seen in lobular carcinoma *in situ*. These cells infiltrate the stroma of the breast in chains or an "Indian file" pattern (Fig. 28.11). The tumor cells ring uninvolved small ducts in a concentric fashion. Despite the higher incidence of bilaterality with lobular carcinomas, the prognosis for both infiltrating lobular and infiltrating ductal carcinoma is similar, and both tend to metastasize initially to axillary lymph nodes.

Risk Factors

Breast cancer is a form of cancer most prevalent in the Western European countries and the United States. The incidence of breast cancer is very low in Japanese women. This geographic distribution of carcinoma of the breast becomes even more interesting when various risk factors are discussed. The most important risk factor for breast carcinoma is a family history of carcinoma of the breast. Women whose mothers had breast cancer are at a 5 times increased risk over

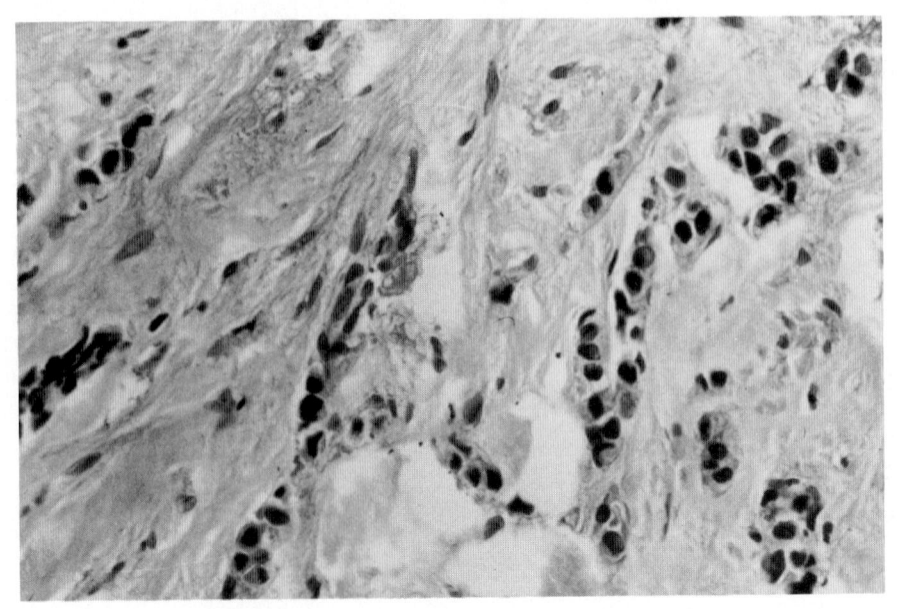

Figure 28.11. Invasive lobular carcinoma. The small darkly staining cells of invasive lobular carcinoma characteristically invade the stroma in single cell chains, the so-called "Indian file" pattern.

women with no family history in a primary relative. Women who have two close family members with bilateral breast cancer have a risk of themselves developing breast cancer approximately 10 times that of the general female population. Most of these increased risks seem to apply to the premenopausal patient, and the risk decreases after menopause to approach more nearly that of the general population. There are several endocrine-associated risk factors for breast cancer. Women who have had their first full term pregnancy after the age of 30 are at greater risk. Early menarche and late menopause, and low parity, are also associated with a slightly increased breast cancer risk; newer studies do not substantiate claims that nursing and lactation decrease risk. Recently, dietary factors have been considered important in the etiology of breast cancer. Several studies have shown that patients with breast cancer may have greater body weight than their noncancer controls, and this has been associated with an increased dietary animal fat intake. This becomes particularly interesting when one considers the low breast cancer rate among Japanese women living in Japan, where diets are traditionally low in animal fats. Women of Japanese birth migrating to the United States have a somewhat increased risk of breast cancer while their children who are of Japanese descent, but born in the United States, have a breast cancer risk similar to other U.S. females.

Patterns of Metastasis in Carcinoma of the Breast

Like all carcinomas, breast cancer metastasizes initially to regional lymph nodes, the ipsilateral axillary nodes for lesions primary in the central regions and the outer quadrants of the breast, and the internal mammary chain for lesions arising in the inner quadrants. The tumors may also metastasize by the bloodstream, primarily to bone, brain, and lung. Breast cancer can metastasize to any organ of the body and some breast cancers metastasize systemically while the primary tumors are still small, and before regional lymph node metastases have occurred. Breast cancer is unusual in that metastases may appear relatively late in the course, 10 to even 20 years after the original diagnosis.

Prognostic Factors in Carcinoma of the Breast

The presence or absence of regional lymph node metastases is the single most important prognostic factor in breast cancer. Patients with no lymph nodes positive at the time of surgery have a good prognosis, with approximately 75% of patients surviving 10 years after surgery. Patients with one to three axillary lymph nodes positive have an intermediate survival with almost 60% of patients surviving 10 years, while patients with four or more axillary lymph nodes positive have a markedly decreased survival rate of approximately 30% at 10 years. In addition to node metastases, other prognostically important factors are the size of the primary tumor (tumors greater than 4 cm have a less favorable prognosis) (Fig. 28.12), the differentiation of the tumor, and the presence of invasion of lymphatic or vascular spaces by tumor cells within the breast itself.

Another important factor is the presence or absence of estrogen receptor protein within the tumor. Estrogen receptor protein is a binding protein for estrogen found within the cytoplasm and also within the nucleus of epithelial cells in the breast. Tumors with a high concentration of estrogen receptor protein within their cells are the only tumors likely to respond to hormone manipulation, and some studies have indicated that these are also tumors with a better

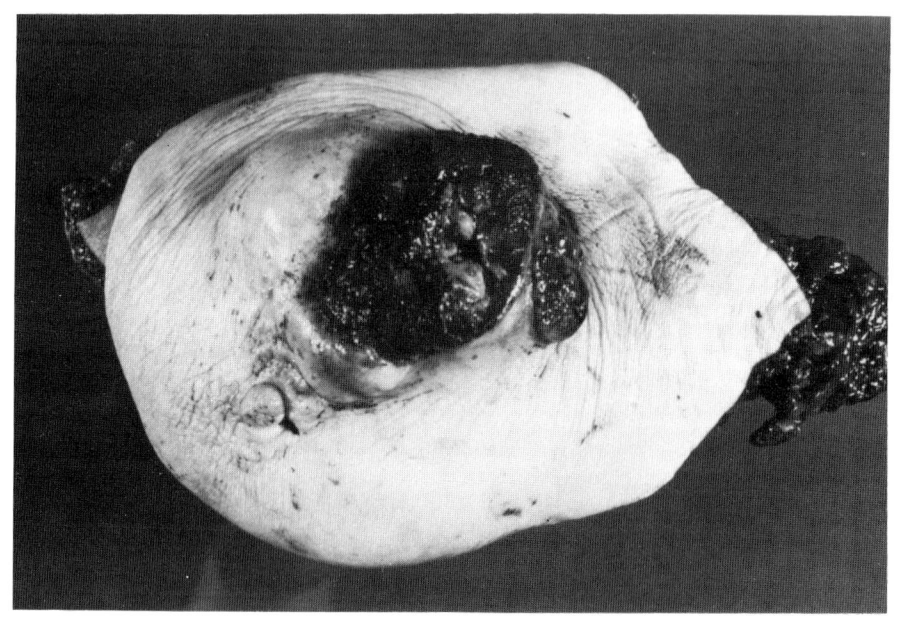

Figure 28.12. Large ulcerating breast carcinoma which has grown through the skin. Tumors of this large size have generally unfavorable prognosis.

404 Pathology: Understanding Human Disease

prognosis. The combination of estrogen and progesterone receptors is thought by some to indicate a better response rate to hormone therapy, as does estrogen receptor production by tumor metastases.

Clinical Manifestations of Breast Lesions

Benign lesions of the breast are more likely to be tender or painful than carcinomas. Benign tumors tend to be freely movable, and have discrete borders, while carcinomas tend to be infiltrative, without discrete borders, and often fix to chest wall or overlying skin (Fig. 28.13). Benign lesions may be multiple while carcinomas are usually solitary. Benign lesions may increase and decrease in size at different times of the menstrual cycle.

Ominous signs of breast cancer include retraction of the nipple, dimpling of the skin, or a peculiar edematous change of the skin with prominent pitting of the epidermal surface, referred to as the orange skin or *peau d'orange* pattern. The edema is due to intramammary lymphatic metastases of a breast tumor, associated with a very poor prognosis.

MALE BREAST DISEASE

Gynecomastia

Gynecomastia refers to enlargement of the male breast and may be either unilateral or bilateral. The etiology of gynecomastia is often related to excess estrogens or gonadotrophins. Patients with severe liver disease may have gynecomastia due to increased circulating estrogen levels. Patients with Klinefelter's syndrome (p. 417) may have increased gonadotrophin levels and patients with

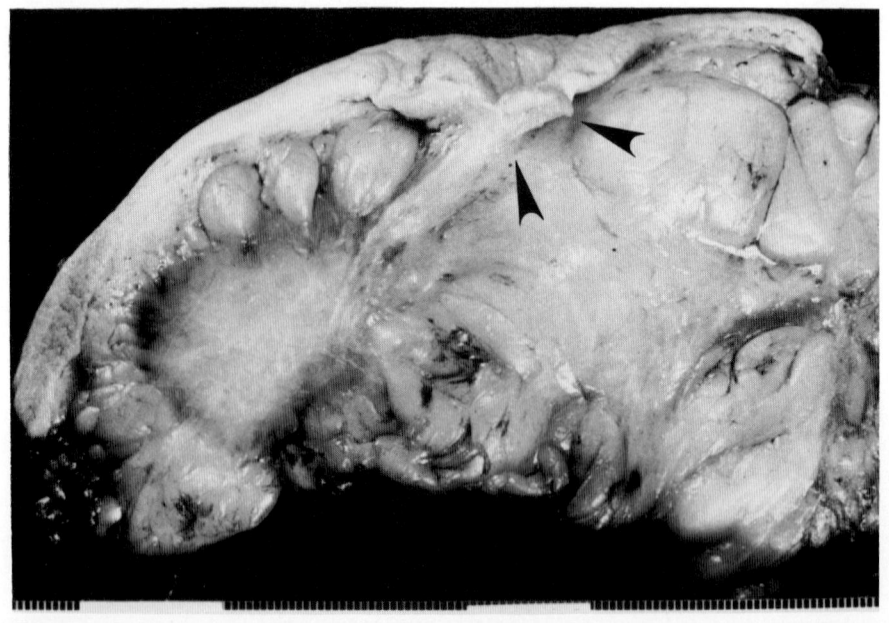

Figure 28.13. Invasive breast carcinoma seen on cut section of the breast shows retraction of the nipple (*arrows*) by the tumor and surrounding fibrosis.

malignant germ cell tumors of testicular or other origin may develop gynecomastia because of high serum levels of chorionic gonadotrophin. Gynecomastia may also be due to such drugs as phenytoin, digitalis, reserpine, and chlordiazepoxide. There may, at times, be no obvious etiology for the enlargement of the breast.

Carcinoma

Carcinoma of the male breast is an extremely rare disease. Since the male breast does not develop true lobules, these carcinomas are virtually always of the ductal variety. Carcinoma of the male breast is usually associated with a less favorable prognosis than female breast cancer because of the large size the tumors reach before diagnosis. Histologically, it resembles ductal carcinoma in the female and the patterns of metastases are the same.

Suggested Readings

Henderson IC, Canellos GP. Cancer of the breast: the past decade. N. Engl. J. Med. *302:* 17, 78, 1980.
McDivitt RW. Breast carcinoma. Human Pathol. *9:* 3, 1978.
Page DL, et al. Relation between component parts of fibrocystic disease complex and breast cancer. J. Natl. Cancer Inst. *61:* 1055, 1978.

Chapter 29

The Urinary Bladder

Discussion in this chapter is confined to infections of the bladder and its important epithelial tumors.

CYSTITIS

Much of what was said about pyelonephritis (p. 195) is applicable to a consideration of infections of the bladder. Most infections are caused by enteric organisms, particularly *Escherichia coli*, although other organisms may be encountered in patients with recurrent infections. They are more common in women than in men. Many infections are relatable to obstructive lesions of the lower urinary tract, particularly in men and children. Bladder neck obstruction caused by hypertrophied musculature is a frequent finding in children with cystitis, and congenital urethral valves frequently cause obstruction in young boys. The principal cause of obstruction in older men is enlargement of the prostate gland. Instrumentation of the lower urinary tract always runs a risk of introducing infection.

The bladder mucosa is inflamed and occasionally ulcerated and hemorrhagic (Fig. 29.1). Inflammation is usually confined to the submucosal tissues and does not extend to the musculature. With repeated infections, the bladder wall may become thin and dilated, or hypertrophy may result in markedly increased trabeculation and diverticulum formation. Stones are not uncommon and usually consist of calcium oxalate, perhaps mixed with calcium phosphate. Struvite (ammonium magnesium phosphate) stones are common in patients with recurrent urinary tract infections due to urea-splitting bacteria.

CARCINOMA

There are some 35,000 new cases of bladder carcinoma reported in this country each year, and some 10,000 deaths are attributable to this disease. There is a marked male predominance (3:1) and a higher incidence in whites than in blacks. Carcinoma of the bladder is the fifth most frequent cause of death in men over 75.

Known risk factors for carcinoma of the bladder include cigarette smoking, exposure to industrial carcinogens (*e.g.*, aniline, β-naphthylamine, and benzidine), abuse of analgesic drugs, pelvic irradiation, and administration of cyclophosphamide and other antimetabolites. Cigarette smoking increases the risk by a factor

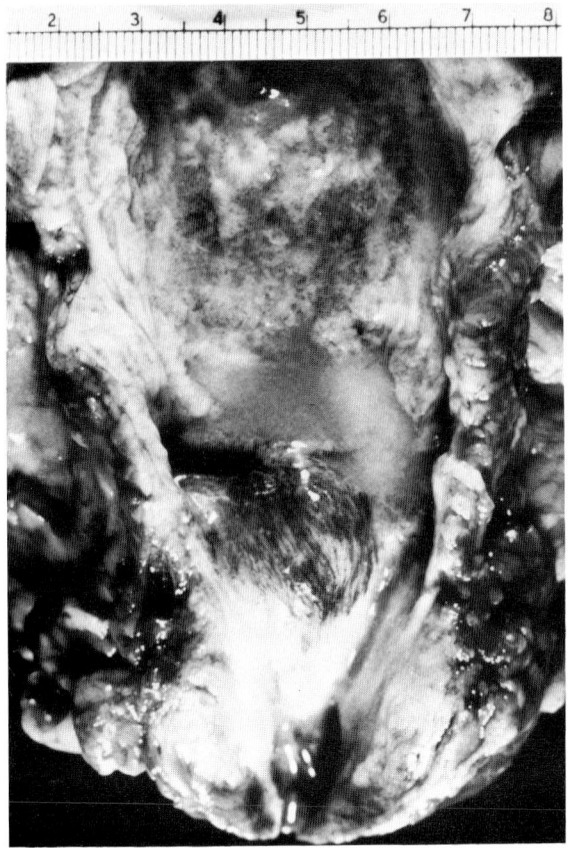

Figure 29.1. Acute cystitis. The bladder mucosa is congested and inflamed, and the small amount of urine at the *center* is grossly purulent. The trigone is at the *lower end* of the photograph.

of 4, cyclophosphamide by 9. Although suspect, studies of the artificial sweetener saccharin have not proven a relationship to carcinoma of the bladder. In the Middle East, particularly Egypt, infestation by *Schistosoma haematobium* is associated with a very high incidence of squamous carcinoma.

Over 90% of bladder tumors are transitional cell carcinomas, some 6% squamous. These tumors are most commonly observed in the trigone area (Fig. 29.2). Transitional cell tumors may have multicentric origin in the urinary tract and involve renal pelves, ureters, and bladder. Adenocarcinomas are uncommon and occur at the fundus, arising from remnants of the urachal glands.

Early transitional cell tumors are usually papillary in configuration (Fig. 29.3), but flat *in situ* lesions may be seen. Transitional tumors are graded on the basis of pleomorphism and anaplasia. Staging is based on invasion of the bladder wall and lymph node metastasis:

---

0   Noninvasive
A   Invasion confined to lamina propria

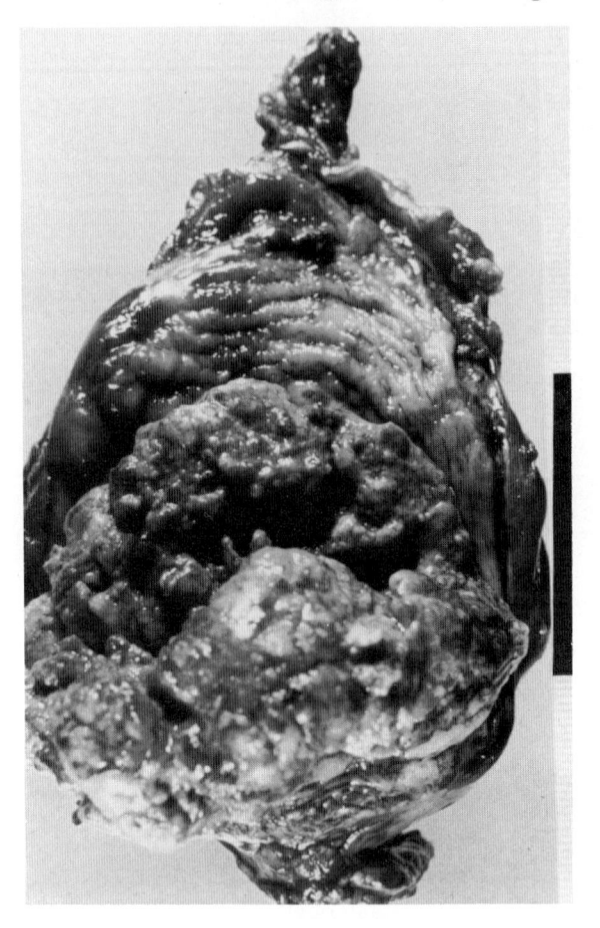

Figure 29.2. Carcinoma of bladder. A large fungating and ulcerated tumor occupies the lower half of the bladder. This tumor was a poorly differentiated transitional cell carcinoma.

B1   Invasion of inner muscle wall
B2   Invasion of outer muscle wall
C   Invasion of perimuscular fat and lymphatics
D   Lymph node metastases

Proper evaluation of transitional carcinoma of the bladder often requires multiple biopsies, particularly in determining the grade and stage of papillary lesions. Not infrequently, the bladder mucosa near a papillary carcinoma will show dysplasia or carcinoma *in situ*, increasing the likelihood of new invasive lesions.

Normal bladder epithelial cells have surface antigens that cross-react with blood group isoantigens. Poorly differentiated transitional tumor cells loose these surface antigens. It is of interest that tumors containing the surface antigens have a recurrence rate of only 10% following removal, whereas 80% of tumors without the antigens recur.

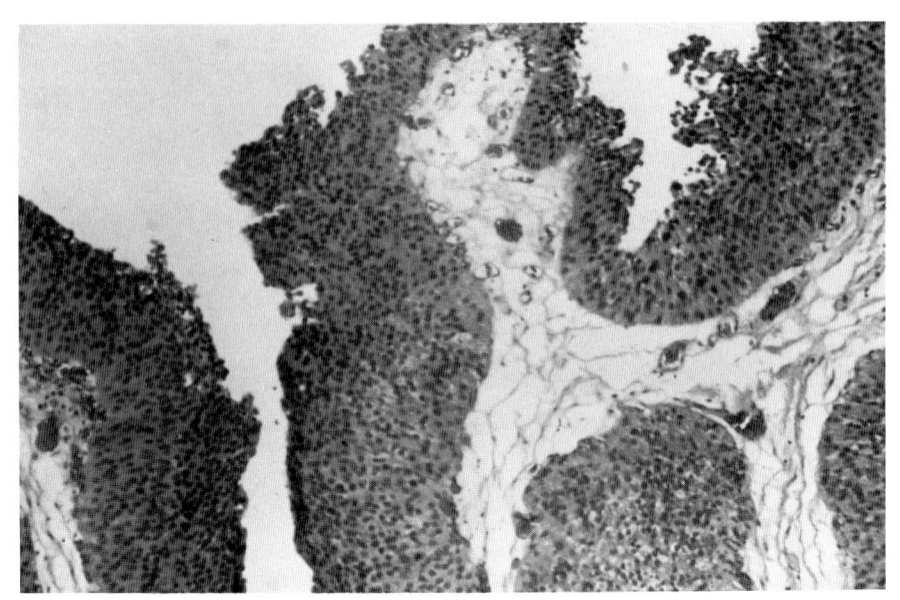

Figure 29.3. Transitional cell carcinoma. This tumor has a papillary configuration. The tumor cells are generally well differentiated, although some nuclear pleomorphism is noted.

Squamous cell carcinomas are not usually papillary; they tend to spread along the surface of the bladder, ulcerate, and invade the wall early in their course.

Suggested Reading

Friedell GH, Jacobs JB, Nagy GK, Cohen SM. The pathogenesis of bladder cancer. Am. J. Pathol. *89:* 431, 1977.

Hoover R. Saccharin—bitter aftertaste? N. Engl. J. Med. *302:* 573, 1980.

Chapter 30

The Male Genital Tract

The principal topics discussed in this chapter include hyperplasia and carcinoma of the prostate and germ cell and stromal tumors of the testis.

HYPERPLASIA OF THE PROSTATE

Prostatic hyperplasia is one of the most common disorders of men, involving a large majority by age 75. Its principal manifestation is urethral obstruction, with difficulty with urination and a predisposition to urinary tract infections. The hyperplasia is both glandular and stromal, although either may predominate (Fig. 30.1), and involves the central, periurethral portion of the gland; the posterior lobe is not affected. The hyperplasia is nodular in configuration (Fig. 30.2). Marked enlargement of the median lobe, together with hyperplasia of bladder neck tissues, can present as a "median bar" that acts as a ball valve and obstructs the bladder outlet.

Hyperplasia of the prostate rarely occurs before age 40 and does not occur in eunuchs. Hyperplasia, in all likelihood, reflects an imbalance between estrogen and testosterone. Both hormones are necessary for the lesion to develop, but the estrogen to testosterone ratio is increased.

Other than requiring a certain age and the presence of testes, there are no known predisposing factors. Although they are often encountered together, hyperplasia is not believed to be a precancerous lesion.

ADENOCARCINOMA OF THE PROSTATE

Adenocarcinoma of the prostate is the second most common malignancy in American men, accounting for 57,000 new cases and some 21,000 deaths each year. If the large numbers of small, localized, occult tumors are included, half of all men have carcinoma of the prostate by age 70.

Adenocarcinomas arise most often in the posterior lobe (Fig. 30.3). They may extend to the lateral lobes and to the periprostatic tissues and may metastasize early to pelvic lymph nodes and to the lumbar vertebral bodies (Fig. 30.4). Most are histologically well differentiated (Fig. 30.5), but some are anaplastic.

There are no known risk factors for prostatic carcinoma. It is rare below age 40, and is androgen-dependent; it does not occur in the absence of testes.

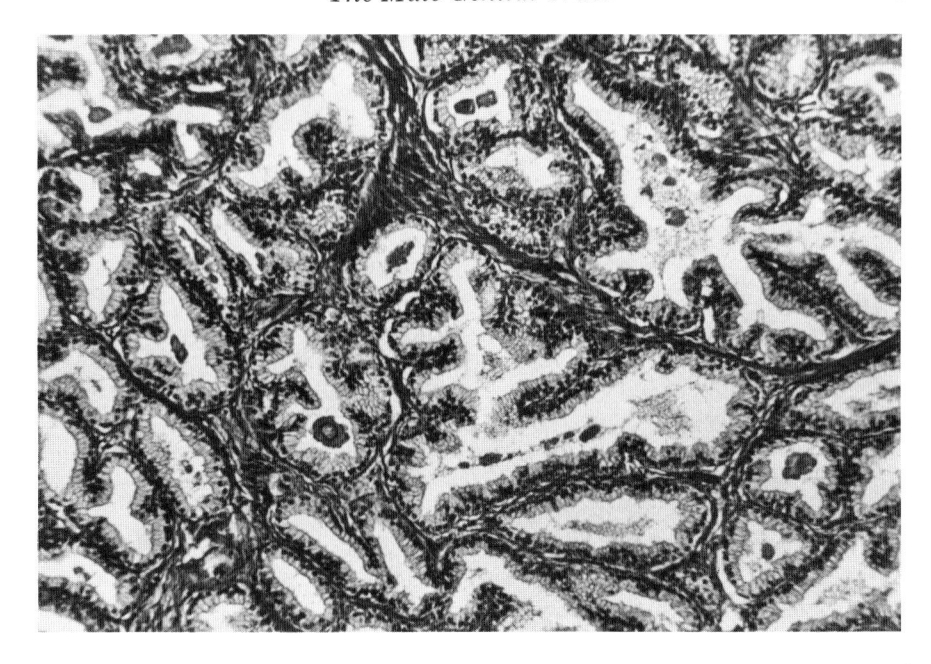

Figure 30.1. Hyperplasia of prostate. This area of glandular hyperplasia shows closely packed glands with tall, often papillary epithelium. The stroma here is very delicate. In other areas, stromal hyperplasia may be the predominant finding.

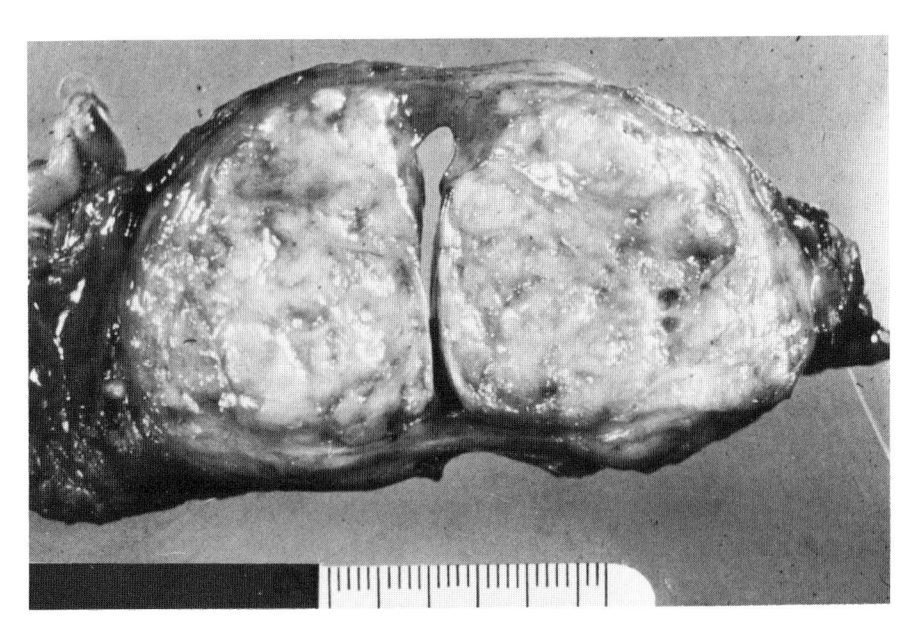

Figure 30.2. Hyperplasia of prostate. The lateral lobes are markedly enlarged, rubbery in consistency, and distinctly nodular. The posterior portion of the prostate is not involved.

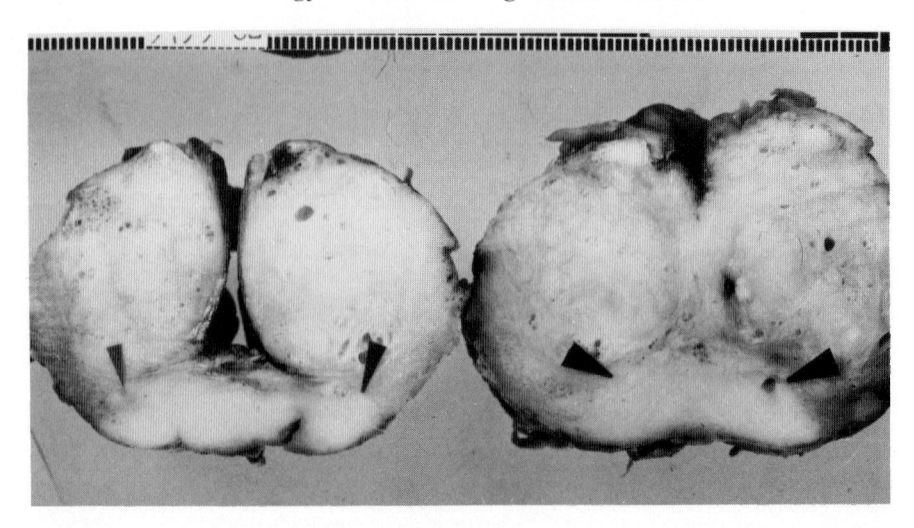

Figure 30.3. Adenocarcinoma of prostate. The *arrows* point to hard grayish white tumor tissue which has enlarged the posterior lobe of the gland. The lateral lobes are enlarged and show invasion by the tumor.

The staging of prostatic carcinoma is:

A Recognizable only on histologic examination
B Palpable on digital rectal examination
C Extension beyond capsule
D Metastases present

The serum acid phosphatase concentration is often elevated in patients with Stage C or D disease and can serve as a marker to follow the effectiveness of therapy. False positive tests can occur, however, particularly in the presence of prostatic infarcts, or following mechanical manipulation of the gland.

Since adenocarcinoma of the prostate is androgen dependent, therapy of Stage C or Stage D disease includes administration of estrogens and, often, orchiectomy.

TESTICULAR TUMORS

Testicular tumors comprise only 1% of neoplasms in males, but a very significant proportion of malignancies in the 15- to 35-year-old group. The vast majority (95%) are of germ cell origin; the others arise principally from Leydig or Sertoli cells.

Germ Cell Tumors

The germ cell tumors are all, to greater or lesser degree, malignant. Their incidence is increased in cryptorchid testes and in the testes of individuals with abnormal or mixed sexual differentiation. There is a question if a history of mumps orchitis constitutes a risk factor.

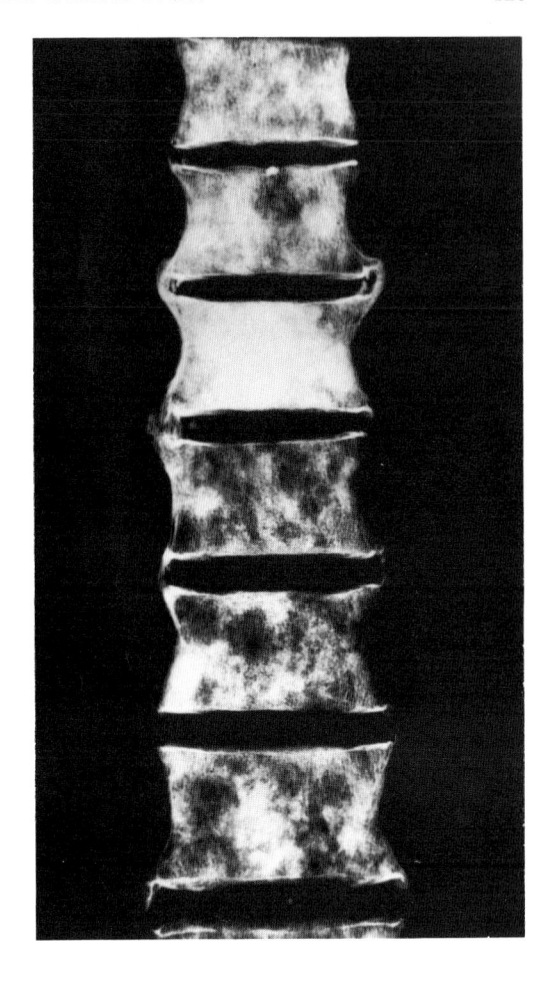

Figure 30.4. Adenocarcinoma of prostate. This x-ray of the lower thoracic and lumbar vertebrae shows multiple areas of lucency, the result of metastases to these bodies. Metastases from prostatic carcinoma may also stimulate new bone formation, appearing as areas of increased density.

All of these tumors arise from pluripotential intratubular germ cells. Most of them consist of a single predominant cell type, but some 40% show mixed cellularity. In addition to the choriocarcinoma, composed entirely of trophoblastic elements, several other tumors may contain syncytiotrophoblastic cells, sufficient to produce detectable quantities of chorionic gonadotrophin.

Seminoma is the most common type of germ cell tumor, and occurs principally in men aged 30 to 50. It may be large and is composed of clear cells with a lymphocytic stroma (Figs. 30.6 and 30.7). The presence of scattered syncytiotrophoblastic cells does not worsen the prognosis, and 95% of patients with seminomas are cured.

Embryonal carcinoma occurs in younger men and is composed of anaplastic cells arranged in glandular or acinar patterns (Figs. 30.8 and 30.9). One-third of patients have metastases to iliac and periaortic lymph nodes, lung, or liver at the time of diagnosis.

Teratomas may contain elements from all three germ layers, including cartilage, neural tissue, and many types of epithelium. It is difficult to predict their

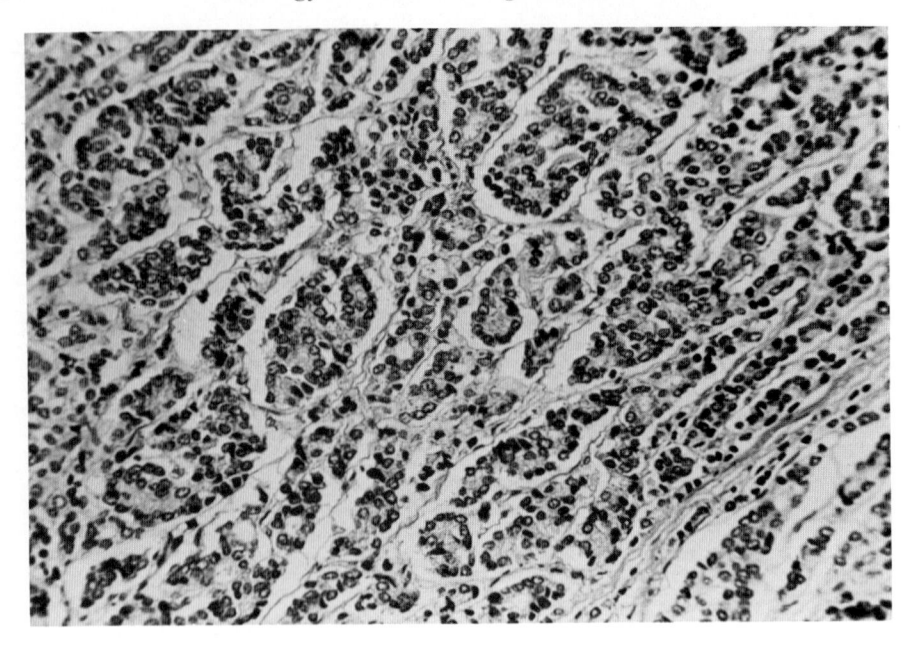

Figure 30.5. Adenocarcinoma of prostate. This is a very well differentiated tumor. The nuclei appear very uniform, and nearly normal appearing glands are formed.

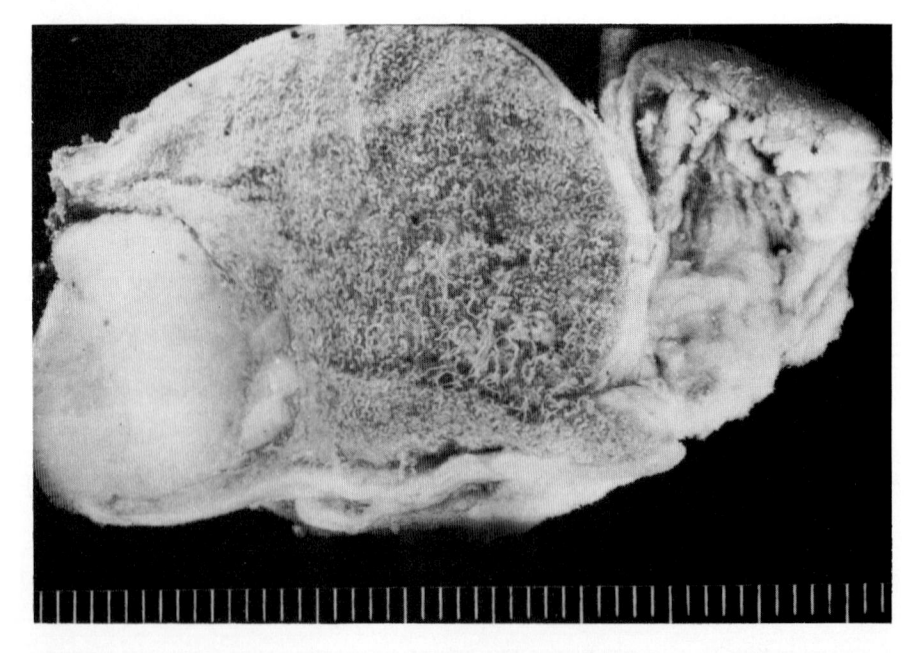

Figure 30.6. Seminoma. The testis has been bisected, revealing a firm grayish white tumor mass at the *left*. It is not clearly demarcated from the normal testicular tissue.

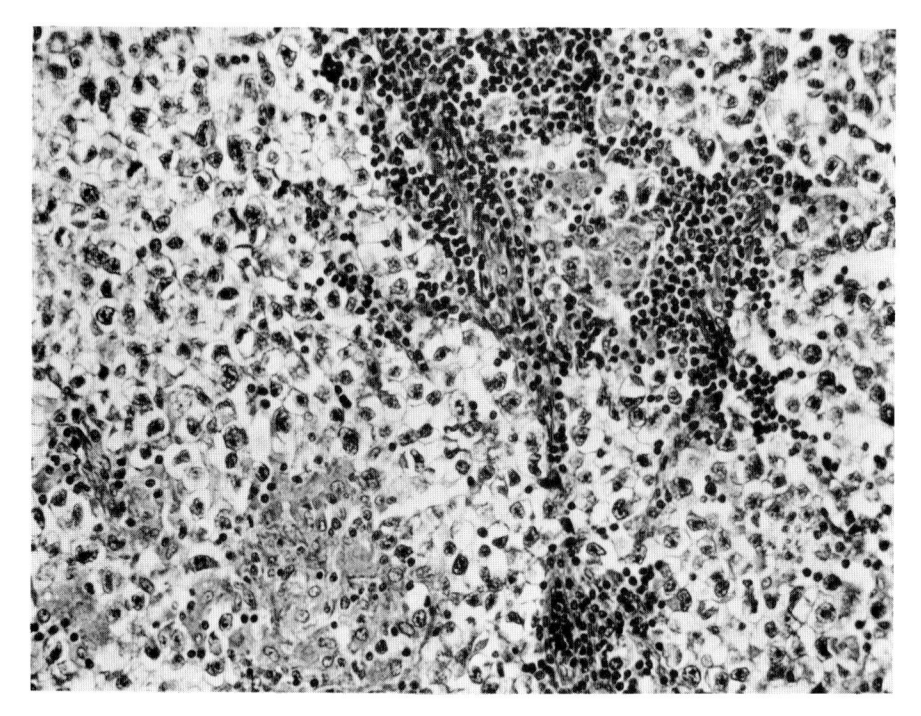

Figure 30.7. Seminoma. The tumor cells are large, with clear glycogen-containing cytoplasm and prominent nuclei and nucleoli. The stroma in many of these tumors is heavily infiltrated by lymphocytes, as shown here.

biologic behavior, and tumors that appear well differentiated may metastasize widely.

Choriocarcinomas comprise only 1% of germ cell tumors. They are usually small and hemorrhagic, composed of both cytotrophoblastic and syncytiotrophoblastic cells. They invade blood vessels and lymphatics and metastasize widely and early. The first symptom is often hemoptysis from pulmonary metastases.

Mixed types are most often composed of embryonal carcinoma and teratoma. The prognosis is determined by the more malignant element.

Some of the germ cell tumors produce substances that can serve as useful markers in following therapy. β-HCG (chorionic gonadotrophin) is secreted by all choriocarcinomas and by some embryonal carcinomas, teratomas, and seminomas. Most embryonal carcinomas produce α-fetoprotein, as do some teratomas. Seminomas and choriocarcinomas do not produce this substance.

The staging of testicular germ cell tumors is:

IA	Tumor confined to one testis
IB	Histologic finding of regional node metastasis
II	Clinical or radiologic evidence of retroperitoneal node metastasis
III	Metastases to mediastinal nodes, lungs, or other organs

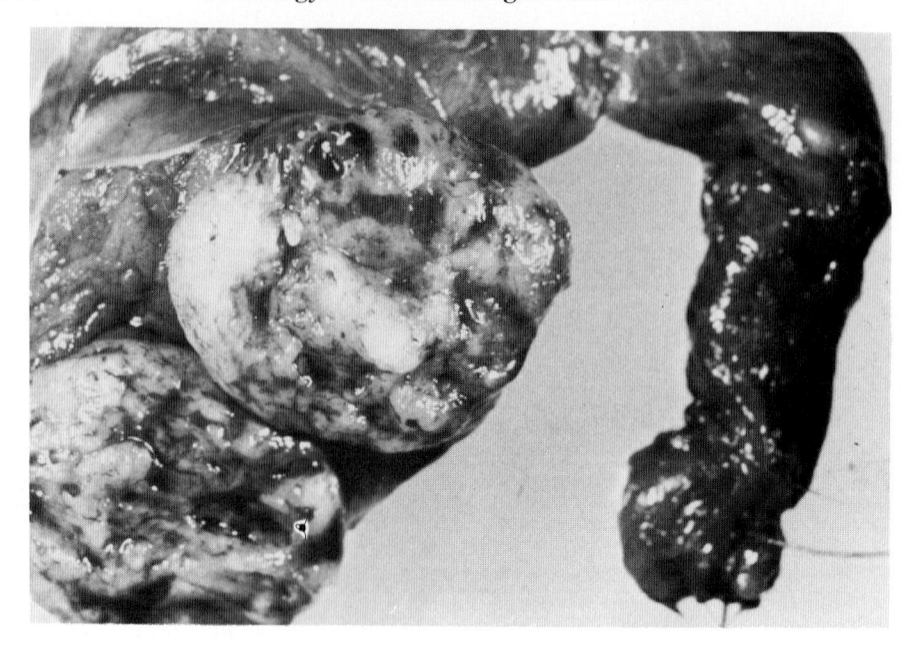

Figure 30.8. Embryonal carcinoma of testis. The tumor mass has replaced a large part of the testis. Its cut surface shows a varied appearance, with areas of hemorrhage and necrosis.

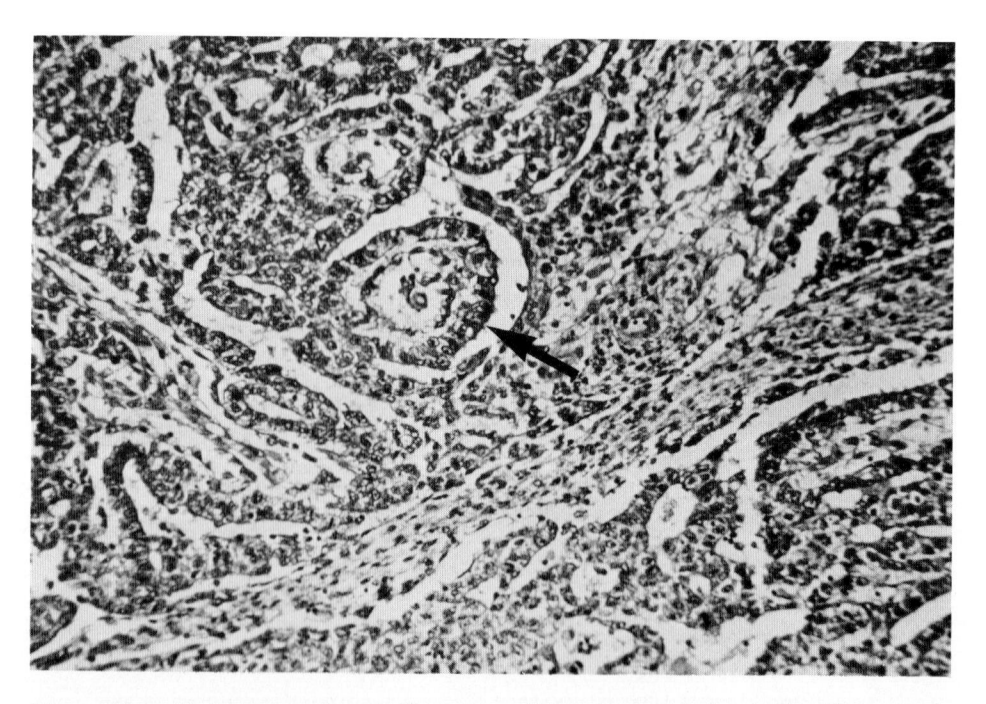

Figure 30.9. Embryonal carcinoma. The tumor cells are large and pleomorphic. They may be arranged in acinar or papillary patterns, sometimes forming glomeruloid structures (*arrow*). The stroma is delicate and highly vascular.

Leydig Cell Tumors

These tumors are composed of cells closely resembling normal interstitial cells. Crystalloids of Reinke are often seen. When these tumors occur in children, they may induce premature puberty. Adults are more likely to manifest gynecomastia.

Leydig cell tumors are usually benign, but a few may show more aggressive behavior.

MISCELLANEOUS DISORDERS

Cryptorchid testes are found in 3 to 6% of prepubertal males. The undescended testis is usually near the inguinal canal. The higher intra-abdominal temperature predisposes the organ to atrophy, and cryptorchid testes also have a higher incidence of germ cell tumors.

Orchitis and *epididymitis* are important lesions. Acute epididymitis may complicate gonorrheal infection and other infections of the prostate and seminal vesicles. The testis is usually spared. Granulomatous epididymitis is a not infrequent consequence of hematogenous dissemination of tuberculosis and may extend into the testis. Syphilis may cause a gummatous orchitis, but does not usually affect the epididymis. Orchitis, usually unilateral, complicates 20% of adult mumps, and atrophy of the testis occasionally follows this orchitis.

Klinefelter's syndrome is characterized by a eunuchoid appearance, infertility, frequent gynecomastia, and mild mental impairment. Pituitary gonadotrophin (FSH) secretion is increased, while testosterone levels are low. The chromosome pattern is 47 XXY. The testes are small and soft and show severe atrophy of the seminiferous tubules. The interstitial cells, however, appear markedly hyperplastic.

Suggested Reading

Fraley EE, Lange PH, Kennedy BJ. Germ-cell testicular cancer in adults. N. Engl. J. Med. *301:* 1370, 1420, 1979.

Murphy GP. Prostatic cancer: progress and change. CA *28:* 104, 1978.

Chapter 31

Disorders of Bone

Major emphasis in this chapter is devoted to a consideration of the metabolic bone diseases, since two of them, osteoporosis and renal osteodystrophy, are assuming ever increasing importance in contemporary medicine. The chapter also includes Paget's disease of bone, osteomyelitis, some examples of bone tumors, and aseptic necrosis.

METABOLIC BONE DISEASE

Bone is a living, actively metabolizing tissue. Throughout life, it is constantly being remodeled by the resorption of existing calcified bone and concurrent new bone formation. These two processes are normally in close balance. Metabolic bone disease represents a significant departure from this balance, resulting in a decrease in skeletal mass (*osteopenia*) or an increase in total mineralized bone (*osteosclerosis*). With few exceptions, metabolic bone diseases affect the entire skeleton, albeit not equally in all parts of the body.

The Remodeling of Bone

Three distinct phases in the remodeling of bone are recognizable: the secretion of bone matrix (osteoid), the accretion of bone salt, and the resorption of mineralized bone. The younger the bone, the more rapid the rate of turnover. In general, there is a net increase in skeletal mass until the age of about 50 years, then a steady decline.

The constant remodeling of bone is in response to the stresses placed on the skeleton. It is also the basis for the development of the Haversian system of secondary osteons that characterize mature compact bone. The significance of stress as the most important, and perhaps the only direct stimulus to new bone matrix formation is illustrated by the rapidity of loss of skeletal mass observed in astronauts during periods of living in a weightless environment. Impairment of osteoblastic collagen secretion (or its maturation) in response to stress is observed in generalized malnutrition, in severe vitamin C deficiency, and in patients with Cushing's syndrome or those receiving prolonged corticosteroid therapy. Each of these conditions is associated with deficient protein synthesis. Growth hormone is essential to normal skeletal development, particularly to epiphyseal growth, and excessive secretion of this hormone leads to giantism or acromegaly. Gonadal hormones, particularly testosterone, generally stimulate new bone formation, although they also hasten the closure of epiphyses, thus limiting longitudinal growth. Thyroid hormone increases the turnover rate of bone and favors resorption. Corticosteroids, in addition to altering collagen synthesis, interfere with mineral absorption from the intestinal tract.

Mineralization of newly formed bone matrix requires certain minimal concentrations of calcium and phosphorus in the extracellular fluid, but it occurs over a rather broad range of values. The mechanism of mineralization of bone is poorly understood. It is not clear why the collagen of bone is normally mineralized, whereas that of other body tissues is not. It is likely that the physical properties of the collagen fibrils themselves, particularly their banding, favor the nucleation of hydroxyapatite. The pattern of mineralization closely follows the organization of collagen fibrils, a prerequisite to the strength of mature bone.

The resorption of bone is intimately related to and dependent upon calcium homeostasis. Since 99% of body calcium is in the skeleton, bone is the only readily available source of mineral to maintain normal levels in the blood and extracellular fluid. Exchanges of mineral between bone and extracellular fluid occur continuously at the interface between bone surfaces and their surrounding hydration shells. This is a simple and rapid physicochemical mechanism. Cellular mechanisms of maintaining calcium homeostasis involve resorption of mineralized bone by osteoclasts and, to a lesser degree, by osteocytes.

Parathyroid Hormone, Calcitonin, and Vitamin D

The several hormones involved in calcium homeostasis invariably affect the structure of bone. *Parathyroid hormone* is rapidly synthesized and secreted in response to a fall in the level of ionized calcium in the circulation. This hormone, which has a half-life of but a few minutes, stimulates osteoclastic and osteocytic resorption of bone, and increases renal phosphate excretion. Since both bone matrix and minerals are resorbed, there is elevation of serum calcium and hydroxyproline, and both may appear in the urine. As soon as the serum ionized calcium level returns to normal, the synthesis and secretion of parathyroid hormone return to baseline levels. *Calcitonin* is secreted by the parafollicular cells of the thyroid gland. Although not directly antagonistic to parathyroid hormone, calcitonin acts on bone so as to inhibit bone resorption. It is secreted in response to an elevation of serum ionized calcium. The serum level of inorganic phosphorus has no direct bearing on the secretion of parathyroid hormone and calcitonin.

Vitamin D is responsible for calcium (and phosphorus) transport from the intestinal tract. It also plays a permissive role in the calcium-mobilizing action of parathyroid hormone on bone, and itself directly stimulates resorption. Before it is biologically effective, however, it must be acted upon by the liver to form 25-hydroxycholecalciferol, and then converted to the hormone 1,25-dihydroxycholecalciferol in the kidney. The rate of secretion of this hormone is regulated by the blood levels of ionized calcium and inorganic phosphorus. Decreased calcium levels lead to an increased synthesis of 1,25(OH)$_2$-cholecalciferol by stimulating secretion of parathyroid hormone. Decreased circulating phosphorus levels also stimulate 1,25(OH)$_2$-cholecalciferol synthesis; this action is unrelated to and independent of the parathyroid glands.

Classification of Metabolic Bone Disease

Most metabolic bone diseases can be regarded as quantitative alterations of one or more of the three component phases of normal bone turnover: osteoid secretion, mineralization of bone matrix, and cellular resorption of mineralized bone. The term *osteopenia* denotes an overall loss of mineralized bone mass, *osteosclerosis* an increase. The former can result from impaired osteoid synthesis, failure to mineralize normal osteoid, or acceleration of resorption. Osteosclerosis can be the product of excessive matrix formation or failure of normal bone resorption.

Osteoporosis designates a group of conditions characterized by atrophy of bone (Fig. 31.1). In many, there is a disorder of connective tissue or protein metabolism reflected in a failure to produce normal bone matrix. That matrix which is formed is normally calcified, and resorption of bone continues at a normal or reduced rate. In others, osteoporosis appears to be the result of a low grade, but persistent, increase in bone resorption. The serum calcium and inorganic phosphorus values are normal. Serum alkaline phosphatase concentration and urinary hydroxyproline excretion are generally normal or slightly reduced, reflecting a low turnover rate of bone.

Osteomalacia results from disordered mineral metabolism such that there is failure of crystallization of bone salt in osteoid. (When this occurs prior to the closure of epiphyses, the term *rickets* is applied.) The resulting weakness of the skeleton makes it highly susceptible to stress, and greatly excessive amounts of osteoid are produced (Fig. 31.2). Serum values are low for calcium, inorganic phosphorus, or both, but alkaline phosphatase concentration is elevated.

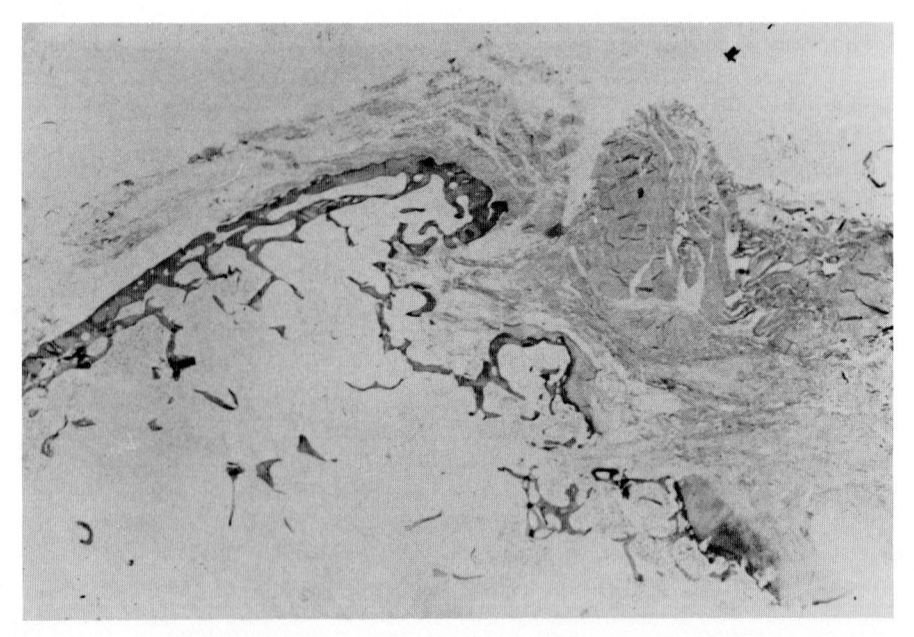

Figure 31.1. Osteoporosis. This low power photograph shows extensive atrophy of both cortical and trabecular bone.

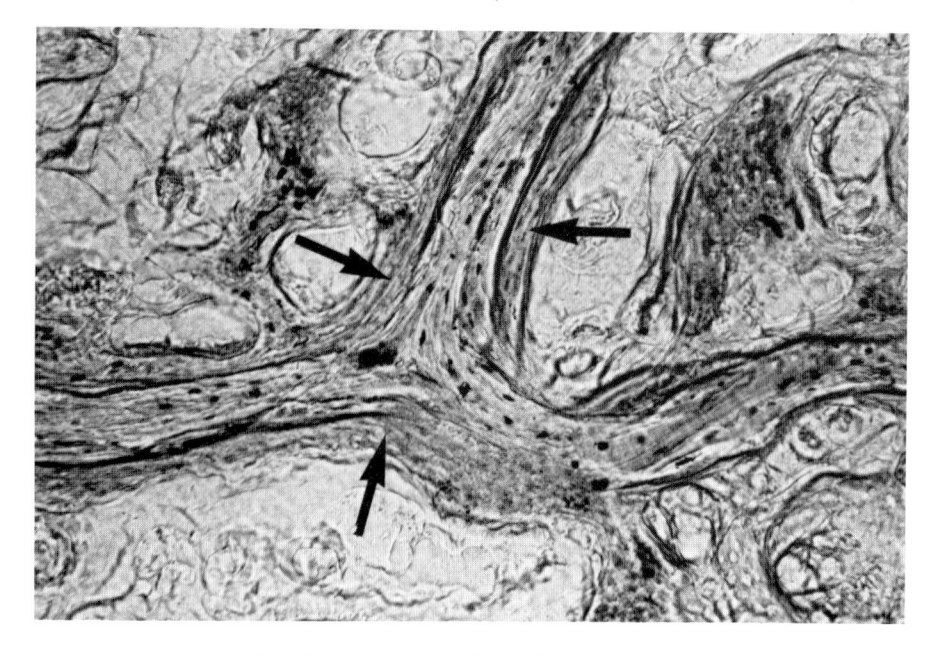

Figure 31.2. Osteomalacia. This section of undecalcified bone shows prominent osteoid seams deposited on the surface of mature bony trabeculae.

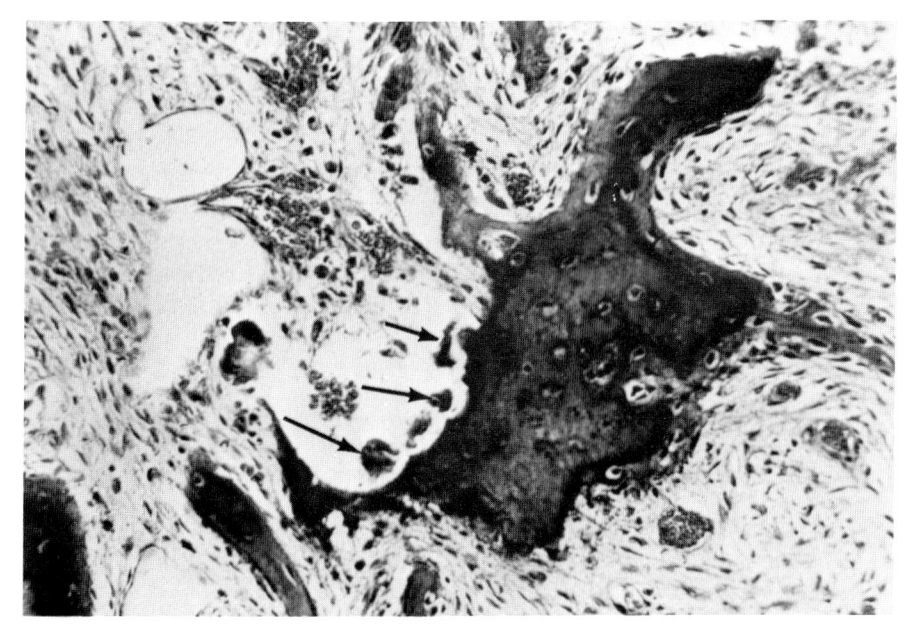

Figure 31.3. Osteitis fibrosa. There is active osteoclastic resorption of woven bone. Some osteoblastic activity can also be noted at the *right*. The marrow spaces show fibrosis, and there is some small cyst formation.

Osteitis fibrosa is the bone disease resulting from a greatly accelerated rate of osteoclastic (and probably osteocytic) resorption of bone (Figs. 31.3 and 31.4). It is almost always relatable to increased secretion of parathyroid hormone. When osteitis fibrosa results from primary hyperparathyroidism (*e.g.*, parathyroid adenoma), the serum calcium is high, the inorganic phosphorus is low, and the alkaline phosphatase concentration is markedly elevated, reflecting acceleration of both new bone formation and resorption. When the bone changes are due to renal failure and secondary hyperparathyroidism, elevation of serum phosphorus and depression of serum calcium concentrations are the rule.

Increased matrix formation is the mechanism leading to osteosclerosis in disorders of growth hormone secretion and in the healing of osteomalacia. Decreased bone resorption is the mechanism in hypoparathyroidism.

Table 31.1 presents a classification of metabolic bone disease. It is not meant to be complete, but rather to illustrate the points made in this chapter. Table 31.2 summarizes the biochemical findings in these disorders and in Paget's disease.

Renal Osteodystrophy

Renal osteodystrophy is a complex metabolic bone disturbance observed in association with chronic renal failure. Now that many patients with end stage kidney disease are kept alive for years on dialysis, this bone disorder has become commonplace, and constitutes one of the most difficult and frustrating aspects of renal failure to manage. It causes severe bone pain, frequently aggravated rather than alleviated by hemodialysis. The findings in bone consist of a variable mixture of osteomalacia, osteitis fibrosa, and osteosclerosis.

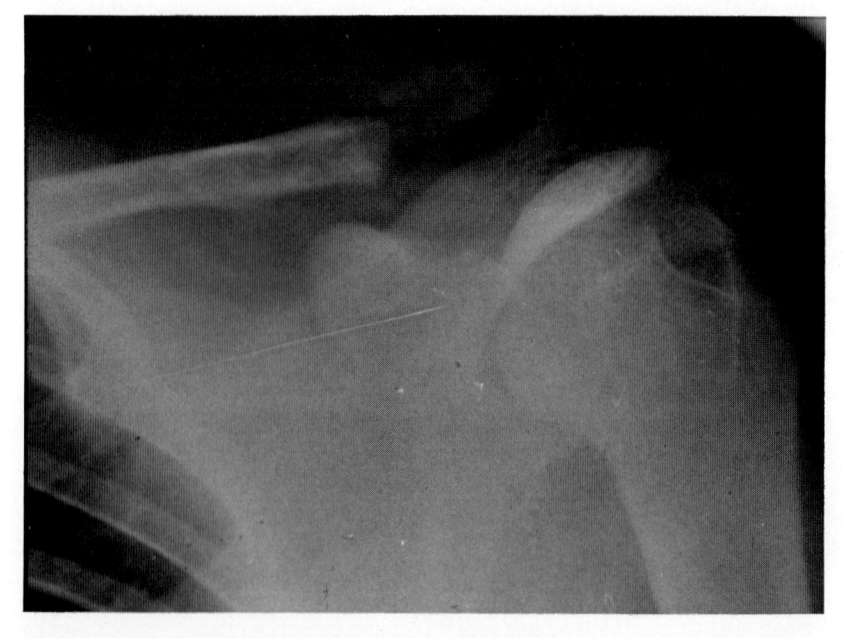

Figure 31.4. Osteitis fibrosa. The distal end of the clavicle has been resorbed in this patient with primary hyperparathyroidism.

Table 31.1
Classification of Metabolic Bone Disease

Osteopenia

Osteoporosis
  "Senile" osteoporosis
  Immobilization
  Shoulder-hand syndrome
  Osteogenesis imperfecta
  Malnutrition
    Scurvy
    Protein deficiency
  Endocrine disorders
    Cushing's syndrome
    Corticosteroid therapy
    Hyperthyroidism
    Ovarian dysgenesis

Osteomalacia
  Renal failure
  Malabsorption syndromes
    Gluten enteropathy
    Nontropical sprue
    Chronic pancreatitis
    Cystic fibrosis
  Vitamin D deficiency
  Renal tubular acidosis
  Anticonvulsant therapy (phenytoin)

Osteitis fibrosa
  Renal failure
  Primary hyperparathyroidism
  Vitamin D intoxication
  ? Bone-resorbing substances secreted by some neoplasms

Osteosclerosis

Increased matrix production
  Acromegaly
  Renal failure
  Osteofluorosis

Reduced resorption
  Hypoparathyroidism
  Osteopetrosis

At least two mechanisms may be involved in the pathogenesis of the bone changes. As nephrons are lost in progressive renal disease, there is retention of inorganic phosphorus which leads indirectly to a decrease in blood calcium. The parathyroid glands secrete increased amounts of parathyroid hormone which returns the blood calcium to normal through resorption of bone and lowers the blood phosphorus by inhibiting its resorption in the proximal renal tubules. A new equilibrium is reached, with essentially normal calcium and phosphorus levels, but at the expense of continuously increased parathyroid function and the development of osteitis fibrosa.

Although the mechanism described above may play a significant role, particularly in early renal failure, a far more important explanation is based on the failure of the chronically diseased kidney to complete the hydroxylation of

Table 31.2
Biochemical Findings in Diseases of Calcium and Skeletal Homeostasis

Disease	Serum or Plasma					Urine	
	Ca	P	Alkaline Phosphatase	Parathyroid Hormone	Ca	P
Hyperparathyroidism	↑	↓→	↑→	↑	↑→	↑→
Hypoparathyroidism	↓	↑	→	↓	↓	↓
Vitamin D intoxication	↑	→↑↓	→↑	↓	↑	→↑
Osteomalacia	↓	↓	↑	↑	↓	→↑
Paget's disease	→↑	→	↑↑	→	↑	→
Renal osteodystrophy	→↓	↑	↑	↑	↓	↓
Osteoporosis	→	→	→	→	→↑	→

cholecalciferol. Loss of this function may be the result of elevated tissue levels of phosphorus in the renal cortex. The result is markedly decreased intestinal transport of calcium and impairment, at least at first, of the calcium mobilizing effect of parathyroid hormone. New osteoid is not mineralized. The bones become more subject to stress, and increasing amounts of osteoid are deposited, appearing as thick seams on the surface of older mineralized lamellae. The bones tend to become bowed and deformed, particularly the long bones of the extremities. When the disorder occurs in children, there is marked disturbance of endochondral bone formation at the epiphyseal plate, with massive accumulation of unmineralized osteoid together with many chondrocytes (Fig. 31.5). Prolonged hypocalcemia leads to secondary hyperplasia of the parathyroid glands, and the bones begin to respond to massive secretion of parathyroid hormone. There is then superimposition of the changes of osteitis fibrosa on those of osteomalacia (Fig. 31.6). Osteoclasts are numerous and actively resorb bone trabeculae, and there is progressive fibrosis of the marrow spaces in areas of resorption. Osteoid remains, however, since osteoclasts cannot resorb the unmineralized matrix. The reason for the development of focal osteosclerosis is not clear.

Problems in Management

Patients with renal osteodystrophy on hemodialysis are very difficult to control. Withdrawal of any calcium from the blood aggravates the bone disease, whereas adding to the calcium level often results in extraskeletal soft tissue calcification. Renal osteodystrophy may remain a serious problem after homotransplantation. The parathyroid glands in renal failure secrete many times the normal amount of

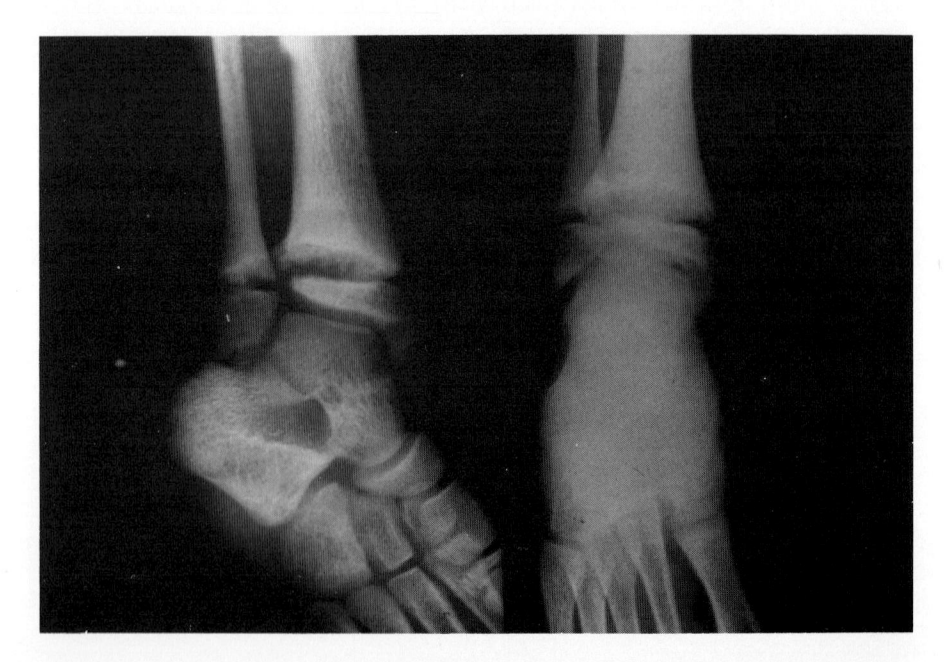

Figure 31.5. Renal osteodystrophy. Accumulation of uncalcified osteoid at the epiphyseal plates has resulted in striking deformity at the lower ends of tibia and fibula in this child.

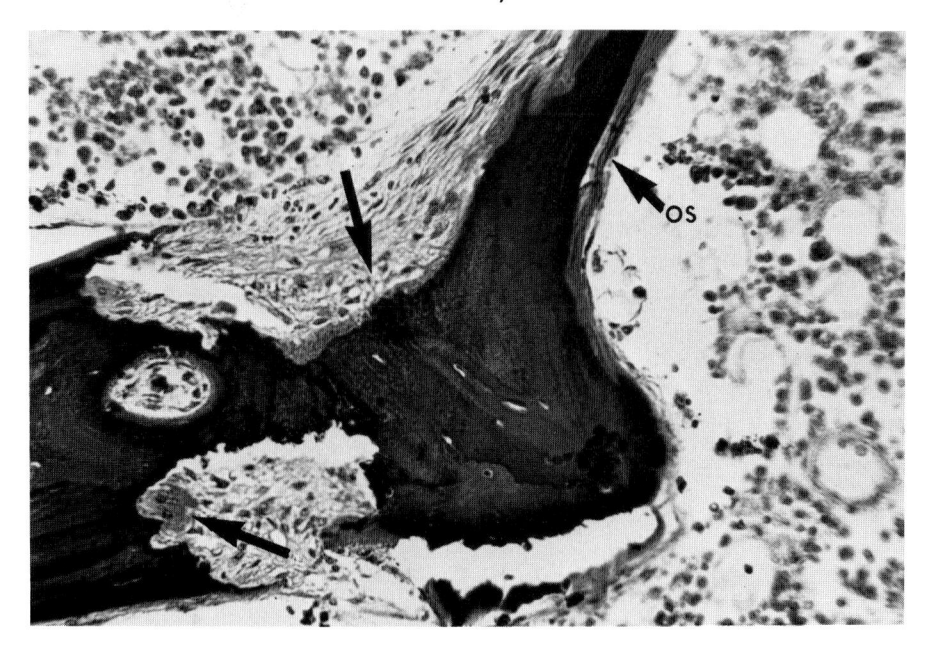

Figure 31.6. Renal osteodystrophy. There is active resorption of trabecular bone, associated with fibrosis (*arrows*). At the same time, there is formation of an osteoid seam (*OS*).

parathyroid hormone, and in time lose their responsiveness to changes in the blood calcium. Following transplantation, the parathyroid glands may continue to secrete excessive amounts of parathyroid hormone for months or years before resuming normal physiologic function. This worsens the osteitis fibrosa and exposes the transplanted kidney to serious injury from excessive calcium excretion, effects that frequently necessitate subtotal parathyroidectomy. Considerable success has attended the administration of $1,25(OH)_2$-cholecalciferol to patients with renal osteodystrophy. There is increased intestinal calcium transport, suppression of parathyroid hormone secretion, and improvement in the morphology of bone.

Osteoporosis

Osteoporosis is atrophy of bone. Cancellous bone becomes porous and consists of markedly thinned bony trabeculae. Cortical bone is also much thinner than normal, the loss taking place from the endosteal surface.

Osteoporosis is undoubtedly the most widespread metabolic bone disease. It has many causes, some of which are included in Table 31.1. The mechanisms of osteoporosis are not well understood. Reduced physical activity may play a role in senile osteoporosis but, in postmenopausal women, the loss of estrogen may make bone more sensitive to parathyroid hormone. There is also need for a higher calcium intake in older individuals. In scurvy, there is deficient osteoid formation to maintain skeletal balance (Fig. 31.7). Loss of the major stimulus to bone formation, *i.e.*, stress, accounts for the osteoporosis of immobilization. In Cushing's syndrome, and in patients receiving corticosteroids, there may also be

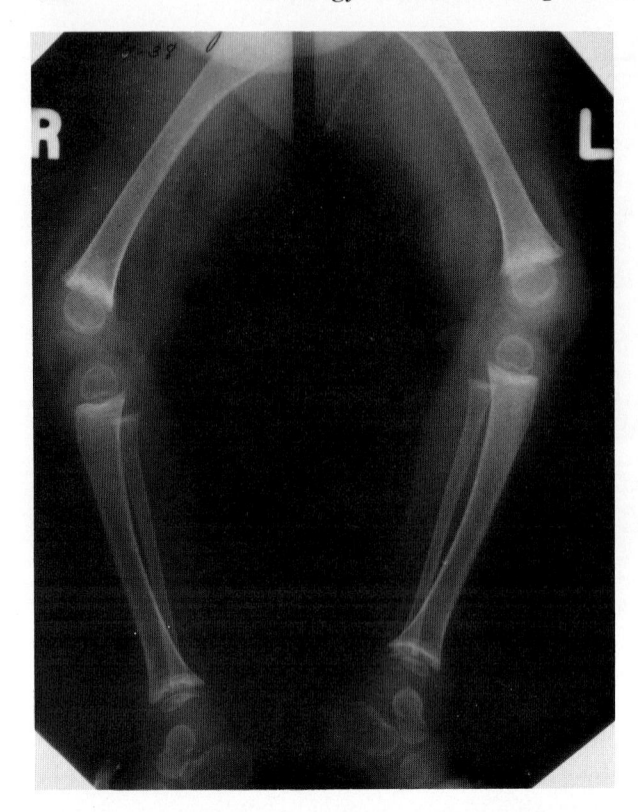

Figure 31.7. Scurvy. The bones, particularly the epiphyses, have a ground glass appearance, due to severe osteopenia. There is bowing of the long bones.

deficient osteoid production, but an increased rate of resorption appears more critical. Increased resorption is also the mechanism of osteoporosis in hyperthyroidism. In these circumstances, the rate of resorption is only slightly increased over normal, and accumulation of osteoclasts is not seen on histologic examination.

Senile Osteoporosis

Senile osteoporosis is the most common form of this disorder. It affects women predominantly, becoming manifest about 10 years after the menopause, but it is also recognizable in some 20% of men over 65 years of age. The lower vertebral bodies are usually most involved, and back pain is a prominent symptom. Changes in long bones, ribs, and pelvis occur later, usually in patients with more severe involvement. Shortening and compression fractures of the spine are frequent. Senile osteoporosis is responsible for 190,000 hip fractures in this country each year and 30,000 deaths. The cost of the acute care of these fractures is over $1 billion per year.

Roentgenographic studies show demineralization and kyphotic deformity of the spine, and the vertebrae assume a "codfish" appearance due to a biconvex expansion of the intervertebral discs (Fig. 31.8).

Senile osteoporosis is resistant to therapy. Although a deficiency of estrogen is commonly accepted as causative in postmenopausal women, the administration

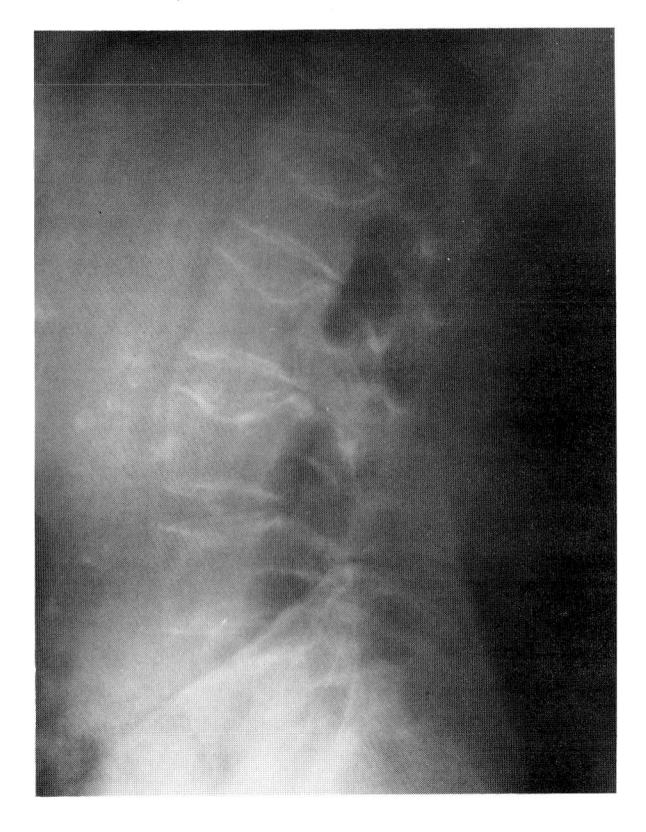

Figure 31.8.– Senile osteoporosis. There is marked demineralization of these vertebral bodies. The biconvex expansion of the intervetebral discs has given the vertebrae a "codfish" appearance.

of anabolic hormones has a questionably beneficial effect. Increasing dietary mineral intake in combination with sodium fluoride has been reported to increase bone mass, and attempts to decrease bone resorption by the therapeutic use of calcitonin may be helpful. Placing normal stress on the skeleton through exercise may prove important, at least in preventing severe disease.

PAGET'S DISEASE OF BONE

Paget's disease of bone (*osteitis deformans*), although of unknown etiology, is probably not a metabolic bone disease. No disturbances of mineral or protein metabolism have been demonstrated. The disease may involve one or many bones, but rarely involves the entire skeleton.

The morphologic findings reflect a greatly accelerated remodeling process. The disorder appears to start as a focal area of osteoclastic resorption and then spreads to involve most or all of an involved bone. Osteoclastic resorption is massive and associated with fibrosis of the marrow space. There is also extensive new bone formation, but the very rapid turnover results in abnormal structure. The trabeculae and cortical bone are thickened and irregular in conformation and present a mosaic appearance on histologic examination due to prominent cement lines (Fig. 31.9). Although quantitatively increased, bone is physically weak, readily fractured, and deformed by stress placed on the skeleton. A

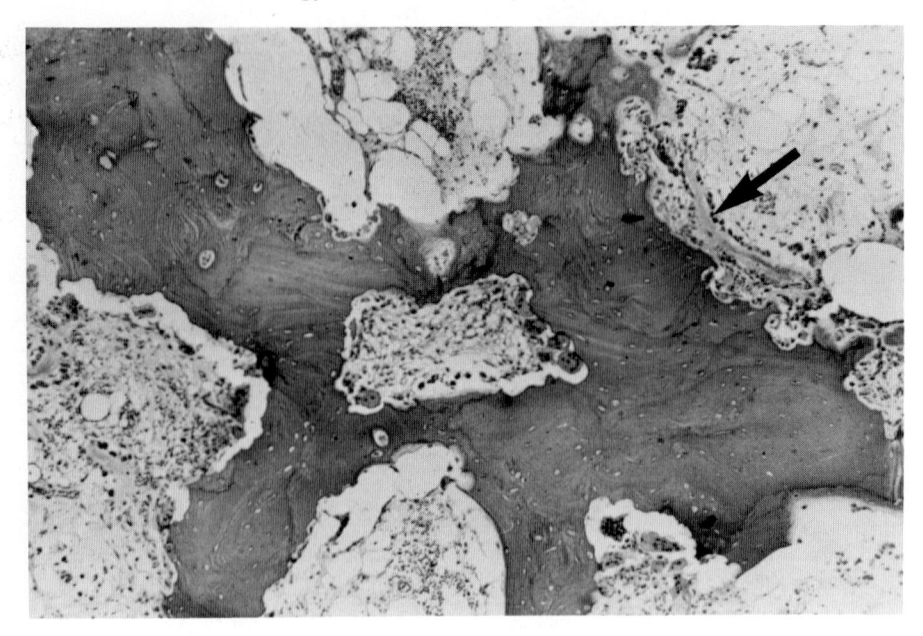

Figure 31.9. Paget's disease. There is very rapid turnover of bone. Active osteoclastic resorption is seen in the *center* of the field and in the *right lower corner*, while active new bone formation is seen at the *upper right (arrow)*. The result of such rapid turnover is the production of bone with irregular structure and weak physical alignment.

prominent finding is greatly increased vascularity, so that an involved bone will be warm to palpation and, with polyostotic involvement, high output congestive heart failure may occur.

Paget's disease is a disorder of middle and advanced age. Some 3% of individuals over 40 years of age have significant disease demonstrable by roentgenographic examination. The bones most frequently involved are those most subject to stress: vertebrae, pelvic bones, long bones of the extremities (Fig. 31.10), and skull (Fig. 31.11). Deafness can result from involvement of the temporal bones and the auditory canals. Patients with Paget's disease usually have normal serum levels of calcium and phosphorus, but the often extreme elevation of serum alkaline phosphatase concentration attests to the rapid turnover of bone.

There are two important complications of Paget's disease. Some 2% of individuals develop malignant bone tumors, most often osteogenic sarcoma. The second complication is related to placing patients with this disorder on bed rest. The reduced stress on the skeleton greatly diminishes new bone formation, but osteoclastic resorption continues apace, and severe, at times fatal, hypercalcemia may result.

OSTEOMYELITIS

Osteomyelitis is an infection of bone and bone marrow. Until recently, it was primarily a disease of children or young adults. The onset of disease was dramatic, with chills, fever, and severe bone pain. The femur and tibia were the bones most

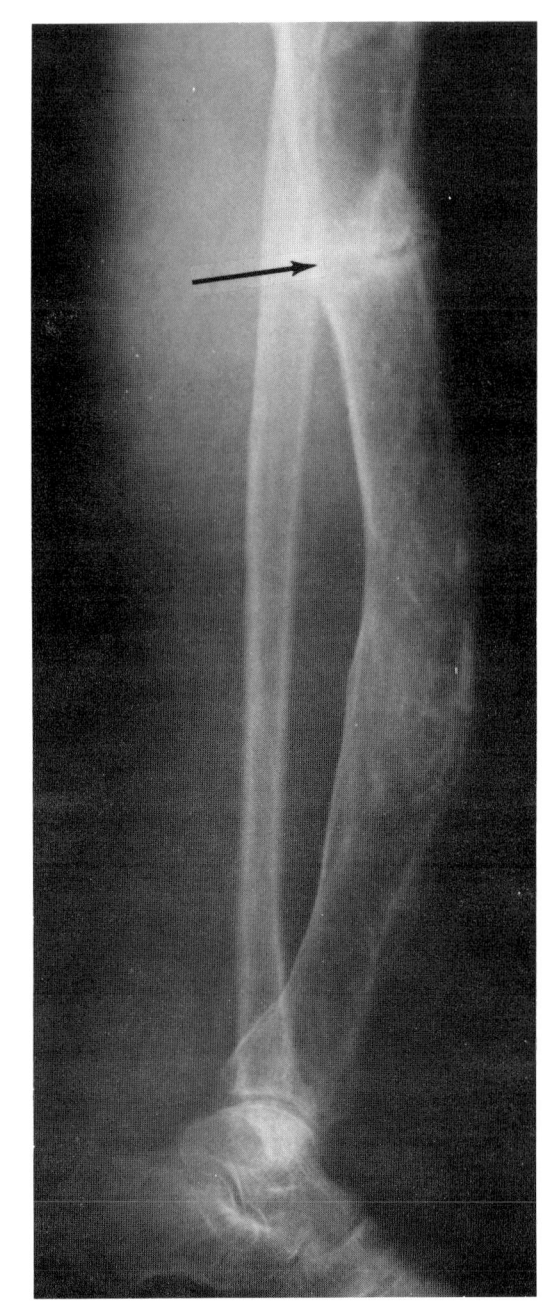

Figure 31.10. Paget's disease. There is striking anterior bowing of the tibia, a very irregular architecture, and a pathologic fracture (*arrow*).

involved, and at least 85% were caused by *Staphylococcus aureus*, reaching bone as part of a hematogenous dissemination from an infection elsewhere, although organisms could also be directly implanted in bone as a result of trauma. Infection most often started at the metaphysis, where terminal nutrient vessels enter large sinusoids and spread to produce extensive necrosis of bone and marrow. It also

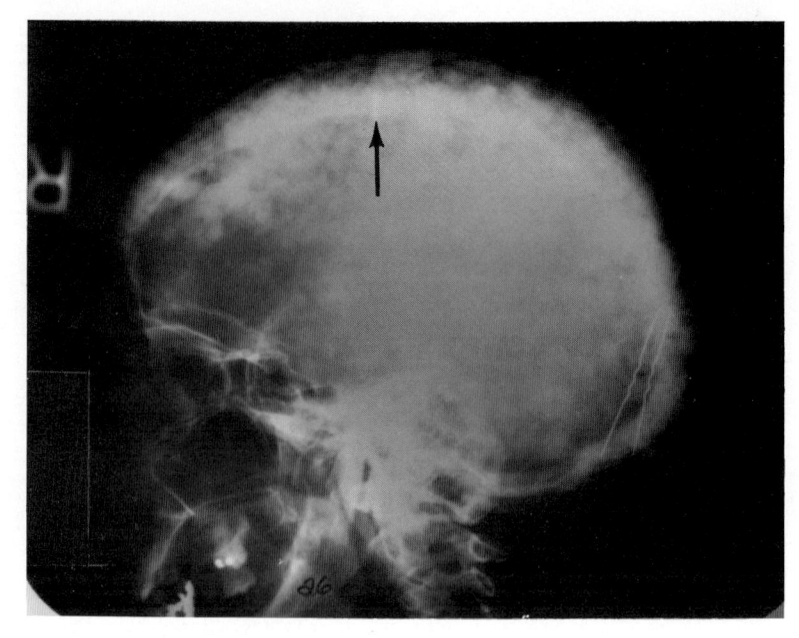

Figure 31.11. Paget's disease. The calvarium is markedly thickened, and calcification of the atypical bone formation is very irregular. The *arrow* indicates the inner table of the calvarium.

spread through cortical bone to soft tissues, elevating the periosteum. The mass of dead bone is called a *sequestrum*, and the new bone formed beneath the elevated periosteum an *involucrum*. The persistence of an infected sequestrum often led to a chronic infection, with formation of sinus tracts to the skin surface. Squamous cell carcinoma, arising in a sinus tract, complicated chronic osteomyelitis in about 1% of patients, and amyloidosis was a not uncommon occurrence.

Antibiotic therapy has changed the pattern of osteomyelitis, although it has not been so successful as in other infections. *Staphylococcus aureus* (occasionally, *Staphylococcus epidermidis*) is still responsible for over 60% of infections, but many other organisms are encountered, including Group B streptococci, *Pseudomonas aeruginosa*, and other Gram-negative organisms, as well as *Candida*, *Aspergillus*, and *Rhizopus* species of fungi. There is an increasing frequency of involvement of vertebral bodies and flat bones and a shift in age groups. There is a high incidence of pseudomonas osteomyelitis in heroin addicts, involving vertebrae and pelvic bones, and nonstaphylococcal vertebral osteomyelitis has become a problem during the seventh and eighth decades. The symptoms are less explosive than in classical osteomyelitis of long bones, and diagnosis is quite difficult.

Despite antibiotic therapy, the persistence of infected necrotic bone can result in the eruption of spreading infection many years after the initial illness. The care of patients with chronic osteomyelitis usually requires surgical removal of all dead bone.

Tuberculosis may involve the vertebral bodies and the bones adjacent to hip and knee joints. This is always a manifestation of hematogenous dissemination

Disorders of Bone 431

and may be apparent at a time when pulmonary disease cannot be detected. Involvement of the lower thoracic vertebrae results in the deformity of *Pott's disease*.

TUMORS OF BONE

Only a few of the many tumors of bone are discussed: osteogenic sarcoma, osteoid osteoma, osteochondroma, enchondroma, chondrosarcoma, giant cell tumor, and Ewing's sarcoma. Multiple myeloma, perhaps the most common primary malignant tumor of bone in older persons, is discussed in Chapter 24 (p. 321).

Osteogenic Sarcoma

Osteogenic sarcoma is the most common primary malignancy of bone. It occurs most frequently in the teens and early twenties, with a male predominance of 2:1, although it can be seen in older individuals as a complication of Paget's disease or exposure to ionizing radiation, particularly through ingestion of radioactive materials that are stored in bone. Children with genetically determined retinoblastoma (p. 466) have an unexplained predisposition to osteogenic sarcoma.

Osteogenic sarcoma most often occurs in the lower femur, upper tibia, upper humerus, or upper femur. It starts at the metaphysis, invades the medullary cavity, destroys the cortex, and invades surrounding soft tissues (Fig. 31.12). It does not usually invade the joint spaces. The tumors are grayish white, with areas of hemorrhage and cyst formation. All osteogenic sarcomas are characterized by tumor cell production of osteoid and, at times, bone. Areas of chondroid differentiation are not uncommon. The tumor cells appear as anaplastic cells resem-

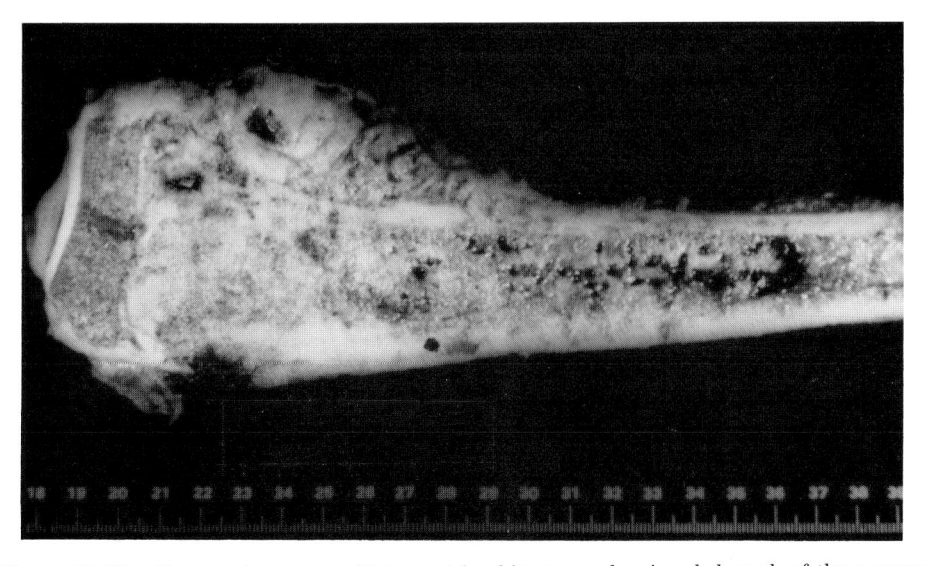

Figure 31.12. Osteogenic sarcoma. This grayish white tumor has invaded much of the marrow cavity, has destroyed the bony cortex, and has extended to the surrounding soft tissues. Although the epiphysis has been invaded, the joint space is uninvolved.

bling fibroblasts, and tumor giant cells may be prominent (Fig. 31.13). Metastases to lung and other viscera may occur quite early, but lymph nodes are spared. Although there has been some improvement in the effectiveness of therapy, the prognosis is still grave.

Osteoid Osteoma

Osteoid osteomas are benign lesions of osteogenic cells, occurring in the diaphysis of long bones of patients below the age of 30. They may cause severe pain. The characteristic x-ray appearance is a lucent center, 1 or 2 cm in diameter, surrounded by a dense halo.

Osteochondroma

Osteochrondromas are benign tumors that project outward from the metaphysis or epiphyseal plate of long bones. They are composed of normal bony architecture covered by mature cartilage (Fig. 31.14). They are the most common benign tumors of bone.

Enchondroma

Enchondromas arise from cartilaginous rests within the substance of bone. They are most often encountered in the bones of the hands and feet. Enchondromas can be multiple and may be familial and hereditary. When this occurs, there is a distinct tendency to malignant change, some 20% of patients developing chondrosarcoma.

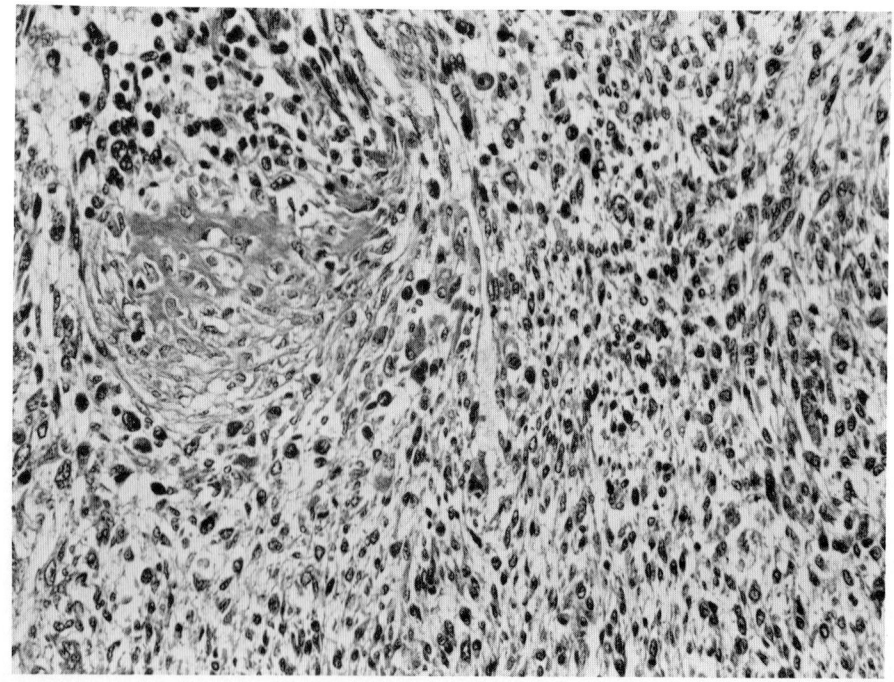

Figure 31.13. Osteogenic sarcoma. The tumor cells resemble fibroblasts but show a striking degree of nuclear pleomorphism. An area of osteoid production by the tumor is seen to the *left of center*.

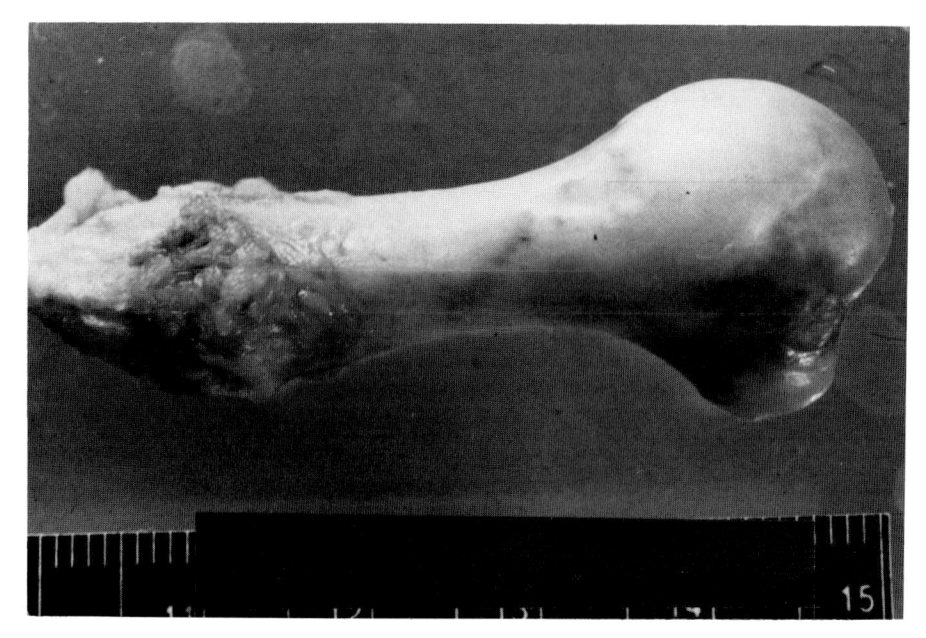

Figure 31.14. Osteochondroma. This surgically removed protrusion from the metaphysis of a long bone consists of normal bony architecture covered by normal mature cartilage.

Chondrosarcoma

Chondrosarcoma is a malignant tumor composed of cartilage-producing cells. It occurs in older individuals than osteogenic sarcoma, most patients being between 30 and 50. The pelvis, ribs, and spine are the bones most often involved. The tumors are destructive and may invade soft tissues. Microscopically, they are composed of chondrocytes of varying differentiation but always showing some areas of anaplasia. Endochondral bone formation may be reproduced by the tumor cells, but this does not indicate osteogenic sarcoma. The outlook, while guarded, is far brighter than for osteogenic sarcoma, and combinations of surgery and chemotherapy have been quite successful.

Giant Cell Tumor

Giant cell tumors occur at the ends of long bones, usually between the ages 20 and 50. They appear multicystic by x-ray and distort, and occasionally rupture, the cortex. The tumors are composed of large numbers of giant cells that appear similar to osteoclasts, embedded in a fibrous stroma. Some 20% behave as malignant tumors, although this is difficult to predict from the morphologic appearance of the individual tumor. It may, at times, be very difficult to distinguish between a malignant giant cell tumor and an osteogenic sarcoma containing many tumor giant cells.

Ewing's Sarcoma

Ewing's sarcoma is a rare tumor of young individuals, aged 10 to 25. It arises in the marrow of the shaft of long bones, pelvis, or ribs and is rapidly destructive and invasive of surrounding tissues. The multiplicity of bone involvement often suggests multicentric origin. Ewing's sarcoma is associated with fever and pain, and the magnitude of symptoms may suggest an infectious disease. The nature of the tumor cells is unknown, although they are felt to arise from primitive bone marrow or other mesenchymal cells. They are small round cells that, to some extent, resemble neuroblasts and show numerous mitoses. There are frequent areas of hemorrhage and necrosis. The prognosis of this tumor is poor, less than 10% of patients surviving for 5 years.

ASEPTIC NECROSIS OF BONE

Aseptic necrosis, or infarction, of bone is not uncommon. It occurs as a complication of disorders that fill the marrow spaces, such as leukemia, lymphoma, or primary or metastatic tumors, presumably by compressing the nutrient vessels. At other times, it occurs without obvious cause, but it can be a complication of glucocorticoid therapy.

The head of the femur and the femoral neck are the most frequent sites of necrosis. Bone necrosis can heal well, particularly in such childhood disorders as *Legg-Perthes disease*, but it can also result in collapse of bone, injury to articular surfaces, and osteoarthritis.

Suggested Reading

DeLuca HF. Vitamin D endocrinology. Ann. Intern. Med. *85:* 367, 1976.
Harris ED, Krane SM. Paget's disease of bone. Bull. Rheum. Dis. *18:* 506, 1968.
Marx JL. Osteoporosis: new help for thinning bones. Science *207:* 628, 1980.
Teitelbaum SL, Bullough PG. The pathophysiology of bone and joint disease (a teaching monograph). Am. J. Pathol. *96:* 279, 1979.
Waldvogel FA, Vasey H. Osteomyelitis: the past decade. N. Engl. J. Med. *303:* 360, 1980.

Chapter 32

The Joints

Arthritis is a major cause of disability throughout the world. Degenerative arthritis (osteoarthritis) is an almost inevitable consequence of the mechanical wear-and-tear of daily life, but it can also be related to pathologic deposition of urate or pyrophosphate crystals. Rheumatoid arthritis is an autoimmune disease, and the joints are prone to involvement in other autoimmune disorders. Injury to the joints may also result from bleeding disorders and disturbances of the nervous system.

RHEUMATOID ARTHRITIS

Rheumatoid arthritis is a relatively new disease, known for only 2 or 3 centuries. It is a disease of young adults, with a 3:1 female predominance, and depending on diagnostic criteria, affects between 1 and 5% of the American population. The involvement is almost always polyarticular and symmetrical, with preference for the wrists and proximal interphalangeal joints. There is a high incidence of HLA Dw4 haplotype in patients with rheumatoid arthritis.

The onset of disease is marked by mild systemic manifestations of fever, anemia, and fatigue, together with painful swelling of joints. The disease may then follow an intermittent course or be relentlessly progressive, at least 10% of patients becoming permanently incapacitated.

Morphologic changes are observed first in the synovium. Congestion and edema are followed by proliferation of granulation tissue and infiltration by lymphocytes and plasma cells. The synovium becomes markedly thickened, with a villous or papillary configuration, hyperplastic lining cells, and formation of lymphoid follicles (Fig. 32.1). In time, granulation tissue extends over the articular cartilages and enzymes released by its cells destroy cartilage and subchondral bone (Fig. 32.2). There is also extension to the joint capsule and supporting ligaments. Destruction of articular surfaces and weakening of joint support results in dislocation (subluxation) and marked deformity. A frequent end result is fusion (ankylosis) of the joint by fibrous tissue or by new bone.

Seventy per cent of patients with rheumatoid arthritis have circulating autoantibodies to the Fc fragment of IgG heavy chains. These antibodies, collectively called *rheumatoid factor*, consist of IgM macroglobulins and, often, IgG and IgA. They are produced by plasma cells of the synovial infiltrate as well as in the lymphoid system.

The proposed pathogenesis of rheumatoid arthritis is that a synovitis, perhaps

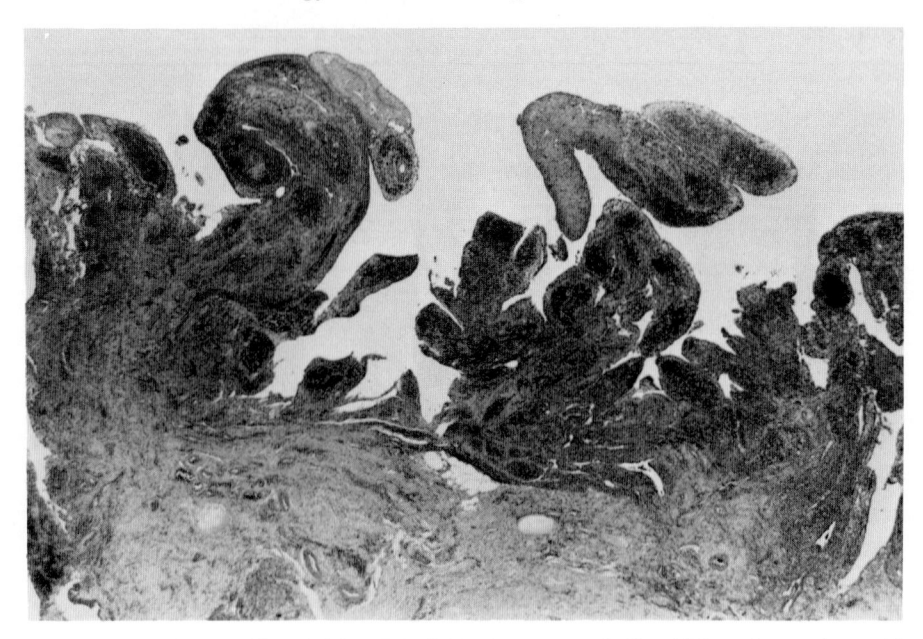

Figure 32.1. Rheumatoid arthritis. This field shows a markedly thickened synovium with a strikingly villous configuration. Many lymphoid follicles are seen within the synovial projections.

of viral origin, stimulates the production of IgG antibodies by the synovium. These antibodies form antigenic aggregates in the joint space and, in turn, result in production of rheumatoid factor. Complexes of rheumatoid factor and IgG activate complement, and the ensuing inflammatory reaction releases the proteolytic enzymes that injure the joint tissues.

Rheumatoid factor produced in the lymphoid system forms complexes with IgG, and these are responsible for an acute vasculitis, observed in many organs. One of the consequences of vasculitis is the subcutaneous *rheumatoid nodule*, observed in some 25% of patients. Rheumatoid nodules vary in size from a few millimeters to 2 cm and are noted over pressure points, such as the olecranon process of the ulna. They consist of a central area of fibrinoid necrosis surrounded by radially arranged, elongated mononuclear phagocytes (Fig. 32.3). Rheumatoid nodules are also seen in the lungs, the myocardium and heart valves, and the gastrointestinal tract. They do not occur in patients who are negative for rheumatoid factor.

Vasculitis may also be the explanation of pericarditis, a frequent systemic manifestation of rheumatoid arthritis.

Amyloidosis, involving liver, spleen, and kidneys, used to be a common complication of severe rheumatoid arthritis. Interestingly, it tends to appear at a time when patients become negative for rheumatoid factor.

ANKYLOSING SPONDYLITIS AND JUVENILE RHEUMATOID ARTHRITIS

Ankylosing spondylitis is not a variant of rheumatoid arthritis. It involves primarily the spine and sacroiliac joints of young adults, and has at least a 10:1

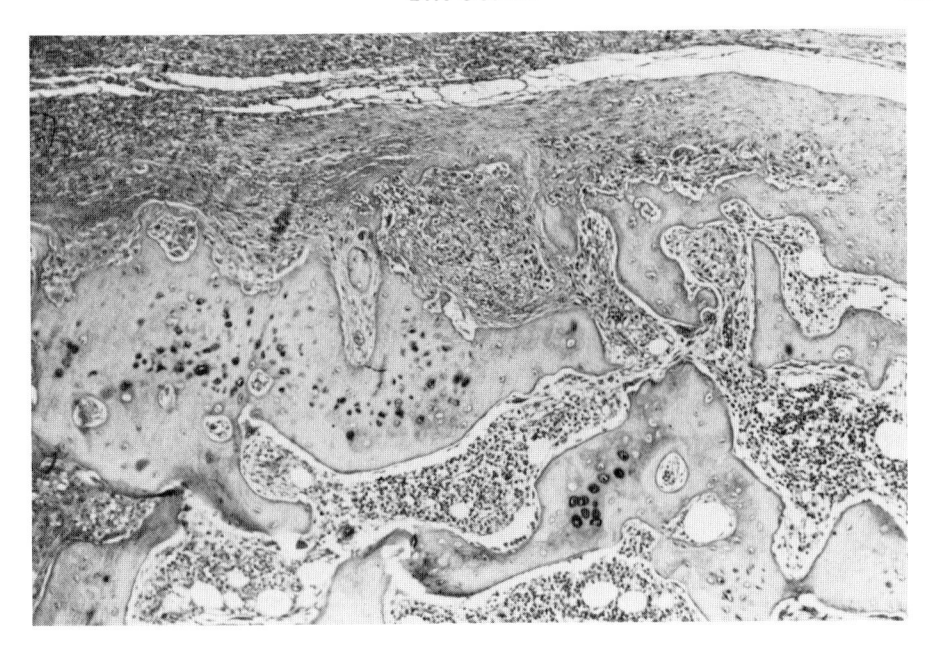

Figure 32.2. Rheumatoid arthritis. The joint surface (*above*) has lost its cartilage and consists of granulation tissue and scar tissue. The subchondral bone shows degenerative changes and areas of necrosis.

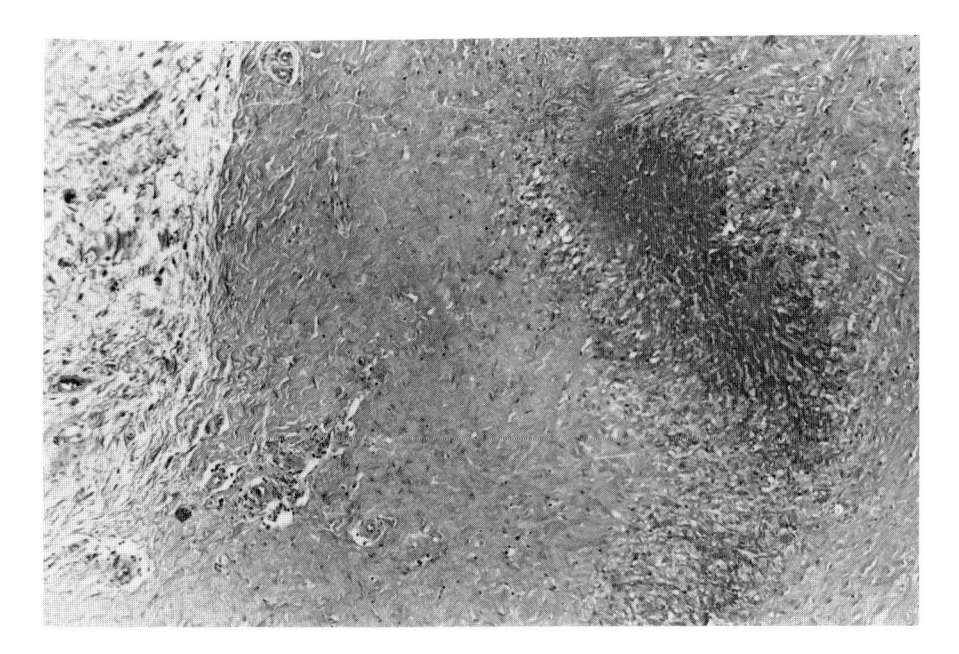

Figure 32.3. Rheumatoid nodule. A dark staining area of fibrinoid necrosis is seen to the *right of center*. It is surrounded by mononuclear phagocytes and dense fibrous tissue.

male predominance. The root of the aorta is altered, resulting in insufficiency of the aortic valve. More than 95% of patients with ankylosing spondylitis have an HLA B27 haplotype.

Juvenile rheumatoid arthritis is also not a rheumatoid arthritis variant. Although the joint involvement resembles rheumatoid arthritis, rheumatoid factor is always negative. Spondylitis, if present, correlates with the presence of HLA B27.

SYSTEMIC LUPUS ERYTHEMATOSUS

The majority of patients with systemic lupus erythematosus complain of joint pains, and a few develop progressive disease similar to rheumatoid arthritis. It is of interest that one-fourth of patients with systemic lupus are positive for rheumatoid factor and one-fourth of rheumatoid arthritis patients have a positive lupus erythematosus cell phenomenon.

SJÖGREN'S SYNDROME

This autoimmune syndrome consists of keratoconjunctivitis sicca (dry conjunctivitis), xerostomia (dry mouth), and an arthritis closely resembling rheumatoid arthritis. Ninety per cent of patients are positive for rheumatoid factor.

OSTEOARTHRITIS

Osteoarthritis, or degenerative joint disease, occurs in virtually all by the age of 50, and it is the principal cause of rheumatic disability. It consists of destruction

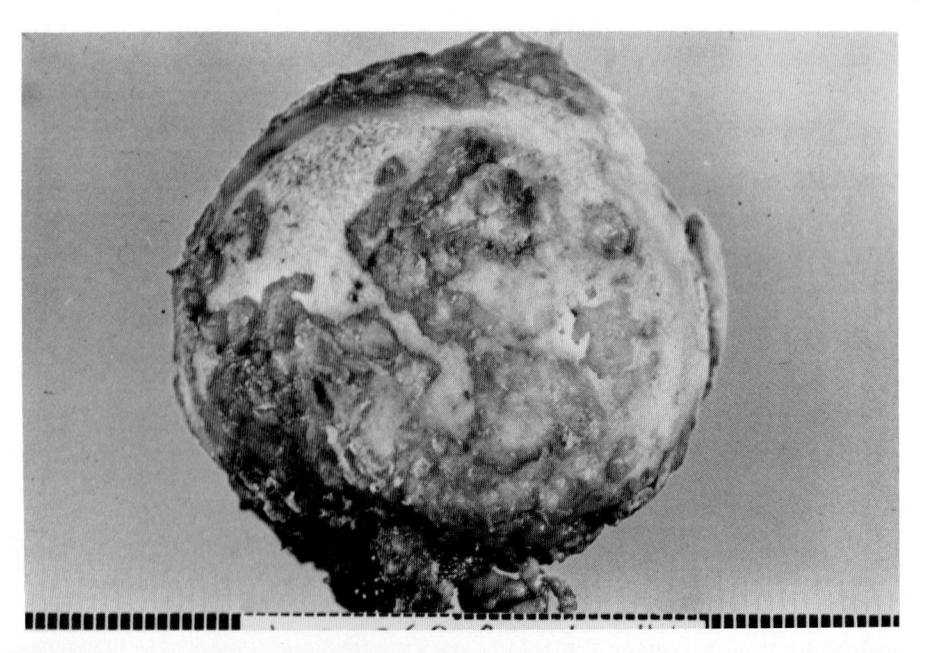

Figure 32.4. Osteoarthritis. This articular surface shows extensive erosion of cartilage and exposure of subchondral bone. In several areas, the bone has become polished and sclerotic.

of the weight-bearing surfaces of articular cartilages and proliferation of new bone surrounding the area of injury.

The initial change is the splitting of articular cartilage, creating a fibrillated surface, and associated with a loss of proteoglycan. There is progressive abrasion of cartilage down to the subchondral bone (Fig. 32.4). The exposed bone becomes polished and sclerotic, resembling ivory (eburnation). There may be some resurfacing with cartilage if the disorder is arrested or stabilized. New bone forms at the margin of articular cartilage, in the non-weight-bearing part of the joint. It forms osteophytes, or spurs, often covered by cartilage, that augment the degree of deformity (Fig. 32.5).

The major weight-bearing joints are most involved: the hips, knees, and spine. The distal interphalangeal joints are also frequently affected and their osteophytes form *Heberden's nodes*.

Osteoarthritis may result from congenital malformations, such as hip joint dysplasia, or from trauma. In most, however, it appears due to the wear-and-tear microtrauma of normal living, possibly abetted by subtle changes of aging.

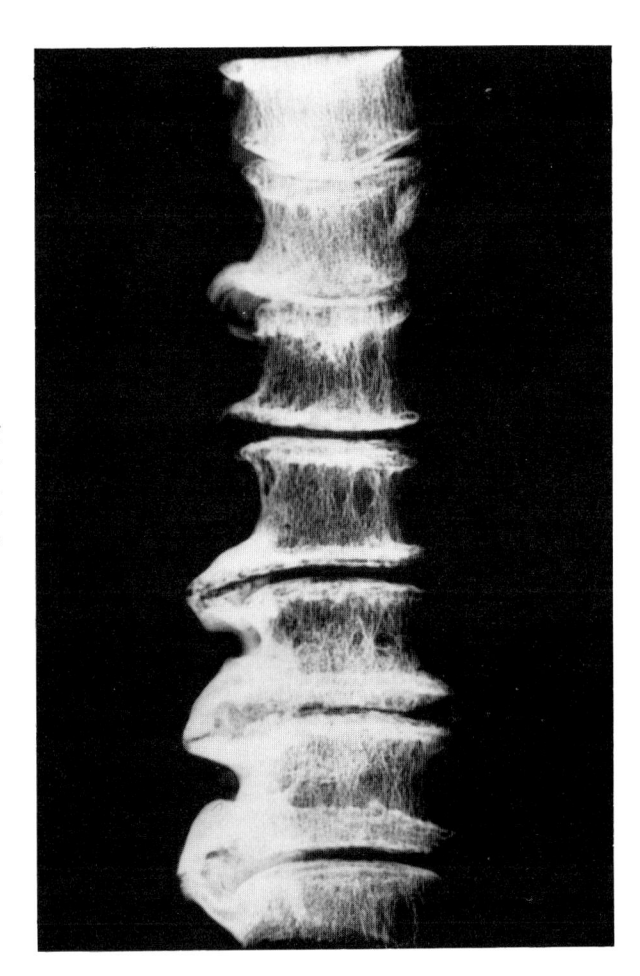

Figure 32.5. Osteoarthritis of spine. There is irregular narrowing of the intervertebral spaces. Striking osteophyte, or spur formation, is noted along the *left-hand margin*.

GOUT

Gout is a disorder, or group of disorders, characterized by the deposition of monosodium urate crystals in synovial fluid, joint tissues, and other body tissues (Fig. 32.6). Its etiology is multifactorial, and there is an association with hypertension, diabetes mellitus, hypertriglyceridemia, and atherosclerosis.

The mechanism of urate crystallization is unknown, but there is a clear relationship to prolonged hyperuricemia. Two-thirds of synthesized urate is excreted in the urine; the remaining third is split by bacterial uricase in the intestines. Hyperuricemia may result from a failure of feedback inhibition of purine synthesis or from inadequate renal excretion.

Acute gouty arthritis is a dramatic event, with severe and painful involvement of a single joint, often the first metatarsophalangeal joint (*podagra*). This is an acute synovitis, associated with crystal deposition in synovial fluid. Crystals are phagocytized by polymorphonuclear leukocytes whose lysosomes initiate the severe inflammatory process. The arthritis subsides, but is recurrent, with increasing frequency and involvement of more joints.

There is progressive formation of chalky deposits of urates in synovial and periarticular tissues. These deposits evoke a foreign body reaction and reparative fibrosis, forming nodular *tophi* around joint structures (Fig. 32.7), in bone, and in such subcutaneous locations as the helix of the ear.

Chronic gouty arthritis is similar to osteoarthritis, but deposits of urate are prominent on the cartilaginous surfaces, and there are destructive deposits in subchrondral bone (Fig. 32.8).

Some 20% of patients with gout develop uric acid stones in the urinary tract.

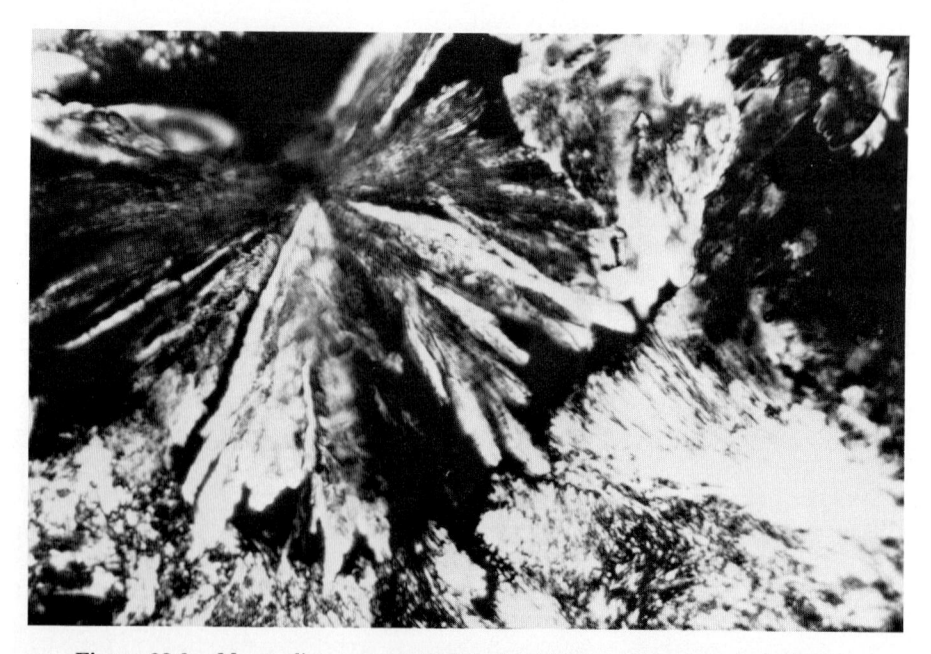

Figure 32.6. Monosodium urate crystals in joint tissue, seen under polarized light.

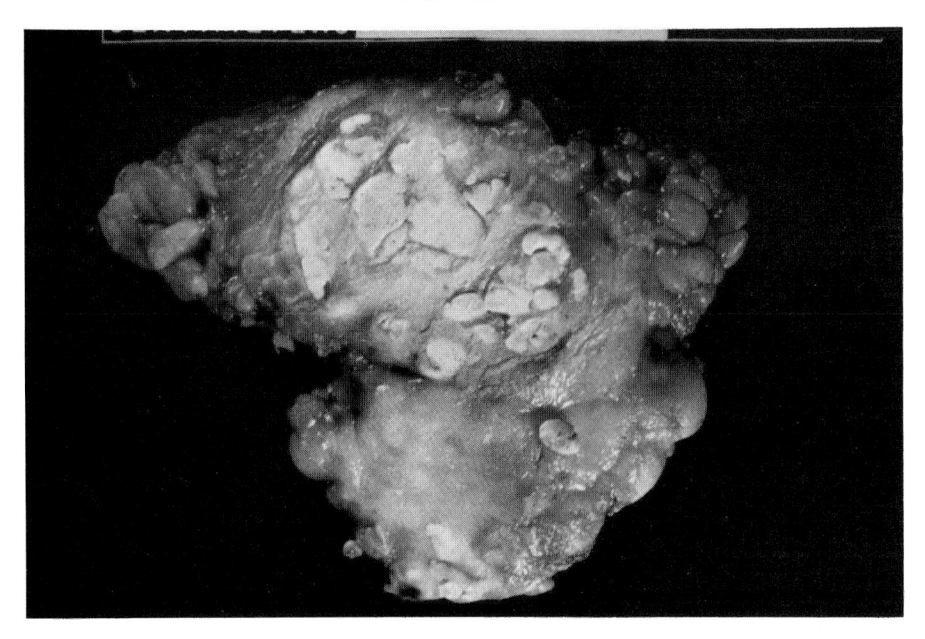

Figure 32.7. Tophus of knee joint. A conglomeration of urate deposits is seen in the soft tissue surrounding the joint.

Small deposits in the renal pyramids evoke a foreign body reaction and serve as intrarenal obstructive lesions that predepose to pyelonephritis (Fig. 32.9).

CHONDROCALCINOSIS

Chondrocalcinosis, or *pseudogout*, consists of the deposition of calcium pyrophosphate crystals in joint cartilages. These deposits tend to rupture into the joint spaces and induce a gout-like acute arthritis. This disorder is seen most in the elderly and can eventually result in osteoarthritis.

MISCELLANEOUS DEGENERATIVE DISORDERS

Hemophilic arthropathy occurs in 90% of hemophiliacs. Bleeding into the synovial cavity, subchondral bone, and periarticular tissues produces a very painful acute arthritis. With repeated episodes, changes similar to osteoarthritis become prominent. Periarticular and periosteal hemorrhages can stimulate formation of tumor-like masses of new bone. These "pseudotumors" may, at times, be difficult to distinguish from true neoplasms.

Neuropathic arthropathy (*Charcot joint*) occurs in disorders such as syphilis, diabetes, and syringomyelia. Loss of pain and proprioceptive senses subjects joints such as the knees to repeated trauma, with tears of the capsule and ligaments. There is a severe osteoarthritis, with many microfractures, and dramatic osteophyte formation.

ARTHRITIS IN INFECTIONS

Acute purulent arthritis can result from seeding of the synovium in the course of gonococcal, staphylococcal, or pneumococcal infections. Some patients with

442   *Pathology: Understanding Human Disease*

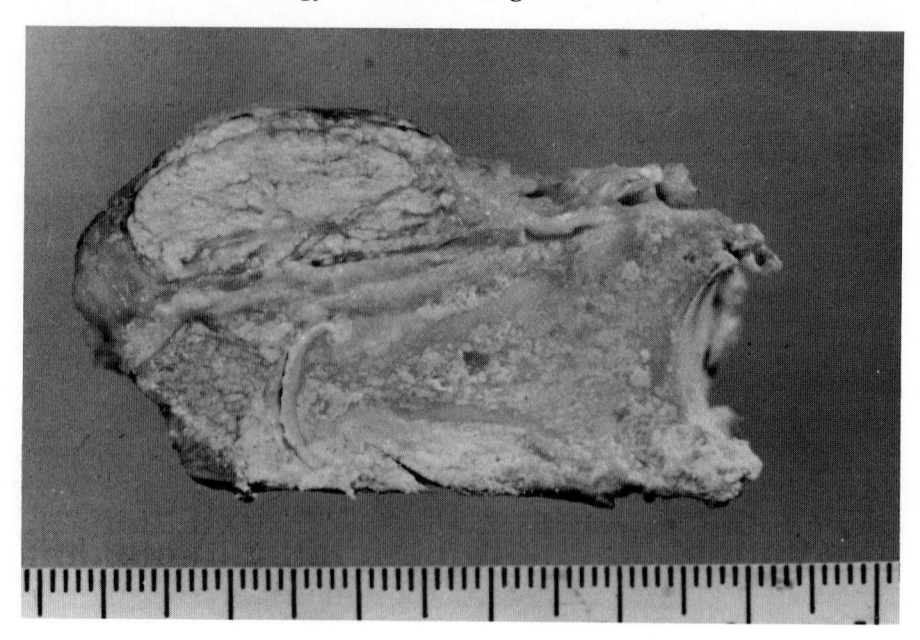

Figure 32.8. Gout. This is a sagittal section of a great toe removed surgically. Massive deposits of urate crystals are seen, destroying and replacing normal structures.

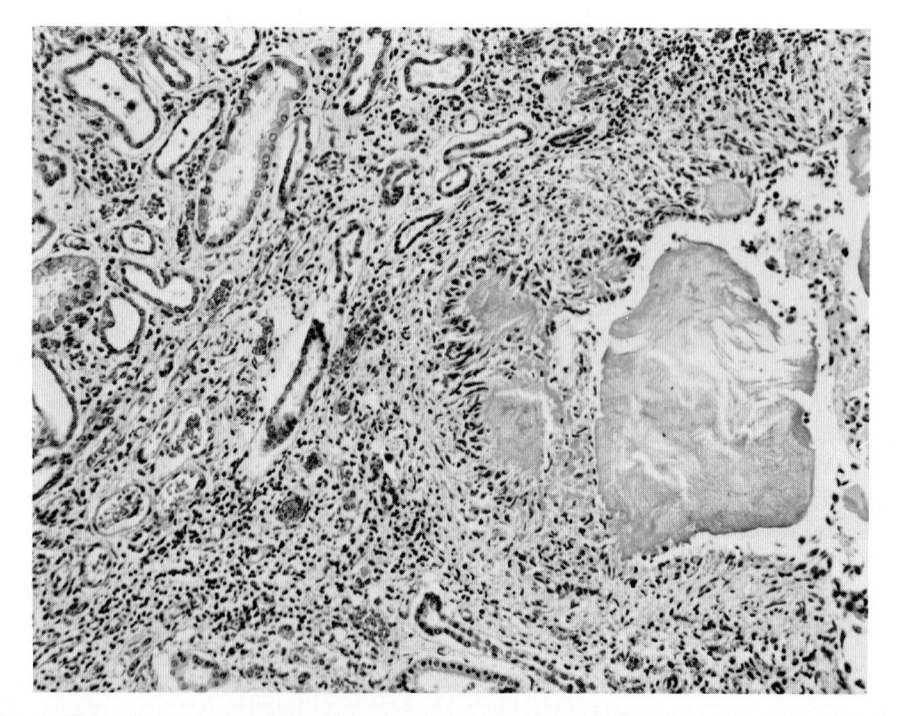

Figure 32.9. Gouty nephropathy. A large medullary urate deposit is seen at the *right*, surrounded by a foreign body reaction. These deposits produce intrarenal obstruction and predispose to pyelonephritis.

meningococcemia may also manifest an arthritis and, for unknown reason, hemolytic anemias predispose to arthritis due to salmonella organisms. Involvement is usually monoarticular and accompanied by severe pain and swelling. The articular cartilages may be destroyed and ankylosis may occasionally result.

Hematogenous dissemination of tuberculosis may result in a destructive arthritis, particularly as a complication of childhood tuberculosis. There may first be a subchondral focus of osteomyelitis which erupts into the joint. Arthritis can also complicate systemic fungus diseases, particularly coccidioidomycosis.

Suggested Reading

Radin EL. Mechanical aspects of osteoarthrosis. Bull. Rheum. Dis. *26:* 862, 1976.
Sokoloff L, Bland JH. The musculoskeletal system. Baltimore, Williams & Wilkins, 1975.

Chapter 33

Diseases of Skeletal Muscle

WILLIAM R. MARKESBERY, M.D.

Pathologists divide muscle diseases into myopathies, in which disease is primarily confined to muscle, and neurogenic atrophies, in which alterations in muscle are caused by disorders in the anterior horn cells, nerve roots, or peripheral nerves.

The major clinical manifestations of muscle disorders are weakness, atrophy, pseudohypertrophy, tenderness, cramps, stiffness, and myotonia. One of the most useful laboratory studies in determining the presence of muscle disease is the serum creatine phosphokinase (CPK) concentration. Muscle contains a large amount of CPK and, when fibers are damaged, it leaks into the serum and can serve as a marker of muscle injury or necrosis. With acute necrosis of muscle fibers, myoglobin is released into the blood and subsequently into the urine. Measurement of urinary myoglobin is an index of acute muscle damage, as in extreme exertion, crush injuries, ischemic disorders, and some inherited diseases. Studies of muscle action potentials (electromyography) and nerve conduction velocities are helpful in determining the presence of muscle diseases and differentiating these from neuropathic disorders. The muscle biopsy is an essential tool in diagnosis. Using histologic, histochemical, and electron microscopic studies, this procedure can differentiate myopathic from neurogenic disorders and establish the presence of some specific diseases not possible by clinical or other laboratory evaluation.

Normal muscle is made up of two major fiber types and several subtypes. *Type 1 (red) fibers* are low in glycogen, phosphorylase, and adenosine triphosphatase (ATPase) activity. They are rich in oxidative enzymes such as nicotinamide adenine dinucleotide (NADH), lipid, and mitochondria and contract slowly. *Type 2 (white) fibers* have sparse oxidative activity, are rich in glycogen, phosphorylase, and ATPase activity, and contract rapidly. In normal muscle, there is a random arrangement of fiber types. It is thought that muscle fibers innervated by the same motor neuron are histochemically similar. Fibers from different motor units overlap, resulting in an irregular and random pattern of the major fiber types.

The myopathies are characterized by random variation in fiber size, scattered splitting and necrosis of fibers, centralization of nuclei, regenerating fibers, an inflammatory reaction, and proliferation of endomysial and perimysial fibrous tissue. Neurogenic atrophy at first shows random fiber atrophy, then atrophy of groups of fibers or fascicles.

MUSCULAR DYSTROPHY

The muscular dystrophies are genetically determined myopathic diseases with progressive degeneration of skeletal muscle.

Duchenne dystrophy, the most common and severe form of dystrophy, is characterized by a sex-linked recessive inheritance pattern (with some sporadic cases because of a high mutation rate), transmission by a relatively unaffected mother, onset by age 3 to 5 years, progressive proximal limb muscle weakness, pseudohypertrophy of calves, cardiomypathy, kyphoscoliosis and joint contractures, marked CPK elevation, and death by age 20 to 25. Muscle biopsies show random variation in fiber size, proliferation of endomysial (Fig. 33.1) and perimysial connective tissue, necrosis and phagocytosis of fibers and regenerating fibers.

Facioscapulohumeral dystrophy, inherited as an autosomal dominant trait, and characterized by progressive weakness of face and shoulder girdle muscles, usually begins in the second or third decade. It often has a slowly progressive course. Muscle biopsy shows many hypertrophied fibers, scattered tiny atrophic

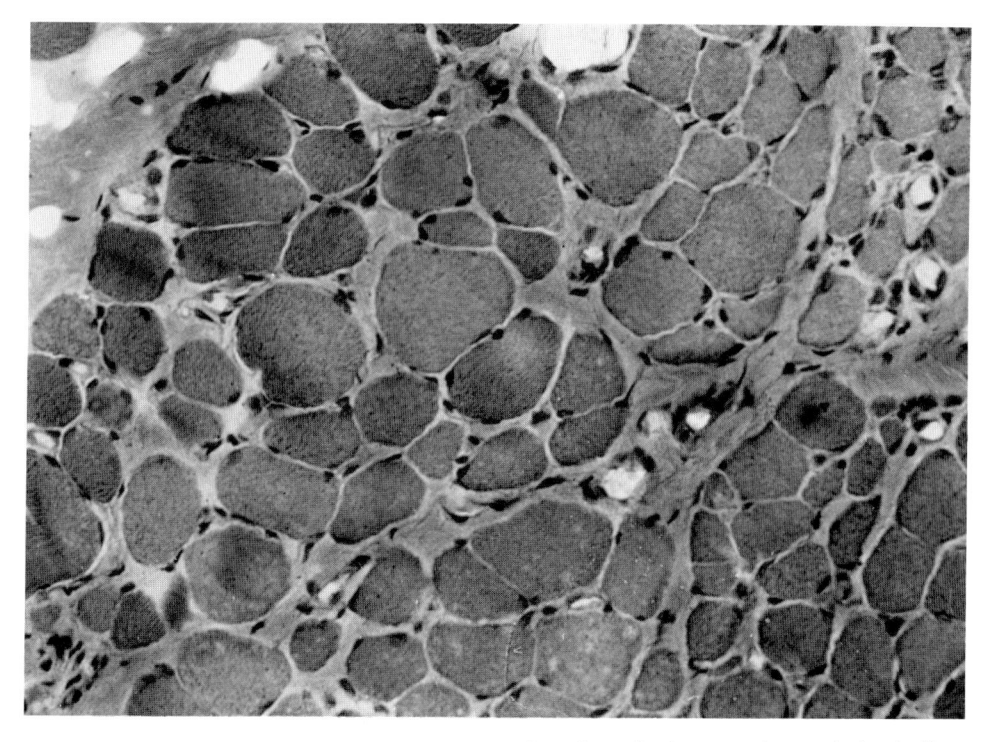

Figure 33.1. Duchenne dystrophy. This cross-section of muscle shows random variation in fiber size with separation of fibers by proliferation of endomysial connective tissue.

fibers, mild to moderate numbers of degenerating fibers, and occasional mononuclear inflammatory infiltrates.

Limb-girdle dystrophy, inherited as an autosomal recessive trait, has a variable age of onset, with proximal shoulder or pelvic girdle muscle weakness as the clinical hallmark. The rate of progression and degree of severity vary considerably. Muscle biopsy shows moderate degenerative changes, marked fiber splitting, and abundant internalization of sarcolemmal nuclei.

Myotonic muscular dystrophy is characterized by an autosomal dominant inheritance pattern, onset in the second to fourth decades, marked myotonia (inability to relax a contracted muscle), distal weakness, frontal balding, hatchet face appearance, cataracts, hypogonadism, cardiomyopathy, and endocrine dysfunctions. Muscle biopsy shows abundant central nuclei, ring fibers, Type 1 fiber atrophy, degenerative changes, and fibrosis. Recent studies have suggested a generalized membrane defect in this disease.

INFLAMMATORY MYOPATHIES

Mild inflammatory changes occur in many muscle diseases, ranging from parasitic, granulomatous, and viral disorders to dystrophies and myasthenia gravis. In polymyositis and dermatomyositis, the inflammatory changes are a prominent part of the histologic picture.

Polymyositis is an acquired disease distinguished by weakness of shoulder and pelvic girdle and neck and swallowing muscles and by muscle and joint pains. When accompanied by a skin rash, it is called *dermatomyositis.* Both may affect any age group or sex and have an acute, subacute, or chronic course. Both may be associated with neoplastic disease and with collagen-vascular disorders, such as systemic lupus erythematosus, polyarteritis nodosa, and rheumatoid arthritis. Neoplasms are not usually found in childhood dermatomyositis, but it is often associated with widespread vascular lesions. Muscle biopsies show diffuse inflammatory infiltrates (Fig. 33.2), perifascicular atrophy, necrotic fibers, and fibrosis. Although the precise etiology is not known, some believe it to be an autoimmune disorder.

MYASTHENIA GRAVIS

Myasthenia gravis is a disease manifest by excessive fatigability and weakness of extremity, trunk, ocular, and bulbar muscles. It can affect any age group but more often affects young women and older men. Common symptoms are diplopia, ptosis, dysphagia, dysarthria, and limb weakness. The course is quite variable but, for most, the disease is most active in the first few years. The disease can only be suspected on clinical grounds and must be confirmed by response to anticholinesterase drugs. Tumors of the thymus gland are found in 10% of myasthenic patients and about 70% have thymic hyperplasia. Some 5% of patients have rheumatoid arthritis, systemic lupus erythematosus, pernicious anemia, or Sjögren's syndrome, underscoring the relationship of myasthenia gravis with autoimmune disorders.

The functional abnormality in this disease is at the neuromuscular junction.

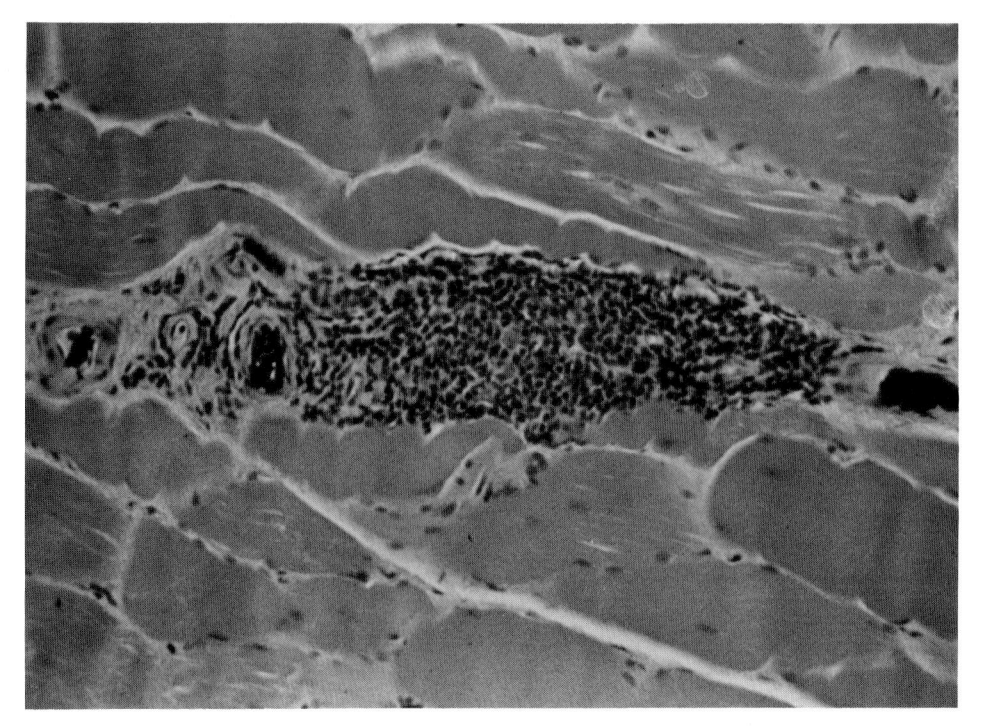

Figure 33.2. Polymyositis. This longitudinal section shows many chronic mononuclear inflammatory cells in a perivascular site.

Recent data indicate decreased postsynaptic receptor binding of acetylcholine and the presence of a serum globulin that inhibits acetylcholine binding. Muscle biopsy is not helpful in making the diagnosis. Type 2 fiber atrophy and some group atrophy may be present. Overemphasis has been placed on small collections of lymphocytes, termed lymphorrhages, which occur in a few patients.

CONGENITAL MYOPATHIES

The congenital myopathies are a relatively new group of disorders in which symptoms are often present at birth, although they can become manifest later in life. Many present as floppy (hypotonic) infants and have a benign, nonprogressive course, while a few have been fatal. Inheritance is often by an autosomal dominant pattern, but sporadic cases are not uncommon. It is not possible on clinical grounds to distinguish among the different congenital myopathies or, in some instances, to distinguish them from other forms of neuromuscular disease. Muscle biopsy, using histochemical techniques and electron microscopy, is required to reach an accurate diagnosis. These disorders have been named after the structural alterations present in the muscle, *i.e.*, central core disease, rod body myopathy, centronuclear myopathy, mitochondrial myopathy, congenital fiber type disproportion, and others.

METABOLIC MYOPATHIES

Metabolic myopathies are a group of disorders associated with known or suspected biochemical abnormalities in muscle. Many present with proximal muscle weakness and a few present with muscle cramps, pain, and fatigue with exercise. The major metabolic myopathies are the glycogen storage diseases, lipid storage diseases, and the periodic paralyses.

Skeletal muscle is involved in four glycogen storage diseases: Types 2, 3, 5, and 7. *Type 2*, or *Pompe's disease*, has a deficiency of α-1,4-glucosidase (acid maltase) activity, and an accumulation of free lying and lysosomal glycogen in skeletal muscle, heart, CNS, kidney, liver, and leukocytes. In its typical form it presents with severe hypotonia, macroglossia, hepatomegaly, and cardiac failure. Muscle biopsy shows an abundance of vacuoles containing glycogen in the fibers. In *Type 3 glycogenosis*, there is a deficiency in amylo-1,6-glucosidase (debranching enzyme). Involvement of skeletal muscle is mild and may cause hypotonia and weakness. The liver, however, can be severely affected and cause hypoglycemia and ketosis. *Type 5*, muscle phosphorylase deficiency, and *type 7*, phosphofructokinase deficiency, present with fatigability, weakness, and muscle cramps with exercise. Venous lactic acid does not rise with exercise. Muscle biopsy shows an increase in glycogen and histochemical stains reveal an absence of the affected enzymes.

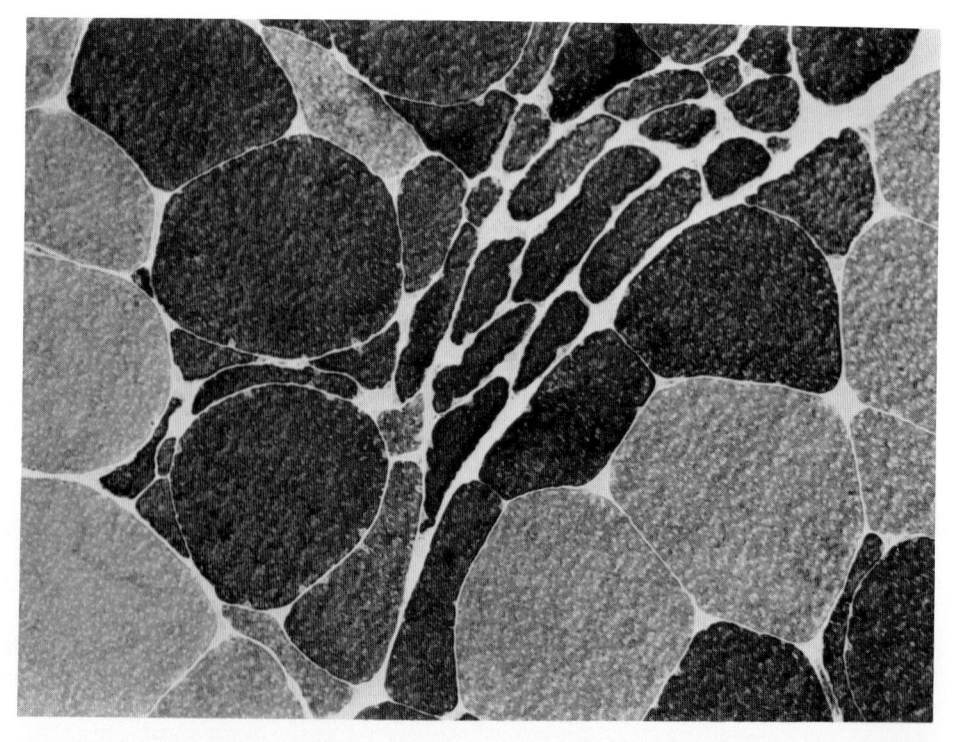

Figure 33.3. Neurogenic atrophy (denervation). Cross-section of muscle showing small group atrophy and scattered angular atrophic fibers (ATPase reaction).

Diseases of Skeletal Muscle

In recent years, a few cases with accumulation of excess lipid in muscle fibers have been reported. These patients have shown a broad spectrum of clinical manifestations, from hypotonic muscles in infants to limb-girdle weakness in adults. All have had multiple small lipid vacuoles in muscle fibers. From this heterogeneous group a few patients with *carnitine deficiency* have been identified. Carnitine, present in high concentrations in muscle, facilitates long chain fatty acid transport across the mitochondrial membrane. Some patients have a generalized deficiency of carnitine. A deficiency of carnitine palmityl transferase, the enzyme responsible for interaction of carnitine and long chain fatty acids, has been described in several patients presenting with myoglobinuria and cramps.

The *periodic paralyses* are a group of inherited disorders with episodic attacks of weakness and flaccidity. They have been classified according to the level of serum potassium during an attack, *i.e.*, hypokalemic, normokalemic, or hyperkalemic periodic paralysis. They primarily affect children and young adults. The severity of attacks varies from almost total paralysis to mild focal weakness. Muscle biopsy shows scattered vacuoles.

DENERVATION OR NEUROGENIC ATROPHY

Disorders affecting the anterior horn cell, nerve root, or peripheral nerve cause similar, relatively specific changes in skeletal muscle, called neurogenic atrophy. Muscle fibers undergoing denervation become shrunken and atrophic. Because

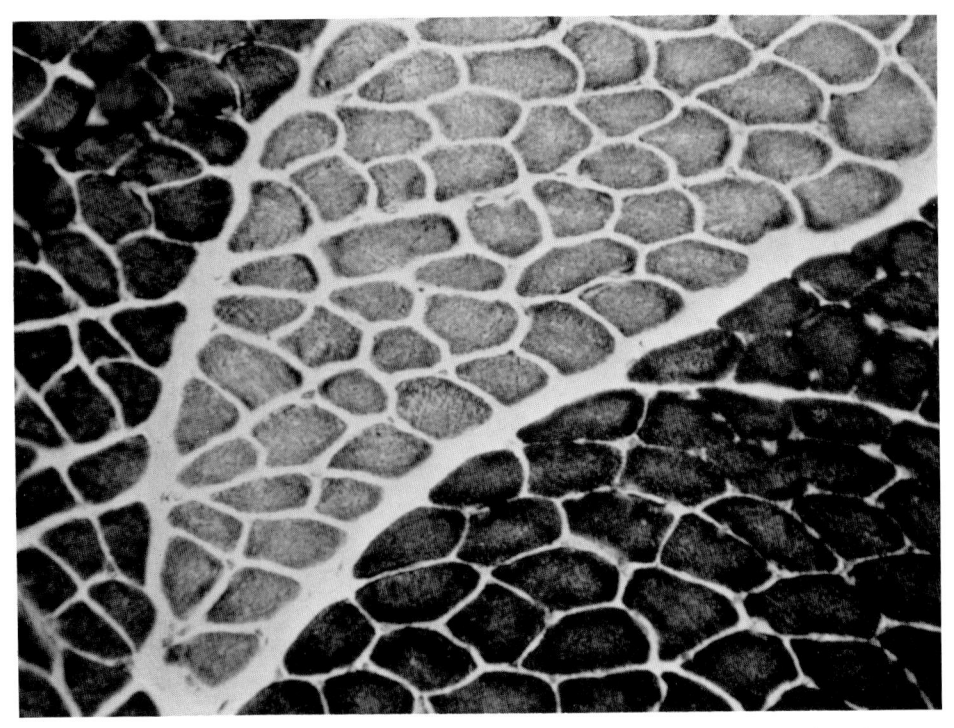

Figure 33.4. Fiber type grouping. Large groups of fibers of one type next to groups of another type indicating denervation and reinnervation (NADH reaction).

individual motor nerves supply many scattered muscle fibers, early denervation causes random atrophy with angular shaped fibers. As denervation progresses, atrophic fibers occur together in groups, referred to as *small group atrophy* (Fig. 33.3). When denervation is severe, whole fascicles may undergo atrophy (*large group atrophy*). Scattered atrophic fibers and small and large group atrophy are the hallmarks of neurogenic atrophy. Target fibers, consisting of central nonreactive zones, surrounded by an area of increased reactivity and a normal staining zone with the NADH reaction, are often seen in denervation. With reinnervation, there is sprouting of terminal axons which convert newly innervated fibers into their respective histochemical type. This leads to groups of fibers of the same histochemical type next to groups of another type referred to as fiber type grouping (Fig. 33.4). Pyknotic nuclear clumps are also typical of neurogenic atrophy.

Suggested Reading

Dubowitz V, Brooke MH. Muscle biopsy: a modern approach. In: Major problems in neurology. London, WB Saunders Co, 1973.

Markesbery WR. Pathology of muscular dystrophy and related disorders. Adv. Neurol. *17:* 175, 1977.

Chapter 34

The Skin

The great multitude of human skin disorders has made dermatopathology a rather complex subspeciality, with its own vocabulary and nomenclature. This chapter includes discussion of the most important skin tumors and a few examples of hypersensitivity dermatoses, autoimmune disorders, and lesions of uncertain etiology.

SKIN TUMORS

The important tumors are squamous cell carcinoma, basal cell carcinoma, and tumors of melanin-producing cells. The many tumors of connective tissue origin and metastatic tumors are not discussed.

Squamous Cell Carcinoma

Squamous cell carcinoma of the skin is probably the most common human malignancy. It occurs predominately in skin areas exposed to the sun and is most likely to affect individuals with fair skin and blue eyes. Squamous cell carcinoma may also occur in areas of chronic inflammation: skin ulcers, sinus tracts, and old burns.

The lesions appear as raised, reddish brown plaques or nodules that frequently ulcerate (Fig. 34.1). They may invade deeply, and some 5% metastasize to regional lymph nodes. Metastasis is more frequent in tumors arising in chronic ulcers and burns.

Squamous cell carcinomas may be well differentiated, with formation of keratinized "pearls," or anaplastic (Fig. 34.2). The prognosis, however, is determined primarily by the extent of invasion. Carcinoma *in situ*, or *Bowen's disease*, appears as a crusted plaque with underlying congestion. Bowen's disease may be associated with internal malignancies, especially of the gastrointestinal tract.

Squamous cell carcinoma is often preceded by *actinic keratosis*, a precancerous epidermal lesion induced by the sun's rays or other radiant energy. There are multiple raised, reddish, often scaly lesions composed of dysplastic epithelium and destruction of dermal elastic tissue with chronic inflammation.

Keratoacanthoma is a rapidly growing tumor-like lesion that may be confused with squamous cell carcinoma. It also occurs in exposed skin, particularly over the temples, and forms a crater-like mass filled with desquamated keratin (Fig. 34.3). Although active squamous cell nests extend into the superficial dermis, keratoacanthomas do not appear to be precancerous, and they show a strong tendency to spontaneous involution.

452   Pathology: Understanding Human Disease

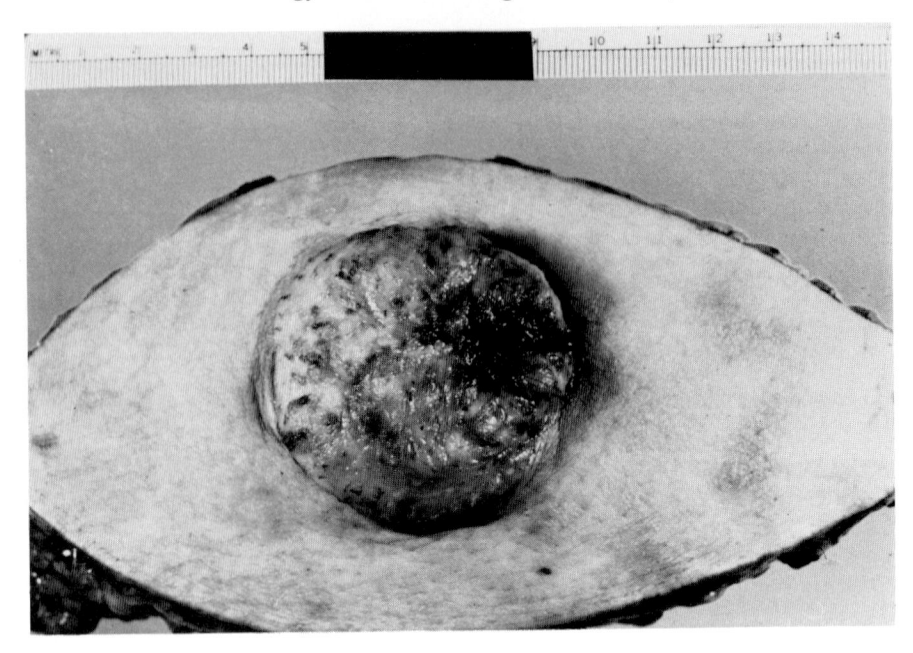

Figure 34.1. Large squamous cell carcinoma removed from the thigh. The lesion is raised and shows extensive surface ulceration. It has a very fleshy appearance.

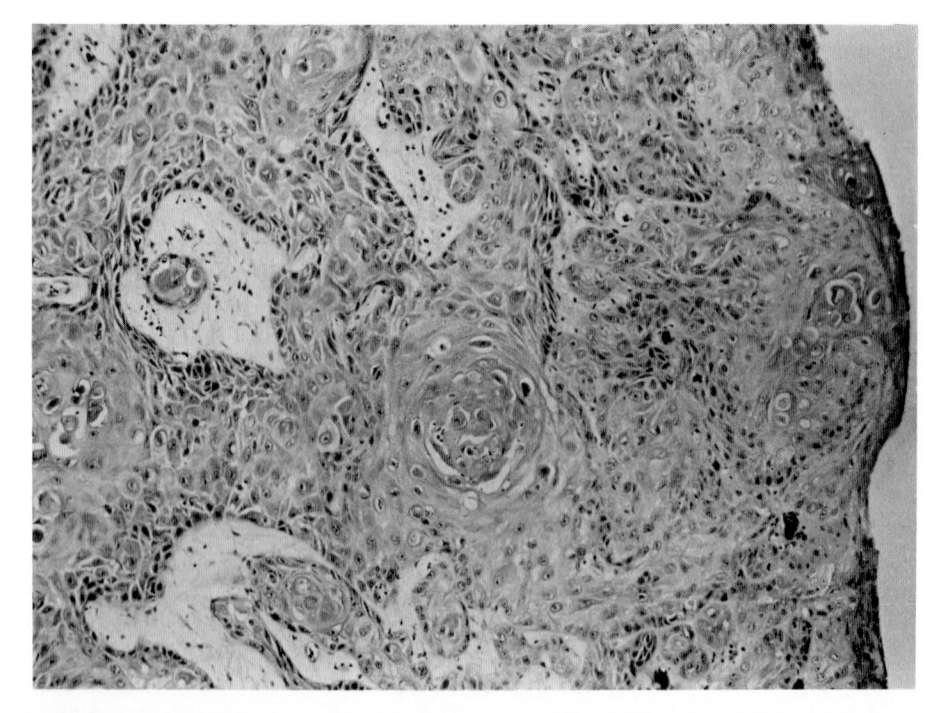

Figure 34.2. Squamous cell carcinoma. This is a well differentiated squamous tumor and shows epithelial "pearl" formation (*center*).

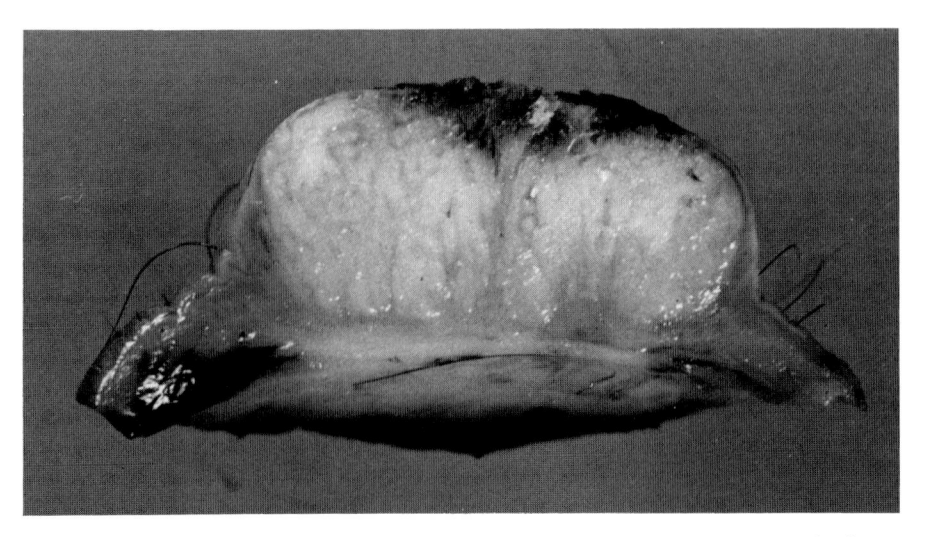

Figure 34.3. Keratoacanthoma. This lesion from the back of the hand measured 2 cm in diameter. The cut surface shows a crater-like structure largely filled with keratinized epithelium. Keratoacanthomas do not show malignant change.

Basal Cell Carcinoma

Basal cell carcinomas arise in exposed skin, particularly on the head, face, and neck. They appear at first as smooth, shiny, nodules, often white, but occasionally pigmented. Later, they ulcerate and tend to invade surrounding tissues and structures. Distant metastases are extremely rare.

Basal cell carcinomas arise from the basal layer of the epidermis or from the skin adnexa. The tumor cells may be arranged in solid groups, or they may replicate the structure of sweat glands and hair follicles (Fig. 34.4). The cells at the periphery of tumor nests show a characteristic palisading.

Although these are slow growing tumors, failure to recognize and remove them early can result in extensive destruction of vital structures of the head.

Tumors of Melanocytes

Benign tumors of melanocytes are called *nevi*. Some are present at birth, but most are acquired during the first several decades. They may appear macular (flat), papular (elevated), nodular, or pedunculated, and are brown or black. They are usually sharply circumscribed. Nevi may be entirely intradermal, or there may be nests of cells within the epidermis at the dermoepidermal junction (*junctional nevus*). *Giant hairy nevi* are congenital raised lesions, often very large and containing many hairs. They are usually intradermal, but may extend quite deeply, and between 5 and 20% of these lesions may eventually show malignant behavior.

There are several types of malignant *melanoma*. *Lentigo maligna melanoma* arises from a premalignant lesion, *lentigo maligna*. The latter is a large, macular lesion with variegated and irregular pigmentation, most often arising on the face. It contains atypical "dendritic" melanocytes that resemble neurons confined to

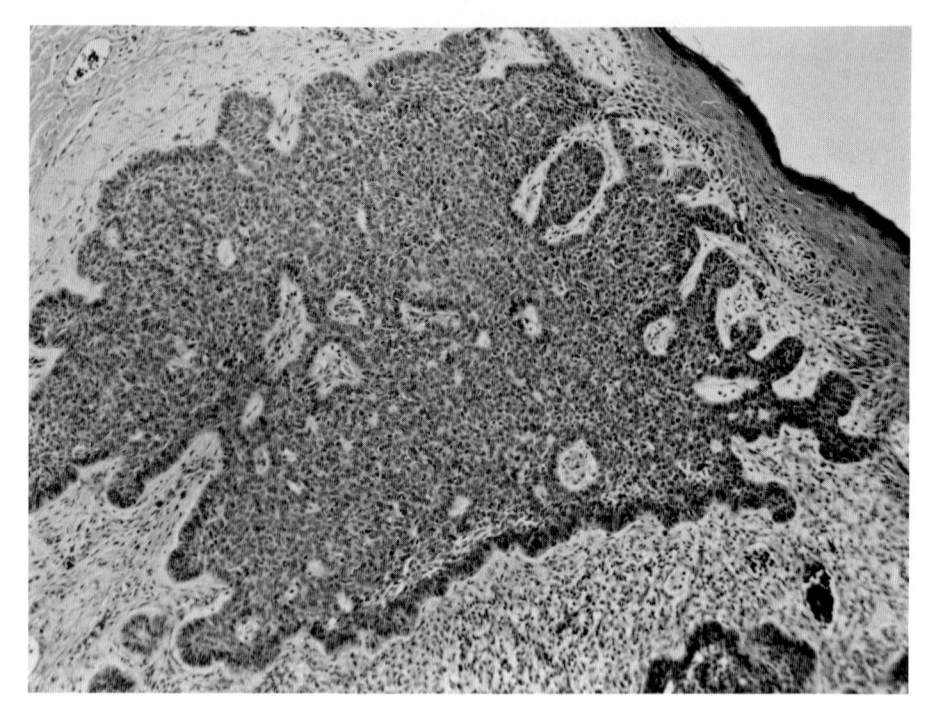

Figure 34.4 Basal cell carcinoma. This tumor, composed of nests of dark staining basal-type cells, appears to arise from the basal layer of the epidermis at the *right*. The cells at the periphery show palisading and club-like extensions.

the basal layer of the epidermis. These lesions may persist for 10 to 15 years, or longer, before becoming frankly malignant. Development of melanoma is usually signaled by a papular change in the lesion. The prognosis of lentigo maligna melanoma is relatively good, but this lesion constitutes only 5% of melanomas.

Superficial spreading melanoma is the most common type of malignant melanocytic tumor. It occurs in young individuals, tending to appear on the backs of men and the thighs and legs of women. The lesions are irregularly pigmented papules and show intraepidermal rounded melanocytes that spread laterally before invading the dermis (Fig. 34.5).

Nodular melanoma presents as a darkly pigmented nodule which is rapidly growing and often ulcerated (Fig. 34.6). It can be seen anywhere on the skin and mucous membranes. The lesion shows invasion, often deep into the dermis and subcutaneous tissues, and there may be small satellite lesions in the surrounding skin. Nodular melanoma has the worst outlook of the three types.

The prognosis of melanoma is determined in part by histologic type, but also in large part by the depth of invasion at the time of surgical removal. Superficial lesions that show only early invasion of the dermis are virtually all curable (Fig. 34.7). If invasion extends through the dermis and into the subcutaneous tissue, there is about a 50% 10-year survival after excision and regional lymph node resection.

HYPERSENSITIVITY DERMATITIS

The hypersensitivity dermatoses are a diverse group of disorders mediated by immunologic reactions to foreign material. *Erythema multiforme* is seen as a manifestation of hypersensitivity to such agents as sulfonamides, penicillin, and barbiturates and in certain fungus and bacterial infections. The lesions may be macular, papular, or vesicular; most characteristic is a raised erythematous lesion with a clear vesicular center. The dermis and epidermis may be separated by edema fluid. Perivascular mononuclear inflammation is present. In the most severe form of this disorder, the *Stevens-Johnson syndrome*, there is extensive involvement of skin and mucous membranes, with extensive exudation and desquamation. Conjunctivitis may be marked, as are systemic manifestations of fever, vomiting, myalgias, and chest pain.

Erythema nodosum presents as swollen, painful nodules over the lower legs, seen particularly in patients with tuberculosis and coccidioidomycosis. It may also be seen in conjunction with certain streptococcal infections and is a manifestation of hypersensitivity to sulfonamides. The lesions consist of a panniculitis of the subcutaneous tissues with marked vasculitis and infiltration of inflammatory cells. Granuloma formation may be seen, but causative organisms are not present. Erythema nodosum is primarily a manifestation of cell-mediated immunity.

AUTOIMMUNE DISEASES

Systemic lupus erythematosus (p. 85) commonly involves the skin, most frequently as an erythematous rash on the face and chest. The facial rash may

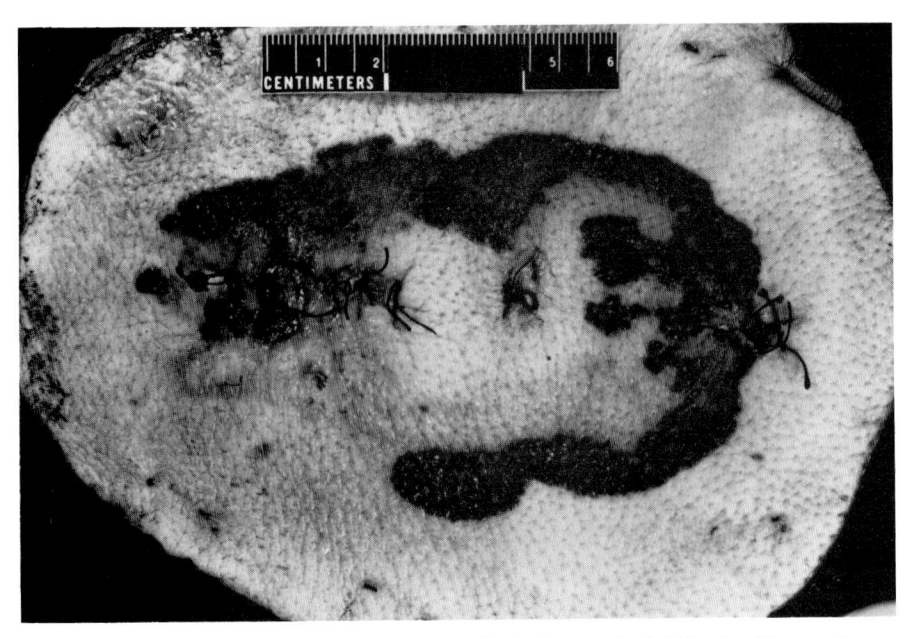

Figure 34.5. Superficial spreading melanoma. This lesion, excised following biopsy, shows an irregular area of pigmentation. The lesion is only slightly raised above the normal skin margin.

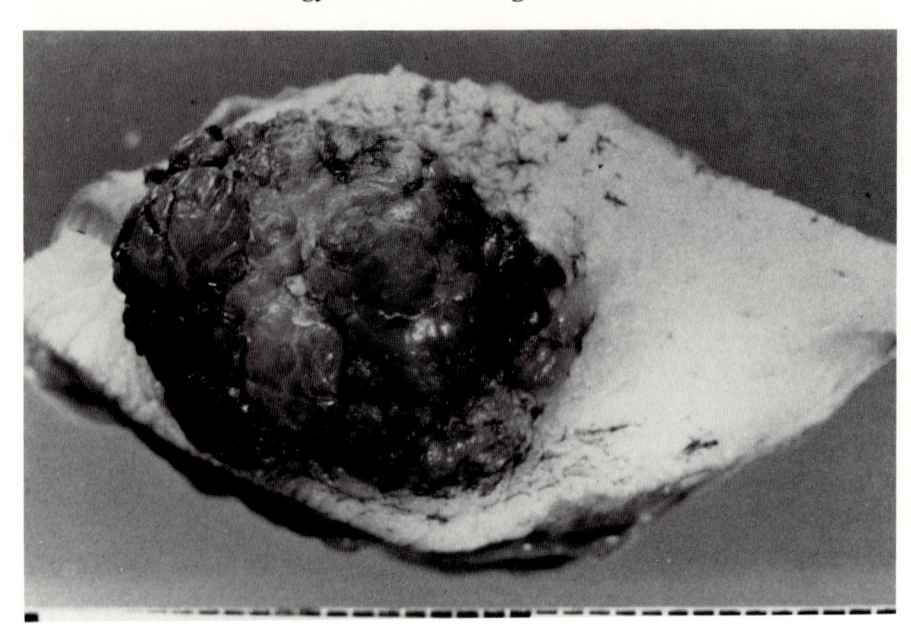

Figure 34.6. Nodular melanoma. This darkly pigmented nodular mass is poorly circumscribed and has invaded deeply into the subcutaneous tissues.

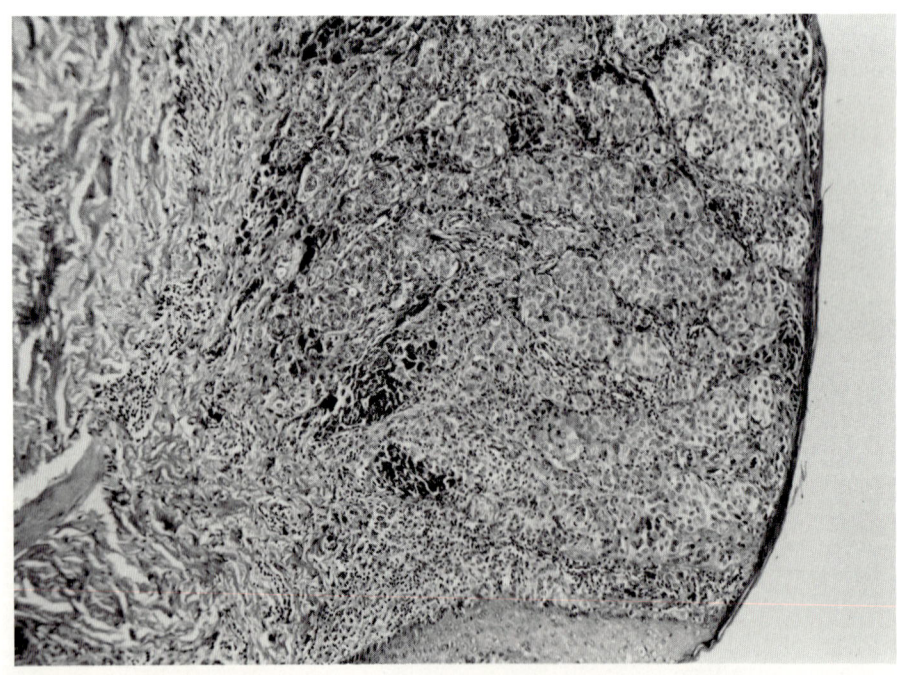

Figure 34.7. Malignant melanoma. The superficial dermis is filled with large irregular melanocytes, arranged in solid nests. The overlying epidermis at the *right* is flattened and atrophic but shows invasion by tumor cells. Deep to the tumor, heavily pigmented macrophages are seen. These are not part of the malignant neoplasm. A superficial lesion such as this carries a good prognosis.

have a butterfly configuration over the bridge of the nose and malar eminences. Histologically, there is marked dermal edema with fibrinoid necrosis, degeneration of basilar epidermal cells, and irregular epidermal atrophy. Perivascular inflammatory infiltration is usually seen, along with a necrotizing vasculitis. Granular antigen-antibody complexes are demonstrable by fluorescent antibody technique in a subepidermal location in the lesions and also in uninvolved but sun-exposed skin.

Discoid lupus erythematosus in an autoimmune disorder in which lesions are characteristically confined to the skin. Some patients, however, may manifest a focal glomerulonephritis. The skin lesions are discrete erythematous plaques, most noted on the face, ears, scalp, or neck. They show epidermal atrophy, keratotic plugging of hair follicles, hydropic degeneration of basal cells, and edema and necrosis of the upper dermis. There is intense lymphocytic infiltration surrounding the dermal appendages. Ten per cent of patients with discoid lupus have circulating antinuclear antibodies. Antigen-antibody complexes are demonstrable in the lesions of discoid lupus, but not in the surrounding skin. A few patients with discoid lupus go on to develop disseminated disease, but most do not.

Pemphigus is a disorder characterized by autoantibodies against the intercellular zone of the epidermis. Destruction of this area results in loss of cohesiveness among epidermal cells (acantholysis) and the accumulation of fluid between epidermal cells (sparing the basal layer), with formation of vesicles and large bullae (Fig. 34.8). They occur throughout the skin and mucous membranes, perhaps stimulated by trauma. The bullae rupture easily and are readily infected.

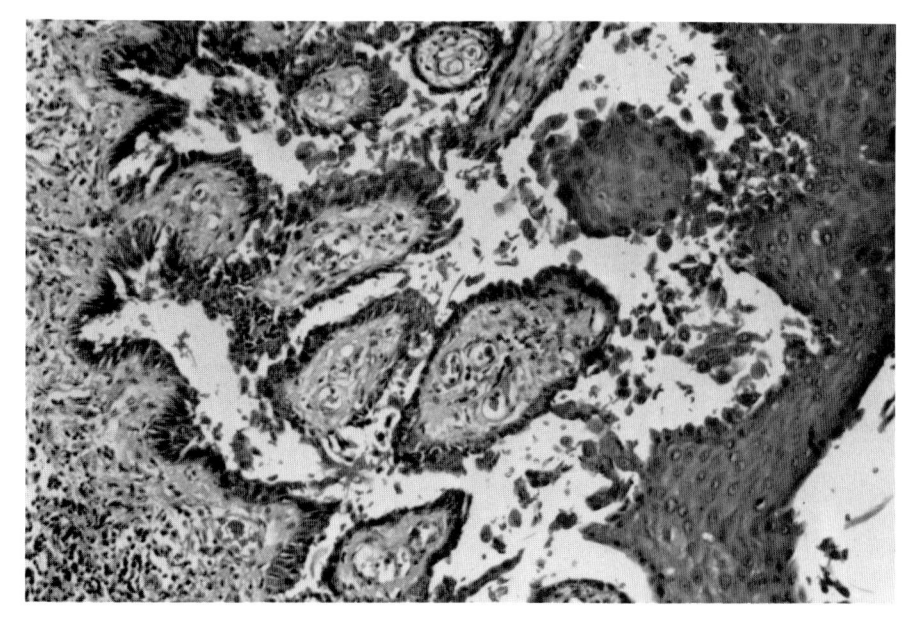

Figure 34.8. Pemphigus. Separation of the epidermis has taken place between the prickle cell layer and the basal cells. The result is formation of a vesicle or bulla, filled with fluid.

The mortality, formerly near 100%, is now about 10%. Immune deposits containing IgG are demonstrable around prickle cells and their intercellular bridges.

In *pemphigoid*, autoantibodies are directed against the epidermal basement membrane. Immunofluorescence demonstrates a ribbon-like distribution of antibody. Subepidermal vesicles are formed, typically over the lower abdomen, groin, and thighs; the mucous membranes are not involved. The bullae in pemphigoid are unlikely to rupture, and the disorder is much less severe than pemphigus.

DISORDERS OF UNKNOWN ETIOLOGY

Psoriasis is a disorder manifested by scaly red plaques on the trunk and extensor surfaces of the arms and legs. Histologically, there is increased thickness of the stratum germinativum (acanthosis), thinning of the epidermis over thickened dermal papillae, delayed keratinization of the horny layer, and microabscesses (of Munro) in the outer epidermis.

Lichen planus is characterized by flat, purplish papules with a ring of peripheral scales. They are frequent around the wrists and elbows and may occur in mucous membranes. There is thickening of the epidermal layers, liquefaction of the basal layer, and an intense band-like infiltration of lymphocytes and mononuclear phagocytes. It has been suggested that the lesions of lichen planus reflect a cell-mediated immune reaction.

Suggested Reading

Clark WH, Mastrangelo MJ, Ainsworth AA, Berd D, Bellet RE, Bernadino, EA. Current concepts of the biology of human cutaneous malignant melanoma. Adv. Cancer Res. *24:* 267, 1977.

Person JR, Rogers RS III. Bullous and cicatricial pemphigoid. Mayo Clin. Proc. *52:* 54, 1977.

Chapter 35

Pediatric Disorders

The pathology of pediatric disorders is a large subject. Rather than listing and characterizing many disease states, a few of the most important have been selected for discussion in some detail. These include the respiratory distress syndrome of the newborn, the sudden infant death syndrome, cystic fibrosis, Reye's syndrome, and several of the tumors peculiar to infants and children.

Although recent years have shown a steady and dramatic improvement, mortality in the neonatal period and early infancy is still high. In 1975, the infant mortality in the United States was 17 per 1000 live births, nearly twice that of Sweden and considerably higher than the mortality in Japan. Immaturity, birth injuries, and the respiratory distress syndrome are important causes of neonatal deaths, and respiratory infections and the sudden infant death syndrome are responsible for many deaths in early infancy. Neoplastic disease accounts for about 8% of deaths between the ages of 1 and 4 years, and 15% of deaths in the 5- to 14-year-old age group. Trauma is responsible for half of all deaths between 1 and 14 years of age. Most traumatic deaths are accidental and related to the automobile, but an unknown number result from child abuse.

THE RESPIRATORY DISTRESS SYNDROME OF THE NEWBORN

The neonatal respiratory distress syndrome, or hyaline membrane disease, accounts for at least 20,000 deaths per year. It is characterized by the appearance of rapidly progressive respiratory difficulty and cyanosis shortly after birth. Although responsive at first to oxygen administration, it often becomes refractory to all therapy, with subsequent apnea and death. The mortality is generally near 25%, but may be as high as 50% in very immature infants.

The lungs are poorly expanded, firm, and meaty in consistency. The principal histologic finding is extensive hyaline membrane formation, reflecting greatly increased permeability of the alveolar septa. There is usually no inflammation.

The neonatal respiratory distress syndrome is observed in some 10% of premature, or low birth weight, infants and is particularly likely to occur after intrauterine hypoxia, in infants of diabetic mothers (23-fold increase), and in infants delivered by Cesarean section before the 38th week of gestation. The pathogenesis of the disorder clearly relates to a deficiency of surfactant production by Type II pneumocytes, so that the lungs tend to collapse completely after each inspiratory effort. The first effective secretion of surfactant occurs at a gestational age of 35 weeks, but it is often not adequate to prepare the lungs for breathing air before 40 weeks. The adequacy of surfactant production can be evaluated by measuring the lecithin/sphingomyelin ratio in amniotic fluid. Although a deficiency of surfactant production is generally accepted as the underlying mechanism of the respiratory distress syndrome, intrapartum aspiration of amniotic fluid may also play a pathogenetic role.

Oxygen therapy of the respiratory distress syndrome may result in severe complications. The alveolar capillaries are injured by high oxygen concentrations and permit increased escape of fluid with high protein content from the capillaries to the alveoli, again resulting in hyaline membrane formation. Necrotizing bronchiolitis may also occur; this tends to heal with an obstructing squamous metaplasia. In the resulting *bronchopulmonary dysplasia*, the lungs show alternating areas of collapse and distension, and there is severe hypoxic respiratory failure (Fig. 35.1). Another serious complication of oxygen therapy is *retrolental fibroplasia*.

THE SUDDEN INFANT DEATH SYNDROME

The sudden infant death syndrome is an unexpected and basically unexplained death in an infant or young child. It occurs once in every 350 to 500 live births, is responsible for between 7,000 and 10,000 deaths each year, and is the principal cause of death in infants between 1 and 6 months of age.

The majority (90 to 95%) of victims of the sudden infant death syndrome die quietly, while asleep. There is no outcry and no evidence of a struggle. One-third have had symptoms of a mild upper respiratory infection. Complete autopsy usually reveals no more than petechial hemorrhages of pleura and pericardium,

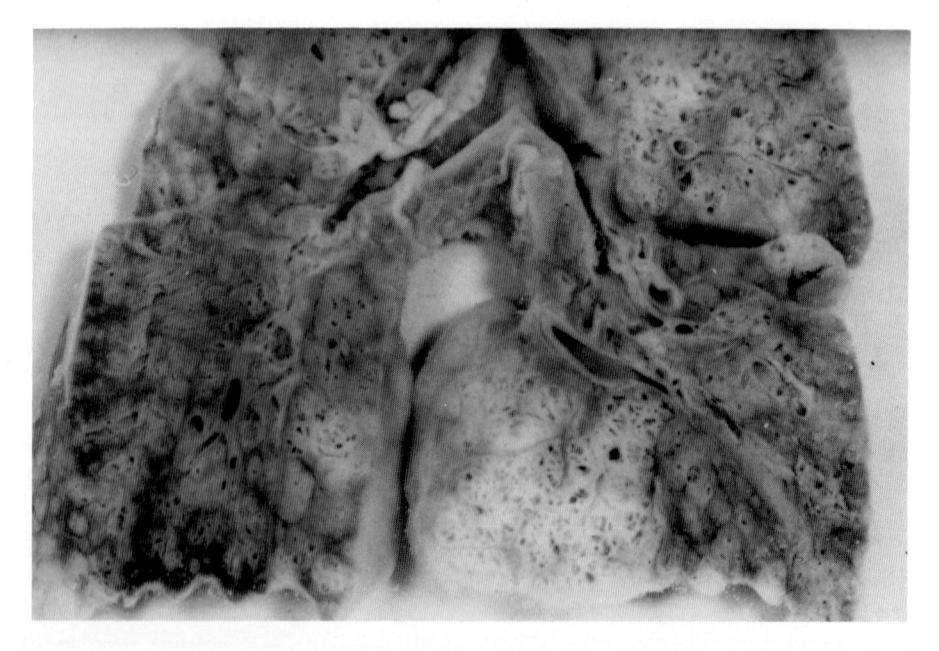

Figure 35.1. Bronchopulmonary dysplasia. Alternating areas of collapse and distension give the lung a very mottled cut surface.

consistant with hypoxia, and slight pulmonary edema. Focal ulcerations of the vocal cords or mild otitis media are very occasionally found.

The peak incidence of the sudden infant death syndrome is between 2.5 and 4 months of age, and almost all cases occur during the first year of life. There is a male predominance of 2:1, and a higher incidence in nonwhites and infants in economically deprived homes. Prematurity is a major risk factor, and the syndrome occurs in 27 of every 1000 premature live births, a 10-fold increased incidence. Other factors that may predispose to the syndrome include blood Type B, infection of the amniotic cavity, maternal anemia, and maternal use of cigarettes and barbiturates.

Although innumerable theories have been proposed to explain the syndrome, the most interesting observations suggest that the victims may have been chronic hypoventilators and suffered earlier episodes of sleep apnea. Related findings include hyperplasia of the media of small pulmonary arteries, persistence of fetal (brown) fat, and underdeveloped carotid bodies. Occasionally, areas of paraventricular brain softening suggest previous episodes of hypoxia. There is evidence in some infants that abnormalities of the cardiac conduction system may also contribute to sudden infant death.

REYE'S SYNDROME

Reye's syndrome tends to occur in the aftermath of virus infections, most often influenza or chickenpox. The onset is heralded by severe and intractable vomiting. This is followed by rapid deterioration of central nervous system function, with disorientation, personality changes, lethargy, and coma. There is evidence of injury to hepatocytes: markedly elevated transaminase enzymes, elevated serum ammonia, and hypoglycemia.

Autopsy findings in fatal cases include small droplet fatty change of hepatocytes and an enlargement of their mitochondria relatable to a deficiency of enzymes of the urea cycle. Similar changes are noted in the mitochondria of central nervous system neurons. Cerebral dysfunction appears to be related primarily to cellular edema, so that therapy consists of monitoring and controlling intracranial pressure. The mortality is about 20%, and another 20% are left with severe and permanent brain damage.

Reye's syndrome was first described in 1963, and its incidence is estimated by the Center for Disease Control to be between 1 and 2 per 100,000 population under 18 years of age. There is some question whether it is a new disease entity, or just a new name applied to a viral encephalitis. Although characterized as a "medical mystery, ... cause and cure unknown," it may be a common symptom complex with multiple causes. Carnitine deficiency, a correctable inherited lipoid storage disease, can present with the picture of Reye's syndrome. Three recent studies have strongly implicated aspirin ingestion in the pathogenesis of many instances of the disorder.

CYSTIC FIBROSIS

The genetic background of cystic fibrosis was discussed in Chapter 10. It is the most common lethal genetic disease of whites. Although it appears to be transmitted as a simple autosomal recessive, the multiplicity of defects that characterize the disease suggests that several inborn errors of metabolism may coexist. There are widespread abnormalities of glandular mucous secretions, disturbed respiratory ciliary function, and altered sodium transport in eccrine sweat glands and salivary glands. Abnormalities of end organ responsiveness to α-adrenergic, β-adrenergic, and cholinergic agents indicate disturbed autonomic nervous system function.

The secretions of many mucous glands are abnormally viscid. In the pancreas, this leads to inspissation, stone formation, and obstruction of pancreatic ducts. The acini undergo cystic dilatation and eventual atrophy, with replacement by fat or fibrous tissue (Fig. 35.2). Thick bronchial secretions tend to obstruct smaller airways. In addition, there is striking asynchrony of ciliary function, related to an abnormal circulating polypeptide, with poor propulsion of mucus to the upper respiratory tree. These abnormalities predispose the lungs to repeated infection and progressive loss of function (Fig. 35.3). Abnormally viscid bile may obstruct the bile ducts and canaliculi, and result in cirrhosis. Stone formation in the biliary tree is frequent.

One of the hallmarks of cystic fibrosis is the high concentration of sodium, potassium, and chloride in sweat and in salivary gland secretions. Hot weather may induce severe electrolyte depletion and hypovolemic shock.

If cystic fibrosis is clinically manifest in the neonatal period, it presents as *meconium ileus*. Abnormally viscid meconium fills the intestine, particularly the distal ileum, and cannot be propelled by peristalsis (Fig. 35.4). There may be an associated ileal stenosis or atresia. Intestinal perforation may occur *in utero* or

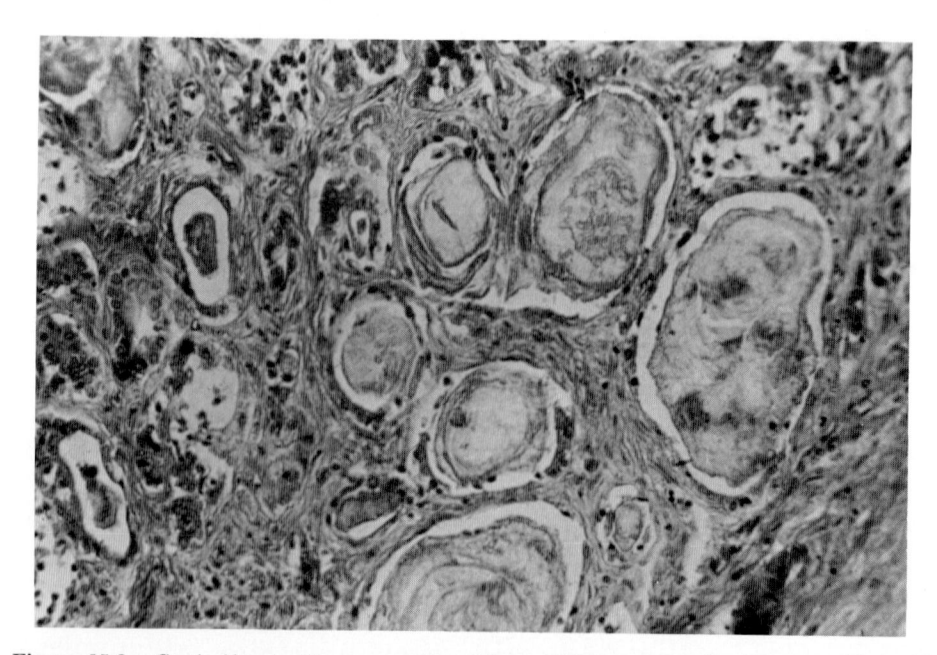

Figure 35.2. Cystic fibrosis. The pancreatic acini are dilated and atrophic. They are filled with inspissated secretions. There is interstitial fibrosis.

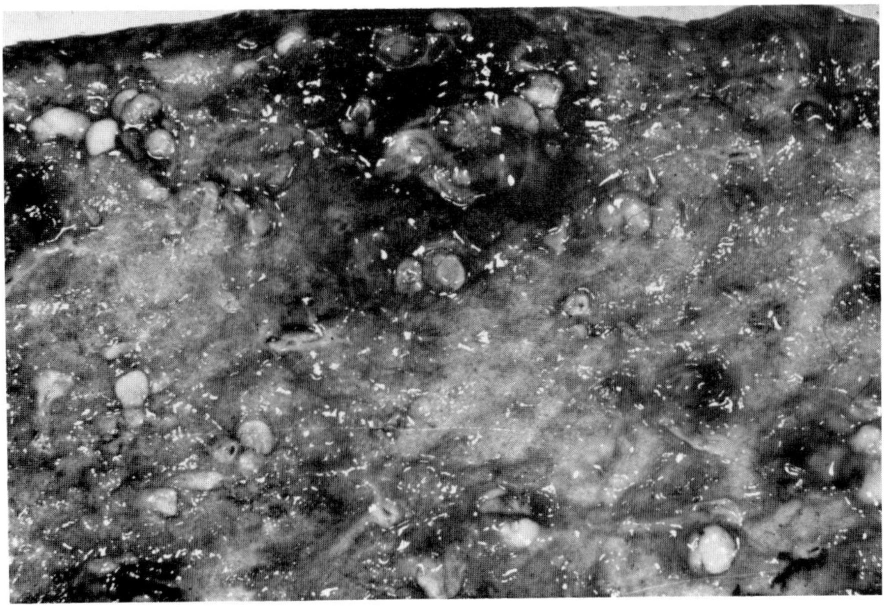

Figure 35.3. The cut surface of the lung shows many small abscesses and bronchi filled with purulent material. There is also a rather generalized increase in fibrous tissue.

during the first few days of life, resulting in a sterile meconium peritonitis. Meconium ileus appears to reflect abnormal intestinal gland function rather than a deficiency of pancreatic enzymes.

Pancreatic insufficiency may become apparent early in infancy, or during the first year or two of life. There is poor weight gain and a severe malabsorption syndrome, with steatorrhea, deficiency of fat-soluble vitamins, and protein deficiency. Rectal prolapse is a frequent, and often frightening, occurrence. Diabetes mellitus is an occasional complication.

Pulmonary infection is the most life-threatening manifestation after infancy. Recurrent episodes of bronchitis and pneumonia, often due to *Staphylococcus aureus* or *Pseudomonas aeruginosa*, eventually lead to bronchiectasis and multiple bronchiectatic abscesses. Pulmonary hypertension may be severe, and many deaths are due to right ventricular cardiac failure. There is a surprisingly high incidence of hypogammaglobulinemia G in children with cystic fibrosis. This appears to be associated with less severe pulmonary disease and suggests that a hyperimmune response may be of pathogenetic significance in the progression of lung disease. Upper respiratory tract findings may be prominent and include acute and chronic sinusitis and nasal polyp formation.

Involvement of the biliary tree may eventuate in cirrhosis, with portal hypertension and esophageal varices.

Intensive therapy with pancreatic enzymes and broad spectrum antibiotics to limit pulmonary complications has achieved considerable success, and more and more victims of cystic fibrosis are surviving into the third and fourth decades. Some women have had successful pregnancies, although abnormally thick vaginal

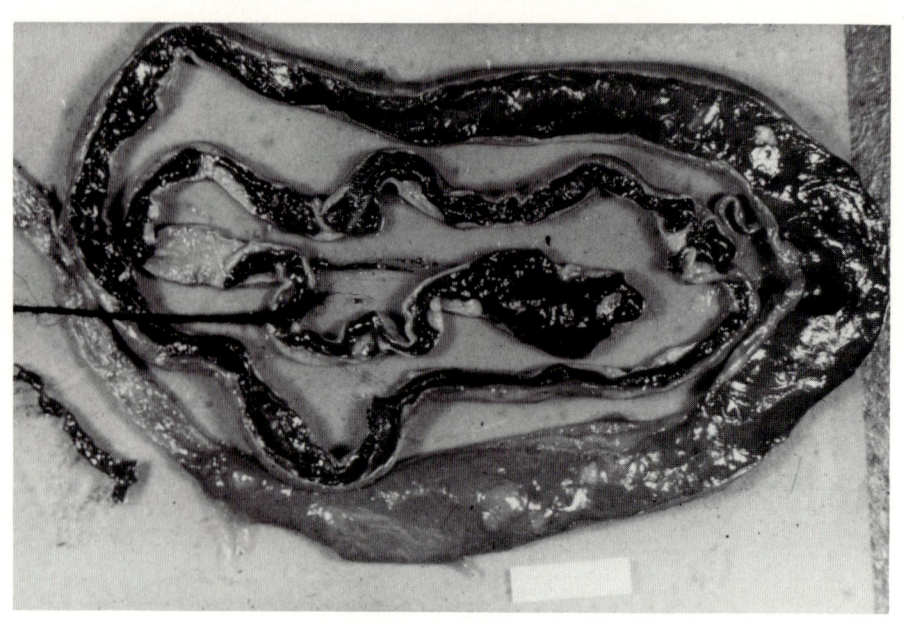

Figure 35.4. Meconium ileus. The intestine is distended and filled with viscid tenacious meconium. The meconium cannot be propelled by peristalsis and produces intestinal obstruction.

secretions decrease fertility. The vast majority of males are sterile, due to failure of normal development of the vasa deferentia.

Identification of individuals heterozygous for cystic fibrosis has been difficult. The most promising results have been reported recently, and are based upon the demonstration of abnormal sodium transport in cultured fibroblasts.

TUMORS IN INFANTS AND CHILDREN

Leukemia accounts for half of all malignant tumors in infancy and childhood. Another 15 to 20% are tumors of the central nervous system. Neuroblastomas comprise 8%, nephroblastoma (Wilms' tumor) 5%, and tumors of bone, muscle, and liver another 7%. These tumors are of great interest; they may demonstrate an inherited pattern, an association with congenital defects, and, occasionally, spontaneous regression. There is a high incidence of leukemia in the presence of chromosome abnormalities (Down's syndrome and the syndrome of chromosomal breakage) and both leukemias and lymphomas are observed in association with immunodeficiency states.

Three of the most interesting tumors in the pediatric age group are neuroblastoma, retinoblastoma, and nephroblastoma.

Neuroblastoma

Neuroblastomas are tumors of neural crest origin. More than half occur in the adrenal medulla, the rest along the sympathetic chain or in locations such as the jaw.

The tumors are soft, fleshy, hemorrhagic, and often contain sufficient calcium

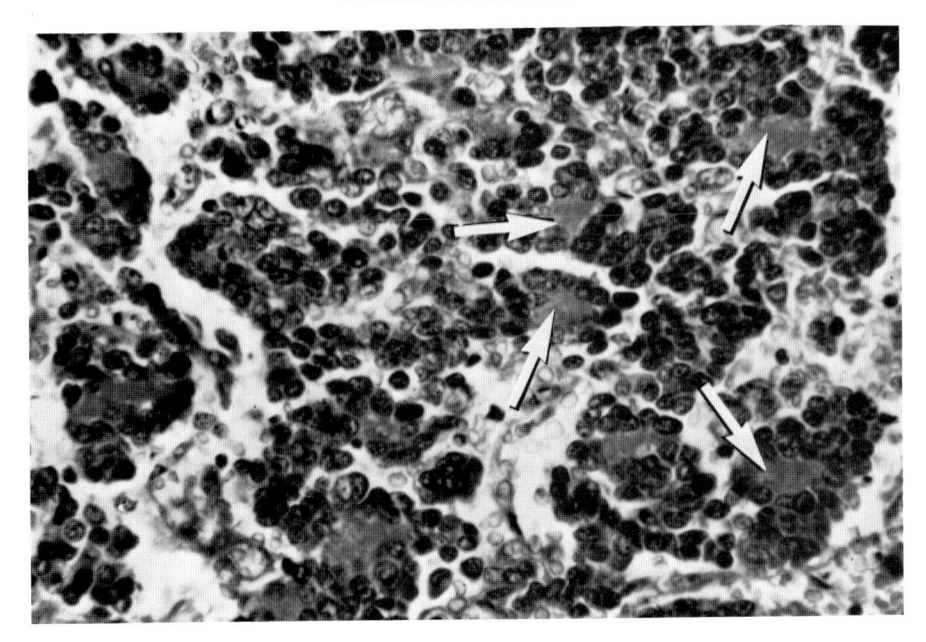

Figure 35.5. Neuroblastoma. The tumor is composed of primitive neuroblastic cells, which tend to arrange themselves in rosettes (*arrows*).

to be visible on abdominal x-rays. The tumor cells are primitive but show some organization into neurofibrillary "rosette" structures (Fig. 35.5). They may secrete catecholamines and, occasionally, other polypeptide hormones, particularly adrenocorticotrophic hormone.

The peak incidence of neuroblastomas is between the ages of 1 and 2. The tumors may grow rapidly, metastasize widely, and cause death in a few months. Neuroblastomas, however, have the highest spontaneous regression rate of any human tumor. They show a distinct tendency to mature; neuroblasts differentiate to ganglion cells and, if maturation is complete, the malignant neuroblastoma will become a benign ganglioneuroma or, occasionally, a neurofibroma.

The single most important factor determining prognosis is the age at which the diagnosis is made. If above 2 years, the tumor follows a highly malignant course and is fatal in 95% of children. If the age at diagnosis is less than 18 months, some 60% survive with therapy, and if less than 12 months as many as 90% appear to be curable. The staging of neuroblastoma is also of prognostic importance:

I	Confined to point of origin
II	Extension in continuity, but not crossing midline
III	Extension in continuity, crossing midline
IV	Remote disease: skeleton, distant nodes, visceral organs, soft tissues
IVS	Metastases to skin, liver, and bone marrow only, and primary tumor like Stage I or II

466 Pathology: Understanding Human Disease

The outlook for Stage I and II lesions is generally very good. Stage IV bears a generally poor prognosis, but Stage IVS follows a course more like Stage I or II. The most dramatic examples of spontaneous regression have occurred in those with Stage IVS tumors. There is no good explanation for these observations, although it has been suggested that Type IVS lesions are not true malignant neoplasms, but collections of neural crest cells that are delayed in maturation.

Neuroblasts are frequently observed in the adrenal medulla during fetal life. Small nodules of these cells, "neuroblastomas *in situ*," are incidental findings at autopsy, many times more frequent than neuroblastomas. These lesions are thought to regress and disappear in the vast majority of instances. Neuroblastomas often have a striking familial incidence and, in studied pedigrees, there is a high frequency of neuroblastoma *in situ*.

Retinoblastoma

Retinoblastoma is a neuroblastic tumor arising in the retina. Its histologic appearance is very similar to that of neuroblastoma, and some retinoblastomas have been shown to secrete catecholamines.

Retinoblastoma may be present at birth, and is usually apparent before the age of 2. There is a familial form that is clearly transmitted genetically as an autosomal dominant. It is often bilateral and has a high association with mental retardation. Survivors reaching reproductive age transmit retinoblastomas to half their offspring. Patients with the familial disease have abnormalities of chromosome 13. The sporadic form of retinoblastoma represents a mutation, and may also be transmissible to children.

With early diagnosis and treatment, some 80 to 90% of patients can be cured,

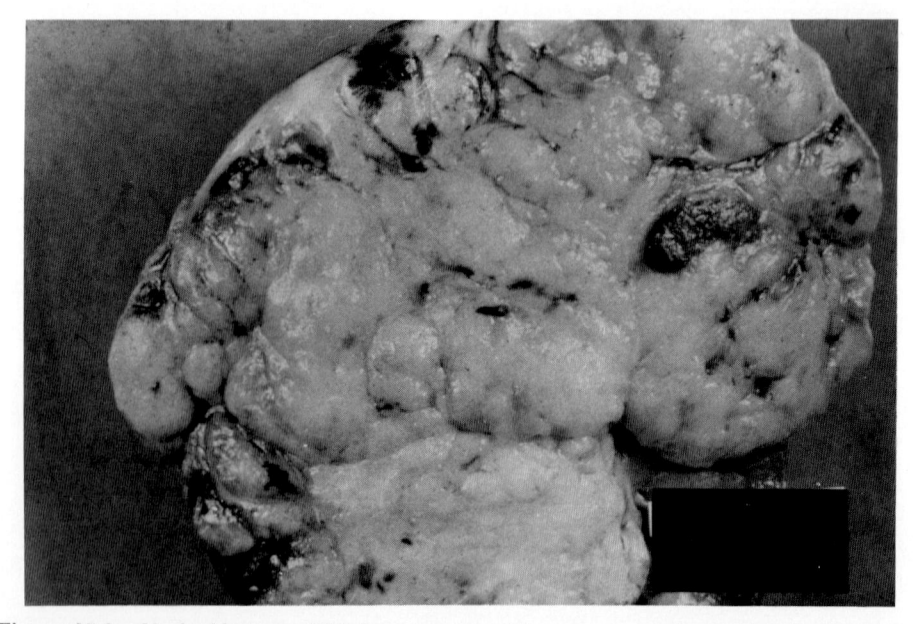

Figure 35.6. Nephroblastoma. This large grayish white tumor mass has replaced most of the kidney. Several areas of hemorrhage are noted.

and rare examples of spontaneous regression have been described. It is of interest that children who have been cured of retinoblastoma subsequently have a higher than normal incidence of osteogenic sarcoma.

Nephroblastoma

Nephroblastoma, or Wilms' tumor, is an embryonal kidney tumor, probably of metanephric origin. The tumor is often large, and consists of soft grayish white tissue that appears to compress the normal kidney (Fig. 35.6). Histologically, there are often tubular structures and abortive attempts at glomerulus reproduction (Fig. 35.7). The stroma appears sarcomatous and often contains striated muscle cells, cartilage, and bone.

Nephroblastoma usually presents as an abdominal mass, with associated pain, nausea, and vomiting. It may be present at birth, and the vast majority are diagnosed before age 6; the peak incidence is at 3. The staging of this tumor is an important determinant of prognosis, but not so clearly as in neuroblastoma:

I	Confined to kidney; completely excised
II	Spread to perinephric tissues, but completely excised
III	Residual tumor confined to abdomen
IV	Hematogenous metastases, *e.g.*, brain, bone, lung, liver
V	Bilateral renal involvement

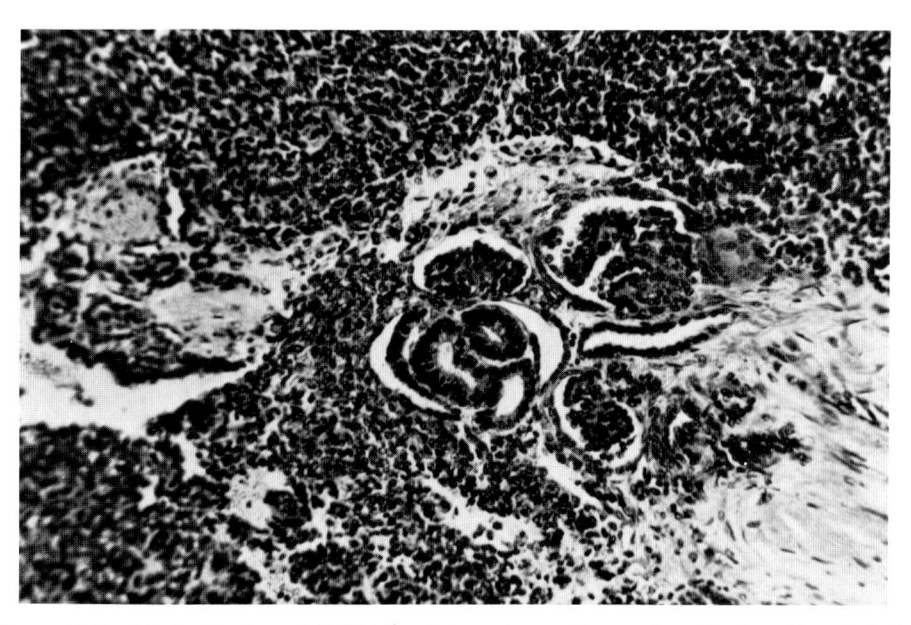

Figure 35.7. Nephroblastoma. This highly cellular embryonal tumor shows the formation of tubules and an attempt at glomerulus production.

Age at diagnosis is also important. Stage I tumors, diagnosed before the age of 2, have a 90% cure rate. Overall, there has been a striking improvement in therapeutic results during the past decade and cure can now be anticipated in 80% of patients.

Nephroblastomas are frequently observed together with abnormalities of somatic growth. The association with aniridia is sufficiently close that individuals with major iris defects are followed closely for evidence of nephroblastoma. There is also an association with horseshoe kidneys, female pseudohermaphroditism, and generalized hemihypertrophy. A few nephroblastomas have been shown to secrete renin and are accompanied by arterial hypertension.

Suggested Reading

diSant'Agnese PA, Davis PB, Research in cystic fibrosis. N. Engl. J. Med. *295:* 481, 534, 597, 1976.
Kolata GB. Reye's syndrome: a medical mystery. Science *207:* 1453, 1980.
Naeye RL. Sudden infant death. Sci. Am. *242:* 56, 1980.

Index

(Page numbers followed by "f" refer to text figures.
Page numbers followed by "T" refer to tables).

Abortion, spontaneous, 379
Abscess, 9, 12f, 31, 33f, 34f
Acid-base balance, 61
Acidosis, metabolic, 62, 62T
Acidosis, respiratory, 63
Acute aortic dissection, 170, 171f
   and medial cystic necrosis, 172
Acute disseminated encephalomyelitis, 253
Acute radiation syndrome, 118
Acute tubular necrosis, 56, 199, 199f
Addison's disease, 344
Adenohypophysis, 332
   (*see also* Hypophysis)
Adenomatous polyps, colon, 305, 306f
Adrenal, 344
   Addison's disease, 344, 345f
      causes, 344
   Conn's syndrome, 348
   cortical insufficiency, 344
   cortical tumors, 346
      adenocarcinoma, 346, 347f
      adenoma, 346, 346f
      manifestations, 346
   Cushing's syndrome, 347
      Crooke's hyaline change in, 347, 348f
      pathogenesis, 347
   hyperaldosteronism, 348
   medullary tumors, 348
      neuroblastoma, 464, 465f
      pheochromocytoma, 348, 349f
Adrenogenital syndromes, 98, 98f
Adult respiratory distress syndrome, 221, 221f, 222T
Age-related diseases, 104
Aging, 104
   age-related diseases, 104
   anatomic changes, 106
   DNA repair in, 105
   mechanisms, 105
   normal lifespan, 104
   physiologic changes, 105
Air pollution, 109, 109T
Alcohol, 110
   alcoholic hepatitis, 269
   as co-carcinogen, 110
   fetal alcohol syndrome, 111
   related disorders of nervous system, 256
Alcoholism, 92
Alkalosis, metabolic, 62
Alkalosis, respiratory, 63

Alport's syndrome, 200
Alzheimer's disease, 248, 249f
Ampulla of Vater
   carcinoma, 278
Amyloidosis, 152, 324f, 325, 325f, 326f
   classification, 325
   kidney in, 194
   rheumatoid arthritis and, 436
Amyotrophic lateral sclerosis, 251, 252f
Analgesic abuse, 112
   nephropathy of, 112, 114f
Anaphylaxis, 77
Anaphylotoxins, 21
Anasarca, 58
Anemia (*see* Blood)
Aneurysms, 167
   atherosclerotic, 169, 170f
   Charcot-Bouchard, 207, 237
   dissecting, 170
   intracranial (berry), 238, 239f
   mycotic, 158
   syphilitic, 174, 175f
Angina pectoris, 148
Anion gap, 62
Ankylosing spondylitis, 436
Anorexia nervosa, 93
Appendicitis, 299
APUD system, tumors of, 350
Arteriolar nephrosclerosis, 208, 208f
Arthritis (*see* Joints)
Asbestosis, 110, 111f, 218, 224
   and mesothelioma, 110, 229
Ascites, 265
Asthma, 217
Astrocytoma, 240
Ataxia telangiectasia, 40, 97T
Atherosclerosis, 167, 168f, 169f
   aneurysms, 169
   fatty streaks and, 168
   high density lipoproteins and, 90
   hyperlipoproteinemias and, 89
   intimal plaque, 167, 169
   nutrition and, 89
   pathogenesis, 168
   risk factors, 167
Atopy, 77
Atrophy, 121
Autoimmune diseases, 82, 84T
   Goodpasture's syndrome, 84
   Graves' disease, 84

Index

Autoimmune diseases—*continued*
  mechanisms, 82
  myasthenia gravis, 84
  pernicious anemia, 84
  progressive systemic sclerosis, 85
  systemic lupus erythematosus, 85

Barlow's syndrome, 157, 158f
Berger's disease, 194
Bladder, urinary, 406
  carcinoma, 406, 408f, 409f
    risk factors, 406
    staging, 407
  cystitis, 406, 407f
Bleeding disorders, 68
  (*see also* Blood)
Blind loop syndrome, 293
Blood
  bleeding disorders, 68
    aspirin, effects of, 69
    hemophilia, 70
    platelet abnormalities, 69
    von Willebrand's disease, 70
  coagulation, 65
    coagulation factors, 65, 65T
    control of, 67
    extrinsic pathway, 66, 66f
    intrinsic pathway, 65, 66f
    lines of Zahn, 67
  erythroblastosis fetalis, 78
  hemoglobin S, 99
  hemolytic anemia, 327
  leukemia, 317
    (*see also* Leukemia)
  partial thromboplastin time, 69
  pernicious anemia, 84, 327
    atrophic gastritis and, 286, 327
    combined system disease, 327
  platelets
    platelet Factor 3, 64, 67
    prostaglandins and, 64
    role in hemostasis, 64
    white thrombus, 64
  prothrombin time, 69
  sickle cell disease, 99
  thrombin test, 69
  thrombosis
    fate of thrombi, 71
  thrombotic disorders, 70
    Virchow's triad, 71
Blood pressure (*see* Hypertension)
Brain (*see* Central nervous system)
Bone, 418
  aseptic necrosis, 434
  metabolic bone disease, 418
    biochemical findings, 423T
    classification, 420, 423T
    osteitis fibrosa, 421f, 422, 422f
    osteomalacia, 420, 421f
    osteopenia, 420
    osteoporosis, 420, 420f, 425, 427f
    renal osteodystrophy, 422, 424f, 425f

    rickets, 420
    scurvy, 426f
  osteomyelitis, 428
  Paget's disease of, 427, 428f, 429f, 430f
  tuberculosis, 430
  tumors, 431
    chondrosarcoma, 433
    enchondroma, 432
    Ewing's sarcoma, 433
    giant cell tumor, 433
    osteochondroma, 432, 433f
    osteogenic sarcoma, 431, 431f, 432f
    osteoid osteoma, 432
Bradykinin, 21
Breast, 391
  carcinoma, 397
    colloid, 400, 400f
    ductal, invasive, 398, 398f, 399f
    estrogen receptor protein in, 403
    intraductal, 397f, 398
    lobular, 400, 401f, 402f
    medullary, 399
    metastasis, 402
    prognostic factors, 403
    risk factors, 401
    scirrhous, 398
  cystosarcoma phyllodes, 395
  fat necrosis, 393
  fibroadenoma, 394, 395f
  fibrocystic disease, 391, 392f
    nonproliferative, 392, 393f
    papillomatosis, 393
    proliferative, 392, 394f
    sclerosing adenosis, 392
  intraductal papilloma, 396f, 397
  male, 404
    carcinoma, 405
    gynecomastia, 404
  Paget's disease, 400
Brenner tumor, 382
Bronchiectasis, 216, 217f
Bronchitis, chronic 216
Bronchogenic carcinoma, 225
Bronchopulmonary dysplasia, 460, 460f
Bruton type agammaglobulinemia, 40
Buerger's disease, 177
Burkitt's lymphoma, 313

Calcific aortic stenosis, 155, 156f, 157f
Candidiasis, 52, 53f
  in familial endocrinopathy, 53
Carcinoembryonic antigen, 141
Carcinoid syndrome, 351
Carcinoid tumors, 351
Cardiomyopathy, 151
  (*see also* Heart)
Caseation necrosis, 9, 12f
Celiac sprue, 291, 292f
Cell(s)
  cloudy swelling, 7, 10f
  degeneration, 8f, 9f
  growth, alterations of, 121

growth, control of, 130
  chalones, 131
  contact inhibition, 131
 hydropic (vacuolar) degeneration, 8
 ionizing radiation, sensitivity to, 119T
 ischemic injury, 3, 6f
 mechanisms of injury, 5, 7
Cell-mediated immunity, 79
Central nervous system, 231
 Alzheimer's neurofibrillary tangles, 232
 aneurysms, intracranial (berry), 238, 239f
 astrocyte reactions, 232
 cerebral edema, 58
 chromatolysis, 231
 concussion, 255
 contusion, 255
 Cowdry A inclusions, 232, 247f
 degenerative diseases, 248
  acute disseminated encephalomyelitis, 253
  Alzheimer's disease, 248, 249f
  amyotrophic lateral sclerosis, 251, 252f
  Friedreich's ataxia, 251, 251f
  Huntington's chorea, 250
  metachromatic leukodystrophy, 254
  Parkinson's disease, 249, 250f
  Werdnig-Hoffman disease, 252
 demyelinating diseases, 252
  globoid cell leukodystrophy, 255
  Krabbe's disease, 255
  multiple sclerosis, 253, 254f
 dural sinus thrombosis, 240
 encephalitis, viral, 246
 encephalomalacia, 233, 234, 235f
 epidural hemorrhage, 255
 gliomas, 240
  astrocytoma, 240
  ependymoma, 241
  glioblastoma multiforme, 240, 241f
  medulloblastoma, 241
  oligodendroglioma, 241
 herniations of brain, 233, 234f, 235f
 infarction (encephalomalacia), 233, 234, 235f
 infections, 243
  brain abscess, 244, 245f
  fungus infections, 246
  meningitis, acute bacterial, 243, 244f
  meningitis, tuberculous, 245
  tuberculosis, 245
  virus infections, 246
 meningioma, 242, 242f
 metastatic tumors, 243
 microglial reactions, 232
 Negri bodies, 232
 neurofibroma, 243
 neuronal reactions, 231
 oligodendroglial reactions, 232
 Schwannoma, 242
 slow virus diseases, 246
  Creutzfeldt-Jacob disease, 247
  kuru, 247
  progressive multifocal leukoencephalopathy, 247

  subacute sclerosing panencephalitis, 247
 subdural hemorrhage, 255, 256f
 tumors, 240
 vascular disease, 234
  cerebral embolism, 236
  Charcot-Bouchard aneurysms, 237
  hypertensive cerebral hemorrhage, 237, 238f
  infarction, 234, 235f, 236f
  intracranial hemorrhage, 237, 237T
  subarachnoid hemorrhage, 238
  Wernicke's encephalopathy, 257
Cerebral embolism, 236
Cervicitis, 360
Cervix uteri, 360
 carcinoma, 363, 363f, 364f
  colposcopy in, 364, 366f
  epidemiology of, 366
  exfolliative cytology in, 364, 365f
  in situ, 361, 362f
  microinvasive, 363, 363f
 cervicitis, 360
 dysplasia, 361, 362f
 Nabothian cysts, 360
 squamous metaplasia, 361
Chalones, 131
 in inflammation, 26
Charcot-Bouchard aneurysms, 207
Chédiak-Higashi syndrome, 26
Chemical carcinogens, 115, 116T
Chemotaxis, 17
Cholecystitis, 277
Cholelithiasis, 276, 276f, 277f
Cholera, 298
Chondrocalcinosis, 441
Chorioadenoma destruens, 377, 377f
Choriocarcinoma, 377, 378f
Chronic glomerulonephritis, 194
Chronic granulomatous disease, 26
Chronic obstructive pulmonary disease, 214
Cigarette smoke, 111
 alveolar macrophages and, 213
 as carcinogen, 112
 cardiovascular disease and, 112
 chronic pulmonary disease and, 111
 squamous bronchogenic carcinoma and, 225
Cirrhosis, 258, 260f, 261f, 262f, 263f, 264f
Cloudy swelling, 7, 10f
Coagulation necrosis, 9, 11f
Coal worker's pneumoconiosis, 219
Colon carcinoma, 304, 304f
 (*see also* Digestive tract)
Combined system disease, 327
Complement, 21, 76
 in inflammation, 21
Congenital heart disease, 160
 (*see also* Heart)
Congestion, passive, 57
Congestive heart failure, 143
 (*see also* Heart)
Conn's syndrome, 348
Cor pulmonale, 148
Craniopharyngioma, 334, 334f

Cretinism, 335
Creutzfeldt-Jacob disease, 247
Crigler-Najjar syndrome, 273
Crohn's disease, 293, 294f
   (*see also* Digestive tract)
Cushing's disease, 333
Cushing's syndrome, 347
   pathogenesis, 347
Cystic fibrosis, 99, 213, 461, 462f, 463f, 464f
   lung infections in, 463, 463f
   meconium ileus, 462, 464f
   pancreatic insufficiency, 463
Cytomegalic inclusion disease, 51

Death, causes of in USA, 129T
Dermatomyositis, 446
Diabetes insipidus, 331
Diabetes mellitus, 90, 353
   adult onset, 90
   cataracts in, 356
   insulin dependent, 90
   juvenile onset, 90, 353
      autoimmune phenomena, 353
      genetic factors, 353
   Kimmelstiel-Wilson disease, 355, 356f
   maturity onset, 354
   and obesity, 354
   microaneurysms, 355, 357f
   microangiopathy, 355
   nephropathy, 355
   neuropathy, 357
   nutrition, and complications of, 91
   retinopathy, 356, 357f
   vascular disease and, 355
Di George syndrome, 40
Digestive tract, 286
   colon, adenomatous polyps, 305, 306f
   appendicitis, 299
      complications, 299
   carcinoembryonic antigen in lesions of, 307
   cholera, 298
   colon carcinoma, 304, 304f, 306f
      and adenomatous polyps, 305
      Duke's classification, 305
      pathogenesis, 305
   Crohn's disease, 293, 294f
      compared to ulcerative colitis, 295T
      granulomatous colitis, 294, 295f
   diverticulosis, 300
   dysentery, 298
   esophageal carcinoma, 300, 301f
   esophageal varices, 265, 266f
   familial polyposis, 307
   gastric carcinoma, 301, 302f, 303f
      and atrophic gastritis, 301
      linitus plastica, 301
   gastric polyps, 302
   gastritis, acute, 286
   gastritis, hypertrophic, 287
      Ménétrier's disease, 287
      Zollinger-Ellison syndrome, 287
   gastritis, chronic atrophic, 286, 287f
      gastric carcinoma and, 286
      pernicious anemia and, 286
   leiomyosarcoma, stomach, 303f
   malabsorption syndromes, 290
      blind loop syndrome, 293
      causes, 290, 290T
      celiac sprue, 291, 292f
      dumping syndrome, 292
      gluten-sensitive enteropathy, 291, 292f
      Whipple's disease, 291, 293f
   peptic ulcer disease, 287, 288, 289f
      complications, 288
      pathogenesis, 289
      risk factors, 288
   pseudomembranous enterocolitis, 298, 298f
      Clostridium difficile in, 299
   ulcerative colitis, 292, 295f, 296f, 297f
      carcinoma of colon and, 297
      compared to Crohn's disease, 295T
      complications, 297
      pseudopolyps, 295
      toxic megacolon, 297
   villous adenoma, colon, 305, 307f
Discoid lupus erythematosus, 457
Disseminated intravascular coagulation, 72
   consumption of coagulation factors, 72
   in Rocky Mountain spotted fever, 50
   in shock, 56
   kidney in, 194
Diverticulosis, colon, 300
Down's syndrome, 101
   heart in, 161, 163f
Doxorubicin toxicity, 112
Dressler's syndrome, 151
Dubin-Johnson syndrome, 273
Duchenne dystrophy, 445, 445f
Dumping syndrome, 292
Dysentery, 298
Dysgerminoma, 382
Dysplasia, 127, 127f

Edema, 58
   cerebral, 58
   hereditary angioneurotic, 26
   in congestive heart failure, 144
   in nephrotic syndrome, 185
   in portal hypertension, 265
Endocrine disorders, 329
   (*see also* Hypothalamus, Hypophysis, Thyroid, Parathyroid, Adrenal, Multiple endocrine lesions)
   autoimmune phenomena in, 330
   general features, 329
   tumors, 330
Environment and health, 108
   air pollution, 109, 109T
   alcohol, 110
   asbestos, 110
   chemical carcinogens, 115, 116T
   cigarette smoke, 111
   drug-related disorders, 112, 113T
      chloramphenicol, 115

methicillin, 115
penicillin, 113
ionizing radiation, 117
acute radiation syndrome, 118
and carcinogenesis, 119
fetal irradiation, 119
lead poisoning, 116
mercury, 117
Embolism, 72
types, 72
Emphysema, pulmonary, 214
Endometrial hyperplasia, 367, 368f
Endometriosis, 373
Endometrium (see Uterus)
Enzymes, tissue (see Tissue enzymes)
Ependymoma, 241
Epidural hemorrhage, 255
Epithelioid cell (see Inflammation)
Erythema multiforme, 455
Erythema nodosum, 455
Esophageal varices, 265, 266f
Esophagus (see Digestive tract)
Exfoliative cytology, 364, 365f
Exudate, 15
Eye
  retinoblastoma, 101, 466

Facioscapulohumeral dystrophy, 455
Fallopian tube, 374
  hydrosalpinx, 375
  pelvic inflammatory disease, 374
  pregnancy, ectopic, 375, 375f
  pyosalpinx, 375
  salpingitis, 374
Familial polyposis, 307
Fat necrosis, 9
  in pancreatitis, 279, 280f, 281f
Fatty change, 3, 6, 7
Female genital tract, 358
  (see also Vulva, Cervix uteri, Uterus, Fallopian tube, Ovary, Trophoblastic disease)
α-Fetoprotein, 141
Fibrinoid necrosis, 79
Fibromuscular dysplasia, 173
Fibrosing lung disease, 218, 218f, 219T
Friedreich's ataxia, 251, 251f

Gall bladder, 276
  cholecystitis, 277
  cholelithiasis, 276, 276f, 277f
  empyema, 277
  hydrops, 276
  tumors of, 277
Gangrene, 3, 5f
Gastric carcinoma, 301, 302f, 303f
Gastrointestinal tract (see Digestive tract)
Genetic disorders, 95
  adrenogenital syndromes, 98, 98f
  autosomal dominant, 96, 96T
  autosomal recessive, 97, 97T
  cri-du-chat syndrome, 101

cystic fibrosis, 99, 213, 461, 462f, 463f, 464f
Down's syndrome, 101
glucose-6-phosphate dehydrogenase deficiency, 100, 115
gonadal dysgenesis, 100
hemochromatosis, 102
hemophilia, 70
HLA linkage, 102, 102T
Klinefelter's syndrome, 101
Marfan's syndrome, 96
multifactorial diseases, 101
Niemann-Pick disease, 97
retinoblastoma, 101, 466
sex-linked recessive, 91, 100T
sickle cell disease, 99
sickle cell trait, 99
Turner's syndrome, 100
vitamin D-resistant rickets, 99
Wilms' tumor, 101, 467, 467f
XYY syndrome, 101
Giant cell arteritis, 176, 176f
Gilbert's disease, 273
Glioblastoma multiforme, 240, 241f
Globoid cell leukodystrophy, 255
Glomerulonephritis, 185, 186T
  (see also Kidney)
Glucose-6-phosphate dehydrogenase deficiency, 100, 115
Gluten-sensitive enteropathy, 291, 292f
Glycogen storage disease, 448
Gonorrhea, 44, 375
Goodpasture's syndrome, 84
Gout, 440, 440f, 441f, 442f
  kidney in, 440, 442f
  podagra, 440, 442f
  tophi, 440, 441f
Granulation tissue, 19
Granuloma, 33, 36
  epithelioid, 36
Granulomatous colitis, 294, 295f
Graves' disease, 84, 334, 335f
Gynecomastia, 101, 404

Hageman factor (XII), 21, 65, 68
Hamman-Rich syndrome, 218
Heart, 143
  amyloidosis, 152
  angina pectoris, 148
  atrophy, 121
  Barlow's syndrome, 157, 158f
  calcific aortic stenosis, 155, 156f, 157f
    causes, 155
  cardiogenic shock, 148
  cardiomyopathies, 151
    alcoholic, 152
    amyloidosis, 152
    classification, 151
    idiopathic congestive, 151
    idiopathic hypertrophic subaortic stenosis, 151
    toxic, 152
  congenital heart disease, 160

Index

Heart—*continued*
  congenital heart disease—*continued*
    atrial septal defects, 161
    coarctation of aorta, 164
    Eisenmenger syndrome, 161
    endocardial cushion defect, 161, 163f
    patent ductus arteriosus, 161
    pulmonary circulation in, 160
    tetrology of Fallot, 162, 163f
    ventricular septal defects, 161, 162f
  congestive heart failure, 143
    cardiac output, 144
    causes, 143
    complicating myocardial infarction, 150
    cor pulmonale, 148
    hemorrhagic enteropathy in, 147
    liver in, 145, 146f
    lungs in, 145, 146f
    manifestations, 144, 145T
    prerenal azotemia, 144
    renal perfusion, 144
    systemic vascular resistance, 144
    thrombo-embolic disease in, 148
  doxorubicin toxicity, 112
  endocardial fibroelastosis, 164
  endocarditis, infective, 157, 159f
    candida, 53
    complications, 158
    microorganisms, 158
    mycotic aneurysms, 158
  endocarditis, marantic, 165
  hypertrophy, 122f, 123
  ischemic heart disease, 148
  mitral valve prolapse, 157, 158f
  myocardial infarction, 4f, 10f, 15f, 16f, 18f, 19f, 20f, 21f, 23f, 24f, 25f, 149
    bypass surgery, 151
    complications, 150
    coronary atherosclerosis and, 149
    Dressler's syndrome, 151
    pericarditis, fibrinous, 165f
    rupture of heart, 149
  rheumatic heart disease, 152
    (*see also* Rheumatic fever)
  syphilis of, 165
  valvular disease, 152
  variant angina pectoris, 149
Heberden's nodes, 439
Hematopoietic and lymphoreticular organs, 308
  (*see also* Lymphoma, Leukemia, Multiple myeloma, Myeloproliferative disorders, Blood)
Hemochromatosis, 102, 271, 272f
Hemolytic anemia, 327
Hemolytic uremia syndrome, 194
Hemophilia, 70, 441
Hemorrhage, intracranial, 237, 237T
Henoch-Schönlein purpura
  kidney in, 191, 195
Hepatic encephalopathy, 265
Hepatitis, 267
  (*see also* Liver)
Hepatocellular carcinoma, 273, 274f, 275f

Hepato-renal syndrome, 265
Hereditary angioneurotic edema, 26
Hereditary nephropathy, 200
Herniations of brain, 233, 234f, 235f
Histamine, 20
Histoplasmosis, 37f
HLA antigens, 102
  genetic linkage, 102, 102T
  hemochromatosis, 102
Hodgkin's disease, 313, 314f, 315f, 316f, 317f
  (*see also* Lymphoma)
Host resistance, 39
  alterations of, 39
Huntington's chorea, 250
Hyaline membrane disease, 459
Hydatidiform mole, 377
Hydrogen peroxide-halide-myeloperoxidase system, 18, 27
Hydronephrosis, 197, 197f
Hydropic degeneration, 8
Hyperkalemia, 60
Hyperlipoproteinemia, 89
Hypernatremia, 59
Hyperparathyroidism, 342
Hyperplasia, 123
  primary, 125
  secondary, 124
  tertiary, 125
Hyperprolactinemia, 333
Hypertension, 203
  acute aortic dissection and, 206
  causes of, 203T
  central nervous system in, 207
  cerebral hemorrhage in, 237, 238f
  classification, 203
  definition, 203
  encephalopathy in, 207
  essential, 203
  heart in, 206
  kidneys in, 208
    (*see also* Kidney)
  malignant, 204, 208
  mechanisms of, 204
  pyelonephritis and, 197
  retina in, 207
  vascular disease in, 205, 205f, 206f
Hypertrophy, 123
Hypokalemia, 60
Hyponatremia, 59
Hypophysis
  adenoma, 332, 332f, 333f
  craniopharyngioma, 334, 334f
  empty sella syndrome, 334
  hyperpituitarism, 332
    Cushing's disease, 333
    hyperprolactinemia, 333
    Nelson's syndrome, 333
  hypopituitarism, 331f, 332
    Sheehan's syndrome, 332
  microadenoma, 333, 333f
Hypothalamus, 330
  diabetes insipidus, 331
  inappropriate ADH secretion, 331

Index

Immune deficiency states, 39
  ataxia telangiectasia, 40
  Bruton type agammaglobulinemia, 40
  Di George syndrome, 40
  Swiss type agammaglobulinemia, 39
  Wiskott-Aldrich syndrome, 40
Immunoglobulins, 75, 76T
  IgA, 76
  IgD, 76
  IgE, 76
  IgG, 75
  IgM, 75
Immunologic cytotoxicity, 78
Immunologically mediated injury, 77, 77T
  anaphylaxis, 77
  atopy, 77
  cell-mediated immunity, 79
  complex-mediated diseases, 78, 80f, 81f
    fibrinoid necrosis, 79
  immunologic cytotoxicity, 78
Infarction, 3
  kidney, 11f
  myocardial, 4f, 10f, 15f, 16f, 18f, 19f, 20f, 21f, 23f, 24f, 25f, 149
Infections
  host resistance, 39
  microbial mechanisms, 38
  nosocomial, 40
Inflammation, 14
  acute, 29, 32, 33, 36
  anaphylotoxins, 21
  bradykinin, 21
  causes, 26
  chalones, 26
  chemotaxis, 17
  chronic, 29, 33, 36
  complement in, 21
  epithelioid cells, 33, 36, 81
  fibrosis, 19
  giant cells, 18
  granulation tissue, 19
  granuloma, 33
  histamine, 20
  leukocyte migration, 16
  lymphocytes, 17
  lymphokines, 22
  mediators of, 20, 22T
  monocytes, 17, 36
  mononuclear phagocytes, 17, 36
  opsonins, 18
  phagocytosis, 18
  plasmin in, 21
  polymorphonuclear leukocytes, 17
  prostaglandins, 24
  repair, 19
  scar formation, 19
  vascular permeability, 15
Injury, reaction to, 14
Interstitial nephritis, 198, 198f
Intestines (*see* Digestive tract)
Ionizing radiation (*see* Environment and health)
Ischemic heart disease, 148
Ischemic injury, 3

Jaundice (*see* Liver)
Joints, 435
  ankylosing spondylitis, 436
  Charcot joint, 441
  chondrocalcinosis, 441
  gout, 440, 440f, 441f, 442f
  hemophilic arthropathy, 441
  juvenile rheumatoid arthritis, 438
  neuropathic arthropathy, 441
  osteoarthritis, 438, 438f, 439f
  rheumatoid arthritis, 435, 436f, 437f
    (*see also* Rheumatoid arthritis)
  Sjögren's syndrome, 438
  systemic lupus erythematosus and, 438

Kidney, 178
  acute tubular necrosis, 56, 199, 199f
    in shock, 56
  Alport's syndrome, 200
  amyloidosis, 194
  analgesic nephropathy, 112, 114f
  Berger's disease, 194
  bilateral cortical necrosis, 56, 56f
  carcinoma, 201
  congenital hypoplasia, 201
  disseminated intravascular coagulation in, 194
  end stage kidney, 179, 181f, 182f, 183f
  focal segmental sclerosis, 192
  glomerulonephritis, 185, 186T
    chronic, 194
    in systemic lupus erythematosus, 194
    membranoproliferative, 190, 190f
    membranous, 192f, 193, 193f
    poststreptococcal, 188, 188f, 189f
    rapidly progressive, 191, 191f
  Goodpasture's syndrome, 84
  hemolytic uremia syndrome, 194
  hereditary nephropathy, 200
  hydronephrosis, 197, 197f
  hypertension and, 208
    arteriolar nephrosclerosis, 208, 208f
    malignant nephrosclerosis, 207f, 209
  infarction, 11f
  interstitial nephritis, 198, 198f
    in analgesic abuse, 198
  lipoid nephrosis, 191
  medullary cystic disease, 200
  medullary sponge kidney, 200
  nephritic syndrome, 185
  nephroblastoma (Wilms' tumor), 467, 467f
  nephrotic syndrome, 184, 184T
  polycystic disease, 200
  pyelonephritis, 42, 43f, 44f, 195, 195T, 196f, 197f
    acute, 42, 43f, 44f, 196
    chronic, 196f, 197
    Escherichia coli, 42
    hypertension and, 197
    mechanisms, 42
    urinary tract obstruction and, 195T
  renal cell carcinoma, 201
  renal failure, 178, 179T, 180f, 198
  renal pelvis carcinoma, 201
  renal vascular hypertension, 209

Kidney—*continued*
  transplantation, 85
  uremic syndrome, 182
  Wilms' tumor, 101, 467, 467f
Kimmelstiel-Wilson disease, 355, 356f
Klinefelter's syndrome, 101, 404, 417
Kruckenberg tumor, 387
Kuru, 247
Kwashiorkor, 93

Larynx, 229
  squamous cell carcinoma, 229
Lead poisoning, 116
Legionnaires' disease, 222
Leriche Syndrome, 169
Leukemia, 308, 317
  acute lymphocytic, 318
  acute myelogenous, 318f, 319, 319f
    aleukemic, 319
    Auer rods, 320
  chronic lymphocytic, 318
  chronic myelogenous, 320, 320f, 321f
  classification, 317
  hairy cell, 320
  in survivors at Hiroshima, 119
  myelomonocytic, 319
  Philadelphia chromosome, 317
Lichen planus, 458
Lines of Zahn, 67
Linitis plastica, 301
Lipoid nephrosis, 191
Liquefaction necrosis, 9, 12f
Liver, 258
  adenoma, 273
  carcinoma, hepatocellular, 273, 274f, 275f
    and hepatitis B virus, 274
  carcinoma, metastatic, 274, 275f
  causes of injury, 259T
  cholangiocarcinoma, 273
  cirrhosis, 258, 260f, 261f, 262f, 263f, 264f
    biliary, 272
    macronodular, 261
    micronodular, 261
  drug-induced injury, 271
  fatty changes, 3, 6, 7
  hemochromatosis, 102, 271, 272f
  hepatic failure, 258, 264
    encephalopathy, 265
    endocrine disturbances, 265
    hepato-renal syndrome, 265
  hepatitis, 267
    acute, 268, 268f
    alcoholic, 269, 270f
    chronic active, 269
    chronic persistent, 269
    hepatitis A, 267
    hepatitis B, 267
    hepatitis C (non-A, non-B), 268
    lupoid, 269
    massive necrosis, 269
    serum enzymes in, 267
  jaundice, 266

Crigler-Najjar syndrome, 273
Dubin-Johnson syndrome, 273
Gilbert's disease, 273
Mallory bodies, 269, 270f
passive congestion, 57, 57f
portal hypertension, 259, 265
  ascites, 265
  esophageal varices, 265, 266f
Wilson's disease, 271
Lung, 211
  abscess, 31, 33f, 34f
  adult respiratory distress syndrome, 221, 221f, 222T
  alveolar macrophages, 213
  asthma, 217
  bronchial adenoma, 228
  bronchiectasis, 216, 217f
  bronchiolar-alveolar carcinoma, 228
  bronchitis, chronic, 216
  bronchogenic carcinoma, 225
    classification, 225
    hormone secretion, 227
  bronchopneumonia, 222
  chronic obstructive pulmonary disease, 214
  distal respiratory unit, 213
  embolism, 4f
  emphysema, 214, 214f, 215f
    centrilobular, 214f, 215
    panacinar, 215f, 216
  fibrosing lung disease, 218, 218f, 219T
  Ghon complex, 46, 47f
  Hamman-Rich syndrome, 218
  hyaline membranes, 221f
  immunologic lung diseases, 219
  infarction, 3
  infections, 222
  Legionnaires' disease, 222
  mesothelioma, 229
  mucociliary apparatus, 213
  mycoplasma pneumonia, 223
  neoplasms, 224
  passive congestion, 58
  pneumococcal pneumonia, 28, 29f, 30f, 31f
  pneumoconioses, 218
    asbestosis, 218, 224
    coal worker's pneumoconiosis, 219
    silicosis, 219
  pneumocystis pneumonia, 53, 54f
  pneumonia, organizing, 32
  pneumonia, viral, 223, 223f
  pulmonary hypertension, 223, 224f
  respiratory failure, 211
    alveolar capillary block, 212
    alveolar hypoventilation, 211
    hypoxic, 212
    ventilation-perfusion imbalance, 212
    ventilatory, 211
  restrictive lung disease, 218, 219T
  sarcoidosis, 220f, 221
  shock lung, 56
  small airways disease, 217
  tuberculosis, 32, 34f, 35f, 46, 47
  tuberculous pneumonia, 47

Lymphokines, 22
Lymphoma, 309
  Hodgkin's disease, 313, 314f, 315f, 316f, 317f
    lymphocyte depletion, 316
    lymphocyte predominant, 315
    mixed cellularity, 314f, 315
    nodular sclerosing, 315, 315f, 316f
    Reed-Sternberg cell, 313, 314f
    staging, 316
  non-Hodgkin's, 309, 310f, 311f
    Burkitt's lymphoma, 313
    classification, 309, 312T
    mycosis fungoides, 313
Lymphoma and leukemia, 308
  environmental factors and, 309
  genetic factors and, 308
  immune deficiency states and, 308
  in transplant recipients, 308
  virus infections and, 308
Lymphoreticular and hematopoietic organs, 308
  (see also Lymphoma, Leukemia, Multiple myeloma, Myeloproliferative disorders, Blood)

Malabsorption syndromes, 290
Male genital tract, 410
  (see also Prostate, Testis)
Mallory bodies, 269, 270f
Marasmus, 93
Marfan's syndrome, 96, 170
  and medial cystic necrosis, 172
Meconium ileus, 462, 464f
Medial cystic necrosis, 172, 173f
  in Marfan's syndrome, 172
Medulloblastoma, 241
Melanoma, 453, 455f, 456f
Membranoproliferative glomerulonephritis, 190, 190f
Membranous glomerulonephritis, 192f, 193, 193f
Meningioma, 242, 242f
Meningitis, acute bacterial, 243, 244f
Meningitis, tuberculous, 245
Metabolic acidosis, 62, 62T
Metabolic alkalosis, 62
Metachromatic leukodystrophy, 254
Metaplasia, 126
  squamous, 126f
Mönckeberg's sclerosis, 173
Multiple endocrine syndromes, 350
  carcinoid tumors in, 351
  pancreatic islet cell tumors in, 350
  Sipple's syndrome, 350
  Wermer's syndrome, 350
Multiple myeloma, 321, 322f, 323f
  Bence-Jones protein, 322
  M protein, 321, 324
Multiple sclerosis, 253, 254f
Muscle, skeletal, 444
  congenital myopathies, 447
  dermatomyositis, 446
  in glycogen storage disease, 448
  muscular dystrophy, 445

  Duchenne dystrophy, 445, 445f
  facioscapulohumeral dystrophy, 445
  limb-girdle dystrophy, 446
  myotonic dystrophy, 446
  myasthenia gravis, 84, 446
    and thymus gland lesions, 446
  neurogenic atrophy, 448f, 449
  periodic paralysis, 449
  polymyositis, 446, 447f
Muscular dystrophy, 445
Myasthenia gravis, 84, 446
Mycosis fungoides, 313
Myeloproliferative disorders, 321
Myocardial infarction, 149
  (see also Heart)

Nabothian cysts, 360
Necrosis, 3
  caseation necrosis, 9, 12f
  coagulation necrosis, 9, 11f
  fat necrosis, 9
  liquefaction necrosis, 9, 12f
Negri bodies, 232
Nelson's syndrome, 333
Neoplastic disease, 128
  anaplasia, 134
  benign, characteristics of, 134
  cancer cachexia, 142
  causes of death, 142
  cell characteristics, 132
  cell karyotypes, 133
  chemical carcinogens, 138
  co-carcinogens, 132
  death rates due to, 128, 129T
  definition, 128
  differentiation, 134
  epigenetic basis, 137
  etiology, 136
  grading, 136
  immune deficiency states and, 141
  immune surveillance, 140
  initiators and promotors, 132
  malignant, characteristics of, 135
  metastasis, 135
  neoplastic transformation, 131
  staging, 136
  tumor-related antigens, 140
  viral oncogenesis, 139
Nephritic syndrome, 185
Nephroblastoma (Wilms' tumor), 101, 467, 467f
  disturbances of somatic growth and, 468
  staging, 467
Nephrotic syndrome, 184, 184T
Neuroblastoma, 464, 465f
  in situ, 466
  spontaneous regression, 465
  staging, 465
Neurofibroma, 243
Niemann-Pick disease, 97
Nosocomial infections, 40
Nutrition and disease, 88
  alcoholism, 92

Nutrition and disease—*continued*
  anorexia nervosa, 93
  atherosclerosis, 89
  breast carcinoma, 91
  colon carcinoma, 91
  diabetes mellitus, 90
  dietary fiber in, 91
  infections, 88
  kwashiorkor, 93
  marasmus, 93
  obesity, 91
  starvation, 93

Obesity, 91
  juvenile and adult onset, 92
  morbid, 92
Oligodendroglioma, 241
Oncofetal antigens, 141
Opsonins, 18
Oral contraceptive pills, 388
  changes in female genital tract, 388
  hepatic adenoma and, 115, 389, 389f
Organization, definition, 19
Osteitis fibrosa, 421f, 422, 422f
Osteoarthritis, 438, 438f, 439f
  Heberden's nodes, 439
Osteomalacia, 420, 421f
Osteomyelitis, 428
Osteoporosis, 420, 420f, 425, 427f
Ovary, 379
  epithelial tumors, 379
    Brenner tumor, 382
    clear cell carcinoma, 381
    endometrioid cystadenoma, cystadenocarcinoma, 381
    mucinous cystadenoma, cystadenocarcinoma, 381
    serous cystadenoma, cystadenocarcinoma, 380, 380f, 381f
  germ cell tumors, 382
    choriocarcinoma, 383
    dermoid cyst, 384
    dysgerminoma, 382
    embryonal carcinoma, 383
    endodermal sinus tumor, 382f, 383, 383f
    teratoma, 383, 384f, 385f
  Kruckenberg tumor, 387
  metastatic tumors, 387
  polycystic ovarian syndrome, 387, 387f
  Stein-Leventhal syndrome, 387
  stromal tumors, 384
    androblastoma, 387
    fibroma, 386
    granulosa cell tumors, 384, 386f
    thecoma, 384, 386f

Paget's disease of bone, 427, 428f, 429f, 430f
Paget's disease of breast, 400
Pancreas, 279
  carcinoma, 283, 284f, 285f
    jaundice in, 284
  islet cell tumors, 350, 350f

pancreatitis, 279, 280f, 281f
  acute, 279
  chronic, 281, 282f
  hemorrhagic, 279, 281f
  pathogenesis, 283
Parathyroid, 342
  hyperplasia, 124, 342
  hypoparathyroidism, 343
  primary hyperparathyroidism, 342
    adenocarcinoma and, 343
    adenoma and, 342, 343f, 344f
    primary hyperplasia and, 343
  pseudohypoparathyroidism, 344
Parkinson's disease, 249, 250f
Partial thromboplastin time, 69
Pediatric disorders, 459
Pelvic inflammatory disease, 374
Pemphigoid, 458
Pemphigus, 457, 457f
Peptic ulcer disease, 287, 288f, 289f
Periodic paralysis, 449
Pernicious anemia, 84, 327
  (*see also* Blood)
Phagocytosis, 18
  chronic granulomatous disease, 26
  opsonins, 18
Philadelphia chromosome, 133, 317
Pituitary, 332
  (*see also* Hypophysis)
Plasmin, 21
Platelet Factor 3, 64, 67
Plummer's disease, 335
Pneumococcal pneumonia, 28, 29f, 30f, 31f
Pneumoconioses, 218
  (*see also* Lung)
Pneumocystis pneumonia, 53, 54f
Podagra, 440, 442f
Polyarteritis nodosa, 174
  kidney in, 191, 195
Polycystic ovarian syndrome, 387, 387f
Polymyositis, 446, 447f
Portal hypertension, 259, 265
Poststreptococcal glomerulonephritis, 188, 188f, 189f
Potassium, disturbances of, 60
Progressive multifocal leukoencephalopathy, 247
Progressive systemic sclerosis, 85
Prostacyclin, 64
Prostaglandins
  in inflammation, 24
  in mediation of platelet function, 64
  prostacyclin, 64
  thromboxane A2, 64
Prostate, 410
  carcinoma, 410, 412f, 413f, 414f
    serum acid phosphatase in, 412
    staging, 412
  hyperplasia, 410, 411f
Prothrombin time, 69
Pseudomembranous enterocolitis, 113, 298, 298f
  clindamycin and, 113,
  Clostridium difficile in, 113,

Index

Psoriasis, 458
Pulmonary embolism, 4f
Pulmonary hypertension, 223, 224f
Pulmonary infarction, 3
Pulseless disease, 176
Pyelonepritis 42, 195
   (*see also* Kidney)
Pyknosis, nuclear, 8
Pylephlebitis, 299
Pyoderma gangrenosum, 297

Rapidly progressive glomerulonephritis, 191, 191f
Reed-Sternberg cell, 313, 314f
Renal osteodystrophy, 422, 424f, 425f
Renal vascular hypertension, 209
Respiratory acidosis, 63
Respiratory alkalosis, 63
Respiratory distress syndrome of newborn, 459
Respiratory failure, 211
Restrictive lung disease, 218, 219T
Retinoblastoma, 101, 431, 466
Retrolental fibroplasia, 460
Reye's syndrome, 461
Rheumatic fever, 152
   heart in, 153
      Aschoff nodule, 153, 153f, 154
      endocarditis, 153
      myocarditis, 153
Rheumatic heart disease, 152
   (*see also* Heart)
   aortic valve in, 155
   mitral stenosis, 155, 155f, 156f
Rheumatoid arthritis, 435, 436f, 437f
   amyloidosis in, 436
   rheumatoid factor, 435
   rheumatoid nodule, 436, 437f
Rickets, 420
Rocky Mountain spotted fever, 48
   disseminated intravascular coagulation in, 50
   endothelial injury, 50f
   glial nodules, 50, 51f

Sarcoidosis, 36f, 37f, 38, 212, 220f, 221
Scleroderma, 85
Serum enzymes
   in hepatitis, 267
   principal sources, 13T
Sheehan's syndrome, 332
Shock, 55
   acute tubular necrosis, 56
   bilateral renal cortical necrosis, 56, 56f
   cardiogenic, 148
   disseminated intravascular coagulation in, 56
   shock lung, 56
Sickle cell disease, 99
Silicosis, 219
Sjögren's syndrome, 438
Skin, 451
   basal cell carcinoma, 453, 454f
   Bowen's disease, 451
   discoid lupus erythematosus, 457
   erythema multiforme, 455

   erythema nodosum, 455
   keratoacanthoma, 451, 453f
   lichen planus, 458
   melanoma, 453, 455f, 456f
   pemphigoid, 458
   pemphigus, 457, 457f
   psoriasis, 458
   squamous cell carcinoma, 451, 452f
   Stevens-Johnson syndrome, 455
   systemic lupus erythematosus, 455
Sodium, disturbances of, 59
Spinal cord (*see* Central nervous system)
Starvation, 93
Stein-Leventhal syndrome, 387
Stevens-Johnson syndrome, 455
Stomach (*see* Digestive tract)
Subacute sclerosing panencephalitis, 247
Subdural hemorrhage, 255, 256f
Sudden infant death syndrome, 460
   risk factors, 461
Swiss type agammaglobulinemia, 39
Syphilis
   aortic aneurysms, 174
   aortitis, 165, 174
   arteritis in, 174
Systemic lupus erythematosus, 78, 85
   joints in, 438
   kidney in, 194
   skin in, 455

Testis
   choriocarcinoma, 415
      and β-HCG, 415
   cryptorchid testes, 47
   embryonal carcinoma, 413, 416f
   epididymitis, 417
   germ cell tumors, 412
      staging, 415
   Klinefelter's syndrome, 417
   Leydig cell tumor, 417
   orchitis, 417
   seminoma, 413, 414f, 415f
   teratoma, 413
   tumors, 412
Tetracycline toxicity, 112
Thromboangiitis obliterans, 177
Thrombocytopenia, 69
Thrombophlebitis, 177
Thrombotic thrombocytopenic purpura, 74, 194
Thromboxane A2, 64
Thrombus, 3, 67
   fate of, 71
Thrush, 52
Thymus (*see* Myasthenia gravis, 446)
Thyroid, 334
   goiter, 339
   Graves' disease, 84
   hyperthyroidism, 334
      adenomas and, 335
      Graves' disease, 334, 335f
      ophthalmopathy in, 335
      Plummer's disease, 335

Index

Thyroid—*continued*
  hypothyroidism, 335
    cretinism, 335
    myxedema, 336
  nodular hyperplasia, 341f
  thyroiditis, 336
    autoantibodies and, 336
    Hashimoto's thyroiditis, 336, 336f, 337f
    subacute thyroiditis, 337
  tumors, 338
    adenoma, 337f, 338
    follicular carcinoma, 338, 339f, 340f
    medullary carcinoma, 338, 340f
    papillary carcinoma, 338, 338f
    undifferentiated carcinoma, 338
Tissue enzymes
  principal sources, 13T
Tissue injury
  release of enzymes, 13T
  systemic manifestations, 9
Tophi, 440, 441f
Toxic megacolon, 297
Transplantation, 85
  kidney, 85
  rejection, 85
Transudate, 15
Trophoblastic disease, 376
  and β-HCG, 378
  chorioadenoma destruens, 377, 377f
  choriocarcinoma, 377, 378f
  complicated, 378
  hydatidiform mole, 377
Tuberculosis, 32, 34f, 35f, 45
  cell-mediated immunity in, 46
  complications, 47
  exudative lesions, 46
  fibro-cavitary, 47, 48f, 49f
  Ghon complex, 46
  hematogenous dissemination, 47
  Langhans giant cells, 45
  meningitis, 47, 245
  miliary, 47
  pneumonia, 47
  proliferative lesions, 46
  tubercle, 45
Turner's syndrome, 100

Ulcerative colitis, 294, 295f, 296f, 297f
Uremic syndrome, 182
Uterus, 366
  abnormal bleeding, 374
  adenoacanthoma, 371, 371f
  adenocarcinoma of endometrium, 369, 370f
  adenosquamous carcinoma, 371
  endometrial hyperplasia, 367, 368f
    adenomatous, 369, 369f
    estrone hypothesis, 368
    cystic, 368
    "Swiss cheese," 368
  endometriosis, 373
    external, 374
    internal, 373
  endometritis, 366
  leiomyoma, 371, 372f
  leiomyosarcoma, 372
  polyps, endometrial, 367, 367f
  sarcoma of endometrium, 373, 373f

Vacuolar degeneration, 8
Vagina, 358
  adenosis, 359, 360f
  clear cell carcinoma, 359, 361f
    DES and, 359
  vaginitis, 358
    atrophic, 358
Vascular disorders, 167
  (*see also* Atherosclerosis, Acute aortic dissection, Mönckeberg's sclerosis, Fibromuscular dysplasia, Vasculitis, Thrombophlebitis)
Vasculitis, 173
  giant cell arteritis, 176, 176f
  hypersensitivity angiitis, 175
  in infections, 174
  polyarteritis nodosa, 174
    and hepatitis B, 175
  pulseless disease, 176
  syphilitic arteritis, 174
  Wegener's granulomatosis, 176, 195, 220
Veins
  thrombophlebitis, 177
Villous adenoma, colon, 305, 307f
Virchow's triad, 71
von Willebrand's disease, 70
Vulva, 358
  Bowen's disease, 358, 359f
  carcinoma, 358

Waldenström's macroglobulinemia, 324
Wegener's granulomatosis, 176, 220
Werdnig-Hoffman disease, 252
Wernicke's encephalopathy, 257
Whipple's disease, 291, 293f
Wilms' tumor, 101, 467, 467f
Wilson's disease, 271
Wiskott-Aldrich syndrome, 40

Xeroderma pigmentosum, 137
XYY syndrome, 101

Zollinger-Ellison syndrome, 287, 350